SURVIVAL OF CANCER PATIENTS IN EUROPE

The EUROCARE Study

INTERNATIONAL AGENCY FOR RESEARCH ON CANCER

The International Agency for Research on Cancer (IARC) was established in 1965 by the World Health Assembly, as an independently financed organization within the framework of the World Health Organization. The headquarters of the Agency are at Lyon, France.

The Agency conducts a programme of research concentrating particularly on the epidemiology of cancer and the study of potential carcinogens in the human environment. Its field studies are supplemented by biological and chemical research carried out in the Agency's laboratories in Lyon, and, through collaborative research agreements, in national research institutions in many countries. The Agency also conducts a programme for the education and training of personnel for cancer research.

The publications of the Agency are intended to contribute to the dissemination of authoritative information on different aspects of cancer research. A complete list is printed at the back of the book.

Front cover: Details from The Athens School, by Raphael (see back cover)

Top left: Plato (depicted as Leonardo da Vinci), pointing towards the sky, and Aristotle, pointing forward.

Top right: Euclid (depicted as Bramante), drawing on a slate, with Zoroaster, holding the sphere of the heavens and Ptolemy, holding the globe of the Earth.

Bottom: Heraclitus (depicted as Michelangelo) on the right and Pythagoras on the left.

WORLD HEALTH ORGANIZATION

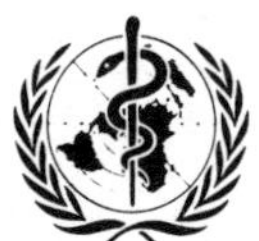

INTERNATIONAL AGENCY FOR RESEARCH ON CANCER

EUROPEAN COMMISSION

SURVIVAL OF CANCER PATIENTS IN EUROPE

The EUROCARE Study

Edited by

F. Berrino, M. Sant, A. Verdecchia, R. Capocaccia, T. Hakulinen and J. Estève

IARC Scientific Publications No. 132

Lyon, 1995

Published by the International Agency for Research on Cancer,

150 cours Albert Thomas, 69372 Lyon cédex 08, France

IARC Library Cataloguing in Publication Data

Survival of cancer patients in Europe : the EUROCARE study /
F. Berrino ... [et al].

(IARC Scientific Publications ; 132)

1. Neoplasms – epidemiology 2. Neoplasms – mortality 3. Europe
I. Berrino, F. II. Series

ISBN 92 832 2132 X (NLM Classification: QZ 200 GA1)
ISSN 0300-5085

Printed in France

Contents

Foreword

The study of survival of cancer patients is essential for monitoring the effectiveness of medical treatment for cancer. To be useful for the purpose of planning more effective health services, however, survival data need to be interpreted, and the first step towards interpretation is to compare the success achieved in different populations. Proper comparison requires population-based data such as only cancer registries can provide, including all the cases that occur in defined populations and time periods. These studies need careful coordination in order to provide reliable results.

The present volume includes survival comparisons based on data from 30 populations in 11 European countries and shows several important differences, both between countries and over time. It is a marvellous product of fruitful cooperation between cancer registries and a notable example of the capability of the European Union to promote international collaborative research in the fields of health care and of cancer control. Together with the achievements of the European Network of Cancer Registries in making available systematic cancer incidence, prevalence and mortality estimates for Europe, this work demonstrates what can be achieved by international coordination of the fight against cancer so as to bring this disease under control.

The differences revealed beween populations will help European countries to establish reasonable and attainable goals for cancer diagnosis and treatment. National health authorities will wish to promote further research in order to understand fully the reasons for differences in survival so that suitable action may be taken to correct them.

P. Kleihues, M.D.
Director, IARC

Preface

A major goal in the fight against cancer is the reduction of cancer mortality rates. This can only be achieved in one of two ways: reducing incidence rates, and increasing the chances of cure. The chances of cancer being cured can be estimated from the probability distribution of survival.

Measures of incidence, survival and mortality are critical to the interpretation of data on progress in the fight against cancer, and in the evaluation of the overall effectiveness of cancer control programmes. Making these data available for study is one of the main reasons for the development of cancer registries and for continuing attempts to improve the quality of the information they provide.

Randomized controlled clinical trials have shown many modern protocols for cancer treatment to be more effective than earlier treatments, but trials rarely include more than a small fraction of the patients with a particular cancer. Only population- based studies, using data from cancer registries, are capable of quantifying the effectiveness of cancer treatments in the population as a whole, allowing survival to be compared between populations, and measuring the extent to which survival has improved. Until now, however, comparable population-based survival figures have rarely been available.

Cancer registries have reached a high standard of comparability for cancer incidence data, largely through the regular compilation of international data sets for *Cancer Incidence in Five Continents,* but a similar standard has not yet been reached for survival figures. This is mainly because of international differences in the definition, classification and grouping of the diseases included in survival analyses, and sometimes also because of differences in follow-up procedures and statistical methods of analysis.

It was in order to overcome these difficulties that in 1988, the EUROCARE project (European Cancer Registry-based Study of Survival and Care of Cancer Patients) was proposed to the European Community's Health Service Research committee (COMAC), which approved it in 1989 and funded it in 1990 (Fracchia & Theofilatou, 1993). EUROCARE is a concerted action among European cancer registries, aimed at estimating and comparing the survival of cancer patients in different European populations. The rationale behind this project is to optimize the comparability of survival data by using an agreed and standard definition of the diseases for which survival is to be compared, and by taking due account of basic demographic variables as confounders in the statistical analysis. A further aim of the project was to describe and compare the patterns of care of cancer patients, both diagnostic and therapeutic, in order to permit appropriate interpretation of differences in survival.

This monograph deals only with the first aspect of the project, that is, variations in cancer patient survival. Patterns of care will be addressed in the next phase of the project.

The first protocol for EUROCARE was drafted by a project management group comprising the following researchers: Franco Berrino (Project Leader, Italy), Jocelyn Chamberlain (UK), Jan Willem Coebergh (Netherlands), Michel Coleman (UK), Alessandro Liberati (Italy), Carmen Martinez (Spain), Mark McCarthy (UK), Hélène Sancho-Garnier (France), Milena Sant (Italy) and Eugène Schifflers (Belgium).

All European cancer registries were then invited to participate in the planning of the study and to contribute data. A first plenary meeting of the EUROCARE Working Group was held in Varese, Italy, in April 1990, at which the potential difficulties of such an endeavour were thoroughly discussed. Provisional consensus was reached on a basic protocol, and all the participating registries agreed to send selected data to establish a communal database for standardized editing, quality control and analysis.

Coordination of the project was undertaken by the staff of the Varese Province Cancer Registry at the National Cancer Institute in Milan (Milena Sant, Gemma Gatta, Andrea Micheli, Livio Dell'Era, Daniele Speciale and Maria Rosa Ruzza) as well as technical support for translation and the organization of meetings and workshops (Emily Taussig and Moira Driscoll), while data management and analysis were carried out by the staff of the Epidemiology Laboratory of the National Institute of Health in Rome (Riccardo Capocaccia, Arduino Verdecchia, Fulvia Valente and Egidio Chessa).

Coordination at IARC was carried out by Jacques Estève and Philippe Damiecki, who worked closely with John Cheney in the preparation of this publication with regard to the statistical and computing aspects, and with Josephine Thévenoux on the typography and presentation.

The EUROCARE Working Group succeeded in collecting, checking and editing data on cancer survival from 30 cancer registries in 11 countries, and established a database covering some 800 000 cancer patients diagnosed in the period 1978–85 and followed up to the end of 1990. This database forms the raw material for this monograph.

The final decision to publish the data in their current form was taken at a meeting in Orta (Novara, Italy) in April 1992. On this occasion, a general policy for publication of material derived from the EUROCARE project was approved, and a formal EUROCARE Steering Committe was elected, comprising representatives of the collaborating cancer registries and of the International Agency for Research on Cancer, Lyon, France. The present composition of the Steering Committee is the following: Franco Berrino (Chairman,Italy), Jan Willem Coebergh (The Netherlands), Michel Coleman (United Kingdom), Jacques Estève (IARC, France), Jean Faivre (France), Timo Hakulinen (Finland), Carmen Martinez (Spain), Milena Sant (Italy), Arduino Verdecchia (Italy) and Sue Wilson (United Kingdom).

The terms of reference of the EUROCARE Steering Committee are to stimulate the use of the EUROCARE database for scientific purposes, to judge the scientific merits of proposals for further analysis of the database put forward by EUROCARE Working Group members or by other scientists, and to ensure respect for the confidentiality and ownership of the data and the appropriateness of its analysis.

The EUROCARE Working Group comprises all the researchers who contributed to the development of the protocol and to the database; it is open to any European population-based cancer registry willing to participate.

The members of the Working Group who have actively contributed to the present monograph are listed on pages xi and xii.

Reference

Fracchia, G.N. & Theofilatou, M., eds (1993) *Health Services Research*. Commission of the European Communities, Directorate-General XII, Science, Research and Development, Amsterdam, IOS Press

Contributors

Aareleid, T., Estonian Cancer Registry, Department of Epidemiology and Biostatistics, Institute of Experimental and Clinical Medicine, Hiiu 42, EE0016 Tallinn, Estonia

Barchielli, A., Tuscany Cancer Registry, Via S. Salvi, 12, 50135 Florence, Italy

Bell, J., Thames Cancer Registry, 15 Cotswold Road, Sutton, Surrey SM 2 5PY, UK

Berrino, F., Lombardy Cancer Registry, Divisione di Epidemiologia, Istituto Nazionale per lo Studio e la Cura dei Tumori, Via Venezian, 1, 20133 Milan, Italy

Black, R.J., Scottish Cancer Registry, Information and Statistics Division, Scottish Health Service, Trinity Park House, Edinburgh EH53 SQ, UK

Bowcock, M., West Midlands Cancer Registry, Queen Elizabeth Medical Centre, Birmingham, B15 2TH, UK

Capocaccia, R., Istituto Superiore di Sanità, Laboratorio di Epidemiologia, Viale Regina Elena, 299, 00161 Rome, Italy

Carli, P.-M., Côte d'Or Malignant Haemopathies Registry, Laboratoire d' Hématologie, Hôpital du Bocage, 2 Blvd Marechal de Lattre de Tassigny, 21000 Dijon, France

Chaplain, G., Côte d'Or Breast and Gynaecologic Cancer Registry, Centre Georges-Francois Leclerc, 1 rue du Professeur Marion, 21000 Dijon, France

Coebergh, J.W.W., Eindhoven Cancer Registry, Comprehensive Cancer Centre South (IKZ), Bogert 55, Postbus 231, 5600AE Eindhoven, The Netherlands and Department of Epidemiology, Erasmus University, P.O. Box 1738, 3000 DR Rotterdam, The Netherlands

Coleman, M.P., Thames Cancer Registry, 15 Cotswold Road, Sutton, Surrey, SM2 5PY, UK

Conti, E.M.S., Latina Cancer Registry, Sezione di Epidemiologia, Istituto Regina Elena per lo Studio e la Cura dei Tumori, Viale Regina Elena 291, 00171 Rome, Italy

Crommelin, M.A., Eindhoven Cancer Registry, Comprehensive Cancer Centre South (IKZ), Bogert 55, P.O. Box 231, 5600AE Eindhoven, The Netherlands

Cummins, C., West Midlands Cancer Registry, Queen Elizabeth Medical Centre, Birmingham, B15 2TH, UK

Estève, J., Special Adviser on Biostatistics, International Agency for Research on Cancer, 150 Cours Albert Thomas, 69372 Lyon, France

Faivre, J., Côte d'Or Digestive Cancer Registry, Faculté de Médecine Inserm SCN N17, 7 Blvd Jeanne d'Arc, 21033 Dijon, France

Gafá, L., Ragusa Cancer Registry, Ospedale Paterno, Piazza Igea 2, 97100 Ragusa, Italy

Galceran, J., Tarragona Cancer Registry, Apartat Correus 1094, 43200 Reus, Spain

Garau, I., Mallorca Cancer Registry, Unitad d'Epidemiologia, Misericordia 2, 07012 Palma de Mallorca, Baleares, Spain

Gatta G., Lombardy Cancer Registry, Divisione di Epidemiologia, Istituto Nazionale per lo Studio e la Cura dei Tumori, Via Venezian, 1, 20133 Milan, Italy

Hakulinen, T., Finnish Cancer Registry, Institute for Statistical and Epidemiological Cancer Research, Liisankatu 21 B, 00170 Helsinki, Finland and Unit of Cancer Epidemiology, Karolinska Institute, Stockholm, Sweden

Kaatsch, P., German Registry of Childhood Malignancies (Mainz), Klinik J. Gutemberg University, Institut für Medizinische Statistik und Dokumentation, Langenbeckstrasse 1, Postfach 3960, 55101 Mainz, Germany

Lawrence, G., West Midlands Cancer Registry, Queen Elizabeth Medical Centre, Birmingham, B15 2TH, UK

Magnani, C., Piedmont Childhood Cancer Registry, Istituto di Anatomia Patologica, Via Santena 7, 10126 Turin, Italy

Martinez, C., Granada Cancer Registry, Escuela Andaluza de Salud Publica, Campus Universitario Cartuja, 18014 Granada, Spain

McCarthy, M., Director of Public Health, 110 Hampstead Road, London NW1 2LJ, UK

Masseling, E., Eindhoven Cancer Registry, Comprehensive Cancer Centre South (IKZ), Bogert 55, P.O. Box 231, 5600AE Eindhoven, The Netherlands

Michaelis, J., German Registry of Childhood Malignancies (Mainz), Klinik J. Gutemberg University, Institut für Medizinische Statistik und Dokumentation, Langenbeckstrasse 1, Postfach 3960, 55101 Mainz, Germany

Micheli, A., Lombardy Cancer Registry, Divisione di Epidemiologia, Istituto Nazionale per lo Studio e la Cura dei Tumori, Via Venezian, 1, 20133 Milan, Italy

Page, M., East Anglia Cancer Registry, Department of Community Medicine, Addenbrookes Hospital, Hills Road, Cambridge CB2 2QQ, UK

Pawlega, J., Cracow Cancer Registry, Pracownia Epidem. Cent. Onckologli, Institute M. Sklodowska-Curie, Garncarskca 11, Krakowie, Poland

Ponz de Leon, M., Colorectal Cancer Registry of Modena, Istituto di Patologia Medica, Policlinico di Modena, Via del Pozzo, 41100 Modena, Italy

Pottier, D., Calvados Digestive Cancer Registry, Faculté de Médecine Niveau 03, Pièce 703 C.H.U., Côte de Nacre, 14044 Caen, France

Raverdy, N., Somme (Amiens) Cancer Registry, CHR Nord Bat. Médecine 4 ème Est, 80054 Amiens Cédex, France

Raymond, L., Geneva Cancer Registry, Médecine Sociale et Préventive, 55 Blvd de la Cluse, 1205 Geneva, Switzerland and Department of Social and Preventive Medicine, CMU, rue Michel Servet 1, 1211 Geneva 14, Switzerland

Rider, L., Yorkshire Cancer Registry, Cookridge Hospital, Leeds LS16 6QB, UK

Robillard, J., Calvados General Cancer Registry, Centre Regional François Baclesse, Route de Lion-sur-Mer, 14021 Caen Cédex, France

Sant, M., Lombardy Cancer Registry, Divisione di Epidemiologia, Istituto Nazionale per lo Studio e la Cura dei Tumori, Via Venezian, 1, 20133 Milan, Italy

Schraub, S., Doubs Cancer Registry, Hôpital Jean Minjoz, Boulevard Fleming, 25030 Besançon Cédex, France

Smith, J., Wessex Cancer Registry, Wessex Cancer Intelligence Unit, Institute of Public Health, Romsey Road, Winchester SO22 5DH, UK

Storm, H.H., Danish Cancer Registry, Division for Cancer Epidemiology, Danish Cancer Society, Strandboulevarden 49, PO Box 839, DK–2100 Copenhagen 0, Denmark

Torhorst, J., Basel Cancer Registry, Institut für Pathologie der Universität Basel, Schönbeinstrasse, 40, 4003 Basel, Switzerland

Tumino, R., Ragusa Cancer Registry, Ospedale Paterno, Piazza Igea 2, 97100 Ragusa, Italy

Valente, F., Istituto Superiore di Sanità, Laboratorio di Epidemiologia, Viale Regina Elena, 299, 00161 Rome, Italy

van der Heijden, L.H., Eindhoven Cancer Registry, Comprehensive Cancer Centre South (IKZ), Bogert 55, P.O. Box 231, 5600AE Eindhoven, The Netherlands

Verdecchia, A., Istituto Superiore di Sanità, Laboratorio di Epidemiologia, Viale Regina Elena, 299, 00161 Rome, Italy

Viladiu, P., Girona Cancer Registry, Hospital S. Caterina, Pl. Hospital, 17001 Girona, Spain

Wilson, S., Centre for Cancer Epidemiology, Christie Hospital NHS Trust, Kinnaird Road, Withington, Manchester M20 9QL, UK

Youngson, J., Mersey Regional Cancer Registry, University of Liverpool, PO Box 147, Liverpool L69 3BX, UK

Ziegler, H., Saarland Cancer Registry, Hardenbergstrasse 3, 66119 Saarbrücken, Germany

PART 1

INTRODUCTION AND METHODOLOGY

CHAPTER 1

Basic issues in estimating and comparing the survival of cancer patients

F. Berrino, J. Estève and M.P. Coleman

Since the earliest days of scientific medicine, the proportion of patients who are cured of a disease has been considered the basic parameter by which to judge the value of prognostic factors and to assess the effectiveness of medical treatment. The complement of this proportion, lethality, usually expressed as cumulative mortality among those with the disease, has also been used (Bernoulli, 1766; Louis, 1835). For chronic illnesses, the proportion of patients who are cured is usually approximated by estimates of the net probability of survival at regular intervals after diagnosis, which provide the distribution of the duration of survival in the absence of other causes of death (Estève *et al.*, 1994).

Mortality from a given disease is a measure of the frequency of death caused by the disease among the entire population at risk, and it is influenced both by the incidence of the disease and by survival from it. By contrast, the probability of survival depends only on the frequency of death from the disease (or from any other cause) among patients who have already developed it, and, in principle, it should not be influenced by the incidence. Progress in the fight against cancer, either through prevention or treatment, should ultimately be reflected in a reduction in mortality, since this is a key overall measure of success, but it is also important to judge separately the effectiveness of prevention and treatment through their respective effects on incidence and survival. The EUROCARE project addresses the issue of survival.

The duration of survival, however, is not a straightforward indicator of the effectiveness of medical treatment. Since it is defined as the time interval between the diagnosis of the illness and the death of the patient, any factor which affects either the definition of the illness, the date of diagnosis or the date of death will also affect the duration of survival. The complexity of the logical structure of survival comparison is shown diagrammatically in Figure 1.1.

The following determinants of the duration of survival, in particular, must be carefully considered when interpreting differences in survival between populations or trends in survival over time, because each of these determinants may vary in space and time:

(1) The nature of the illness and the criteria used for diagnosing it; the latter in turn depend on the availability of diagnostic technology and equipment;

(2) The distribution of demographic and socio-economic characteristics in the population from which the cancer patients are drawn, and possible selection with respect both to these same characteristics and to the distribution of stage of disease in the patients whose survival is being estimated and compared;

(3) The availability of methods for early diagnosis and the existence of screening programmes, which bring forward the date of diagnosis but may also delay the date of death by increasing the effectiveness of standard therapies;

(4) The availability of effective therapeutic procedures, which affect the date of death by increasing the probability of cure or the length of time for which an incurable illness can be kept in check;

(5) The age distribution of the patients, which may modify the natural history of the illness and both the availability of treatment and the patient's response to it; in the present monograph, whenever possible, age-specific or age-adjusted survival proportions are presented;

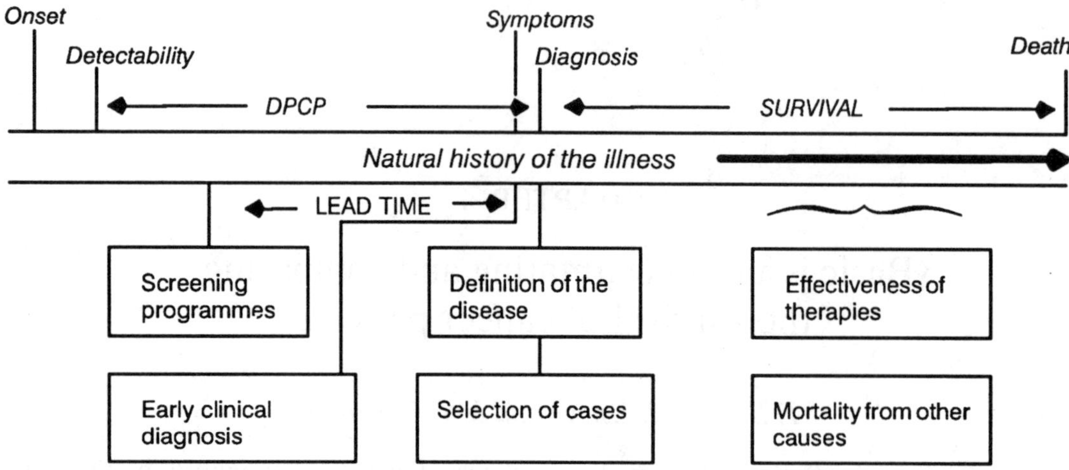

Figure 1.1. Natural history of chronic illnesses and major determinants of survival time.
DPCP = Detectable Pre-Clinical Phase

(6) The force of mortality from other causes, to which cancer patients are also subject, must be taken into account. The extent of mortality from causes other than cancer varies substantially between populations. Evaluating the excess mortality of cancer patients over that of a comparable population without cancer is therefore essential in analysing the duration of survival. The need to estimate this excess led to the concept of relative survival. The methodology for controlling for competing causes of death is considered in Chapters 3 and 4.

All these factors are capable of modifying the true survival of cancer patients. Other factors may lead to artefactual changes in estimated survival. These include the definition of the index date for survival comparison (date of diagnosis or date of start of follow-up) and differences in follow-up procedures (reviewed in Chapter 2) and in statistical methodologies (reviewed elsewhere, Estève *et al.*, 1994).

The basic issue in the interpretation of differences in survival between populations and of changes in survival over time is to determine the respective contributions of earlier diagnosis and postponement of death to any such differences or improvements. Earlier diagnosis will automatically prolong the observed duration of survival by the addition of lead time (i.e. by a backward shift of the 'zero' time from which survival is computed). Postponement of death, on the other hand, can only be produced by advances in therapy, or by more effective management of the disease resulting from earlier diagnosis. Early diagnosis without postponement of death carries no advantage for the patient; it may in fact be a serious disadvantage, in that it creates a longer period of morbidity.

In the first part of this chapter we consider how the major structural determinants mentioned above can affect the duration of survival. This discussion is limited to the first four factors (definition of the disease, selection of patients, early diagnosis and the effectiveness of treatment), because differences in the age distribution of cancer patients and their mortality from other causes can be controlled by conventional statistical analysis, and these issues are dealt with in Chapters 3 and 4. We then consider how the interpretation of population-based survival statistics could be improved by the collection of properly standardized data on the stage of disease and the procedures used to determine stage. In the second part of the chapter we present the rationale of the current EUROCARE study and its advantages and limitations.

The nature of the disease and its definition

When survival probabilities are compared between different populations or in successive time periods, the disease under study should be defined in exactly the same way in all groups. For instance, when studying malignant neoplasms (codes 140–208 of the 9th revision of the International Classification of Diseases (ICD-9); WHO, 1977), tumours classified as benign, uncertain whether benign or malignant, or *in situ* should be carefully excluded.

When a malignant neoplasm occurs in an existing premalignant condition, e.g. an invasive carcinoma arising in a previously diagnosed in situ carcinoma, the index date from which survival should be computed is the date of diagnosis of the malignant condition and not the date of the precursor. For several cancers, however, the distinction between the two conditions may not be straightforward.

Transitional cell carcinoma of the urothelial lining, for instance (ICD-9 188, bladder, and 189.1–189.2, renal pelvis and ureter), is frequently diagnosed from small biopsy fragments that do not allow the pathologist to establish unequivocally whether the tumour is invasive or *in situ*. Several cancer registries, therefore, include invasive, *in situ* and unspecified transitional cell tumours in the same category when publishing incidence data (Muir *et al.*, 1987; Parkin *et al.*, 1992). The proportion of bladder tumours explicitly indicated as non-invasive is likely to vary considerably depending on the attitude of the surgeons and of the pathologists, but also on cancer registration practice. For instance, among cancer registries that included non-invasive tumours in their incidence data for bladder cancer in the sixth volume of *Cancer Incidence in Five Continents* (Parkin *et al.*, 1992), the proportion of non-invasive cases varied from about 50% in Denmark to 2% in South Thames, UK, but most cancer registries were not able to provide valid figures. In practice, there is little prospect of reliable comparison of survival for bladder cancer patients outside specially designed trials. Bladder cancer incidence is also difficult to compare between populations and over time.

Multiple myeloma provides another example. This syndrome has a somewhat arbitrary definition (Salmon & Cassady, 1989), requiring at least two of the following: (*a*) a serum electrophoretic peak of monoclonal immunoglobulins above a predefined level; (*b*) biopsy evidence of bone marrow colonization by plasma cells greater than a predefined percentage; and (*c*) multiple lytic bone lesions. Various diagnostic protocols incorporate different threshold levels for immunoglobulins and plasmacytosis, however. Multiple myeloma is sometimes preceded by an asymptomatic monoclonal gammopathy of uncertain clinical significance, a condition that may last for many years before eventually evolving to meet the above requirements. The diagnosis of this condition is frequently made incidentally, during a routine blood examination, and it usually gives rise to regular follow-up examinations during which, rarely, myeloma may eventually be detected. Unfortunately, there is an overlap between the presenting clinical features in patients with monoclonal gammopathy of uncertain significance and those in patients with stage I myeloma, resolution of which frequently requires serial follow-up of the patient. The clinical use of such terms as 'indolent' or 'smouldering' myeloma reflects the diagnostic difficulty. It is clear that even if standard diagnostic criteria were universally recognized, the date of diagnosis of myeloma would depend heavily on the extent to which the relevant symptoms and signs are actively sought and on the follow-up policy for patients with monoclonal gammopathy. The attempts which have been made to interpret trends in survival (Black *et al.*, 1993), incidence and mortality (Coleman *et al.*, 1993; Cuzick, 1990; Schwartz, 1990) from multiple myeloma suggest that artefacts due to variations in the manner in which the disease is sought and diagnosed cannot be excluded.

Like multiple myeloma, many clinically malignant tumours are preceded by an asymptomatic phase in which the abnormality is morphologically indistinguishable from that seen in clinically overt disease, but the clinical evolution of which is unpredictable. Perhaps the best example of this problem is provided by focal prostatic carcinoma (variously called 'incidental', 'silent', 'microscopic', 'latent' or 'dormant') diagnosed either at screening or incidentally, on microscopic examination of a prostatic gland removed surgically for benign hyperplasia . The prevalence of this condition is very high: according to some autopsy studies it increases exponentially from about 10% at 55 years of age to 20% at age 65 and 40% at age 75 (Gittes, 1991; Yatani *et al.*, 1982). Incidence trends for prostatic cancer can be markedly influenced by the frequency of surgical resection for hyperplasia (Potosky *et al.*, 1990), which in turn depends on the cultural attitude of both patients and physicians more than on objective clinical criteria. Comparison of the survival of patients with prostatic cancer would make little sense without strictly standardized criteria for inclusion of patients in the series to be compared.

These problems were judged likely to invalidate any attempt to estimate and compare survival probabilities for myeloma and cancers of the bladder and prostate. To a lesser extent, however, the same type of problem arises for several other cancers included in this monograph. The relevance of the problem is well described in the context of cancer screening, where a certain degree of over-diagnosis is to be expected.

For example, in a randomized trial of screening for lung cancer (Fontana, 1984), about 10 000 heavy smokers were randomized to receive either chest X-ray and sputum cytology every four months or just a recommendation for an annual X-ray. After nine years, 167 lung cancers had been diagnosed in the intervention group versus 131 in the comparison group. Five-year survival was significantly higher in the intervention group (35% against 15%) but the cumulative mortality from lung cancer (30/1000) was the same in each group. The excess of cancer in the intervention group was confined to epidermoid carcinoma. A similar number of cases had probably also arisen in the comparison group without being detected. Their detection in the intervention group explains why observed survival for this group was better. They were all successfully operated, but the patients apparently obtained no mortality advantage from the trial intervention, at least within the first nine years of follow-up. Some of these clinically silent tumours might well have persisted for the rest of the patient's life and never have been detected if left unscreened. It is questionable if these cases, albeit histologically indistinguishable from those diagnosed clinically, can be considered to belong to the same disease entity. It is possible, therefore, that part of the international variation in the survival of lung cancer patients reported in this monograph is ascribable to international variation in the frequency of detection of such asymptomatic lesions.

Very small lesions detected at screening may also pose serious diagnostic problems. Out of 506 'minimal breast cancers' (tumours less than 1 cm in diameter) detected with mammography within the framework of the Breast Cancer Detection Demonstration Project in the USA, 48 (9.5%) were not subsequently confirmed as malignant tumours by a panel of pathologists reviewing the histological slides (Bears & Smart, 1979). In the absence of extensive screening programmes, however, it is unlikely that diagnostic uncertainties of this type will materially affect international comparison of the survival of cancer patients. The period covered by the data in this monograph precedes that of the national breast cancer screening programmes in the UK and in the Netherlands, which began in 1988 and 1990, respectively.

Patient selection

Compared with the more usual hospital-based studies of cancer survival, the major advantage of population-based studies such as EUROCARE is the avoidance of selection bias. Patients seen in any one hospital department are unlikely to be representative of all cancer patients with respect to age, clinical features and, perhaps, wealth or other socio-demographic factors. Avoidance of this selection bias was the main reason why a cancer registry-based study was proposed for international comparison of cancer survival. Other forms of selection bias may affect cancer registries, however, particularly if incidence registration is not exhaustive.

Many cancer registries have access to death certificates as a systematic source of information; this guarantees that almost all cancer deaths are registered sooner or later. Cases known to the cancer registry only from their death certificate, usually referred to as DCO (death certificate only) cases, are generally integrated in incidence data, but they cannot be included in survival estimates, because the actual date of diagnosis is not known. Some of these cases may have escaped the cancer registry information network because they were too ill to be hospitalized or to undergo surgical biopsy: their exclusion may therefore result in the selective exclusion of very poor survivors. Long-term survivors may also be lost, however, since a high proportion of DCO cases also suggests that the routine data collection system does not adequately cover all the clinics and pathology laboratories. With incomplete registration, therefore, both long-term and short-term survivors may be under-represented in the data. The direction of the resulting bias in survival statistics is unpredictable; in principle, however, long-term survivors have a greater chance of being notified while still alive, just because they live longer. The selection bias caused by incomplete notification is likely to be more serious for older patients, among whom DCO cases are more frequent. The proportion of DCO cases reported by cancer registries contributing to the EUROCARE study ranges from none to about 15% (see Chapter 2).

Cases first discovered from a death certificate are usually followed back by cancer registries through family doctors or hospital files to trace clinical information (at least the date of diagnosis) which would enable them to be included in survival statistics. In the Danish Cancer Registry, for instance, about 10% of the incident cases are first notified from a death certificate, but the eventual proportion of DCO cases is only about 1% after follow-back procedures are completed (see Chapter 5). In the Lombardy Cancer Registry (Varese Province, Italy) the corresponding figures are 3% and 2%, respectively (Gafà *et al.*, 1992).

Cases first notified to the cancer registry from a death certificate are sometimes referred to as DCI (death certificate initiated) cases; they are an indicator of the timeliness and exhaustiveness of the other sources of cancer registration. By contrast, DCO cases, i.e. those included in incidence statistics with a death certificate as the only source of information, are more an indicator of the quality of incidence data, since diagnostic details on death certificates are scanty. The extent to which follow-back procedures are successful may affect survival comparisons. The theoretical relationships between the proportion of cases registered either initially (DCI) or only (DCO) from a death certificate and the reliability of cancer incidence and survival estimates are summarized in Table 1.1.

A high proportion of DCI cases suggests that routine sources of registration during life are less reliable than sources of death certificates; this implies that some long-term survivors are likely to be missed too, and, therefore, incidence rates will be underestimated. Thus, if most DCI cases are successfully traced back, enabling them to be included in survival analyses (high proportion of DCI but low proportion of DCO), the data are likely to be defective mainly in long-term survivors, and survival would be underestimated. If, on the other hand, the date of diagnosis of most DCI cases cannot be traced, forcing their exclusion from survival computation as DCO cases (high DCI and high DCO), the series of patients used for estimating survival most likely also selectively lacks some very poor survivors (Lourie, 1964), making the direction of any bias in survival estimation unpredictable.

Unfortunately, the information currently available does not usually allow the effect of different proportions of DCI and DCO cases on survival to be precisely evaluated, because most cancer registries do not keep records of the follow-back operations. To provide an estimate of the effect of tracing back DCI cases on the estimation of survival, the Thames Cancer Registry (UK) conducted a special search to obtain the date of diagnosis of DCO cases who died in 1992, using a source of information never previously used, the Family Health Service Authorities, which receive the patient's medical record from the general practitioner within a few weeks of death, and normally retain it for a few years. More than 90% of the 6000 records actually sought were obtained for review. Survival distributions of the 1992 DCO cases by site, sex and age were then applied to the DCO cases of the most recent incidence period that was available for survival computation, namely 1986–87. For this period, as for the period included in this monograph (1978–84), little active tracing-back had been performed. The analysis, shown in Table 1.2 and in Figure 1.2, incorporates the working assumptions that

Table 1.1. Theoretical relationships between the proportion of registrations initiated by a death certificate (DCI), the proportion of cases registered from death certificate only (DCO), and the reliability of cancer incidence and survival statistics

DCI cases	Proportion of DCO cases	Effect on incidence	Effect on survival
High	High	Underestimate	Unpredictable bias
High	Low	Underestimate	Underestimate
Low	Low	Accurate	Accurate

Table 1.2. Effect of excluding cases known from death certificate only (DCO) on estimates of survival in the Thames Cancer Registry (South Thames Region only)

	Cancer site		
	Lung	Breast	Colon
Cancer incidence in 1986–87 by registration status in 1994:			
DCO cases	2670	906	997
Non-DCO cases	7802	6743	3535
DCO (% of total incidence)	25.5	11.8	22.0
Crude survival (%) at five years:			
Conventional (without DCO)	6.4	60.1	33.3
Adjusted (including DCO[a])	4.8	54.1	26.6
Reduction (%)	25	10	20

[a] whose survival distribution has been estimated by tracing back DCO cases registered in 1992 (1719 cases for lung, 308 for breast and 491 for colon)

DCI cases for which the date of diagnosis could not be traced have the same survival distribution as those that were successfully traced, and that the survival distribution of cases which escape registration in life has not changed substantially between 1986–87 and 1992. Results are presented here for cancers of the lung, colon and female breast; these cancers were chosen because they are all common, and because they represent a wide range of survival, from poor (lung) to moderate (colon) to fair (breast).

Table 1.2 and Figure 1.2 show the conventional estimate of the survival distribution, which excludes all DCOs, and an adjusted estimate, which includes them as if they had all been successfully traced back. The adjusted survival figures, shown by the bold lines in Figure 1.2, are systematically lower than the conventional ones, shown with a thin line. The absolute difference in survival estimates introduced by tracing back DCI cases is likely to be relatively minor for highly lethal cancers, i.e. those with survival of 10% or less at five years, such as lung cancer, but it may be important if the prognosis is relatively good. In the case of breast cancer, for example, excluding all DCI cases, which comprise about 12% of the 1986–87 incidence, the five-year crude survival estimate would be 60.1%; while if all of them were successfully traced back and included in the survival analysis, the corresponding figure would be 54.1%, that is 10% less. Note that the percentage reduction in survival is similar to the proportion of DCO cases in the whole case series (Table 1.2). It should be stressed that the proportion of DCO cases in the Thames Cancer Registry in this period was quite high; if the estimates of bias obtained here were to apply to other populations, for which the percentage of DCO cases is often in the range 2–5%, it is unlikely that the conventional estimates of survival would be substantially overestimated by the exclusion of DCO cases. However, a low proportion of DCO may indicate either a small number of DCI cases, in which case the survival estimate would be unbiased, or a successful trace-back of a substantial number of DCI, which may imply that survival is underestimated because all short-term survivors have been included while long-term survivors may not (Table 1.1). The latter may be the case, for instance, for the Mersey Cancer Registry, where the proportion of DCI cases is brought down to 0% DCO by tracing them back to clinical notes (J. Youngson, personal communication).

Early detection

The issue of screening and its effect on survival has already been mentioned in the section on the definition of the disease. The effect depends on the detectability of the lesion before symptoms appear (i.e. the length of the detectable pre-clinical phase, see Figure 1.1), which, in turn, depends on its natural history, the sensitivity of the screening test and the frequency of screening.

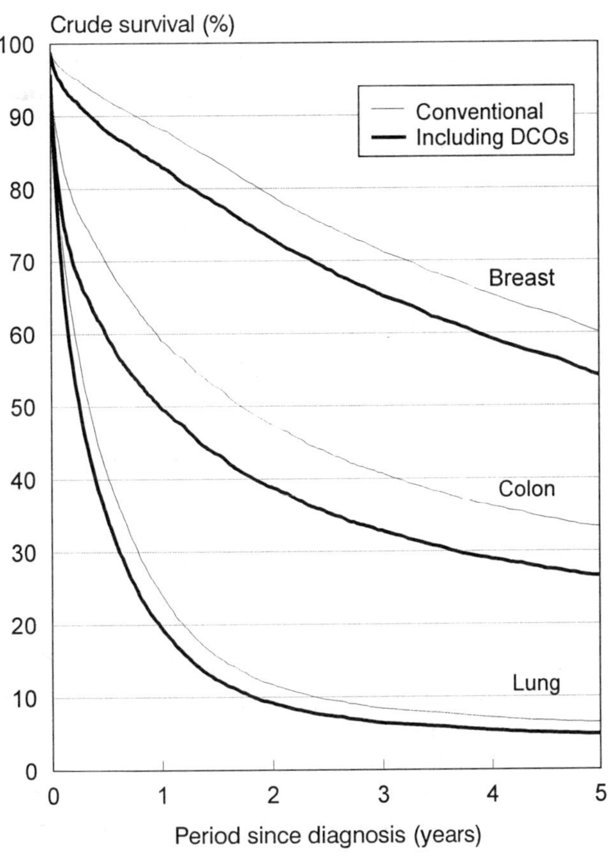

Figure 1.2. Estimated effect of tracing back DCO cases and including them in survival computation. South Thames, 1986–87 cases.

Several cancer registries collect some information on how the diagnosis was made, whether as a result of symptoms, as a result of a screening or a check-up examination, or incidentally during investigation for other diseases. In the absence of organized screening programmes, however, this information may be quite subjective, and in practice there are few reliable data to quantify the level of opportunistic screening (i.e. screening investigations done outside the control of an organized programme) in the populations covered by cancer registries. Indirect information on screening activity may be provided at the population level by the frequency of *in situ* carcinoma and, for large bowel cancer, by the frequency of adenocarcinoma arising in an adenomatous polyp. The relative frequency of *in situ* breast carcinoma, for instance, increased from about 3% to 8% between 1973 and 1987 in Detroit (Michigan, US), where mammographic screening was rapidly expanding (Simon *et al.*, 1992), while it remained at around 3% in Varese province (Italy), where there was no significant screening activity. *In situ* carcinomas are usually excluded from survival analyses, but a high proportion of *in situ* cases in the registry data would also suggest that a substantial proportion of invasive cases may have been detected preclinically.

Randomized trials have proved that mammographic screening for breast cancer can reduce mortality rates, but it is difficult to quantify the extent to which the effect on survival is due to advancing the date of diagnosis, or to an actual postponement of the date of death. These effects are very specific to each programme, and they change over time as screening techniques and schedules evolve. In the Swedish Two-County trial of mammographic screening for breast cancer, which showed a substantial reduction in mortality rates for screened women, the mean lead time was estimated to be about three years, and the improvement in survival was due both to the addition of lead time and to postponement of death (Tabàr *et al.*, 1992). There are instances, however, in which the effect of screening is to produce a substantial increase in survival solely by the addition of lead time, without any effect on the length of life (or before any such effect is apparent). In the Canadian National Breast Screening Study of women aged 50–59 years, which did not show any advantage of annual mammographic screening over and above annual physical examination in reducing breast cancer mortality, "...18 (47%) of the 38 women who died in the group randomized to undergo annual mammography had tumours detected at the first screening, as compared with only 8 (20%) of the 39 women who died in the physical examination only group". Thus, "the use of mammography advanced the time of detection by at least a year for about a quarter of the women who died of breast cancer in the mammography group..." (Miller *et al.*, 1992).

A further reason why the duration of survival may be increased by screening is the increased detection of slow-growing tumours, i.e. those with a long detectable preclinical phase, some of which might never be diagnosed as clinical cancers if left unscreened. In the Swedish Two-County trial, for instance, long-term survival of patients whose cancer was detected at the first screen was significantly higher than in the control group, even after careful adjustment for tumour size, nodal involvement and grade (Tabàr *et al.*, 1992). This kind of effect of screening on survival will be expected to vary over time (Saxen & Hakama, 1964). When an organized screening programme begins, survival will be expected first to increase, due to the detection of slow-growing tumours, then to decrease, when the prevalent slow-growing tumours have already been detected, before eventually reaching a new steady state. For example, a decreasing trend in survival for cervical cancer has been reported by the Saarland Cancer Registry (Germany) between 1972–76 and 1977–81 (Wiebelt *et al.*, 1991), and such a change is also seen in this monograph for a few other countries, particularly Switzerland. This decreasing trend may be due to a progressive decline in the proportion of slow-growing tumours among the incident cases of cervical cancer in the age range of screening.

The problem of early detection is not restricted to cancers detected in screening programmes, however. For cancers detected clinically, the interval between the onset of symptoms and the diagnosis is also a major determinant of survival, at least in the short term. This interval has probably declined substantially in the past few years, at least for some cancer sites, since a shift in stage distribution towards less advanced tumours has been a common clinical experience, even in the absence of screening programmes (Bergman *et al.*, 1992; Sue-Ling *et al.*, 1993).

A trend towards early diagnosis would be expected to lead to a more favourable distribution of clinical stage, which is the major prognostic factor associated with the time of diagnosis. Unfortunately, the definition and recording of cancer stage are not standardized among cancer registries (nor indeed among clinicians), and, still worse, information on stage is not systematically available to tumour registrars from the clinical records. As we shall see, however, even if all cases were staged and the information on stage systematically recorded, stage-specific comparisons of survival between populations covered by different cancer registries would not be easily interpretable, and stage-adjusted comparisons would be biased: additional data are needed to resolve this problem (see below).

The effectiveness of treatment

Retrospective comparisons of the efficacy of cancer treatment are well known to be unreliable. Except in the context of randomized trials, cancer patients undergoing a given therapeutic regimen are likely to be different from those receiving other regimens. Patients may be excluded from receiving a given treatment either because they are too ill, or are judged to be too old, or because they refuse treatment, or a concomitant illness contraindicates it. In this respect, clinical judgement has important subjective components, and depends on cultural and social factors. Treatment-specific or treatment-adjusted survival comparisons, therefore, would not be easily interpretable, because patients receiving a given treatment may differ quite widely between populations, or over time within a population, as a result of national or regional differences in the accepted indications for that treatment, or changes in the indications over time.

If, for example, the development of new treatment techniques (or just a change in the attitude of clinicians) enables more successful treatment than was previously possible of patients with advanced disease, then—even if the overall survival of all cancer patients increased—one might observe a drop in survival among both treated and untreated patients, the former because they would now include additional advanced cases, previously untreated, and the latter because they would now include only the very advanced, untreatable cases. Such a phenomenon has recently been described in the comparison of survival of patients with lung cancer, excluding small cell lung cancer, in three French regions covered by population-based cancer registries (Grosclaude *et al.*, 1994). The highest proportion of patients treated surgically was in Tarn (37%) and the lowest in Calvados (21%). After adjusting for age and morphology with the Cox model, 18-month survival was slightly better in Tarn. When treatment was included in the model, however, both resected and unresected patients in Calvados appeared to survive better than those in Tarn. As the authors point out, this effect is analogous to the stage migration phenomenon (Feinstein *et al.*, 1985; see below); it illustrates the point that adjusting for therapeutic procedures when comparing survival in different populations may be misleading.

Several registries collect more or less detailed information on therapy, but this information is far from being standardized or exhaustive. Therapies performed during hospital stay are usually reliably recorded, but treatment made on an outpatient basis (frequently the case for chemotherapy) is more likely to be missed. The exact intent of therapy, whether curative or palliative, or whether or not it is judged radical by the treating physician, is also difficult or impossible to establish. These definitions are quite subjective even in clinical practice. Even if cancer registries were able to collect detailed, exhaustive and standardized information on treatment, however, it would not usually be possible to judge the effectiveness of treatment from survival analysis alone, because the choice of treatment is based on the stage of disease and on the general condition of the patient.

Several studies have provided evidence of longer survival for cancer patients treated in specialist centres, where therapeutic protocols are more likely to be applied, than for patients treated at other hospitals (Stiller, 1989). Most of these studies could not exclude the possibility that the patients treated in specialist centres were selected according to stage of disease or other prognostic factors, particularly general health at diagnosis. A few studies showed that the better prognosis persisted after adjustment for stage of disease, but diagnostic procedures to establish the stage are likely to vary between centres, specialist centres being more likely to perform more thorough staging investigations. Proper comparison would require adjustment for diagnostic procedures as well (see below).

Despite these difficulties, it would be important to check whether international differences in the pattern of treatments were consistent with differences in survival; but again the issue would arise whether a greater frequency of treatments with curative intent were just a consequence of a more favourable stage distribution, and, therefore, whether longer survival simply reflected earlier diagnosis (i.e. lead time) rather than true prolongation of life.

Improving the interpretation of survival statistics

Advances in diagnostic technology such as ultrasonography, magnetic resonance imaging and cancer biomarkers allow the detection of smaller or less advanced lesions than was possible even quite recently. To the extent that these advances change the biological spectrum of malignant disease that is actually diagnosed, and because they are not yet uniformly available, such technological advances actually complicate the interpretation of geographical differences in survival and of trends in survival over time.

In principle, in order to disentangle whether longer survival is due to better treatment (which actually prolongs the life of the patient), or to earlier diagnosis (by the addition of lead time or because it makes conventional treatment more effective), or both, one might wish to compare stage-specific survival: if survival were increasing in both localized and advanced stages of disease, one would conclude that therapy had improved; if stage-specific survival did not change, one would conclude that it had not, and that any increase in overall survival was due to the shift towards earlier stages of disease.

Such a simple stage-specific analysis, however, would be misleading, because the specific content of a stage category varies with time and place, depending on geographical differences in diagnostic technology and medical practice with respect to stage, or changes in these factors over time.

Today, we classify as 'advanced' a significant proportion of cases that yesterday would have been labelled as 'localized' just because early metastases were not discovered, and could not have been detected with the techniques available at the time. This constitutes the stage migration phenomenon, by which cases with intermediate survival 'migrate' from the localized to the advanced stage as medical technology improves, thus apparently improving the prognosis of cases in both categories (Feinstein *et al.*, 1985). By the same token, when survival figures for the same time period in different countries are compared, countries where more advanced staging technologies are available would show better stage-specific or stage-adjusted survival, even if there were no difference in overall survival. To proceed safely to stage-adjusted or stage-specific analysis, one should guarantee that stage categories are comparable, that is, defined on the basis of the same diagnostic procedures. An unbiased comparison can also be achieved by adjusting not only for stage but also for the relevant diagnostic determinants of stage. Within any given stage, in fact, those cases that have undergone more thorough diagnostic investigation are likely to be less advanced and to have a better prognosis. Adjustment for the staging procedure, however, would require that registries collect standardized information not only on stage but also on the examinations made to determine the stage, which is not normally done.

A recent study from the National Cancer Institute in Milan, Italy, showed that breast cancer patients treated surgically in the late 1970s had a significantly better prognosis than patients treated in the early 1970s: 66% versus 60% observed ten-year survival (Cascinelli *et al.*, 1991). In particular, among women with positive axillary lymph nodes the age-adjusted risk of death was 18% lower in the later period (relative risk 0.82, $p < 0.03$). Adjusting for the number of positive nodes in the axilla increased the apparent prognostic advantage of the second period still further (RR = 0.73, $p < 0.001$). This was clearly a stage migration effect. The mean number of axillary lymph nodes examined in each patient was much higher in the more recent period (15 vs 6); thus, for any given stage of disease (as defined by the number of involved lymph nodes), it is likely that cases in the earlier period were, on average, more advanced than those in the later period, simply because microscopic metastases were less likely to have been discovered, leaving the tumour misclassified to a lower stage. Adjustment for the number of lymph nodes examined made the period effect almost disappear (RR = 0.94, $p = 0.79$). Appropriate adjustment for stage of disease, therefore, showed that almost all of the improvement in survival in the later period was due to earlier diagnosis.

The above example shows that correction for stage migration bias is theoretically possible, provided the relevant information has been collected. Such information was not available for the analyses presented in this monograph, however, and no attempt has been made to adjust for stage. In the EUROCARE-2 study, a concerted action among European cancer registries approved by the European Community in 1993, a standardized description of the stage at diagnosis and of a few key diagnostic determinants of stage will be collected on samples of incident cases. The stage determinants will include, for example, the number of axillary nodes examined for breast cancer and the availability of liver imaging data for colorectal cancer. This is a wider range of data than is usually collected by cancer registries, and it will require modification of their information pathways, but it should permit adjustment for stage migration bias in the comparison of survival statistics. If it should prove feasible to collect and analyse these data on a regular basis, the value of cancer registries for monitoring progress against cancer would be greatly enhanced, but this extension of cancer registry activity will require additional resources, since trained staff are needed to collect data according to a strictly standardized protocol from medical records.

The EUROCARE monograph

A pioneering effort to compare survival data from six countries was carried out in the early 1960s (Cutler, 1964).

In the above discussion we have introduced the major difficulties encountered in estimating and comparing relative survival in different populations. Some of these difficulties cannot be resolved with the existing data sets held by most cancer registries. In effect, the current practices of cancer registries are being challenged by more precise questions about cancer survival, and by the demand for more wideranging analyses. In this context, the EUROCARE-1 study (carried out in 1991–93) has helped to define the improvements required to enable some of these questions to be addressed, while EUROCARE-2 (planned for 1994–96) is expected to provide reliable information to quantify these biases in survival comparison, and to enable them to be corrected in the future for several cancer sites. The present monograph provides the largest international set of population-based estimates of cancer survival ever published.

Despite the difficulties in the estimation and comparison of cancer survival, it was considered that analyses based on the data currently available would be informative. In particular, the EUROCARE Working Group judged that it would be possible to estimate survival for selected sites of cancer in a number of well defined populations, and to provide a starting point for more detailed investigation of any observed differences in survival between them. The major aim of EUROCARE-1, therefore, was to establish a database suitable for carrying out these basic analyses. First, the Working Group decided to make available sex- and age-specific survival probabilities for each contributing country, as well as, whenever the sample size made it possible, age-standardized survival rates. Although examination of trends in cancer survival was not a major aim in this study, results are also given for three successive time periods. More detailed analyses are now in progress for some frequent cancers, but we are confident that the main information of the database is included in the analyses presented here.

A number of specific warnings have been highlighted in the presentation of the tables, in order to avoid misinterpretation (see Chapter 16), and further commentary, in Chapter 18, gives various possible explanations of the observed differences. In addition, however, some of the choices made in analysis of the data and presentation of the results need discussion here, since, in order to produce such a comprehensive picture of survival among cancer patients in Europe, we were obliged to adopt a number of simplified procedures.

First, for some analyses, we pooled data from different cancer registries in the same country, despite the fact that there were some regional differences in survival; in general, however, regional differences within a country were not large, and they were usually smaller than international differences.

Second, in the absence of better information, we assumed that the available registry data for a given country, sometimes derived from only a small fraction of the national population, could be used to obtain an estimate of cancer survival in the nation as a whole, in order to compute a weighted European average survival. It is unlikely, for instance, that the data for Geneva and Basel comprise a representative sample of all cancer patients in Switzerland. Nevertheless, since they were the only data from Switzerland available to EUROCARE, it was considered reasonable to give them the appropriate national weight in a European pooled estimate of survival. Whenever survival figures are compared between countries, however, it is indicated that the comparison refers to the populations actually covered by the cancer registries, not necessarily the countries in which they operate.

Third, we sometimes pooled data from registries whose periods of activity did not precisely coincide. Under the EUROCARE protocol, survival data were requested for patients diagnosed in 1978–84, but a number of registries were not able to provide data for the whole period; in order to increase the size of the study in some countries, cases diagnosed in 1985 were also accepted from a few registries. In Italy, for instance, the cancer registry of Varese Province covered the whole period 1978–84 , but the cancer registry of Ragusa Province (1981–84) and the Modena colo-rectal cancer registry (1983–84) were added, and the cancer registry of Florence Province was also accepted, even though it had data only for 1985. Similar situations exist for France and Switzerland (Chapter 2). In such circumstances, geographical differences in survival within a country could influence the estimation of survival trends. To check whether survival trends were confounded by geographical variability, the pooled national estimates of trends in survival were systematically compared with the trends in each constituent registry. No major difference was detected, with the following exceptions:

Cervical cancer in Switzerland, where the Geneva Cancer Registry covered the entire period 1978–84 and the Basel registry only 1982–84. In the pooled overall trend, survival fell from 71% in 1978–80 to 67% in 1981–82 and 55% in 1983–84, but the trend in Geneva was more pronounced: 71%, 52% and 50%.

Testis cancer in France, where the registry of Doubs covered 1978–85 but the registry of Amiens only 1983–84. The pooled overall trend was 75%, 83%, 83%, but the trend in Doubs continued to increase up to 96% in 1983–85.

Leukaemia in Italy, where the significant decreasing trend reported for the combined leukaemia analysis (30%, 28%, and 22% in the three successive periods) was not apparent in Varese Province (30%, 33%, and 30%); the decreasing trend of survival for chronic myeloid leukaemia, however, was present both for Varese Province and in the pooled national analysis.

Fourth, we decided to present survival data by ICD-9 three-digit cancer site, even though substantial international differences are known to exist in the frequency of cancers at subsites within a single site defined at the three-digit level (e.g. glottis, ICD-9 161.1, and supraglottis, ICD-9 161.0, within larynx, ICD-9 161), and cancers in these subsites may have quite different survival probabilities. This issue is especially relevant for cancers of the head and neck, but also for large bowel, and for sites that group different tissues and organs, such as ICD-9 189 (kidney, pelvis and ureter). The distribution by relevant fourth-digit subsites and by country is given in Chapter 2.

Cancers of the head and neck, for example, show a typical dichotomy between Latin and Anglo-Saxon countries, the former showing a clear excess of alcohol-related cancers at subsites such as the base of the tongue, oral mucosa other than cheek and palate, oropharynx other than tonsil, pyriform sinus, and supraglottis (Tuyns *et al.*, 1988). Since the prognosis is worse for cancer at most of the subsites which are more frequent in Latin countries (Gatta *et al.*, 1994), several international comparisons are affected; it is likely, for instance, that the relatively poor survival recorded for cancers of the head and neck in Italy, France and Switzerland, compared with the United Kingdom, Denmark and the Netherlands, is at least partially ascribable to this bias. Unfortunately, the high proportion of cases for which the subsite was not known made it impossible to carry out more specific analyses.

Similar problems may arise for colon cancers, for which the distribution by subsite varies considerably between populations. The proportion of cancers of the left side (descending colon and sigmoid), which have a slightly better prognosis than those in the right hemicolon, ranges from 61% in Estonia to 44% in the Netherlands; it is relatively high also in Scotland (57%) and France (55%) and low in England (46%). From a detailed analysis of EUROCARE data, however, the survival advantage of left-sided cancers appears to be limited to the first 4–5 years after diagnosis, after which the survival curves overlap (data not shown), suggesting that long-term survival comparisons for all colon cancers combined are not likely to be biased by differences in the distribution of cancers within the colon.

Under the heading 'Kidney' the frequency of cancer coded to ICD-9 189.1 and 189.2 (renal pelvis and ureter) varies substantially among countries, from 3% to 26%. The issue is relevant because these organs give rise to urothelial tumours of the same types as those of which the uncertain definition led to the exclusion of bladder cancer from this monograph. Unfortunately a variable proportion of renal pelvis cancers may also have been coded to 189.0 (renal parenchyma, and kidney, not otherwise specified), which would make fourth-digit-specific analyses as uncertain as global analyses.

Fifth, a relevant factor that has not been considered in this monograph is the histological classification. Although for most cancer sites one histological type dominates the picture, it is also true that for almost every site there are other histological types with different known or suspected causes and, frequently, different prognosis, which, if differently distributed in different populations, might blur survival comparison. Unfortunately, little testing has ever been done on either the reproducibility or coding of histological diagnoses, and cancer registry data on histology are not yet suitable for international comparisons. This is a general problem of cancer epidemiology (Berg, 1985): although the ICD-O morphology code (WHO, 1976) is a standard, internationally accepted and widely used code for cancer histology, much material has been coded and little has ever been retrieved.

Despite these caveats to the interpretation of the results, the EUROCARE data indicate that there are international differences in the survival of cancer patients which seem too large to be explained solely by uncontrolled methodological differences in cancer registration and follow-up procedures between the various participating countries. We are confident, in particular, that the observed differences cannot be explained by such factors as differences in the index date from which survival is computed, nor by different follow-up procedures, which, as shown in Chapter 2, introduce only minor biases. The study was restricted to ICD categories that are likely to be defined in the same way in different populations, and, apart from head and neck cancers, and, possibly, kidney cancer, differences in the distribution of anatomical subsites are unlikely to explain any major survival difference. A somewhat larger bias may arise from the incompleteness of cancer registration: we cannot exclude the possibility that some of the observed differences in survival may be due to the selective loss of some longterm or short-term survivors. The simulation carried out in the Thames Cancer Registry, however, suggests that even differences in survival due to the exclusion of some short-term survivors are likely to be smaller than the observed differences in survival between countries. For some cancers there are also large differences in survival between populations for which cancer registration is likely to be virtually complete. Many of the differences in cancer survival between populations reported in this monograph, therefore, are likely to depend largely on differences in access to health systems and in cancer care.

References

Bernoulli, D. (1766) *Essai d'une nouvelle analyse de la mortalité causée par la petite vérole, et des avantages de l'inoculation pour la prevenir.* Memoires de mathématiques et de physique tirées des registres de l'Académie Royale des Sciences de l'année MDCCLX, Paris

Bears, O.H. & Smart, C.M. (1979) Diagnosis of minimal breast cancer in the BCDDP: the 66 questionable cases. *Cancer*, **43**, 848–850

Berg, J.W. (1985) Problems in classification of cancer for epidemiologic research. In: Garfinkel, L., Ochs, O. & Mushinski, M., eds, *Selection, Follow-up and Analysis in Prospective Studies: a Workshop* (Natl. Cancer Inst. Monogr., No. 67), Washington, DC, US Government Printing Office, pp. 123–127

Bergman, L., Kluck, H.M., van Leeuwen, F.E., Crommelin, M.A., Dekker, G., Hart A.A.M. & Coebergh, J.W.W. (1992) The influence of age on treatment choice and survival of elderly breast cancer patients in South-eastern Netherlands: a population-based study. *Eur. J. Cancer*, **28A**, 1475–1480

Black, R.J., Sharp, L. & Kendrick, S.W. (1993) *Trends in Cancer Survival in Scotland, 1968–1990.* Edinburgh, ISD Publications

Cascinelli, N., Greco, M., Morabito, A., Bufalino, R., Testori, A., Baldini, M.T., Andreola, S., Leo, E., Galluzzo, D. & Rilke, F. (1991) Comparison of long-term survival of 1986 consecutive patients with breast cancer treated at the National Cancer Institute of Milano, Italy (1971 to 1972 and 1977 to 1978). *Cancer*, **68**, 427–434

Coleman, M.P, Estève, J., Damiecki, P., Arslan, A. & Renard, H. (1993) *Trends in Cancer Incidence and Mortality* (IARC Scientific Publications No. 121), Lyon, IARC

Cutler, S.J., ed. (1964) *International Symposium on End Results of Cancer Therapy* (Natl. Cancer Inst. Monogr. No. 15), Washington, DC, US Government Printing Office

Cuzick, J. (1990) International time trends for multiple myeloma. *Ann. N.Y. Acad. Sci.*, **609**, 205–214

Estève, J., Benhamou, E. & Raymond, L. (1994) *Statistical Methods in Cancer Research*, Vol. IV, *Descriptive Epidemiology* (IARC Scientific Publications No. 128) Lyon, IARC

Feinstein, A.R., Sosin, D.M. & Wells, C.K. (1985) The Will Rogers phenomenon: stage migration and new diagnostic techniques as a source of misleading statistics for survival in cancer. *New Engl. J. Med.*, **312**, 1604–1608

Fontana, R.F. (1984) Early detection of lung cancer: The Mayo lung project. In: Prorok, P.C. & Miller, A.B., eds, *Screening for Cancer. I – General Principles on Evaluation of Screening for Cancer and Screening for Lung, Bladder and Oral Cancer* (UICC Technical Report Series Vol. 78), Geneva, International Union Against Cancer

Gafà, L., Viganò, C. & Pavone, G. (1992) Treatment of DCO: two examples. In: Zanetti, R. & Crosignani, P., eds, *Cancer in Italy*, Turin, Lega Italiana per la Lotta contro i Tumori, Associazione Italiana di Epidemiologia, pp. 69–72

Gatta, G., Sant, M., Micheli, A., Capocaccia, R., Verdecchia, A., Barchielli, A., Gafà, L., Ramazzotti, V. & Berrino, F. (1994) La sopravvivenza per tumori dell'apparato digerente: Dati italiani su base di popolazione e confronti internazionali. *Ann. Ist. Super. Sanità* (in press)

Gittes, R.F. (1991) Carcinoma of the prostate. *New Engl. J. Med.*, **324**, 236–245

Grosclaude, P., Gallat, J.P., Mace-Lesech, J., Machelard-Roumagnac, M., Schraub, S. & Robillard, J. (1994) Traitements et survie des cancers du poumon à petites cellules dans trois départements français. In: *Epidémiologie dans les pays de langue latine* (IARC Technical Reports No. 20), Lyon, IARC, pp. 57–67

Louis, P.C.A. (1835) *Recherches sur les effets de la saignée dans quelques maladies inflammatoires, et sur l'action de l'émetique et des vésicatoires dans la pneumonie*, Paris, Baillière

Miller, A., Baines, C.J., To, T. & Wall, C. (1992) Canadian national breast screening study: 2. Breast cancer detection and death rates among women aged 50 to 59 years. *Can. Med. Ass. J.*, **147**, 1477–1488

Muir, C.S., Waterhouse, J.A.H., Mack, T., Powell, J. & Whelan, S., eds (1987) *Cancer Incidence in Five Continents,* Volume V (IARC Scientific Publications No. 88), Lyon, IARC

Parkin, D.M., Muir, C.S., Whelan, S., Gao, Y.-T., Ferlay, J. & Powell, J., eds (1992) *Cancer Incidence in Five Continents*, Volume VI (IARC Scientific Publications No. 120), Lyon, IARC

Potosky, A.L., Kessler, L., Gridley, G., Brown, C.C. & Horm, J.W. (1990) Rise in prostatic cancer incidence associated with increased use of transurethral resection. *J. Natl Cancer Inst.*, **82**, 1624–1628

Salmon, S.E. & Cassady, J.R. (1989) Plasma cell neoplasms. In: DeVita, V.T., Jr., Hellman, S. & Rosenberg, S.A., eds, *Cancer, Principles & Practice of Oncology*, 3rd edition, Philadelphia, Lippincott, pp. 1853–1887

Saxén, E. & Hakama, M. (1964) Cancer illness in Finland, with a note on the effect of age adjustment and early diagnosis. *Ann. Med. Exp. Biol. Fenn.*, **42** (suppl. 2), 1–28

Schwartz, J. (1990) Multinational trends in multiple myeloma. *Ann. N.Y. Acad. Sci.*, **609**, 215–224

Simon, M.S., Schwartz, A.G., Martino, S. & Swanson, G.M. (1992) Trends in the diagnosis of in situ breast cancer in the Detroit metropolitan area, 1973 to 1987. *Cancer*, **69**, 466–469

Stiller, C.A. (1989) Survival of patients with cancer. Those included in clinical trials do better. *Br. Med. J.*, **299**, 1054–1059

Sue-Ling, H.M., Johnston, D., Martin, I.G., Dixon, M.F., Lansdown, M.R.J., McMahom, M.J. & Axon, A.T.R. (1993) Gastric cancer: a curable disease in Britain. *Br. Med. J.*, **307**, 591–596

Tabàr, L., Fagerberg, G., Duffy, S.W., Day, N.E., Gad, A. & Gröntoft, O. (1992) Update of the Swedish Two-County program of mammographic screening for breast cancer. *Radiol. Clin. North Amer.*, **30**, 187–210

Tuyns, A.J., Estève, J., Raymond, L., Berrino, F., Benhamou, E., Blanchet, F., Boffetta, P., Crosignani, P., del Moral, A., Lehmann, W., Merletti, F., Péquignot, G., Sancho-Garnier, H., Terracini, B., Zubiri, A. & Zubiri, L. (1988) Cancer of the larynx/hypopharynx, tobacco and alcohol: IARC international case–control study in Turin and Varese (Italy), Zaragoza and Navarra (Spain), Geneva (Switzerland) and Calvados (France). *Int. J. Cancer*, **41**, 483–491

Wiebelt, H., Hakulinen, T., Ziegler, H. & Stegmaier, C. (1991) Leben die Krebspatienten heute länger als früher? Eine Überlebenszeitanalyse der Krebspatienten im Saarland der Jahre 1972 bis 1986. *Soz. Präventivmed.*, **36**, 86–95

WHO (World Health Organization) (1976) *International Classification of Diseases for Oncology (ICD-O),* Geneva

WHO (World Health Organization) (1977) *International Classification of Diseases, Manual of the International Statistical Classification of Diseases, Injuries, and Causes of Death*, 9th revision, Geneva

Yatani, R. Chigusa, I., Akazaki K., Stemmerman, G.N., Welsh, R.A. & Correa, P. (1982) Geographic pathology of latent prostatic carcinoma. *Int. J. Cancer*, **29**, 611–616

CHAPTER 2

The EUROCARE database

M. Sant and G. Gatta

Although the biological and clinical information recorded by cancer registries is much less detailed than that collected in clinical studies, the information that is collected pertains to all the cancer cases occurring in a given population, which is often a large region or an entire country, and can thus provide an indication of the overall effectiveness of health care measures and their impact on the population of that region. Furthermore, population-based cancer registry information is eminently suited for effecting comparisons between one population and another and for revealing changes in cancer incidence, survival and other parameters over time.

Unfortunately, however, survival analyses published by individual cancer registries have not in the past adopted a standardized methodological approach, and have usually not provided sufficient details of their methodology to permit valid comparisons between registries to be made. One of the reasons for setting up the EUROCARE project was to collect cancer survival data from cancer registries across Europe, for analysis according to standardized procedures, in order to be able to make reliable comparisons of survival between different European populations.

The validity of survival estimates calculated from cancer registry data depends on the quality (accuracy and completeness) of the incidence data; it also depends on the thoroughness of the follow-up procedures. Problems relating to the quality of incidence data have been discussed in Chapter 1. This chapter describes the EUROCARE database and the checks performed on it to assess information quality. The results of an analysis of the completeness of follow-up procedures are also presented.

Participating centres, study period and inclusion criteria

Registries

Figure 2.1 shows the locations of the 30 cancer registries participating in EUROCARE. European Community countries are particularly well represented (United Kingdom, Denmark, the Netherlands, Germany, France, Italy and Spain); participating countries not belonging to the European Community are Switzerland, Finland, Poland and Estonia.

Table 2.1 (a and b) lists the 30 participating cancer registries together with the period of incidence covered by each and the total number of cases contributed by tumour site, coded according to the first three digits of the ninth revision of the International Classification of Diseases (ICD-9) (WHO, 1977). The EUROCARE database contains information on about 800 000 patients.

The registries of Denmark, Estonia and Finland have nationwide coverage. Much of the United Kingdom is also covered: the six English cancer registries participating in EUROCARE cover 46% of the population of England (Thames, Mersey, Yorkshire, East Anglia, West Midlands and Wessex), while the Scottish Cancer Registry covers the whole of Scotland. Italy, France, Switzerland and Spain are each represented by more than one cancer registry, but much lower proportions of the population are covered by cancer registration in these countries. Finally, the Netherlands, Poland and Germany are each represented by a single centre covering only a small fraction of their respective national populations.

A number of registries only provide information on certain tumour sites, as reported in Table 2.1. A number of specialized registries have contributed to the study: the digestive tract cancer registries of Calvados

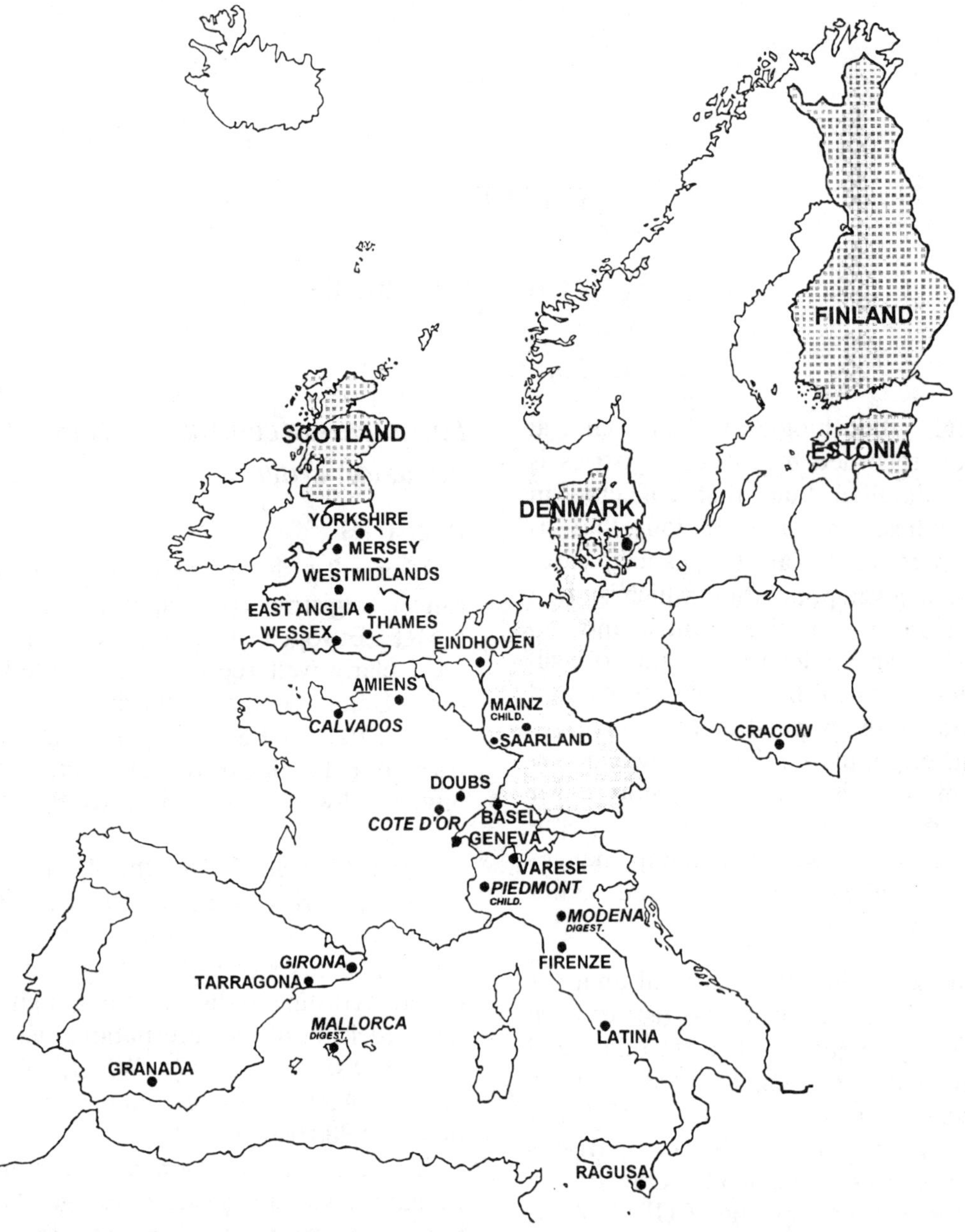

Figure 2.1. European cancer registries participating in the EUROCARE survival study. National registries are indicated in capitals. Registries covering a single region or town are in small capitals, specialized registries in italics.

and Côte d'Or in France, Modena in Italy and Mallorca in Spain, and the registry of haematological malignancies and of breast cancer, Côte d'Or. The Cooperative Childhood Registry of Malignancies of Germany (referred to in this book as the Mainz Childhood Cancer Registry) and that of Piedmont in Italy, which have national and regional coverage, respectively, allowed special analyses on tumours of infancy.

Tumour sites

All major cancer sites are included; except those for which diagnostic, classification and registration criteria are not sufficiently standardized. Sites not included are non-Hodgkin lymphomas (ICD−9 codes 200 and 202), multiple myeloma (ICD−9 203), bladder tumours (ICD−9 188), prostate tumours (ICD−9 185), skin tumours, melanoma (ICD−9 172) and non-melanoma (ICD−9 173), liver tumours (ICD−9 155) and gallbladder tumours (ICD−9 156). Non-Hodgkin lymphomas were excluded because variability of diagnostic criteria among pathologists and changes in histological classification over the last two decades

Table 2.1 (a). Cancer registries participating in the EUROCARE study: incidence period and number of cases by site included in the study

Registry	Country	Period (year)	ICD–9 code[a] 141	143	144	145	146	147	148	150	151	153	154	157	161	162
Amiens	F	83–84	43	2	20	28	64	7	62	131	195	267	210	76	107	459
Basel	CH	81–84	30	7	10	10	27	2	22	48	298	462	311	132	54	737
Calvados	F	78–85	0	0	0	0	0	0	0	798	765	794	700	277	0	0
Côte d'Or	F	78–85	0	0	0	0	0	0	0	292	604	1037	764	359	0	0
Cracow	PL	78–84	40	17	27	19	48	20	20	132	1061	441	432	354	283	2035
Denmark	DK	78–84	362	204	189	406	460	209	173	1180	6380	12229	9440	4728	1604	18905
Doubs	F	78–85	180	9	86	65	226	25	187	316	589	886	671	173	279	1181
East Anglia	ENG	79–84	133	37	52	60	75	56	109	961	2443	3681	2382	1374	398	8281
Eindhoven	NL	78–85	57	9	34	30	34	21	19	131	1147	1610	940	425	241	3381
Estonia	EST	78–84	88	34	43	31	65	34	40	210	3573	1213	1171	812	406	3232
Finland	FIN	78–84	317	..	141[b]	156	113	100	135	1349	7546	4743	3860	3538	927	14219
Geneva	CH	78–84	56	14	44	50	91	10	59	132	337	687	442	240	141	1141
Girona	E	80–85	0	0	0	0	0	0	0	0	0	0	0	0	0	0
Granada	E	85	0	0	0	0	0	0	0	0	0	0	0	0	0	170
Latina	I	83–84	9	1	3	12	5	3	0	15	144	106	83	39	40	258
Mainz Child.	D	80–84	1	0	0	6	0	15	0	0	0	2	1	2	1	2
Mallorca	E	82–84	0	0	0	0	0	0	0	0	0	246	203	0	0	0
Mersey	ENG	78–84	209	43	124	129	149	59	136	1578	4136	4650	3260	1710	676	12977
Modena	I	83–84	0	0	0	0	0	0	0	0	0	73	59	0	0	0
Piedmont Child.	I	78–84	0	0	0	0	0	5	0	0	0	0	0	1	0	0
Ragusa	I	81–84	13	2	1	4	6	6	0	25	246	192	111	79	70	307
Saarland	D	78–84	179	23	71	60	117	26	84	275	1885	2200	1800	477	343	3262
Scotland	SCO	78–82	288	89	217	216	146	103	201	2415	5762	8082	4260	2856	950	20493
Tarragona	E	85	7	1	7	5	5	8	3	23	94	100	84	29	33	159
Thames	ENG	78–84	534	112	188	273	274	160	323	3380	9112	13082	8077	5526	1447	32744
Tuscany	I	85	0	0	0	0	0	0	0	0	693	0	0	0	0	682
Varese	I	78–84	128[c]	23[c]	62[c]	57[c]	167[c]	58[c]	107[c]	249	1992	1503	879	458	596[c]	2841
Wessex	ENG	83–84	70	14	23	24	17	26	39	511	1006	1992	994	617	185	3383
West Midlands	ENG	79–84	289	65	154	138	213	114	281	1963	6769	7738	5888	2693	881	18519
Yorkshire	ENG	78–84	283	64	156	204	168	68	203	1920	5899	7082	5251	2805	977	18055

[a] For tumour sites corresponding to the ICD–9 code, see Table 2.2

[b] This figure for Finland corresponds to ICD–9 codes 143+144

[c] Incidence period 1978–85

Table 2.1 (b) Cancer registries participating in the EUROCARE study: incidence period and number of cases by site included in the study

Registry	Country	Period (Year)	ICD–9 code[a] 170	174	180	182	183	184	186	187	189	191	201	204–8	Total
Amiens	F	83–84	12	397	106	89	90	19	21	9	85	64	32	94	2689
Basel	CH	81–84	16	845	87	207	126	35	64	13	149	81	40	158	3971
Calvados	F	78–85	0	0	0	0	0	0	0	0	0	0	0	0	3334
Côte d'Or	F	78–85	0	762[b]	0	0	0	0	0	0	0	0	58[c]	311[c]	4187
Cracow	PL	78–84	42	1090	618	317	322	65	69	9	279	214	130	276	8360
Denmark	DK	78–84	320	17508	4199	4404	3987	829	1589	317	3603	2519	862	3973	100528
Doubs	F	78–85	26	1339	278	0	213	74	80	18	221	197	93	324	7736
East Anglia	ENG	79–84	96	5702	914	1078	1196	274	273	81	770	664	334	1070	32494
Eindhoven	NL	78–85	49	2653	249	410	427	70	115	26	462	272	141	407	13360
Estonia	EST	78–84	91	2387	1095	873	956	184	66	37	620	317	227	820	18625
Finland	FIN	78–84	275	11123	1290	2867	2322	510	290	96	2636	1906	812	2610	63881
Geneva	CH	78–84	18	1398	146	272	227	45	74	8	187	132	65	262	6278
Girona	E	80–85	0	734	97	173	100	27	0	0	0	0	0	0	1131
Granada	E	85	0	154	0	0	0	0	0	0	0	0	0	0	324
Latina	I	83–84	7	203	56	57	23	7	5	6	36	39	12	67	1236
Mainz Child.	D	80–84	313	0	0	0	26	6	16	14	307	441	295	1848	3296
Mallorca	E	82–84	0	0	0	0	0	0	0	0	0	0	0	0	449
Mersey	ENG	78–84	107	7223	1752	976	1338	268	323	128	831	758	400	1348	45297
Modena	I	83–84	0	0	0	0	0	0	0	0	0	0	0	0	132
Piedmont Child.	I	78–84	42	0	0	0	4	0	1	0	40	166	37	258	554
Ragusa	I	81–84	10	353	74	98	57	11	10	7	23	44	32	93	1874
Saarland	D	78–84	74	3360	713	965	544	139	204	42	694	381	175	471	18564
Scotland	SCO	78–82	220	11263	1955	1368	2143	497	571	165	1706	1294	728	1985	69973
Tarragona	E	85	1	156	29	43	24	13	3	7	10	25	14	34	917
Thames	ENG	78–84	350	20839	2900	3749	4465	837	741	230	2600	2612	1182	3670	119407
Tuscany	I	85	0	595	0	0	0	0	0	0	0	0	0	49	2019
Varese	I	78–84	54	2447	349	518	419	108	98	32	431	301	202	534	14474
Wessex	ENG	83–84	47	2688	426	432	553	124	107	36	361	332	125	533	14665
West Midlands	ENG	79–84	235	13264	2435	2279	2551	549	515	232	1484	1353	757	2303	73662
Yorkshire	ENG	78–84	202	10997	2382	1655	2047	499	475	186	1448	1318	669	2036	67049

[a] For tumour sites corresponding to the ICD–9 code see Table 2.2

[b] Incidence period 1982–85

[c] Incidence period 1980–84

rendered the groups of cases from different cancer registries difficult (if not impossible) to compare. Multiple myeloma was also excluded because of lack of standardized criteria for determining onset of malignant disease. Neoplasms of the bladder were excluded as standardized rules for inclusion of papillomas and non-invasive transitional cell carcinoma have not been adopted by the registries. Prostatic tumours were excluded because levels of both incidence and survival are heavily dependent on active search for asymptomatic disease. Skin cancers, both non-melanoma and melanoma, were excluded because the working group determined that many cancer registries have incomplete incidence data. Liver and gallbladder tumours were excluded because it was not always possible to reliably distinguish primary from metastatic lesions: distinction depends mainly on the use of diagnostic equipment (computerized tomography, ultrasonography, biopsy under sonographic or radiographic control) which was neither universally available nor as highly developed as now, during the study period. These problems have been outlined more fully in Chapter 1.

Study period

The study protocol originally stipulated inclusion of cases occurring during 1978–84. The incidence period was then extended to 1985 in order to include data from registries (for example in France and Spain) which had started activity more recently. For this reason there is some variation in the study period between registries.

Cohort definition

All cases diagnosed during the study period were recruited, whether or not they were hospitalized or microscopically (histologically or cytologically) verified. Only malignant tumours were included. All cases with ICD–O (WHO, 1976) behaviour code 0, 1 or 2 (benign, uncertain whether benign or malignant, or *in situ*, respectively) were excluded from the database. Cases incidentally discovered at autopsy were also excluded, as were those known to registries from the death certificate only (DCO cases). The implications of excluding DCO cases from the survival analysis have been discussed in Chapter 1.

In cases of multiple metachronous tumours, only the first-diagnosed tumour was registered, subsequent tumours being ignored. Bilateral breast cancers were considered as a single disease, with the date of diagnosis corresponding to that of discovery of the first tumour. For multiple synchronous tumours, the one at the most advanced stage was registered.

The minimum length of follow-up required by the study protocol was five years, but in fact the shortest follow-up always exceeded six years.

Database description

A minimum core of information, necessary to analyse survival and available from all registries, was selected for inclusion in the EUROCARE database: sex, date of birth, date of diagnosis, date of death or end of follow-up, living/dead status at the end of follow-up, ICD–9 code for the tumour site, microscopic confirmation or not, ICD–O morphology code with behaviour code, broad stage category and, when available, additional dates recorded by the registry for computing incidence and survival. Data were collected anonymously and date coding omitted the day of the month, to prevent identification of individual patients. The only exception to this was for childhood tumours, when the day of birth, etc., was recorded in order to compute age in the first year of life.

Tumour site

During the study period, most registries were using the ninth revision of ICD for coding tumour site, or provided their data coded according to this classification. For the Finnish Cancer Registry (which used ICD–7), the Danish Cancer Registry, and the Piedmont childhood and Côte d'Or haematological cancer registries (which sent ICD–O codes), data were converted to ICD–9 with the aid of the morphology codes also supplied. Table 2.2 reports the ICD–9 codes, the short description of the cancer site adopted in this monograph and the full description taken from the ICD–9 manual.

The fourth digit of the ICD–9 code was required for head and neck, colorectal and urogenital tumours. The distribution of these cancer sites by subsite and country is given in Tables 2.3–2.5. A few cancer registries, however, were not able to provide fourth-digit

Table 2.2. ICD−9 code, short description adopted in this monograph and full description in ICD manual

ICD−9 code	Short description	ICD−9 description
141	Tongue	Tongue
143−145	Oral cavity	Gum, floor of mouth, other and unspecified parts of mouth
146	Oropharynx	Oropharynx
147	Nasopharynx	Nasopharynx
148	Hypopharynx	Hypopharynx
141, 143−148	Head & neck	Tongue, gum, floor of mouth, other and unspecified parts of mouth, oropharynx, naso-pharynx, hypopharynx
150	Oesophagus	Oesophagus
151	Stomach	Stomach
153	Colon	Colon
154	Rectum	Rectum, rectosigmoid junction, anal canal and anus
157	Pancreas	Pancreas
161	Larynx	Larynx
162	Lung	Trachea, bronchus and lung
170	Bone	Bone and articular cartilage
174	Breast	Female breast
180	Cervix uteri	Cervix uteri
182	Corpus uteri	Corpus uteri
183	Ovary	Ovary and other uterine adnexa
184	Vagina & vulva	Other and unspecified female genital organs
186	Testis	Testis
187	Penis	Penis and other male genital organs
189	Kidney	Kidney and other and unspecified urinary organs (excluding urinary bladder)
191	Brain	Brain
201	Hodgkin's disease	Hodgkin's disease
204.0	Acute lymphatic leukaemia	Acute lymphatic leukaemia
204.1	Chronic lymphatic leukaemia	Chronic lymphatic leukaemia
205.0	Acute myeloid leukaemia	Acute myeloid leukaemia
205.1	Chronic myeloid leukaemia	Chronic myeloid leukaemia
204−208	Leukaemia	Leukaemia

information. The implications of differing fourth-digit subsite distribution in the comparison of survival figures between countries have been discussed in Chapter 1.

Microscopic confirmation

Table 2.6 shows the percentage of cases confirmed either histologically or cytologically for all sites and for colon, lung and breast cancers; the data are divided into two age groups (0−64 and 65+). Cytological and histological confirmations are presented together (as 'microscopic' confirmation), because some registries cannot distinguish between them. Combining ages, the proportion of microscopic confirmations ranges from 65% to 96% according to registry, but it should be noted that the sites included are not the same for each registry (see Table 2.1). The proportion of cases confirmed by microscopic examination is higher among younger than older patients. Table 2.6 illustrates

Table 2.3. Upper aerodigestive tract cancers by anatomical subcategory (ICD−9 fourth digit) and country

Site (ICD−9 code)[a]	Denmark		England		Estonia		France		Germany		Italy		Netherlands		Scotland		Switzerland	
	No.	%[b,c]	No.	%	No.	%	No.	%	No.	%	No.	%	No.	%	No.	%	No.	%
TONGUE, Total (141.0−141.9)	362	(10.7)[b]	1515	(15.3)	88	(12.4)	223	(16.4)	179	(20.4)	150	(11.5)	57	(13.5)	288	(13.6)	86	(14.0)
Tongue, base (141.0)	70	39.1[c]	241	31.3	14	23.7	21	52.5	61	70.9	44	37.0	16	30.2	48	37.5	28	36.8
Tongue, OSS (141.1−141.8)	109	60.9[c]	530	68.7	45	76.3	19	47.5	25	29.1	75	63.0	37	69.8	80	62.5	48	63.2
GUM, Total (143.0−143.9)	204	(6.0)	335	(3.4)	34	(4.8)	11	(0.8)	23	(2.6)	26	(2.0)	9	(2.1)	89	(4.2)	21	(3.4)
FLOOR OF MOUTH (144.0−144.9)	189	(5.6)	696	(7.0)	43	(6.1)	107	(7.9)	71	(8.1)	66	(5.0)	34	(8.0)	217	(10.3)	54	(8.8)
MOUTH, OTHER PARTS Total (145.0−145.9)	406	(11.9)	828	(8.3)	31	(4.4)	93	(6.9)	60	(6.9)	73	(5.6)	30	(7.1)	216	(10.3)	60	(9.7)
Cheek mucosa (145.0) and palate (145.2−145.5)	174	90.6	599	83.9	21	77.8	16	44.4	38	100.0	41	67.2	21	77.7	150	87.2	38	76.0
Mouth, OSS (145.1 & 145.6−145.8)	18	9.4	115	16.1	6	22.2	20	55.6	0	0.0	20	32.8	6	22.2	22	12.8	12	24.0
OROPHARYNX, Total (146.0−146.9)	460	(13.5)	896	(9.0)	65	(9.2)	290	(21.3)	117	(13.3)	178	(13.6)	34	(8.0)	146	(7.0)	118	(9.2)
Tonsil (146.0)	286	81.0	610	80.9	24	51.1	26	40.6	90	79.6	64	37.9	15	46.9	77	74.0	42	43.8
Oropharynx, OSS (146.1−146.8)	67	19.0	144	19.1	23	48.9	38	59.4	23	20.4	105	62.1	17	53.1	27	26.0	54	56.3
HYPOPHARYNX, Total (148.0−148.9)	173	(5.1)	1091	(11.0)	40	(5.7)	249	(18.3)	84	(9.6)	107	(8.2)	19	(4.5)	201	(9.5)	81	(13.2)
Postcricoid region (148.0)	1	2.0	354	38.3	2	8.3	3	5.5	0	0.0	2	2.3	2	15.4	59	35.8	0	0.0
Pyriform sinus (148.1)	41	80.4	516	55.8	17	70.8	47	85.5	7	58.3	59	67.8	8	61.5	96	58.2	46	86.8
Hypopharynx, OSS (148.2−148.8)	9	17.7	55	5.9	5	20.8	5	9.1	5	41.7	26	29.9	3	23.1	10	6.0	7	13.2
LARYNX, Total (161.0−161.9)	1604	(47.2)	4564	(46.0)	406	(57.4)	386	(28.4)	343	(39.1)	706	(54.1)	241	(56.8)	950	(45.1)	195	(31.7)
Glottis (161.0)	781	63.1	2127	68.9	106	65.8	29	36.3	155	77.5	255	45.4	124	59.3	371	72.9	92	52.0
Supraglottis (161.1)	386	31.2	706	22.9	34	21.1	45	56.3	35	17.5	242	43.1	64	30.6	112	22.0	77	43.5
Larynx, OSS (161.2−161.8)	70	5.7	256	8.3	21	13.0	6	7.5	10	5.0	65	11.6	21	10.0	26	5.1	8	4.5
Total no. of head and neck cases	3398	(100%)	9925	(100%)	707	(100%)	1359	(100%)	877	(100%)	1306	(100%)	424	(100%)	2107	(100%)	615	(100%)

[a] OSS=Other specified sites

[b] (within brackets): Percentage over the total number of head and neck cases

[c] without brackets: Percentage over the total number of specified anatomic subcategories within each three-digit anatomical site

Table 2.4. Colon and rectum cancer by anatomic subcategory (ICD−9 fourth digit) and country

Site (ICD−9 code)	Denmark		England		Estonia		France		Germany		Italy		Netherlands		Scotland		Switzerland	
	No.	%[b,c]	No.	%	No.	%	No.	%	No.	%	No.	%	No.	%	No.	%	No.	%
COLON, Total (153.0−153.9)	12229	(56.4)[b]	38225	(59.7)	1213	(50.9)	2984	(56.0)	2200	(55.0)	1874	(62.3)	1610	(63.1)	8082	(65.5)	1149	(60.4)
Caecum (153.4)	2006	17.6[c]	7512	23.6	60	6.6	301	14.4	202	15.6	162	9.3	295	18.7	885	16.9	229	20.2
Appendix (153.5)	172	1.5	228	0.7	4	0.4	21	1.0	20	1.5	7	0.4	54	3.4	55	1.1	9	0.8
Ascending colon (153.6)	1662	14.5	3146	9.9	57	6.2	238	11.4	165	12.7	217	12.4	183	11.6	478	9.1	172	15.2
Hepatic flexure of colon (153.0)	228	2.0	1129	3.5	28	3.1	85	4.1	80	6.2	90	5.1	89	5.6	148	2.8	22	1.9
Transverse colon (153.1)	1378	12.1	3229	10.1	194	21.2	195	9.3	143	11.0	183	10.5	141	8.9	428	8.2	128	11.3
Splenic flexure of colon (153.7)	252	2.2	1607	5.0	12	1.3	83	4.0	40	3.1	89	5.1	81	5.1	216	4.1	30	2.7
Descending colon (153.2)	856	7.5	2426	7.6	53	5.8	196	9.4	80	6.2	183	10.5	89	5.6	519	9.9	87	7.7
Sigmoid colon (153.3)	4713	41.3	12198	38.3	502	55.0	969	46.2	532	41.1	752	43.0	606	38.3	2467	47.1	452	40.0
Overlapping subcategories (153.8)	157	1.4	402	1.3	3	0.3	8	0.4	33	2.5	67	3.8	43	2.7	40	0.8	2	0.2
Colon, NOS (153.9)	805		6348		300		888		905		124		29		2846		18	
RECTUM,Total (154.0−154.8)	9440	(43.6)	25852	(40.3)	1171	(49.1)	2345	(44.0)	1800	(45.0)	1132	(37.7)	940	(36.9)	4260	(34.5)	753	(39.6)
Rectosigmoid junction (154.0)	1341	14.2	3131	12.1	62	5.3	503	21.5	280	15.6	327	28.9	246	26.2	553	13.0	172	22.8
Rectum, NOS (154.1)	7766	82.3	21833	84.5	1069	91.3	1065	45.4	1493	82.9	745	65.8	678	72.1	3578	84.0	493	65.5
Anal canal (154.2)	149	1.6	406	1.6	37	3.2	62	2.6	9	0.5	41	3.6	5	0.5	83	1.9	68	9.0
Anus, NOS (154.3)	140	1.5	320	1.2	1	0.1	42	1.8	14	0.8	8	0.7	5	0.5	25	0.6	12	1.6
Other parts of rectum (154.8)	44	0.5	162	0.6	2	0.2	673	28.2	4	0.2	11	1.0	6	0.6	21	0.5	8	1.1
Total number of colon and rectum																		
(153.0−153.9 & 154.0−154.8)	21669	100.0	64077	100.0	2384	100.0	5329	100.0	4000	100.0	3006	100.0	2550	100.0	12342	100.0	1902	100.0

[b] (within brackets): Percentage over the total number of colon and rectum cases (153.0−153.9 & 154.0−154.8)

[c] without brackets: Percentage over the total number of specified anatomic subcategories (153.0−153.8 and, respectively,154.0−154.8)

Table 2.5. Urinary and genital cancer by anatomical subcategory (ICD–9 code) and country

Site (ICD–9 code)[a]	Denmark		England		Estonia		Germany		Italy		Netherlands		Scotland		Switzerland	
	No.	%[b]	No.	%	No.	%	No.	%	No.	%	No.	%	No.	%	No.	%
Kidney, parenchyma & NOS (189.0)	2832	73.1	6042	82.3	596	96.7	584	91.1	403	83.6	358	77.5	1433	86.2	251	75.4
Renal pelvis (189.1)	755	19.5	673	9.2	10	1.6	35	5.5	44	9.1	59	12.8	120	7.2	61	18.3
Ureter (189.2)	267	6.9	439	6.0	9	1.5	20	3.1	29	6.0	36	7.8	96	5.8	15	4.5
Urinary organs, OSS (189.3–189.8)	21	0.5	190	2.5	1	0.2	2	0.3	6	1.3	9	1.9	14	0.8	6	1.8
Total[c] (189.0–189.9)	3603		7494		620		694		490		462		1706		336	
Vagina, NOS (184.0)	196	25.8	448	18.0	40	21.9	30	25.4	26	23.9	16	23.5	132	28.4	26	35.1
Vulva (184.1–184.4)	564	74.2	2043	82.0	143	78.1	88	74.6	83	76.1	52	76.5	333	71.6	48	64.9
Total[c] (184.0–184.9)	829		2551		184		139		126		70		497		80	
Penis (187.1–187.4)	263	90.4	728	86.6	32	88.9	32	94.1	37	100.0	21	87.5	106	80.3	19	95.0
Scrotum (187.7)	28	9.6	113	13.4	4	11.1	2	5.9	0	0.0	3	12.5	26	19.7	1	5.0
Total[c] (187.0–187.9)	317		893		37		42		45		26		165		21	

[a] OSS=Other specified sites

[b] Percentage over the total number of specified anatomic subcategories

[c] Including other and unspecified

inter-registry variability of microscopic confirmation for tumours which have high, medium and low frequencies of such confirmation (breast, colon and lung cancers, respectively). The highest percentages of microscopic verification were from Switzerland, the Netherlands, Germany, Denmark and Finland. Countries with the lowest proportions of microscopic verification were the United Kingdom, Italy, Estonia and Poland. The Piedmont Childhood Registry is an exception for Italy, reporting 90% microscopically verified cases, compared to 75% from the Mainz Childhood Cancer Registry.

Table 2.6. Percentages of microscopic verification for all cases and for colon, lung and breast cancer by age and registry

		All cases		Colon cancer		Lung cancer		Breast cancer	
	Age:	<65	≥65	<65	≥65	<65	≥65	<65	≥65
Registry	Country								
Amiens	F	96.9	85.5	97.8	82.7	96.7	84.5	96.1	84.4
Basel	CH	98.6	93.5	100.0	92.8	97.2	91.9	99.6	96.7
Calvados	F	–	–	96.3	91.2	–	–	–	–
Côte d'Or	F	93.8	84.1	95.3	86.6	–	–	100.0	100.0
Cracow	PL	80.0	52.8	66.5	39.7	95.3	46.5	89.0	77.6
Denmark	DK	97.0	90.0	95.9	88.9	95.3	86.8	98.6	92.6
Doubs	F	NA	NA	NA	NA	NA	NA	NA	NA
East Anglia	ENG	87.3	64.8	92.2	74.1	75.3	51.4	91.6	66.8
Eindhoven	NL	93.7	85.9	96.7	92.5	89.7	79.6	98.6	94.4
Estonia	EST	79.6	57.3	87.6	68.5	61.7	28.2	89.4	71.4
Finland	FIN	94.5	83.3	98.0	90.7	85.1	65.5	99.4	97.0
Geneva	CH	99.0	94.3	100.0	90.6	99.2	96.5	99.3	96.7
Girona	E	95.1	85.1	–	–	–	–	92.8	78.5
Granada	E	90.8	66.8	–	–	81.1	57.5	98.5	83.7
Latina	I	74.3	63.2	70.0	59.1	47.7	36.2	87.4	83.8
Mainz Child.	D	75.3	–	–	–	–	–	–	–
Mallorca	E	96.9	91.7	94.9	88.5	–	–	–	–
Mersey	ENG	78.3	52.2	81.6	60.8	59.8	32.7	89.5	64.3
Modena	I	72.1	69.7	73.7	66.7	–	–	–	–
Piedmont Child.	I	90.4	–	–	–	–	–	–	–
Ragusa	I	80.7	52.3	79.6	53.6	44.3	21.6	91.9	82.4
Saarland	D	95.9	86.9	98.2	92.4	91.4	67.7	98.9	95.1
Scotland	SCO	83.7	69.0	88.0	76.5	66.5	52.3	93.8	81.4
Tarragona	E	97.4	85.5	96.8	91.3	94.6	87.1	100.0	82.2
Thames	ENG	82.1	58.9	87.2	69.7	67.1	39.9	88.4	66.0
Tuscany	I	82.1	61.3	–	–	74.7	47.9	92.4	81.2
Varese	I	87.1	68.5	90.8	71.5	60.2	34.0	96.6	81.5
Wessex	ENG	NA	NA	NA	NA	NA	NA	NA	NA
West Midlands	ENG	85.9	66.6	90.3	74.1	70.6	49.6	92.1	73.3
Yorkshire	ENG	85.0	62.7	88.5	71.5	68.9	46.0	94.3	71.2
Median		87.3	69.0	90.8	76.5	74.7	52.3	94.3	82.2

NA=Not available

In Mainz, however, it is likely that the actual percentage of microscopically confirmed cases is about 95%, as the exact modality of diagnosis was not recorded in all cases (Parkin *et al.*, 1988).

Tumour morphology

Morphology codes were requested to distinguish broad histological categories (e.g. carcinomas from sarcomas) and to perform quality checks on the whole database. Registries were not asked to check the reliability of this information, nor to enquire into the intra- and interobserver repeatability of histological examinations; for these reasons, morphology was not used for detailed analysis of the prognostic significance of histotype. All registries except Finland provided histological data classified according to ICD–O (WHO, 1976), as required by the protocol. The Finnish Cancer Registry uses its own classification system, but it proved possible to convert their codes to main ICD–O categories.

Tumour stage

Registries usually record stage information in broad categories, but between- and within-registry comparability of data on stage is low, since it depends on both the thoroughness of the diagnostic investigation and on registration procedures. Furthermore, because of stage migration (Feinstein *et al.*, 1985), stage-specific comparisons between countries and over time are difficult to interpret (see Chapter 1). For these reasons, stage was not analysed as a prognostic factor, although this variable was required by the EUROCARE protocol to facilitate data-quality checks (e.g. to validate data on long-term survivors with metastases at diagnosis).

Additional dates

The definition of the date of incidence and the date from which survival was calculated varied somewhat between registries; for example, survival could be calculated from the date of hospital admission, the date of diagnostic confirmation or the date of beginning therapy.

The extent to which the adoption of different index dates influences survival estimates has not been investigated before in population-based survival studies. In EUROCARE, when more than one index date was available in the data from a given registry, its effect on survival was evaluated. Table 2.7 reports observed survival rates for lung and colon cancer (two tumours with markedly different prognoses) using three different index dates: hospital admission, confirmation of diagnosis and start of therapy, for data from the Geneva, Amiens, Calvados and Mallorca cancer registries. Short-term survival is slightly lower when the second or third dates are taken as the beginning of follow-up, but from the third year of follow-up onwards, no major survival differences are evident.

Comparability of incidence data

In Table 2.8, additional characteristics of the cancer registries participating in EUROCARE are summarized: method of case collection, index date adopted for computing incidence and survival, follow-up method, percentage of cases known only by death certificate and percentage of the national population covered.

Cases are recorded actively in France, Italy and Spain by means of direct access to relevant information sources by registry personnel. In the United Kingdom the method of case collection varies, some registries collecting information actively and some receiving passive notification from the primary sources. In Denmark and Finland, data collection is mainly based on statutory or voluntary notification of cases to the registries by health or administrative authorities and by doctors treating the patients. 'Passive' and 'active' case collection does not necessarily imply differences in data quality. Generally speaking, in countries where cancer registration is long established (mostly northern European countries), the process of routine notification ensures that registry information is relatively accurate and complete, relying on multiple reporting.

The percentages of cases known only from death certificates are given in Table 2.8, divided into two age groups (<65 and 65+ years). For all registries for which this information was available, the percentage of DCO cases was always greater among older (ranging from 19% to <1%) than younger patients.

The percentage of the national population covered by cancer registries ranged from 100% (countries with national registries) to less than 1% (Italian and French registries).

Table 2.7. Effects of variation of definition of date of diagnosis on survival estimates: example of observed survival of lung and colon cancer patients in selected European cancer registries (Date 1=hospital admission; Date 2=diagnostic confirmation; Date 3=start of treatment)

GENEVA, CH	Lung cancer % survival at:					Colon cancer % survival at:			
	1yr	2yrs	3yrs	5yrs		1yr	2yrs	3yrs	5yrs
Males, N=606					Males, N=268				
Date 1	44.7	26.7	18.6	13.8	Date 1	75.6	65.6	55.9	44.8
Date 2	42.9	25.7	18.3	13.7	Date 2	74.8	64.4	55.9	44.6
Date 3	40.3	24.9	18.0	13.6	Date 3	74.8	64.4	55.9	44.1
Females, N=120					Females, N=287				
Date 1	45.8	26.6	23.2	19.7	Date 1	75.0	65.8	60.4	52.0
Date 2	45.8	26.6	23.2	19.7	Date 2	74.7	65.8	59.7	51.5
Date 3	43.3	26.6	23.2	19.7	Date 3	74.7	66.2	59.7	51.4
AMIENS, F	Lung cancer % survival at:					Colon cancer % survival at:			
	1yr	2yrs	3yrs	5yrs		1yr	2yrs	3yrs	5yrs
Males, N=157					Males N=54				
Date 1	50.1	26.0	17.6	12.4	Date 1	63.0	46.3	40.7	29.6
Date 2	46.1	25.3	17.5	12.4	Date 2	63.0	46.3	40.7	29.6
Females, N=10					Females, N=47				
Date 1	60.0	40.0	30.0	30.0	Date 1	71.7	67.1	55.5	55.5
Date 2	60.0	40.0	30.0	30.0	Date 2	71.3	69.0	55.2	55.2
CALVADOS, F	Colon cancer % survival at:				**MALLORCA, E**	Colon cancer % survival at:			
	1yr	2yrs	3yrs	5yrs		1yr	2yrs	3yrs	5yrs
Males, N=506					Males, N 120				
Date 1	68.5	55.0	48.2	39.2	Date 1	66.7	55.8	46.2	38.8
Date 2	68.5	54.3	47.7	39.2	Date 2	66.7	55.8	46.3	38.9
Females, N=538					Females, N=125				
Date 1	63.6	50.5	43.3	38.4	Date 1	60.6	54.5	46.7	37.7
Date 2	63.2	49.9	43.3	38.4	Date 2	60.7	53.8	46.8	36.9

Table 2.8. Selected data on cancer registries participating in EUROCARE

Registry	Country	Collection of cases (1)	Index date (2)	Follow-up method (3)	% DCO(4) <65yrs	≥65yrs	% of total population (5)
Amiens	F	A	D	A	NA	NA	1.1
Basel	CH	P	D	M	0.0	0.0	7.1
Calvados	F	A	D	A	NA	NA	1.2
Côte d'Or	F	A	D	A	NA	NA	0.9
Cracow	PL	A	H	A	2.0	12.7	2.0
Denmark	DK	P	H,D	A	0.5	2.5	100
Doubs	F	A	D	A	NA	NA	0.9
East Anglia	ENG	A	T	A	0.03	0.4	4.1
Eindhoven	NL	A	D	A	NA	NA	7.0
Estonia	EST	P	D	A	NA	NA	100
Finland	FIN	P	D	A	0.1	0.7	100
Geneva	CH	A	H,D	A	0.2	1.5	6.3
Girona	E	A	D	A	5.7	5.8	1.4
Granada	E	A	D	A	2.3	17.4	2.1
Latina	I	A	H	A	2.0	1.8	0.8
Mainz Child.	D	P	D	A	0.0	.	100
Mallorca	E	A	D	M	4.9	13.9	1.6
Mersey	ENG	A	T	P	0.0	0.2	4.9
Modena	I	A	H	A	0.0	0.0	0.5
Piedmont Child.	I	A	D	A	0.0	.	6.5
Ragusa	I	A	H	M	0.0	2.5	0.5
Saarland	D	P	D	P	3.0	12.5	1.7
Scotland	SCO	P	T	P	2.6	7.6	100
Tarragona	E	A	D	M	2.8	7.0	1.3
Thames	ENG	A	H	P	7.5	19.0	13.6
Tuscany	I	A	H,D	A	1.0	6.5	2.1
Varese	I	A	H	A	0.5	3.2	1.4
Wessex	ENG	P	D	P	4.1	12.4	6.1
West Midlands	ENG	A	T	P	0.8	3.2	10.4
Yorkshire	ENG	P	T	M	1.7	5.2	7.3

(1) Collection of cases:

A=Data collection mainly based on active solicitation of information by the registry personnel.

P=Data collection mainly based on compulsory/statutory or voluntary notification of cases to registry by sources of information.

(2) Preferred index date for computing incidence and survival:

H=Date of hospital admission; D=Date of diagnostic confirmation; T=Date of start of therapy; H, D = H or D, whichever was first

(3) Method of follow-up:

A=Active, by linkage to population files or active inquiry into patients living/dead status; P=Passive notification of death certificates; M=Mixed, i.e. passive follow-up complemented by active enquiry into living/dead status if a death certificate does not arrive after a given period.

(4) Percentage of patients known to the registry by death certificate only, by age group (0–64, 65+). Source: *Cancer Incidence In Five Continents*, Vol. VI (Parkin *et al.*, 1992) for registries included; otherwise source is respective registry.

(5) Percentage of national population covered by the registry.

Checks on data quality

General validity checks

The data-set sent by each registry was systematically checked at the data analysis centre by means of a computer program developed for this purpose. In addition to common consistency checks for acceptable range and value of variables (including non-acceptable missing values), logical verifications were carried out for sex–site and site–histotype combinations. The errors discovered were referred back to the registries for correction. Table 2.9 lists the types of error found and Table 2.10 summarizes the results of the check, showing the number of incongruences found and records excluded by registry. For some registries it was not possible to correct any record. All records with errors remaining were excluded from the study. After this editing phase, 95–100% of cases from each registry were available for analysis.

Validity of living/dead status assessment

The methods adopted by cancer registries for following up patients can be distinguished as active or passive: active follow-up implies regular comparison of registry records with other files of data on the population and/or direct contact with hospitals, physicians or patients' relatives; passive follow-up relies largely on notification of death by administrative authorities. The follow-up methods used by the EUROCARE registries are indicated in Table 2.8. Passive follow-up may lead to overestimation of survival, due to incomplete matching of registry and administrative authority death records.

The registries using mainly passive follow-up methods were requested by EUROCARE to check the reliability of their procedures for tracing patients. The study protocol recommended checking the living/dead status of a sample of lung cancer patients recorded as still living five years after diagnosis. The lower the proportion of dead patients revealed by the exercise, the more efficient the follow-up system. A highly lethal cancer was chosen in order to reduce the sample size required to estimate the error. Assuming that the efficiency of the living/dead verification procedure was the same, in a given registry, for all cancer sites, knowledge of the error for one site allows correction of survival figures for other sites.

Table 2.9. Incongruences tested for by EUROCARE systematic data check

Sex out of range 1 (= male) – 2 (= female)
Birth month out of range 1–12
Birth year earlier than 1850
Diagnosis month out of range 1–12
End of follow-up month out of range 1–12
End of follow-up year greater than 1991
Living/Dead status out of range 1–2
ICD–9 out of range 140.0–239.9
ICD–9 code unknown
Microscopic confirmation out of accepted range 1(=Yes)–2(=No)
Morphology code out of range 8000.0–9940.0
Morphology code unknown
Age out of range 0–100
Follow-up interval (years) out of range 0–15
Unusual sex–site association
Unusual site–morphology association

Table 2.10. Results of systematic data quality check by registry

Registry	Country	No. of errors found	No. of excluded records	Cases in study after check	No. accepted (%)
Amiens	F	88	73	2616	(97.3)
Basel	CH	251	230	3741	(94.2)
Calvados	F	233	223	3111	(93.3)
Côte d'Or	F	155	116	4071	(97.2)
Cracow	PL	111	14	8346	(99.4)
Denmark	DK	179	112	100416	(99.9)
Doubs	F	59	59	7677	(99.8)
East Anglia	ENG	28	0	32494	(100.0)
Eindhoven	NL	1	1	13359	(100.0)
Estonia	EST	32	12	18613	(99.9)
Finland	FIN	9	9	63872	(100.0)
Geneva	CH	10	9	6269	(99.9)
Girona	E	38	38	1093	(96.6)
Granada	E	1	0	323	(100.0)
Latina	I	144	65	1171	(94.7)
Mainz Child.	D	196	188	3108	(94.3)
Mallorca	E	3	0	449	(100.0)
Mersey	ENG	216	216	45081	(99.5)
Modena	I	0	0	132	(100.0)
Piedmont Child.	I	28	19	535	(97.6)
Ragusa	I	1	0	1874	(100.0)
Saarland	D	6	0	18564	(100.0)
Scotland	SCO	183	60	69913	(99.9)
Tarragona	E	5	5	912	(99.5)
Thames	ENG	716	509	118898	(99.6)
Tuscany	I	5	3	2016	(99.8)
Varese	I	125	109	14365	(99.3)
Wessex	ENG	508	508	14157	(96.6)
West Midlands	ENG	1415	48	73614	(99.9)
Yorkshire	ENG	134	113	66936	(99.8)

Most registries using passive follow-up performed some checks on the efficiency of these procedures; five registries provided a formal analysis which permitted evaluation of the effect of living/dead status corrections on survival. One registry has published the results of its work (Wilson *et al.*, 1992). Table 2.11 summarizes the results of the EUROCARE analysis of follow-up quality for the Thames, West Midlands, Yorkshire, Basel and Saarland registries, which use mainly passive procedures. The first two columns show the registries and the number of lung cancer patients believed to be alive five years after diagnosis according to the usual procedures; columns B, C and D report the results of active checking: the number that could not be traced, the number found to be dead, and the number

Table 2.11. Results of survey on quality of passive follow-up: long-term surviving lung cancer patients

Registry	A No. of cases recorded as alive	B No. lost to follow-up	C No. dead	D No. actually alive	E % error among live cases	F EUROCARE % 5-year observed survival	G Corrected % 5-year observed survival	H % Dead cases registered living
Thames	175	39	18	118	13.2	3.9	3.4	0.5
West Midlands	121[a]	14	25	77	24.5	5.5	4.1	1.4
Yorkshire	111	49	10	52	16.1	4.4	3.7	0.7
Basel	180	–	35	147	19.2	13.2	10.7	2.8
Saarland	38	–	18[c]	20	47.4[d]	7.5[d]	3.9[d]	3.7[d]
All registries	587[b]		88	394	18.3	7.2	5.9	1.4

[a] Includes five cases that proved not to have a cancer of the lung.
[b] Excluding the Saarland Cancer Registry.
[c] For Saarland, this category includes B+C, as legislation prevents distinction between lost and dead patients.
[d] Maximum error: Figures computed assuming all patients lost to follow-up are dead.
E=Proportion of dead patients among those recorded as alive following the usual cancer registry practice: C/(D+C)
G=Corrected five-year observed survival: F−(F*E/100)
H=Proportion of dead patients erroneously considered alive: (F−G)*100/(100−G)
Note that G=(F−H)*100/(100−H)

confirmed as still alive. Column E reports the proportion of cases actually dead among those believed alive from the usual procedures, excluding those who could not be traced in the checking exercise; columns F and G report, respectively, the EUROCARE estimate of five-year observed survival and the corrected estimate taking into account the errors in determining living/dead status. The last column, that of greatest interest, shows the proportion of dead patients erroneously considered alive relative to the total number of dead subjects. This was computed as the ratio of the difference between the EUROCARE estimate and the corrected estimate of five-year survival over the cumulative risk of death at five years (computed as the complement of corrected survival). This figure ranged from 0.5% in Thames to a potential maximum of 3.7% in Saarland; the latter is an overestimate, however, because national legislation did not permit the Saarland Cancer Registry to distinguish between dead patients and those lost to follow-up. The mean error (excluding Saarland) was 1.4%.

Assuming that the probability of not obtaining news of a patient's death, over five years, is the same for all types of cancer, the figures in last column of Table 2.11 can be used to correct five-year survival estimates for other cancers by means of the following formula:

$$S_c = (S_o - H)*100/(100 - H)$$

where S_o is the observed survival, S_c the corrected survival and H is the percentage of dead cases considered alive.

The results of this analysis demonstrate that with passive methods a certain proportion of errors in determining living/dead status is probably unavoidable. The investigation was carried out on long-term survivors of a highly lethal cancer, where even a small percentage error may substantially affect survival estimates. For example, with reference to the data shown in Table 2.11, the five-year observed pooled survival is 7.2%, while the corrected figure would be 5.9% — a 22% overestimate. For less lethal tumours, errors of this magnitude would affect survival estimates to only a minor extent, and can be considered acceptable in most cases. In support of this conclusion, it may be noted that the results of survival analysis by United Kingdom registries, which rely almost entirely on passive follow-up, do not suggest that survival has been overestimated. Another point is that the percentage of errors found for lung cancer may not apply for less lethal cancers. It must be remembered, however, that the analysis shown in Table 2.11 is restricted to patients successfully traced; further studies are evidently necessary to improve our knowledge of the completeness of follow-up procedures.

Among the registries that actively follow up their patients (and are not therefore included in the above analysis), the Estonian cancer registry investigated the error in determining living/dead status among long-term lung cancer survivors. The proportion dead was 1% of a sample of 196 patients, leading to an overall observed eight-year survival of 6.0% instead of 6.1%. In the Varese Cancer Registry, of the 82 patients apparently alive five years after diagnosis, only one was found to be dead (Sant *et al.*, 1992).

Most registries do not follow up patients who migrate abroad; these are considered censored observations from the date of migration. Generally this is a minor problem, but in registries covering populations with a high proportion of foreigners, such as the Swiss registries, it can be a major issue. Survival estimates in Geneva, for instance, are systematically higher for foreigners than for the Swiss, especially for males (see Chapter 14). This is probably because foreign residents with incurable cancer tend to return to their native country, removing poor survivors from observation. The overestimation of survival for foreign residents in Switzerland affects overall estimates to various extents depending on cancer site.

References

Feinstein, A.R., Sosin, D.M. & Walls, C.E. (1985) The Will Rogers' phenomenon: stage migration and new diagnostic techniques as a source of misleading statistics for survival in cancer. *New Engl. J. Med.*, **312**, 1604–1606

Parkin, D.M., Muir, C.S., Whelan, S., Gao, Y.T., Ferlay, J. & Powell, J., eds (1992) *Cancer Incidence in Five Continents*, Vol. VI (IARC Scientific Publications No. 120), Lyon, IARC

Parkin, D.M., Stiller, C.A., Draper, G.J., Bieber, C.A., Terracini, B. & Young, J.L., eds (1988) *International Incidence of Childhood Cancer* (IARC Scientific Publications No. 87), Lyon, IARC

Sant, M., Gatta, G., Capocaccia, R., Verdecchia, A., Micheli, A., Speciale, D., Pastorino, U. & Berrino, F. (1992) Survival for lung cancer in northern Italy. *Cancer Causes Control*, **3**, 223–230

Wilson, S., Prior, P. & Woodman, C.B.J. (1992) Use of cancer surveillance data for comparative analyses. *J. Public Health Med.*, **14**, 151–156

WHO (World Health Organization) (1976) *International Classification of Diseases for Oncology* (ICD–O), Geneva

WHO (World Health Organization) (1977) *Manual of the International Statistical Classification of Diseases, Injuries, and Causes of Death*, Geneva

CHAPTER 3

Methods of data analysis

A. Verdecchia, R. Capocaccia and T. Hakulinen

Introduction

Time to occurrence of some event or response, such as death of cancer patients, is the basic data item for survival analysis. Let **T** be a non-negative random variable representing the response time of an individual from a homogeneous population, i.e. the time to death for cancer patients in a study group. The probability distribution of **T** can be specified in many ways, three of which are particularly useful in survival applications: the survival function, the probability density function, and the hazard function.

The survival function is defined as the probability that **T** has at least a value t; that is,

$$S_t = \mathrm{P}\ (\mathbf{T} \geq t) \quad 0 < t < \infty$$

The survival function S is based on the cumulative distribution function and gives the probabilities in the right tail of the distribution.

Information on the cause of death of patients is often vague or unavailable. Instead of using information on an individual's cause of death, in medical follow-up studies survival times are generally defined with respect to death without regard to the specific cause. However, deaths from causes other than the disease of interest may influence the observed survival, for example by reducing the survival rate from what it would be if the disease of interest were the only cause of death to a greater extent for old than for young patients, or differently in heterogeneous groups of patients. In order to eliminate the effect of mortality from other causes on survival rates, the concept of relative survival has been introduced (Berkson & Gage, 1950). Relative survival has been defined as the ratio of the observed survival rate in the group of patients to the survival rate expected in a group of people in the general population, who are similar to the patients with respect to all the possible factors affecting survival at the beginning of the follow-up period, except for the disease under study.[1] The variables usually taken into consideration are demographic variables such as sex, age, calendar time and geographical area.

In principle, relative survival should represent the survival rate if the disease of interest were the only cause of death, i.e. accounting for the extra risk of dying in sick people compared with the general healthy population. Its value is not restricted to the range 0–1. If the patients' observed survival is higher than expected because the cancer patients are a selected sample of population which is heterogeneous for the determinants of survival, relative survival will be greater than unity. After several years of follow-up, risk of death in patients who are still alive can reduce to the same level or lower than that expected for the general population. It has been shown by Hakulinen (1977, 1982) that this may occur in long-term relative survival as the consequence of selection biases in heterogeneous populations. Due to these biases, relative survival computed as the ratio of observed to expected survival cannot be strictly interpreted as survival probability. If relative survival is depicted graphically as if it were a real cumulative survival curve, it may happen that the curve increases after some years of follow-up. Thus, analysing and plotting curves for homogeneous subgroups is generally recommended, supplemented when appropriate, by suitable statistical modelling (Hakulinen *et al.*, 1987, Estève *et al.*, 1990).

---

[1] The expression 'survival rate' is used in this chapter as meaning survival probability, as is current practice among clinicians, despite the fact that rate and probability are different concepts in theory.

Estimation of relative survival

The present results of the EUROCARE cancer survival study were obtained using the statistical package for relative survival constructed by Hakulinen and Abeywickrama (1985). First the entire follow-up period is divided into shorter (e.g. annual) subintervals. Relative survival from the beginning of the follow-up to the end of the ith subinterval is expressed as:

$$R_i = S_i / S_i^* \qquad (1)$$

where S_i represents the observed survival rate and S_i^* the corresponding expected survival. The quantity S_i is estimated by the life table method (e.g. Chiang, 1968). Several methods exist for deriving the expected survival rate (Ederer & Heise, 1959; Ederer *et al.*, 1961; Hakulinen, 1982).

Selection bias is usually important when the follow-up is longer than ten years. Its effect can be reduced by deriving the expected survival rate from an expected life table that allows the potential follow-up times to be taken into account and precludes the expected survival rate being dependent on the fatality of the disease of the patients (Hakulinen,1982). Let us designate by L_i the subset of all patients with a potential follow-up time greater than or equal to the starting point of the ith interval, and let n_i be their number, which is defined by the structure of the study. A subset L_{i+1} of these patients will have a potential follow-up time great enough to reach the $(i+1)$th interval. Therefore $n_i - n_{i+1}$ patients are potential withdrawals during the ith interval; the set of such patients will be designated C_i. The expected number of patients alive and under observation at i is given by:

$$l_i = \sum_{h \in L_i} {}_hS_i^*$$

where the index h indicates patients, and summation over h is extended to all patients belonging to L_i. The expected cumulative survival ${}_hS_i^*$ is obtained by the expression:

$${}_hS_i^* = \prod_{m=0}^{i-1} {}_hp_m^* \qquad (2)$$

where ${}_hp_m^*$ is the expected probability of surviving the mth subinterval for the hth patient, normally obtained from population life tables.

The expected number of patients with potential complete follow-up during the ith subinterval, here denoted by $[i, i+1]$, and dying during the same subinterval, is given by:

$$d_i = \sum_{h \in L_{i+1}} {}_hS_i^*(1 - {}_hp_i^*)$$

where each term summed represents the expected probability of dying during $[i, i+1]$, subject to still being alive at i. The expected number of patients withdrawing while alive during $[i, i+1]$ is given by:

$$\omega_i = \sum_{h \in C_i} {}_hS_i^*({}_hp_i^*)^{\frac{1}{2}}$$

where the square root of ${}_hp_i^*$ represents the expected probability of surviving half of the ith interval, i.e. the average time of observation for patients withdrawing during the interval. The expected number of patients dying during $[i, i+1]$, with potential follow-up time ending during the same interval, is given by:

$$\delta_i = \sum_{h \in C_i} {}_hS_i^*[1 - ({}_hp_i^*)^{\frac{1}{2}}]$$

The expected interval-specific survival rate is then derived as:

$$p_i^* = 1 - (d_i + \delta_i)/(l_i - 1/2\omega_i)$$

and, finally, the expected survival rate from 0 to i is obtained by calculating:

$$S_i^* = \prod_{m=0}^{i-1} p_m^*$$

which is similar to equation (2) stated for an individual patient h.

Alternative methods are simpler than the one outlined here, but they do not allow for the possibility that the potential follow-up times of patients are of unequal length (Ederer *et al.*, 1961), or they accommodate for heterogeneous potential follow-up times in a way that leads expected survival to depend on the fatality of the disease under study (Ederer & Heise, 1959). As shown by Hakulinen (1982), using expected survival computed by both of these two alternative methods will result in a biased estimate of relative survival.

The standard error of the estimated survival rate S_i is obtained using Greenwood's formula (Greenwood, 1926). Confidence intervals for R_i are computed as the roots of the second-degree equation in ϕ:

$$(S_i - S_i^* \phi)^2 = (1.96)^2 S_i^* \phi (1 - S_i^* \phi)/n_i^*$$

where n_i^* is the effective sample size at the start of the ith subinterval, estimated as:

$$n_i^* = [S_i\ (1 - S_i)]/[\mathrm{SE}(S_i)]^2$$

Confidence intervals for R_i computed in this way are constrained within the range between 0 and $1/S_i^*$, as it should be, since the survival rate must be in the range of 0–1.

The European pool: rationale and definitions

In order to complement the results from the single areas or registries and to provide a basis for overall comparisons with other data, such as those from the SEER program, it was decided to present in addition summary survival figures, derived from the whole set of available data. Pooled survival statistics also give a set of reference figures with which to compare the results from each single area. Furthermore, pooling the available information is the only way to perform a standard survival analysis on very rare cancer sites, profiting from the existence of a sufficient number of cases that would never be available in a single registry or country.

Pooled survival figures and their standard errors have been calculated according to the following expression:

$$\mathrm{PR}_{ij} = \sum_k (w_{jk}\ /\ W_j) R_{ijk}$$

$$\text{where} : W_j = \sum_k w_{jk}$$

$$\mathrm{SE}\ (\mathrm{PR}_{ij}) = [\sum_k (w_{jk}\ /\ W_j)^2 (\mathrm{SE}(R_{ijk}))^2]^{\frac{1}{2}}$$

where R_{ijk} indicates the relative survival up to subinterval i estimated for age class j (j=1,...,a) and population k (k=1,...,c), and w_{jk} is a set of weights to be chosen. Confidence intervals for pooled survival probabilites have been computed by assuming the Normal approximation on the logistic scale. According to specific choices of w_{jk}, pooled survival figures assume different meanings.

One possible set of weights consists of the annual numbers of sex- and site-specific cases observed or estimated at the national level in each country. In this case, assuming that relative survival in each region is representative of survival at the national level, the pooled survival figures can be interpreted as estimating the relative survival of the totality of cases diagnosed in all the countries considered. Here, age-dependent weights based on total estimated numbers of all ages combined have been used, both for practical (availability of data, ease of presentation) and for theoretical (comparability of results, stability of estimates) reasons. The resulting pooled survival figures are still fairly sensitive to the uncertainty coming from large countries represented by small registries, such as Spain, France, Germany and Italy. As a consequence, this definition of weights has been used only for the analysis of frequent cancer sites, for which survival of the (weighted) European pool is presented. The annual numbers of cancer patients were directly derived from our data for countries covered by national cancer registries (Denmark, Estonia, Finland and Scotland), and taken from previously published estimates (Jensen *et al.*, 1990) for other countries (England, France, Germany, Italy, the Netherlands and Spain). For Poland and Switzerland, not included in the reference cited, weights were estimated on the basis of the average incidence rates from cancer registries in those countries (Muir *et al.*,1987).

An alternative set of weights for the pooled analysis is provided by the numbers of patients at the start of follow-up belonging to the jth age class and the kth population. In this case, the first of the above expressions automatically gives the crude pooled survival, and the results are exactly the same as would have been obtained by analysing the whole set of data without taking into account the different areas. The use of this particular definition of weights presents, in our case, the serious disadvantage that the resulting values are heavily biased towards the UK relative survival, since the great majority of cases available to us derive from UK registries. On the other hand, this choice leads to the smallest standard errors, since each area is weighted proportionally to the precision of the corresponding survival estimates. This second set of weights, i.e. site-specific numbers of patients actually observed in each area as given by sex, age and period, was therefore chosen for calculating crude (unweighted) pooled survival figures for infrequent or rare cancer sites.

Example

An example of the pooling procedure, using both definitions of weights and considering only four countries, is shown in Table 3.1 for head and neck cancer. In columns 1 and 2, five-year relative survival estimated for the 15–99-year age class and the corresponding standard error are presented, respectively. Column 3 reports the first set of weights, based on the mean annual estimated numbers of head and neck cancers at the national level. The second set of weights, given by the actual numbers of cases available for the analysis in the age class considered is shown in column 4. The last two rows report the pooled survival and its standard error calculated using the first and second sets of weights.

The first set of weights, i.e. the expected number of cases in the country, gives a more central estimate for the relative survival in the pool of the four countries, with respect to the second estimate, which is based on available cases, at the price of a much greater statistical error.

Standardized survival

Most biological phenomena are related to age: there is therefore no reason to expect that survival is not. This is obvious for observed survival, which is affected by the force of mortality from all causes, but it is in general true for relative survival as well. On the other hand, the age distribution of both the general population at risk and cancer patients varies substantially between different areas. Comparing relative survival between different populations would require, therefore, either age-specific or age-adjusted survival rates to be considered. Comparisons between countries in this study are presented in terms of age-adjusted survival, computed by the direct method, using the population of cases from the whole set of data, for given site, as a standard. Formally we have therefore:

$$\mathrm{ASR}_{ik} = \sum_{j} (M_j/M)R_{ijk}$$

$$\text{where} : M = \sum_{jk} m_{jk} \text{ ; and } M_j = \sum_{k} m_{jk}$$

$$\mathrm{SE}\ (\mathrm{ASR}_{ik}) = \Big[\sum_{j} (M_j/M)^2\ (\mathrm{SE}\ (R_{ijk}))^2\Big]^{\frac{1}{2}}$$

where m_{jk} indicates the number of patients at the beginning of follow-up for age class j and population k. Confidence intervals for age-standardized relative survival probabilities, similarly to the case of pooled relative survival probabilities, have been computed by assuming the Normal approximation on the logistic scale.

Table 3.2 reports site-specific values of M_j and M used for computing age-standardized relative survival figures. Male and female relative survival figures were adjusted using the same standard population in order to allow the reader to look at gender differences in addition to differences between countries.

Age-standardized survival is a synthetic index whose validity may depend in a crucial way (as for all standardized measures) upon the consistency of risk differentials across age strata. Detailed comparisons between age-specific survival rates are therefore recommended whenever a suspicion about non-persistence of these differences arises.

Table 3.1. Comparison of pooled five-year relative survival rate estimated using two different definitions of weights

Country		$R_{5,15-99}$	SE	w(1)	w(2)
England		39	1.3	1079	2267
Netherlands		60	7.5	180	66
Italy		55	6.1	123	90
Pool	w(1)	47	2.6		
	w(2)	40	1.3		

Table 3.2. Site-specific number of cancer cases in the EUROCARE European pool, in each age stratum, M_j, and in all ages combined, M

(*a*) Adult cancer cases

Site	Age 15–44	45–54	55–64	65–74	75–99	All
Tongue	244	539	871	877	768	3299
Oral cavity	261	678	1170	1206	1067	4382
Oropharynx	158	515	729	657	398	2457
Nasopharynx	190	189	288	261	150	1078
Hypopharynx	102	360	661	628	448	2199
Head & neck	956	2282	3720	3631	2833	13422
Oesophagus	403	1586	4105	5923	5991	18008
Stomach	1929	4905	11561	21585	22620	62600
Colon	2643	5794	13732	24220	28437	74826
Rectum	1531	4411	10823	17768	17268	52161
Pancreas	661	2132	6021	10431	10488	29733
Larynx	440	1722	3508	3304	1638	10612
Lung	3172	15337	45629	64593	38355	167086
Bone[a]	496	185	267	332	280	1560
Breast	15603	23256	27397	28376	24507	119139
Cervix uteri	6376	3835	5195	4318	2395	22119
Corpus uteri	767	3690	7502	6466	4343	22768
Ovary	2481	4368	6375	6250	4556	24030
Vagina	233	367	791	1569	2211	5171
Testis	4394	608	323	180	110	5615
Penis	137	186	347	554	446	1670
Kidney	1077	2503	4940	5876	3850	18246
Brain	3241	2451	3552	3129	945	1331
Hodgkin's disease	3694	738	846	882	568	6728
Acute lymphatic leukaemia	604	86	159	211	187	1247
Chronic lymphatic leukaemia	124	501	1335	2454	2637	7051
Acute myeloid leukaemia	1013	650	1023	1623	1513	5822
Chronic myeloid leukaemia	473	361	508	764	788	2894
Leukaemia	2707	1970	3686	6287	6710	21360

(*b*) Childhood cancer cases

Site	Age 0–1	2–4	5–9	10–14	All
Brain	177	365	563	539	1644
Leukaemia	432	1370	1036	880	3718

[a] First age class: 20–44 years.

References

Berkson, J. &. Gage, R.P. (1950) Calculation of survival rates for cancer. *Proceedings of the Staff Meetings of the Mayo Clinic,* **25**, 270–286

Chiang, C.L. (1968) *Introduction to Stochastic Process in Biostatistics*, New York, John Wiley

Ederer, F. & Heise, H. (1959) Instructions to IBM 650 programmers in processing survival computations. Methodological Note No. 10, End Results Evaluation Section, Bethesda, MD, National Cancer Institute

Ederer, F., Axtell, L.M. & Cutler, S.J. (1961) The relative survival rate: A statistical methodology. In: *End Results and Mortality Trends in Cancer* (Natl. Cancer Inst. Monogr. No. 6), Washington DC, US Government Printing Office, pp. 101–121

Estève, J., Benhamou, E., Croasdale, M. & Raymond, L. (1990) Relative survival and the estimation of net survival; elements for further discussion. *Stat. Med.*, **9**, 529–538

Greenwood, M. (1926) The natural duration of cancer. *Reports on Public Health and Medical Subjects 33*, London, HMSO

Hakulinen, T. (1977) On long-term relative survival rates. *J. Chronic Dis.*, **30**, 431–443

Hakulinen, T. (1982) Cancer survival corrected for heterogeneity in patient withdrawal. *Biometrics*, **38**, 933–942

Hakulinen, T. & Abeywickrama, K.H. (1985) A computer program package for relative survival analysis. *Computer Prog. Biomed.*, **19**, 197–207

Hakulinen, T. & Tenkanen, L. (1987) Regression analysis of relative survival rates. *Appl. Stat.*, **36**, 309–317

Jensen, O.M., Estève, J., Møller, H. & Renard, H. (1990) Cancer in the European Community and its member states. *Eur. J. Cancer,* **26**, 1167–1256

Muir, C., Waterhouse, J., Mack, T., Powell, J. & Whelan, S. , eds. (1987) *Cancer Incidence in Five Continents.*, Vol V (IARC Scientific Publications No. 88), Lyon, IARC

Summary of symbols used

h index of patient

i,j,k indices of follow-up interval, age class and country, respectively

R relative survival rate

S observed survival rate

S^* expected survival rate

n observed number of patients at the start of each interval

n^* effective number of patients at the start of each interval

m number of patients at the start of follow-up

N sum of n over countries and/or age classes

l expected number of patients at the start of each interval

p^* expected probability or rate of surviving during an interval

d expected number of deaths among patients with potential follow-up extending over the interval

ω expected number of patients withdrawing alive during the interval

δ expected number of deaths with potential follow-up ending within the interval

w weight

W sum of weights over countries

PR pooled relative survival

ASR age standardized relative survival

M_j European pool number of cases in age class j

M European pool number of cases over all ages

CHAPTER 4

General mortality and its effect on survival estimates

A. Micheli and R. Capocaccia

Introduction

In this monograph, survival is expressed as either observed or relative survival. Observed survival is the cumulative probability of surviving for a given time after diagnosis, irrespective of the cause of death. It measures the actual phenomenon of death as it occurs in a specific group of patients. In this study, case populations consist of all cases of a given cancer occurring in a well defined geographical area in a given calendar period.

Relative survival is calculated as the ratio of observed survival to the survival that the patients would have experienced if they had had the same probability of dying as the general population having the same age and sex. However, it is an estimate which is valid only under certain conditions (Estève *et al.*, 1994; see also Chapter 3) of the survival probability in the absence of mortality from causes of death other than the illness of interest (that is in the absence of competing mortality).

Figure 4.1, derived from Lopez (1990), presents sex- and age-standardized death rates for the countries participating in the EUROCARE study. In 1986–88, the age-adjusted death rates per 100 000 ranged from 700 in Switzerland to 1100 in Poland and the USSR, with a ratio between these extreme values of 1.6. These figures indicate that general mortality is very different in different countries; it is necessary to take this into account when comparing survival from cancer.

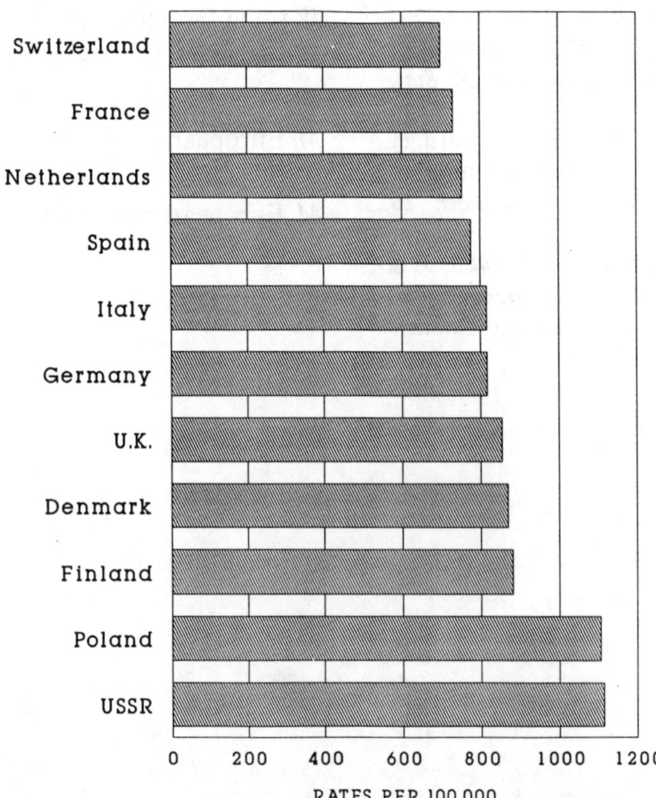

Figure 4.1. Sex- and age-standardized death rates in selected countries, 1986–88 (European standard population) (Lopez, 1990)

Table 4.1. Available and estimated general mortality data for each cancer registry population

Registry	Country	Available mortality data			Estimated mortality data		
		Age interval	Up to age of	Period[a]	Age interval	From age .. to age	Periods year by year
(1)	(2)	(3)	(4)	(5)	(6)	(7)	(8)
Amiens	F	5 yrs[b]	89	1974–76 1982	1 yr	90..99	1978..1981 1983..1990
Basel	CH	5 yrs	99	1981..90	1 yr	–	1978..1980
Calvados	F	5 yrs[b]	89	1974–76 1982	1 yr	90..99	1978..1981 1983..1990
Côte D'Or	F	5 yrs[b]	89	1974–76 1982	1 yr	90..99	1978..1981 1983..1990
Cracow	PL	5 yrs	99	1976–81 1982–85 1986–90	1 yr	–	–
Denmark[d]	DK	1 yr	99	1978..90	–	–	–
Doubs	F	5 yrs[b]	89	1974–76 1982	1 yr	90..99	1978..1981 1983..1990
East Anglia	ENG	10 yrs	99	1979 1981 1989	1 yr	–	1978..1990
Eindhoven	NL	5 yrs	99	1976–80 1981–85 1986–90	1 yr	–	–
Estonia[d]	EST	1 yr	99	1978..84			1985..1990
Finland[d]	FIN	1 yr	99	1976–80 1981–85	–	–	1986..1990
Florence	I	1 yr	99	1978..88	–		1989..1990
Geneva	CH	1 yr	99	1978–83	–	–	1984..1990
Girona	E	5 yrs	94	1983–90	1 yr	95..99	–
Granada	E	1 yr	99	1980–81	–	–	1982..1990
Latina	I	1 yr	99	1978..88	–	–	1989..1990
Mainz, Germany	D	5 yrs[c]	90	1981..84	1 yr	–	1978..1980 1985..1990
Mallorca	E	5 yrs	99	1985–87	1 yr	–	1978..1984 1988..1990
Mersey	ENG	10 yrs	99	1979 1981 1989	1 yr	–	1978..1990
Modena	I	1 yr	99	1978..88	–	–	1989..1990
Piedmont	I	1 yr	99	1978..88	–	–	1989..1990
Ragusa	I	1 yr	99	1978..88	–	–	1989..1990
Saarland	D	1 yr	99	1978..84	–	–	1985..1990
Scotland	SCO	1 yr	99	1980–82	–	–	1978..1979 1983..1990
Tarragona	E	5 yrs	99	1985..89	1 yr	–	1978..1984 1990
South Thames	ENG	10 yrs	99	1979 1981 1989	1 yr	–	1978..1990

Table 4.1. (contd)

Registry	Country	Available mortality data			Estimated mortality data		
		Age interval	Up to age of	Period[a]	Age interval	From age .. to age	Periods year by year
(1)	(2)	(3)	(4)	(5)	(6)	(7)	(8)
Varese	I	1 yr	99	1978..88	–	–	1989..1990
Wessex	ENG	10 yrs	99	1979 1981 1989	1 yr	–	1978..1990
West Midlands	ENG	10 yrs	99	1979 1981 1989	1 yr	–	1978..1990
Yorkshire	ENG	10 yrs	99	1979 1981 1989	1 yr	–	1978..1990

[a] When a hyphen links two years, it means that the available datum is the mean of all the years included in the interval. When there are dots between two years, it means that all individual included years were available.
[b] The age interval for first classes were: 0, 1–4; after that by 5 years.
[c] The age interval for first classes were: 0, 1, 2–4; after that by 5 years.
[d] National registry

The statistical methods used in this monograph for analysing survival data and adjusting for general mortality are described in detail in Chapter 3. The present chapter illustrates the general mortality data used to compute relative survival and provides broad guidelines to aid the interpretion of survival figures taking into consideration the effects of general mortality.

Estimation of general mortality data in the populations of the EUROCARE study

All registries participating in the EUROCARE project were invited to provide life tables for the corresponding geographical area by sex, age (from 0 to 99 years) and calendar year (from 1978 to 1990, to cover the entire period of follow-up). Unfortunately, complete statistics with the requested details were not obtainable for all registries; therefore missing data had to be estimated. Table 4.1 presents, for each participating registry, available and estimated general mortality data. When only five-year age-specific mortality rates were available, the one-year age-specific mortality rates were calculated presuming a constant mortality increase by age within each five-year age-class (see columns 3 and 6 in Table 4.1). The French registries could not provide mortality data for ages above 89; the missing figures were estimated assuming the age trend of the Italian mortality rates at same ages (see columns 4 and 7). However, it must be remembered that at advanced ages even official data are rather imprecise, due to the well known inaccuracy in determining the death risk in the last decades of life. For those registries where the available vital statistics did not cover the entire calendar-year period, the probability of dying in each missing year was estimated (see columns 5 and 8). The trend by calendar period was assumed to be linear and independent of age. The coefficient of the linear trend was calculated by fitting the age-standardized national mortality rates for the relevant period, derived from WHO data. The registry population life tables for the entire period were calculated applying the estimated linear trend to the area-specific mortality figures.

For English registries, whose mortality data were available only for 10-year age classes, the following method was used: a single complete life table (showing the one-year age classes) referring to the whole of England in 1981 was taken as the basis for the construction of the vital statistics for the individual English registries. The mortality trend for England was estimated from WHO data according to the general procedure described above. Area- and sex-specific relative risks of death were estimated by comparison of available local age-standardized mortality rates with those at national level. These relative risks were then applied to the national life table, so as to obtain registry-specific life tables.

In order to reduce the computing time required, the 1979 general mortality data were used for the calculation of relative survival in the years 1978–80; those of 1982 for the years 1981–83; those of 1985 for the years 1984–86; those of 1988 for the years 1987–89; the last interval included the 1990 data only.

Variability of general mortality

Tables 4.2 and 4.3 show the cumulative general mortality of each registry population by sex and age interval computed from (observed or estimated) mortality data for 1979 and 1988. Table 4.2 shows data up to 75 years and Table 4.3 from 75 to 99 years of age. Cumulative general mortality expresses the probability, at a given year of age, of dying before the end of the age-span considered.

Considering all ages, variability between registries was higher for females than for males (see the gap between the minimum and maximum values in Table 4.2). Estonia had the highest cumulative mortality risk for almost all age-classes, for both males and females. Cracow, particularly for males, was another area with a high death risk. The other northern European areas showed intermediate mortality figures. In contrast, the southern areas (in Italy and particularly Spain) generally presented the lowest levels of mortality. The picture was less clear for childhood mortality, for which some southern areas (e.g. Ragusa) showed a much high risk. In 1988, cumulative mortality in the first year of life ranged from 6 per 1000 in Tarragona to 19 per 1000 in Estonia for males, and from 5 in Calvados to 14 per 1000 in Amiens for females. In the same calendar year, the ratio between the highest and lowest cumulative death rates from 55 to 64 years was 2.4 for males (244 per 1000 in Estonia versus 100 per 1000 in Tarragona) and 2 for females (99 per 1000 in Cracow versus 49 per 1000 in Girona).

In all registries but Estonia and, for females only, Denmark, mortality decreased over the ten-year period. The decreasing trend was very marked for females in Germany, Finland and Switzerland, where mortality decreased by about 20% or more. In Italy, Spain, the United Kingdom and Finland, the mortality for males and females combined decreased by 10–15%; in the Netherlands by 5–10%; in Poland and Denmark (males) by 1–3%.

The effect of competing causes of death on survival from cancer

In order to illustrate the effects of competing mortality on cancer patients' survival, an example is given showing the five-year survival of patients suffering from colon cancer in Swiss and German populations (Table 4.4). In all areas the differences between observed and relative survival are nil or very slight for the youngest patients (15–44 years) but increase with age. For patients of both sexes combined, aged 65–74 years, for instance, relative survival is 17% higher than the observed survival in Switzerland and 28% in Germany. Germany shows the largest difference because it has the highest risk of death.

Among males, the differences between observed and relative survival are more pronounced than among females. For males aged 65–74 relative survival is 24% and 37% more than observed survival, as compared with 12% and 20% for females, in Switzerland and Germany, respectively. This is due to the higher risk of mortality for all causes in males compared with females. In all countries participating in the EUROCARE project, in fact, life expectancy at birth for females is higher than that for males, the difference between sexes ranging from 5.7 (United Kingdom) to 8.6 years (Poland) (Lopez, 1990).

The risk of dying changes over time, affecting the differences between observed and relative survival in different periods. In Switzerland, colon cancer five-year relative survival for both sexes is 27% greater than the observed survival for 1978–80, 30% for 1981–82 and 28% for 1983–85. For the same periods the figures are 32%, 29% and 26% in Germany, where the general mortality decreased dramatically.

Table 4.2. Cumulative general mortality risk per 1000 for various age-classes by registry area[a] in 1979 and 1988: mortality data used in EUROCARE study

a. Males

	Country	1979							1988						
		0–1	0–14	15–44	45–54	55–64	65–74	0–74	0–1	0–14	15–44	45–54	55–64	65–74	0–74
Amiens	F	15	18	70	102	184	338	557	13	16	63	92	167	309	518
Basel	CH	14	18	43	51	145	318	480	7	**9**	38	43	125	302	442
Calvados	F	9	14	61	94	179	358	558	8	12	51	80	153	311	496
Côte D'Or	F	10	16	60	79	151	325	511	8	14	51	68	130	283	455
Cracow	PL	22	25	63	95	207	421	621	17	20	62	97	213	406	612
Denmark	DK	11	16	46	62	159	355	522	10	14	48	60	157	335	505
Doubs	F	10	17	54	73	153	324	506	9	15	47	63	134	286	456
East Anglia	ENG	13	17	35	59	166	377	536	11	14	**29**	49	138	320	466
Eindhoven	NL	14	18	37	54	155	376	528	12	14	31	46	135	351	488
Estonia	EST	**23**	**31**	**117**	**124**	**224**	**429**	**668**	**19**	**27**	**106**	**125**	**244**	**439**	**677**
Finland	FIN	10	15	63	91	206	415	610	7	10	50	68	168	350	526
Florence	I	14	19	38	56	145	332	491	9	12	31	**42**	125	285	426
Geneva	CH	11	16	47	54	142	326	487	9	13	40	45	121	282	429
Girona	E	ne	ne	ne	ne	ne	ne	ne	ne	ne	ne	ne	ne	ne	ne
Granada	E	ne	ne	ne	ne	ne	ne	ne	16	21	43	55	131	304	464
Latina	I	17	21	**35**	59	149	348	507	10	13	32	43	133	293	440
Mainz, Germany	D	16	20	55	73	172	394	569	10	13	40	56	137	315	472
Mallorca	E	15	20	53	74	172	347	536	12	16	44	61	142	291	462
Mersey	ENG	16	20	41	68	190	424	592	13	17	33	56	159	362	519
Modena	I	14	18	43	62	153	343	510	10	13	38	42	131	286	436
Piedmont	I	16	20	44	70	166	365	539	10	12	38	52	142	306	464
Ragusa	I	22	27	35	**51**	128	312	466	13	16	34	42	114	278	417
Saarland	D	22	26	57	77	184	**433**	608	10	13	45	57	151	348	508
Scotland	SCO	14	19	49	81	205	432	612	12	16	40	67	172	371	542
Tarragona	E	**6**	**10**	43	54	**110**	**265**	**414**	**6**	9	44	46	**100**	**260**	**398**
South Thames	ENG	14	18	36	60	170	384	545	11	15	29	50	141	327	474
Varese	I	14	18	45	81	194	406	588	8	10	40	54	160	331	495
Wessex	ENG	14	18	35	60	168	380	540	11	14	**29**	49	139	323	470
West Midlands	ENG	15	20	39	67	186	415	582	12	16	33	55	155	354	509
Yorkshire	ENG	15	20	40	68	189	421	588	13	16	33	56	157	359	515

b. Females

	Country	1979							1988						
		0–1	0–14	15–44	45–54	55–64	65–74	0–74	0–1	0–14	15–44	45–54	55–64	65–74	0–74
Amiens	F	16	20	30	43	68	171	297	**14**	16	25	36	57	145	254
Basel	CH	6	8	24	28	70	219	317	8	9	22	25	54	147	238
Calvados	F	7	11	26	33	67	172	279	**5**	9	21	26	53	139	229
Côte D'Or	F	8	11	26	29	65	167	271	6	8	19	22	49	**128**	212
Cracow	PL	**17**	20	25	42	98	252	382	13	16	23	40	**99**	245	372
Denmark	DK	8	11	26	41	89	202	328	8	11	25	42	96	202	333
Doubs	F	10	15	22	30	63	180	282	8	12	18	25	51	148	236
East Anglia	ENG	11	14	22	38	96	225	350	9	11	18	31	79	187	295
Eindhoven	NL	9	12	21	29	69	198	299	10	13	20	28	73	169	276
Estonia	EST	17	**23**	**33**	44	100	245	387	13	**19**	**35**	**45**	85	**269**	**395**
Finland	FIN	8	11	22	30	78	222	327	6	**8**	18	24	65	186	276
Florence	I	13	16	18	25	62	168	265	7	9	**16**	**21**	55	139	223
Geneva	CH	8	11	22	29	67	174	276	7	9	18	24	55	145	233
Girona	E	7	8	19	24	56	**150**	**237**	8	10	20	25	**48**	146	231
Granada	E	ne	ne	ne	ne	ne	ne	ne	12	15	20	26	63	177	275
Latina	I	13	16	18	28	69	197	298	8	10	17	24	59	161	251
Mainz, Germany	D	13	16	27	37	85	223	344	8	10	19	27	65	170	267
Mallorca	E	12	16	25	32	75	201	313	9	11	18	23	55	151	240
Mersey	ENG	13	17	26	45	113	263	402	11	13	21	37	93	219	341
Modena	I	11	14	20	27	67	184	284	8	10	20	24	59	140	234
Piedmont	I	14	17	21	32	76	204	314	7	9	18	26	61	161	254
Ragusa	I	16	20	19	31	76	210	319	10	12	16	24	63	179	269
Saarland	D	14	18	26	42	94	253	380	9	11	24	26	71	195	297
Scotland	SCO	12	15	27	**50**	**121**	**272**	**416**	9	11	20	38	94	215	337
Tarragona	E	**6**	**8**	**15**	**16**	**54**	173	247	7	9	20	**21**	54	144	230
South Thames	ENG	11	14	22	38	96	227	352	9	11	18	31	79	188	297
Varese	I	12	15	19	32	79	207	317	8	9	17	25	62	161	253
Wessex	ENG	11	14	21	37	95	223	346	9	11	18	30	78	185	292
West Midlands	ENG	12	16	24	42	107	250	384	10	13	20	35	88	209	326
Yorkshire	ENG	12	16	25	43	109	254	390	10	13	20	35	90	212	331

[a] The minimum and maximum values for each age-class are printed in bold type

ne, not estimated (the registry of Girona sent data for females only and the registry of Granada for only 1985)

Note: Both minimum and maximum values were chosen before eliminating decimal digits.

Table 4.3. Cumulative mortality risk per 1000 for various age-classes of older people by registry area[a] in 1979 and 1988: mortality data used in the EUROCARE study

	Country	MALES 1979			MALES 1988			FEMALES 1979			FEMALES 1988		
		75–79	80–89	90–99	75–79	80–89	90–99	75–79	80–89	90–99	75–79	80–89	90–99
Amiens	F	**347**	775	975	316	**735**	975	203	672	954	172	602	954
Basel	CH	353	804	**881**	281	757	945	204	**660**	955	166	**589**	922
Calvados	F	362	859	999	313	801	999	204	786	999	166	699	999
Côte D'Or	F	321	841	999	279	785	999	**188**	748	**999**	**145**	638	**999**
Cracow	PL	416	804	971	386	804	971	279	738	945	269	738	945
Denmark	DK	338	792	969	325	779	979	215	689	956	200	654	959
Doubs	F	341	857	**999**	301	809	999	207	778	999	171	699	999
East Anglia	ENG	370	827	967	313	757	967	238	723	940	198	644	940
Eindhoven	NL	355	808	958	348	806	958	220	703	**912**	209	671	900
Estonia	EST	**422**	865	978	**401**	**965**	993	**301**	783	964	**302**	**801**	987
Finland	FIN	387	834	979	332	777	980	254	750	954	214	684	948
Florence	I	316	847	948	283	758	994	201	735	956	165	650	923
Geneve	CH	327	808	975	281	745	975	208	702	963	174	625	963
Girona	E	ne	ne	ne	ne	ne	ne	208	712	938	168	653	893
Granada	E	ne	ne	ne	307	776	928	ne	ne	ne	211	699	916
Latina	I	347	834	942	302	793	**1000**	230	747	964	190	693	997
Mainz, Germany	D	397	856	ne	322	783	ne	264	779	ne	200	673	ne
Mallorca	E	357	832	978	299	758	978	233	753	961	176	634	961
Mersey	ENG	418	875	967	355	811	967	278	**788**	940	232	711	940
Modena	I	345	847	948	287	754	990	218	737	953	167	636	922
Piedmont	I	365	838	941	310	775	993	229	762	959	184	667	939
Ragusa	I	320	825	934	292	781	994	244	786	943	210	725	996
Saarland	D	409	839	974	349	782	963	287	759	947	207	638	943
Scotland	SCO	414	863	975	354	800	975	272	757	944	215	655	944
Tarragona	E	**303**	**764**	943	**259**	728	**914**	207	748	949	169	664	**891**
South Thames	ENG	377	835	967	319	766	967	240	726	940	199	646	940
Varese	I	384	**965**	919	319	781	998	241	762	951	186	666	938
Wessex	ENG	373	831	967	316	761	967	235	718	940	195	639	940
West Midlands	ENG	409	867	967	347	802	967	265	768	940	220	690	940
Yorkshire	ENG	**414**	871	967	352	807	967	269	774	940	224	697	940

[a] The minimum and maximum values for each age-class are printed in bold type

ne, not estimated (the registry of Girona sent data for females only and the registry of Granada for only 1985; the registry of Mainz, Germany is a childhood national cancer registry)

Table 4.4. Comparison of five-year observed and relative survival (%) for colon cancer in Swiss and German registries, by age classes and by period of diagnosis

	Age class						Period		
	15–44	45–54	55–64	65–74	75–99	All (15+)	1978 –80	1981 –82	1983 –85
	obs rel	obs rel	obs rel	obs rel	obs rel	obs rel	obs rel	obs rel	obs rel
Swiss registries									
Males	45 45	58 60	48 53	42 52	25 45	39 51	39 50	40 53	38 50
Females	66 67	63 64	54 56	50 56	35 55	44 57	40 53	46 59	46 58
All	53 53	60 62	51 54	46 54	31 51	42 54	40 51	43 56	42 54
German registry									
Males	62 63	58 61	40 44	35 48	19 39	36 48	32 44	35 48	40 54
Females	56 57	48 50	44 46	35 42	21 33	33 42	31 39	35 43	36 44
All	59 60	54 56	42 45	35 44	20 35	34 45	31 41	35 45	38 48

In order to quantify the effect on relative survival that might derive from errors in estimating general mortality trends, an exercise was carried out on colon cancer survival of patients from four Italian registries: Varese, Latina, Florence and Ragusa. In Italy, during the EUROCARE study period (considering both recruitment and follow-up periods: 1978–90), overall mortality rates decreased by 3% each year, which may be an important factor in computing relative survival. This is one of the fastest decreases observed in Europe.

Figure 4.2 compares six-year colon cancer relative survival computed using the 1982 general mortality over the entire period (shaded bars) versus a precise correction which considered the decreasing calendar-year specific general mortality (black bars). Comparisons were performed for the patients diagnosed in 1978–79, 1980–81, 1982–83 and 1984–85. The analyses were carried out according to Hakulinen's method and program (Hakulinen, 1982; Hakulinen & Abeywickrama, 1985). The error is higher for the last two periods, both for males and females, because the 1982 general mortality overestimates the actual mortality in more recent years. The Italian general mortality, in fact, decreased over these years; the resulting higher general survival leads to a lower relative survival, as shown in the lower black bars. The maximum error in computing six-year relative survival, using a stable intermediate mortality instead of a proper calendar-year-specific mortality is approximately 4% of the correct figure. In this monograph, the errors are likely to be largely below this level, because the mortality trend has been systematically considered, at least so far as it could be estimated using the data at the national level.

References

Estève, J., Benhamou, E. & Raymond, L. (1994) *Statistical Methods in Cancer Research*, Vol. IV, *Descriptive Epidemiology* (IARC Scientific Publications No. 128), Lyon, IARC

Hakulinen, T. (1982) Cancer survival corrected for heterogeneity in patient withdrawal. *Biometrics*, **38**, 933–942

Hakulinen, T. & Abeywickrama, K.H. (1985) A computer program package for relative survival analysis. *Computer Prog. Biomed.*, **19**, 197–207

Lopez, A.D. (1990) Who dies of what? A comparative analysis of mortality conditions in developed countries around 1987. *Wld. Hlth. Statist. Quart.*, **43**, 105–114

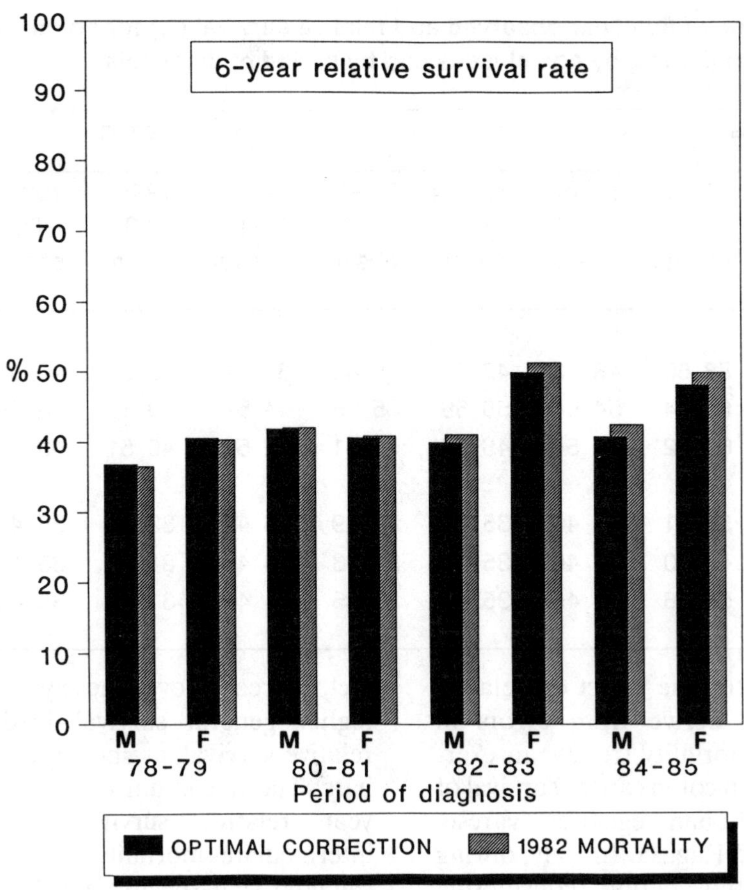

Figure 4.2. Comparison between relative survival figures for colon cancer using stable general mortality (1982) and decreased general mortality (optimal correction). Italian data

PART 2

CONTRIBUTING CANCER REGISTRIES AND RESULTS

CHAPTER 5

Health care system, cancer registration and follow-up of cancer patients in Denmark

Hans H. Storm

Denmark covers 43 080 km^2 and had a population of 5.1 million at 1 January 1987 (density: 118 per km^2). The majority (65%) live in urban areas. Since 1968 all inhabitants have been allocated unique personal identification numbers; a central computerized population registry keeps a continuously updated file on all inhabitants. From this file, annual life tables of the general population by age, sex, county and commune are published. The unique ID number is widely used for registration purposes (e.g. health care, cancer registration, mortality).

Health care in the kingdom of Denmark is provided free of charge to all inhabitants and funded by state and county taxes. Health care is organized regionally under the auspices of the regional governments (counties), supervised by the Ministry of Health and the National Board of Health. For Greenland and the Faroe Islands, which are not included in this monograph, health care is the sole responsibility of the local government, but specialist care, such as radiotherapy is provided by the University Hospital in Copenhagen (funded nationally).

Primary health care is delivered by private physicians under contract to regional governments. Hospital care is provided in 127 hospitals, of which one or two are major hospitals in each of the 16 regions of Denmark. A total of 39 273 hospital beds and 13 144 physicians were available in 1989 (Tulinius *et al.*, 1992). During the study period, no small private hospitals were in operation.

Dental care is, by and large, private, but operates under contract to regional health authorities with part of the cost covered by public health insurance.

Drugs are dispensed through pharmacies, also under contract to the health authorities, and medication for which a medical or dental prescription is necessary is subsidized to varying degrees. Medication in hospitals is supplied at no charge to the patient.

Initial cancer diagnosis and treatment is predominantly carried out at surgical departments, both at peripheral and central hospitals. Oncological service, including radiotherapy — is delivered by five highly specialized and well equipped oncological centres located at the four university hospitals (two in Copenhagen and in Odense and Aarhus) and one in the north of Jutland. In addition haematological malignancies are treated at haematology departments outside the centres, and some cytotoxic treatment for non-haematological cancer is also given in non-specialized centres. Furthermore, childhood cancers are treated at major paediatric departments, often located in the same hospitals as the oncological centres.

Aftercare and control may be carried out both at the central or the peripheral levels of the health care system. Terminal care is usually provided in hospitals, but support for home care can be obtained if so desired. There were no hospices in Denmark during the study period.

In principle, cancer treatment has been coordinated between the centres via coordination boards. These were established in the late 1970s in order to provide the best possible treatment and make maximal use of resources, in particular for rare cancers. A national clinical trial for breast cancer has been in operation since 1977 (Andersen & Mouridsen, 1988). Nationally agreed protocols for treatment of cancers of the head and neck, urinary bladder, colon and rectum, Hodgkin and non-Hodgkin lymphomas, testis and ovary lymphomas, melanoma and recently lung cancer have been or are applied, and may have influenced survival over the last few decades (Carstensen *et al.*, 1993; Andersson & Hansen, 1992).

Screening activity was carried out in many counties for pre-cancerous lesions of the cervix uteri during the study period, and population-based screening has recently been initiated on a trial basis in a few counties, for breast cancer (mammography) and for colon cancer (hemocult and colonoscopy).

The Danish Cancer Registry

The Danish Cancer Registry was established in May 1942, and has had all new cases of malignant diseases on file since 1943. Since 1987 reporting has been mandatory for physicians undertaking treatment or care of cancer patients. The registration system is 'passive', relying on multiple reports from hospitals, pathology institutes and practising physicians (accounting for 5% of all non-skin cancer, and 50% of skin cancer incidence; Storm *et al.*, 1992). These reports together with annual record linkage to the National Patient Discharge Registry and linkage and cross checks to all death certificates in Denmark, constitute the backbone of the registration system. An element of active registration relates to follow-up procedures on cases reported only by means of discharge registers and death certificates. From the Discharge Registry only verified cases are included in the database. The registration system and quality control procedures have been described in detail by Storm (1991).

Although the incidence publications present the data by the 7th revision of the International Classification for Diseases (Storm *et al.*, 1990; 1992), the Registry has used the ICD–O (WHO, 1976) classification for all cases since 1978 and converted to the ICD–7 for presentation purposes to allow for temporal comparisons. For the purpose of this study, data were submitted using the original ICD–O codes including behaviour. It should be noted that for sites where the Registry accepts and includes tumours reported by pathologists as benign, such as urothelial tumours of the renal pelvis, and brain tumours, the EUROCARE study population deviates from that covered by other publications from Denmark (Storm *et al.*, 1990; Carstensen *et al.*, 1993) by excluding such cases.

For survival analysis, data quality and other possible sources of incomparability should be kept in mind, especially comparing survival between registries and across national boundaries. Access to death certificates (Coleman & Démaret, 1988) and how follow-up procedures are employed are important. In Denmark, only 1.2% of all cancers are based on death certificate alone (Storm *et al.*, 1992) and thus excluded from survival analysis. However, about 10% of the annual incidence in the study period comprises cases first reported to the Registry by means of a death certificate, with notification and date of diagnosis obtained by follow-back procedures. Such cases may represent poor survivors and add only few months of observation, as outlined in the Danish survival publication (Carstensen *et al.*, 1993). Furthermore, cases reported by practising physicians (general practitioners) only (Storm *et al.*, 1992) may also represent cases with poor survival not referred to hospital care, and in some registries that do not use general practitioners as a data source would be excluded, as is the case for death certificate only cases. For such registries, survival would be artificially improved.

The index date for computing incidence and survival is that of diagnosis, which is either the date of first hospital admission or the date of first outpatient visit (either at hospital or in general practices) where the diagnoses were established.

Completeness of follow-up, vital status and date of death are equally important. In Denmark, as in other Nordic countries having computerized population-based monitoring with unique ID numbers, no patients have been lost in the study period, and patients migrating from Denmark or dying have not contributed after their date of departure.

References

Andersen, K.W. & Mouridsen, H.T. (1988) Danish Breast Cancer Cooperative Group (DBCG). A description of the register of the nationwide program for primary breast cancer. *Acta Oncol.*, **27**, 627–647

Andersson, M. & Hansen, O. (1992) Klinisk Cancerforskning i Danmark. Cancer, status over dansk onkologi. *Månedsskrift for praktisk laegegerning*, Suppl. **122–130** (in Danish)

Carstensen, B., Storm, H.H. & Schou, G., eds (1993) Survival of Danish cancer patients 1943–1987, *Acta Pathol. Microbiol. Scand.*, **101**, Suppl. 33

Coleman, M.P. & Démaret, E. (1988) Cancer registration in the European Community. *Int J. Cancer*, **42**, 339–345

Storm, H.H, Manders, T., Sprøgel, S., Bang, S. & Jensen, O.M. (1990) *Cancer Incidence in Denmark 1987*, Copenhagen, Danish Cancer Society

Storm H.H. (1991) The Danish Cancer Registry, a self-reporting national cancer registration system with elements of active data collection. In: Jensen, O.M., Parkin, D.M., MacLennan, R., Muir, C.S. & Skeet, R.G., eds, *Cancer Registration: Principles and Methods* (IARC Scientific Publications No. 95), Lyon, IARC, pp. 220–236

Storm, H.H., Manders, T., Friis, S. & Bang, S. (1992) *Cancer Incidence in Denmark 1989*, Copenhagen, Danish Cancer Society

Tulinius, H., Storm, H.H., Pukkala, E., Andersen, A. & Ericsson, J. (1992) Cancer in the Nordic Countries 1981–86, a joint publication of the five Nordic cancer registries. *Acta Pathol. Microbiol. Scand.*, **100**, Suppl. 31

WHO (World Health Organization) (1976) *International Classification of Diseases for Oncology (ICD–O)*, Geneva

CHAPTER 6

Health care system, cancer registration and follow-up of cancer patients in Estonia

Tiiu Aareleid

During the period included in this study, Estonia was a part of the USSR, and its National Health System (NHS) was similar to that of other republics of the USSR.

The Ministry of Health coordinated health services throughout Estonia. The NHS was organized by region: fifteen rural counties (rayons) and six urban areas aimed to provide the full range of primary and secondary health services to the local population. Two large centres, Tallinn and Tartu, served different parts of the country in terms of tertiary care.

The centralized system was financed from the State budget. A limited number of facilities was also financed and partly controlled by State enterprises. All health services were free as well as all drugs administered to hospital inpatients. Outpatient drugs were provided free of charge for some disease categories.

Since the dissolution of the Soviet Union and Estonia's re-establishment of complete independence in 1991, the NHS has been undergoing a process of change from a centralized state-controlled system towards a decentralized health-insurance-based system.

Before the changes in the NHS, there were about 120 hospitals in Estonia, including small first-level care centres, county and town hospitals providing secondary care and national and university hospitals providing tertiary services. The latter group consists of 30 units.

There are two specialized cancer hospitals (Estonian Cancer Centre and Tartu University Radiology and Oncology Clinic) responsible for diagnosis and treatment of the majority of cancer patients. No organized mass screening programmes for early detection of cancer have been introduced in Estonia (Aareleid *et al.*, 1993).

The Estonian Cancer Registry

Cancer registration in Estonia dates back to 1953, when compulsory registration of incident cases of cancer was introduced in the USSR. The Estonian Cancer Registry was officially established in January 1978 and is now run by the Estonian Cancer Centre and the Department of Epidemiology and Biostatistics of the Institute of Experimental and Clinical Medicine. The Registry's records are reasonably complete since 1968, when the level of cancer registration in Estonia reached a satisfactory level for calculating reliable incidence and survival rates (Karjalainen *et al.*, 1989).

The Estonian Cancer Registry covers the whole of Estonia (territory 45 215 km^2; population 1 565 662 according to the 1989 census; density: 34.6 per km^2). About 33% of the working population is employed in industry.

Every health-care institution where cancer has been diagnosed is obliged to send a notification form to one of the 17 local cancer registries in the catchment area where the patient lives. A special follow-up card is prepared in duplicate: one copy is kept in the local registry, another at the Estonian Cancer Registry (Rahu, 1992).

The date of diagnosis of cancer is used as the index date for computing incidence and survival. The follow-up is mixed. On a quarterly basis the registrars of the local registries visit the Estonian Cancer Registry to check the follow-up cards for completeness and to update them. If the information received by the Estonian Cancer Registry is incomplete, inquiries are made to the relevant health-care institution or population registry.

At monthly intervals, all death certificates kept in the Estonian State Department of Statistics are checked manually. The relevant information is copied from each certificate mentioning cancer, and is used to update the Estonian Cancer Registry's follow-up cards for patients' vital status. Additionally, the lists of deaths are sent to local cancer registries in order to match them against the lists made there by regional civil registration offices.

The ICD−O classification is used for coding cancer diagnoses. For statistical purposes, these codes are converted to ICD−9 codes. The Registry has provided annual reports to the Ministry of Health (now the Ministry of Social Affairs) since 1968. Detailed incidence and survival statistics are available from 1978 (Rahu & Aareleid, 1990; Aareleid & Rahu, 1991).

References

Aareleid, T. & Rahu, M. (1991) Cancer survival in Estonia from 1978 to 1987. *Cancer*, **68**, 2088−2092

Aareleid, T., Pukkala, E., Thomson, H. & Hakama, M. (1993) Cervical cancer incidence and mortality trends in Finland and Estonia: a screened vs. an unscreened population. *Eur. J. Cancer*, **29A**, 745−749

Karjalainen, S., Aareleid, T., Hakulinen, T., Pukkala, E., Rahu, M. & Tekkel, M. (1989) Survival of female breast cancer patients in Finland and in Estonia: stage at diagnosis important determinant of the difference between countries. *Soc. Sci. Med.*, **28**, 233−238

Rahu, M. (1992) Estonia. In: Parkin, D.M., Muir, C.S., Whelan, S.L., Gao, Y.T., Ferlay, J. & Powell, J., eds, *Cancer Incidence in Five Continents*, Vol. VI (IARC Scientific Publications No. 120), Lyon, IARC, pp. 569−573

Rahu, M. & Aareleid, T. (1990) *Cancer in Estonia 1978−1987. Diagrams.* Cancer Society of Finland Publication No. 44. Helsinki, Estonian Cancer Registry and Finnish Cancer Registry

CHAPTER 7

Health care system, cancer registration and follow-up of cancer patients in Finland

Timo Hakulinen

According to the Sickness Insurance Act, every Finnish resident was, during the period covered by this study, entitled to consult a physician at a municipal health centre free of charge. The costs incurred in consultations with private physicians or in purchasing medicines were partly reimbursed. More than 90% of the costs incurred during hospital stays were covered. In larger towns or cities especially, the private sector occupied an important position complementing the services offered by the municipal authorities. Regional differences in the availability of medical care and diagnostic facilities were small. In 1988, Finland had 9600 active physicians and 67 000 hospital beds.

The Central Population Register is able to give estimates of the population size, age and sex structure at any given point in time. Between 1982 and 1986, the average population of Finland was 4.89 million, with more than 60% living in urban municipalities. The Central Statistical Office of Finland provides population life tables based on linkage between the file of annual deaths and that of the entire population.

The proportion of the active population working in various sectors in 1988 was as follows: services 29%, industry 24%, commerce, banking and insurance 22%, agriculture and forestry 9% and transport and communications 7%.

The 460 municipalities of Finland are responsible for the local organization of public health and medical services. The country is divided into 22 health care districts, five of which (Helsinki, Kuopio, Oulu, Tampere and Turku) include university hospitals and medical faculties. The five university hospitals serve as regional cancer centres with specialized diagnostic, treatment and research facilities. However, the diagnosis and treatment of cancer are only partly centralized. Four other hospitals have oncological units, and cancer surgery is practised in all central hospitals of the health care districts. There are about 50 pathology laboratories in Finland: hospital departments, laboratories run by the Cancer Society of Finland and private laboratories. In the study period, countrywide mass screening for early detection of cervical cancer was conducted over the entire country.

The Finnish Cancer Registry

Finland has been covered by a national cancer registry since 1952. The Registry was founded and subsequently supported by the Cancer Society of Finland. In the study period, about two thirds of the expenses were covered by state-controlled funds arising from legalized small-scale gambling. The Finnish Cancer Registry receives reports from physicians, hospitals, institutes with hospital beds, and pathology and cytology laboratories as well as death certificates; on average, there are five notifications per case. Notification has been compulsory since 1961. No marked changes in incidence or incidence trends were noticed at or immediately after that year (Hakulinen *et al.*, 1986).

The death certificates provided by the Central Statistical Office of Finland are used to complete the series of incident cancer cases and in following up patients. The registry makes regular checks against files of persons who have emigrated from Finland and against the Central Population Register. Registration and comparisons are greatly facilitated by the use of the unique personal identification number. No patients were lost to follow-up in this study.

If a cancer case is notified from a pathology or cytology laboratory or known from a death certificate alone, or if the information received is incomplete or contradictory, further information is requested from hospitals and other institutions. Patients and their relatives are never contacted for the purpose of routine registration or patient follow-up. The index date for computing incidence and survival is the date of diagnosis. All medical coding is supervised by a physician. A slightly modified version of the ICD−7, expanded to include histology and certain information on tumour behaviour, is employed.

In addition to preparing the official cancer statistics for Finland, the Finnish Cancer Registry also provides data for planning purposes, clinical and pathology studies and for follow-up of cancer patients. It is also engaged in active research, particularly in cancer epidemiology, survival analysis and health care evaluation.

Reference

Hakulinen, T., Andersen, A., Malker, B., Pukkala, E., Schou, G. & Tulinius, H. (1986) Trends in cancer incidence in the Nordic countries. A collaborative study of the five Nordic cancer registries. *Acta Pathol. Microbiol. Scand.*, **94**A, Suppl. 288

CHAPTER 8

Health care system, cancer registration and follow-up of cancer patients in France

Jean Faivre, Paule-Marie Carli, Gilles Chaplain, Didier Pottier, Nicole Raverdy, Jean Robillard and Simon Schraub

The French National Health System (Sécurité Sociale) is funded by citizens' and employers' contributions, representing 21% and 42% respectively of the gross salary. Many institutions are entirely financed by the Health System. It provides health assistance for all citizens, even those without resources. Expenses in relation to diagnosis, treatment and surveillance of cancer are 100% paid directly by the Health System. Patients may be treated in either public or private health facilities under the same conditions. About half of the patients are treated in public hospitals (including some cancer centres) and half in the private sector.

The French cancer registries

Cancer registration started in France in 1975 in the Bas-Rhin. Despite the absence of a national policy, many cancer registries were established between 1975 and 1985, as a result of particular interest of clinicians or researchers. In 1986, a National Committee of Population-Based Registries was set up. During the period 1987–91, 11 cancer registries were funded at the national level. They include six general registries (Bas-Rhin, Calvados, Doubs, Isère, Martinique, Tarn) and five specialized registries, for digestive tract cancers (Côte d'Or and Calvados), childhood cancers (Lorraine, Provence-Côte D'Azur) and malignant haemopathies (Côte d'Or). The scientific quality of registration was recognized for five other registries, but they did not receive any funding; these were two general cancer registries (Herault and Somme [Amiens]) and three specialized registries: digestive tract cancers (Haute-Garonne), buccal cavity and pharynx cancers (Nord-Pas de Calais), and breast and gynaecological cancers (Côte d'Or). Representatives of the registries meet three to four times a year to coordinate their activities at both scientific and political levels.

Registration is active in all French cancer registries. Reports of all histological examinations with a cancer diagnosis are collected from public and private pathology laboratories. The registry staff visits all wards in public and private hospitals and makes enquiries to practitioners. Because of their poor quality, death certificates are not used to register patients, but serve to verify the completeness of registration and to identify cases not reported to the registry.

Seven cancer registries contributed to the present volume: the general ones of Doubs, Calvados and Somme (Amiens) and the specialized ones of Côte d'Or (digestive tract cancers, breast and gynaecological cancers and malignant haemopathies) and Calvados (digestive tract cancers). In all these registries, follow-up of patients is both active and passive. Death certificates are collected regularly at the département level. Other sources of information are municipalities of birth and residence, general practitioners and specialists.

The General and the Digestive Tract Cancer Registries of Calvados were set up in 1978 and cover the département of Calvados, an area of 5548 km^2 with 618 700 inhabitants (1990 census) (density: 112 per km^2). The registry is situated in Normandy in the northwest of France. The département of Calvados includes 631 rural communes (37% of the population) and 73 urban communes. 43% of the population is active and 6.9% of the active population works in agriculture.

There are 22 health care centres, including one university hospital and 2 radiotherapy units. In 1992 there were 1398 medical practitioners including 557 general practitioners.

The index date for computing incidence and survival is the date of the first histological examination or the date of the examination confirming the diagnosis. Regularly, every two to three years, a letter is sent to the mayor's office to assess the patient's status (dead or alive).

The Digestive Cancer Registry, the Malignant Haemopathies Cancer Registry and the Breast and Gynaecologic Cancer Registry of Côte d'Or were established in 1976, 1980 and 1982, respectively. The département of Côte d'Or, situated in the centre-east of France, has an area of 8733 km^2, and its capital is Dijon. The population covered is 493 931 (1990 census) (density: 56.6 per km^2). Overall 11% of the active population works in agriculture and 36% in industry.

In the département there are 11 hospitals, including one university hospital, one anti-cancer centre and five private hospitals, and two radiotherapeutic facilities. Date of diagnosis is the index date for computing incidence and survival. Death certificates mentioning digestive tract cancer are collected every month. For patients not identified as being dead, an active search of vital status is performed every year, using both the registries of the municipality of birth and medical practitioners.

The Doubs Cancer Registry was set up in 1976. It covers the 484 770 resident population (1990 census) (density: 92.2 per km^2) of the département of the Doubs, in the east of France not far from the Swiss border. It covers 5260 km^2, including two industrial areas: one in the northern part of the département, where the Peugeot factory is located, and the other at Besançon, the capital city, with a range of light industry.

There are three public hospitals (one a university hospital), five private clinics and two radiotherapeutic facilities in this area.

The index date for computing incidence and survival is the day of diagnosis. All death certificates are collected, and an active search of vital status is performed using records of the municipality of birth and general practitioners.

The Somme Cancer Registry (referred to here as Amiens) has been active since 1982. It covers the département of the Somme, in the north of France. The département has an area of 6170 km^2 with a population of 545 060 inhabitants (1990 census) (density: 90.1 per km^2). It is a relatively industrialized area (the percentage of those who work in industry is 32.6%). In the area covered by the Registry, there are ten hospitals, one of which is a university hospital, and five private hospitals. There are four radiotherapy centres.

Registrars contact pathology laboratories, specialized centres in the district and a general hospital outside the area limits.

Date of diagnosis is the index date for computing incidence and survival. Cases are followed up through access to death certificates with cancer notification and enquiries to physicians or to the mayor's office.

CHAPTER 9

Health system, cancer registration and follow-up of cancer patients in Germany (West)

Hartwig Ziegler, Peter Kaatsch and Jörg Michaelis

The health care system in Germany (West) comprises all services and persons contributing to the health of the population by treating patients, promoting their physical and mental well-being and rehabilitating them. A multitude of governmental and non-governmental institutions directly employing nearly one million people are involved in these activities.

The functioning of the health system is closely linked to the organization of the State. The authorities responsible for public health services are the Bund, Länder and Gemeinden or other institutions incorporated under public law. Nevertheless, this is not a state-administered public health system, but a collaboration of health insurance companies, health professionals, hospitals and other service facilities.

The statutory health insurance funds are obliged by law to ensure comprehensive health protection services for their members. The major schemes are local compulsory sickness funds, insurance schemes for industrial workers and public service employees, as well as voluntary health insurance. Approximately 90% of all citizens are covered by the statutory sickness funds. Membership in the health schemes is mandatory up to a certain income level, while higher-income employees may continue as voluntary members or entrust their medical care to private funds (as self-employed citizens do). Insurance companies receive a fixed percentage of the salaries of all employees, paid in equal amounts by the employers and employees. Retired people also have to pay regular contributions to meet at least a small part of their medical costs. Only 0.2% of the population is estimated to have no health insurance at all.

Benefits include medical and dental fees, hospital payments, prescriptions, laboratory tests, rehabilitation measurements and medical appliances. The expenses for cancer treatment and after-care are also fully covered.

Cancer treatment is carried out by both hospitals and private physicians. Since 1971 the German Social Security System has offered free and voluntary cancer screening for women over 30 (and since 1982 over 20) and men over 45.

Since 1980 treatment of cancer at the hospital level has been coordinated under a government programme structured on several levels:

(*a*) The 'Tumorzentren' cover large regional areas and are connected with big university hospitals. They are involved in both research and treatment.

(*b*) A series of regional hospitals dedicate considerable personnel and funds to cancer treatment.

(*c*) A still small number of private oncological practices provide diagnostic and after-care structures.

The ultimate aim of the German Health Security System is to provide all citizens with equally good health services without consideration of their financial situation, position in society or place of residence.

The Saarland Cancer Registry

In Germany, apart from the nationwide registry for childhood malignancies at the University of Mainz (see below) and the registry of the former German Democratic Republic, population-based cancer registries operate in the regions of Saarland, Hamburg, Münster and Baden-Württemburg. Only the 'Krebsregister Saarland' provides reliable incidence data for the entire area of a federal State, the others being still in an initial phase or having an inadequate level of completeness for incidence data (Hamburg).

The Saarland Cancer Registry is an integrated unit of the State Statistical Office and is based on the Saarland Law of Cancer Registration (SKRG), which came into force in 1979. Since its inception, it has been financed by the Government of Saarland and by regular subsidies from the Federal Ministry of Health.

Located in the south-west of Germany bordering France and Luxembourg, Saarland is the second smallest State in the Federal Republic, covering an area of 2600 km^2. The population monitored by the Registry is 1.07 million (in 1990) (density: 417 per km^2) or 1.3% of the whole German population. Some 55% live in communities with more than 20 000 inhabitants.

About 48.1% of the surface of Saarland is used for agricultural purposes, 33.2% is forest, and the remaining 18.7% includes housing, industrial areas, water and recreational areas. The active population is 40.9% of the total (1990) of which 41.9% is employed in industry, 18.7% in commerce and transport, 1.3% in agriculture and 38.1% in other services.

The basic system of the Saarland Cancer Registry is a centralized registration of individual records including personal identifiers which do not require the consent of registered patients. Notification is voluntary. Hospitals, physicians and persons acting on their behalf have a right, not a duty, to report cancer cases without violating their professional obligations.

The main suppliers of information are hospitals, outpatient departments, pathology and radiotherapy departments and private practitioners. To minimize under-registration, death certificates are also used as data sources.

There are 30 hospitals including four radiotherapeutic departments and seven institutes of pathology in the registration area. About 50% of all new reports of cases come from pathologists.

The first date of cancer diagnosis is taken as the index date for computing incidence and survival rates, without regard to the type of diagnostic verification. It may, but does not necessarily, coincide with the date of histological diagnosis.

Due to very restrictive legal framework, the follow-up of patients is largely passive. Though all physicians treating cancer patients are generally requested to report any serious change in the state of a patients' health, the registry is not allowed to conduct further enquiries. The files of registered cases are linked annually with all death certificates, but there is no regular matching with migration data for people leaving the Saarland region.

The German Registry of Childhood Malignancies (The Mainz Cancer Registry)

The nationwide Registry of Childhood Malignancies was initiated by the German scientific society for paediatric oncology and haematology. The registry is run at the Institut für Medizinische Statistik und Dokumentation at the University of Mainz. Its first five years were funded by the Volkswagenwerk Foundation. It is now financed by the Federal Ministry of Health and the Ministry of Labour, Social Affairs, Family and Health of Rhineland-Palatinate via the Regional Cancer Centre.

From 1980 to 1990, all incident cases of childhood malignancies in the former Federal Republic of Germany (FRG) were reported to the Registry. During the first five years of operation, which was the study period of the EUROCARE project, about 80% of the incident cases in the former Federal Republic were reported. Thereafter, completeness increased to an estimated 95%. During the EUROCARE study period, the annual population of children averaged 10 376 000. Since 1991, cases from the former German Democratic Republic have also been included. There are about 8500 municipalities in this area.

The German Childhood Registry combines features of a population-based and a hospital-based registry. The Registry is run without any specific legal basis in accordance with existing legislation on data privacy and security. Information is provided on a voluntary basis by physicians who obtain informed consent from the patients' parents.

More than 100 paediatric hospitals and centres for paediatric oncology report their cancer patients to the registry. About 70% of all diseased children are participating in clinical trials, and an integrated documentation sequence and information flow between the cancer registry, treating hospitals, and trial study centres has been established.

To calculate incidence and survival rates, the index date is the date of taking histological material to verify diagnosis. The precise basis of diagnosis is not recorded by the registry for all cases, but for cases enrolled in clinical trials histological data are always available. The percentage of cases with microscopic verification is possibly as high as 95%.

An individual active follow-up is performed according to a set procedure. Annually each participating hospital receives a list of all patients for whom no information has reached the Registry during the previous 12 months, requesting a few data items describing the patient's current status. If a major event like relapse or death has occurred, this is reported in greater detail. The quality of follow-up data is further improved by the close cooperation with clinical trials.

CHAPTER 10

Health care system, cancer registration and follow-up of cancer patients in Italy

Milena Sant, Gemma Gatta, Alessandro Barchielli, Ettore M.S. Conti, Lorenzo Gafá, Corrado Magnani and Maurizio Ponz de Leon

The Italian National Health System (NHS) provides health assistance for all citizens, covering the entire population of the country, with very few exceptions. The NHS is funded by State and Regional administration and by contributions from all citizens. A fixed percentage from salaries of all employed people is retained for this purpose.

The Italian NHS is organized in local Health Units, covering areas of variable size (mostly with about 100 000 inhabitants), which administer all the health facilities in their areas, with a few exceptions, e.g. university and research clinics.

There is a mixture of public and private facilities, with 85.5% of hospitals public and 16.5% private; most private health facilities however, are partially supported economically by the NHS, directly or through reimbursements to the patients.

Drugs are dispensed within the NHS, with 30–40% of the total price paid by the patient, with some exceptions for people with low income, who pay nothing. The same applies for diagnostic tests and outpatient therapy.

Hospitalization in public hospitals is free, as are all examinations and drugs administered during a stay in hospital.

The Italian cancer registries

Approximately 10% of the Italian population is covered by nine active cancer registries which started their activity in the 1970s or early 1980s (Zanetti & Crosignani, 1992). Many cancer registries were established because of a particular interest of researchers and have subsequently been funded at least partially by local authorities. National coordination of working practices is achieved through annual meetings of the working group of the Italian Cancer Registries within the Italian Association of Epidemiology. A number of minor differences persist, however, for example in the definition of index dates to compute incidence and survival.

In all the Italian registries, cases are sought actively by the registry's personnel, through consultation of clinical notes in hospitals and in pathology and haematology departments.

Six cancer registries have contributed to the present volume: the general ones of Lombardy, Tuscany, Latina and Ragusa and the specialized ones of Piedmont (childhood) and Modena (colorectal).

Every year estimates of the resident population by sex and age are provided by the Istituto Superiore di Sanità for each province, on the basis of an update of the latest national census. Annual life tables of the general population by age, sex, and province are also produced by the same institute, on the basis of the national mortality data.

In most registries, follow-up of patients is mixed active and passive, including an active search for cases who have migrated out of the area. All the registries participating in EUROCARE have established formal contacts with the municipalities of their area, to collect the death certificates of individual patients. In Italy the death certificates provided by the municipalities are nominative, allowing the identification of patients and their cause of death. In addition, other procedures for following up cases are adopted locally by the registries.

The *Lombardy Cancer Registry* is run by the Division of Epidemiology at the Istituto Nazionale Tumori in Milan. It has been active since 1976, covering the province of Varese in

Lombardy region, northern Italy, on the border with Switzerland. It is a highly industrialized and wealthy area, and 60% of the active population works in industry. It covers approximately 1200 km^2, with a population of about 800 000 (density 657 per km^2). There are 144 municipalities.

In the province there are 12 hospitals, of which one is a university hospital and three are private clinics. Two radiotherapeutic facilities exist in the area.

The index date for computing incidence and survival is the date of first hospital admission or, if the case is diagnosed and treated as an outpatient, the date of diagnostic confirmation.

Follow-up is mixed: the 144 municipalities of the province send all death certificates to the registry, where they are linked to the registry's files. An active search of vital status is then automatically performed through the NHS population files, which cover all the resident population and are updated every few months. Whenever an inconsistency is found, for example in the case of death outside the province, it is resolved through active contact with the relevant administration.

The *Tuscany Cancer Registry* was set up in 1984 and is run by the Centro per lo Studio e la Prevenzione Oncologica, at the Florence Local Health Unit. It covers the province of Florence, of approximately 3800 km^2, in central Italy, with 1 174 000 inhabitants (density: 308 per km^2). Of the employed population, 49% works in industry. There are 51 municipalities.

There are 12 public hospitals and 13 private clinics in the province, and a university clinic is located at the main public hospital. One radiotherapeutic centre is present within the province.

Date of hospital admission is the index date for computing incidence and survival. If the patient is not hospitalized or if histological verification precedes hospital admission, the index date is that of diagnostic confirmation as an outpatient. For breast and cervix cancers, for which a screening programme covers the province, the index date is that of diagnosis made following screening detection, regardless of hospitalization.

Follow-up is mixed active and passive, the latter through automatic linkage of regional mortality data with the registry's files. For all people identified as not dead by this check, a manual active search in the municipalities' population files is performed.

The *Latina Cancer Registry* was established in 1981 and is supported by the local League Against Cancer and the Regional Epidemiological Observatory; it is run at the Oncological Centre of the Latina General Hospital together with the National Cancer Institute in Rome.

The registry area covers the province of Latina, in the Latium region of central Italy, at the border with the province of Rome, covering a surface of about 2200 km^2, of which 90% is agricultural. The area has approximately 450 000 inhabitants (density 193 per km^2). There are 33 municipalities.

There are nine public and five private hospitals in the area, with one radiotherapy department in the main hospital.

The index date for computing incidence and survival is that of hospital admission or of diagnostic confirmation in the case of outpatients.

Follow-up of patients is performed through linkage with the death certificates collected in the framework of the MONICA project (which includes the Latina province) and the registry of deaths managed by the Regional Epidemiological Observatory of Latium. The vital status of patients who are not traced in the list of deaths is checked in the municipalities' files of the resident population. For patients who have migrated out of the region, direct contact with the new municipalities of residence is performed. These checks are performed at anniversary dates, every five years.

The *Ragusa Cancer Registry*, established in 1979 as a section of the Epidemiological Observatory of Sicily, is sponsored by the Italian League against Cancer. It covers the whole of Ragusa province, about 1600 km^2, with approximately 280 000 inhabitants (density: 177 per km^2). There are 12 municipalities. Twenty-six per cent of the active population is employed in farming and 26% in industry.

There are six hospitals in the area, but no radiotherapeutic facilities are available and patients requiring radiotherapy are treated in larger towns, such as Catania.

The index date for computing incidence and survival is that of hospital admission, except for cases diagnosed as outpatients.

Follow-up is mixed: all death certificates of the 12 municipalities of the province are checked periodically by the registry's personnel. Contact is made with general practitioners and relatives of the patients not identified as dead or if the diagnosis is not clear.

The *Colorectal Cancer Registry of Modena* has been active since 1984 and is run by clinicians of the University Hospital in Modena. It was established as a result of a clinical and etiological research interest in colorectal cancer, particularly on familiality for these tumours.

The province of Modena is a flat area covering about 580 km^2 and having approximately 260 000 inhabitants (density: 450 per km^2) located in the north-central area of Italy. It is one of the richest and most industrialized provinces in Italy, and 60% of the active population works in industry. There are 10 municipalities in the province.

There are four public hospitals (including the University one) and two private hospitals in the area. Radiotherapeutic facilities are available at the University.

The index date for computing incidence and survival is that of hospital admission or of diagnostic confirmation in the case of outpatients.

Follow-up of patients is mixed active and passive. The registry receives all death certificates from the municipalities' data files; active contact is made with clinicians and families of patients, also in pursuance of the study of familial cancers.

The *Piedmont Childhood Cancer Registry*, established in 1967, is run by the Cancer Epidemiology Unit of Turin (Local Health Unit and University of Turin) and collects cases from the whole region of Piedmont, in north-western Italy. The region covers 25 000 km^2, and has approximately 4 500 000 inhabitants (density: 177 per km^2), of whom 800 000 are children under 15 years of age. Approximately 55% of the active population is employed in industry. There are 1209 municipalities in the area.

There are 60 hospitals in the region, including one paediatric hospital in Turin. At least three major radiotherapy units are located in Turin, and other radiotherapeutic facilities are available in peripheral hospitals.

Cases are collected actively by the Registry's personnel, who every two years visit all hospitals in the region where patients are likely to be treated, in order to collect the relevant clinical documentation. Also, specialized hospitals in other Italian regions are checked, as well as the Institut Gustave Roussy in Villejuif (France), where children may be treated.

The index date for computing incidence and survival is that of histological or cytological verification. If no microscopic verification is performed, the date of hospital admission is taken as the reference date.

Follow-up is active: every two or three years the vital status of every registered patient is checked in the population files of the municipality of residence by the personnel of the registry.

Reference

Zanetti, R. & Crosignani, P. (1992) *Cancer in Italy*, Turin, Lega Italiana per la lotta contro i Tumori, Associazione Italiana di Epidemiologia

CHAPTER 11

Health care system, cancer registration and follow-up of cancer patients in The Netherlands

Jan Willem W. Coebergh, Mariad A. Crommelin, Erica Masseling and Louis H. van der Heijden

Access to medical care in the Netherlands is good, as a result of the relatively short distances to hospitals (universally less than 40 km), the ample supply of the various health services and a health insurance system that poses no major financial obstacle.

Some 40% of the population have private insurance, mostly through their employers, and 60% of the population are covered by the Sickness Benefit Fund, a compulsory social insurance policy for people with lower incomes and those on welfare. Less than 1% of the population is uninsured.

In the area covered by the Eindhoven Cancer Registry (the south-eastern Netherlands), virtually all specialized clinicians, who are consulted mainly through referral from general practitioners (about one for every 2500 inhabitants), work in community hospitals. The hospitals have declined in number from 12 to 8 through mergers and now offer about 3.5 beds per 1000 inhabitants, allowing larger numbers of medical staff with increasing specialization in, for example, oncology. By 1980, most modern diagnostic techniques including endoscopy, echography and cytology, were amply available, except for computerized tomographic scanning. Few patients were referred to the eight university hospitals and the two cancer hospitals in Amsterdam and Rotterdam. Radiotherapy is delivered in one regional institute that serves the community hospitals. Pathologists work in three regional laboratories, which assemble all their diagnoses in a national database (PALGA), which, since 1988, has also notified the Cancer Registry.

Although the number of beds in nursing homes has increased markedly since 1970 to about 3 per 1000 people, the confirmation of a cancer diagnosis still generally occurs in a hospital.

To coordinate cancer care, nine Comprehensive Cancer Centres (CCCs) were founded between 1977 and 1983, paid for by health insurance. In addition to developing a nationwide system of cancer registries, they arrange regular oncological consulting services in specialized hospitals and community hospitals, support regional tumour study groups, provide data management for clinical research and arrange postgraduate education. Increasingly they foster the development of psychosocial services for cancer patients, palliative and home care and (since 1990) breast cancer screening, in collaboration with the regional public health services. A cervical screening programme was carried out between 1975 and 1983 for about 70% of women between 35 and 55 years of age. This was restarted in 1988, and there is also a considerable level of spontaneous cervical smear taking by gynaecologists.

The Eindhoven Cancer Registry

The Eindhoven Regional Cancer Registry began operation in 1955 as part of a programme for nationwide cancer registration. It started as a system of clinical documentation in three hospitals in Eindhoven, collecting data on new cancer patients during the consultants' weekly meetings and, subsequently, directly from pathology reports and patient records, including all radiotherapy files. Registration activities expanded in parallel with the decentralized consulting services of radiotherapists from Eindhoven, where megavoltage facilities were concentrated. More systematic registration procedures were developed according to international guidelines in the 1960s. By the early seventies, the registry served 13 hospitals in an area consisting of south-eastern North Brabant and middle and northern Limburg.

In 1979 a regional organization, the Cooperative Association of Hospitals in Oncology (SOOZ) was established. In 1980 it compiled an evaluation of completeness. The evaluation was based on the analysis of referral patterns and registration procedures, including the collection of data on patients directly referred to specialized centres elsewhere. For most tumours, the registration was judged complete since 1970 in a core area containing 85% of the population covered by the registry. Due to a strict interpretation of privacy regulations on the access to the causes of deaths register of the Central Bureau of Statistics, the proportion of death-certificate-only cases could not be computed. The ratio between mortality and incidence rates, however, was higher than one only for elderly patients with highly lethal cancers (oesophagus, stomach, pancreas and lung) (Coebergh *et al.*, 1990).

The registry serves an area of about 2500 km^2, with almost 1 million inhabitants or 7% of the Dutch population in 1985 (density: 400 per km^2; roughly the national average). Annual population data are derived from the Central Bureau of Statistics, which holds demographic data from municipalities. Forty-seven per cent of the population-at-risk lived in urban, 41% in suburban and 12% in rural municipalities.

Mortality rates for major causes of death, except cancer, are declining, especially in the elderly. The population was still relatively young in 1985, in part due to immigration related to economic development.

During the period 1978–87, registration procedures remained unchanged, depending upon multiple sources, that varied according to local circumstances and consisted of:

— routine reports for all patients, provided by departments of pathology and radiotherapy;

— regular active and direct collection of data from patient records in all hospitals, in cooperation with the medical records offices and supported by regular contacts with consultants and outpatient clinics (including dermatology);

— annual cross-checks with data from specialized departments and hospitals as well as periodically with the Committee for the Diagnosis of Bone Tumours and the Dutch Childhood Leukaemia Study Group.

At the registration office, data were coded according to ICD–8 until 1978 and ICD–9 since that year. Follow-up of date of death consisted of systematic checks of the vital status of patients diagnosed since 1975, both through hospitals and in municipal population registers as of 1988. Less than 1% of these patients proved to be lost to follow-up (Coebergh *et al.*, 1991a; Coebergh & van der Heijden, 1991b).

The registry still operates on a voluntary basis, but within a newly developing national scheme of cancer registration, that has been gradually evolving since 1984 (Netherlands Cancer Registry, 1992). In this scheme, the same procedures are followed and have proved to lead to reasonable completeness (Berkel, 1990; Schouten *et al.*, 1993).

References

Berkel, J. (1990) General practitioners and completeness of cancer registry. *J. Epidemiol. Commun. Health,* **44**, 121–124

Coebergh, J.W.W., Verhagen-Teulings, M.Th., Crommelin, M.A., Bakker, D. & van der Heijden, L.H. (1990) Trends in incidence of cancer in southeastern North Brabant and northern Limburg in the period 1975–1986. *Ned. Tijdschr. Geneeskd*, **134**, 754–760

Coebergh, J.W.W. & van der Heijden, L.H., eds (1991b) *Cancer Incidence and Survival 1975–1987.* Eindhoven: Comprehensive Cancer Centre South, Eindhoven Cancer Registry Publications, No. 2

Coebergh, J.W.W., Crommelin, M.A., van der Heijden, L.H., Hop, W.C.J. & Verhagen-Teulings, M.Th. (1991a) Survival of cancer patients in southeastern Netherlands. *Ned. Tijdschr. Geneeskd,* **135**, 938–943

Netherlands Cancer Registry (1992) *Incidence of Cancer in the Netherlands, 1989*, Utrecht, Coordinating Council of Comprehensive Cancer Centres, No. 1

Schouten, L.J., Höppener, P., van den Brandt, P.A., Knottnerus, J.A. & Jager, J.J.(1993) Completeness of cancer registration in Limburg, The Netherlands. *Int. J. Epidemiol.*, **22**, 369–376

CHAPTER 12

Health care system, cancer registration and follow-up of cancer patients in Poland

Janusz Pawlega

Under the present system of health care, Poland is divided into 11 regions, each with a medical school. The population of these regions ranges from 2 to 5 million. All 11 regions have either specialist regional cancer hospitals or regional cancer centres. The most advanced diagnostic facilities are usually housed in the medical schools, while radiotherapy equipment is concentrated in the regional cancer hospitals or centres, enabling them to provide facilities for treatment over the entire region.

The basic administrative units of the country, called voivodships, have cancer outpatient clinics and diagnostic facilities.

In Poland the majority of patients with more common cancers are treated in general hospitals. However, most patients with leukaemia and childhood tumours are treated in the clinical departments of medical schools, while a large proportion of patients with lung cancer are treated in specialist hospitals for pulmonary diseases and tuberculosis. These were established shortly after the Second World War, when tuberculosis was still a major health problem. The specialist oncological hospitals and centres are equipped with comprehensive facilities for treatment with radiotherapy and other combined treatments, employing the majority of medical oncologists in the area. The oncological network is largely responsible for:

— promoting standards of modern cancer treatment and care;

— health education and professional training;

— providing the facilities for treatment of about 50% of cancer patients requiring radiotherapy, combined treatment or intensive chemotherapy, either directly or in cooperation with other hospitals.

The M. Sklodowska-Curie Memorial Cancer Centre and Institute of Oncology in Warsaw, with branches in Cracow and Gliwice, is responsible for coordination of all activities related to cancer control.

Each year an estimate of the resident population by age and sex is provided, based on the latest national census, by the main Statistics Office in Warsaw. Life tables of the general population by age, sex, five-year period and voivodship are published by the same institution.

The Cracow Cancer Registry

In Poland, nationwide reporting of cancer has been compulsory since 1952. However, with the resources that were provided, it proved impossible to obtain data of a good and uniform standard from the central registration scheme covering the whole country. To improve the quality of registration, a few selected areas of Poland were chosen, where reporting of cancer was based on active registration. One of these was Cracow, where the cancer registry was set up in 1965.

Cracow, the third largest city in Poland, is situated on the Vistula River, at 50° 4′ N. and 19° 58′ E. and is 220 metres above sea level. The surface area is 321.7 km^2 and the population about 700 000.

The main occupational groups are: industry (about 30%), construction (about 18%), science and education (about 13%), trade (9%), health care (6%) and transport (about 6%). The number of physicians is about 2500 and the number of hospital beds about 8000, including 220 beds in the Cracow branch of the Centre for Oncology and 40 beds in the Department of Oncology at the Medical Academy.

The Registry is housed in the Cracow branch of the M. Sklodowska-Curie Memorial Cancer Centre and Institute of Oncology. Because of its location, the Cancer Registry has direct access to medical records of patients who are treated and followed up in the Cancer Centre. These constitute about 50% of all cancer patients in Cracow, of whom about 90% require radiotherapy and about 75% need complex treatment. The remaining 50% of Cracow cancer patients are treated in the departments of the Medical Academy or in general hospitals. Examinations as well as hospital care and drugs are free.

Almost all lymphoma patients, over 75% of head, neck, breast, corpus and cervix uteri cancer patients, about 30% of lung and urological cancer patients and 15% of digestive tract cancer patients in the Cracow area are treated at the Cracow Cancer Centre or the Department of Oncology of the Cracow Medical Academy.

By Administrative Order, all hospitals and outpatient clinics have to report cancer cases to the registry. This information is completed and checked against data from pathology departments and death certificates. Cases are filed in alphabetical order by year and new reports are checked for duplicates.

Follow-up of patients is carried out by annual check-ups of medical records, death certificates and information from local statistics offices. Each death from cancer in Cracow must be reported to the registry. Follow-up is, therefore, both active and passive.

The most common index date for computing incidence and survival is the date of diagnosis. If this information is unavailable (for about 12% of cases), date of the first hospital admission or the date of filing of the first notification card is used.

CHAPTER 13

Health care system, cancer registration and follow-up of cancer patients in Spain

Carmen Martinez, Jaume Galceran, Isabel Garau and Pau Viladiu

Spain has 38 million inhabitants and is organized administratively into Comunidades Autonomas (CCAA), each with its own parliament and local government. Within each, there is an organization called the "Consejeria de Salud" that is responsible for health issues. The size of each CCAA varies from 300 000 to 7 million people. The strength of the links between the Consejeria and the central Ministry of Health varies from one Community to another.

Some of the characteristics of the Spanish National Health System (SNHS) are: universal coverage, a majority of public funding and the provision of mostly public services. The SNHS is approximately 70% funded by the State and 30% by a fixed contribution from workers' salaries.

Hospital beds are 70% public and 30% private (15% of them are funded by charity). Most private hospitals are also funded by the SNHS through reimbursement procedures.

Medication is free of charge for 'pensionistas' (retired and disabled people) and for widows. For the rest of the population it is partially funded by the SNHS, while 40% is paid by the citizens except for long-term treatments, where payment is 10% if the sum does not exceed a certain limit. There is no charge for examinations, diagnostic tests or hospitalization, including medication administered during hospital stay.

The Spanish cancer registries

In Spain there are eight active general registries that cover 20% of the population, and two specialized ones, one for childhood cancers and one for female breast and gynaecological cancers. Two were set up in 1960 and 1970, and the others in the 1980s.

Most registries are linked to the local administration, and only three are partially funded by other sources. No national coordination scheme exists, and the main links between registries are common research projects.

In all registries, cases are actively sought by registry personnel, within hospitals and health services.

Four cancer registries have contributed to the present volume: the general ones of Granada, Tarragona and Mallorca (which specialized in colorectal cancers during the EUROCARE study period) and the Female Breast and Gynaecological Cancer specific registry of Girona.

Periodically, the departments of statistics in every Comunidad Autonoma provide annual estimates of the resident population in each province, as well as life tables of the general population by sex, age and province, on the basis of national mortality data.

In most registries, follow-up is mixed passive and active, through searches in hospitals and municipalities' population files. The death certificates provided by the municipalities are nominative, allowing identification of patients and their cause of death.

The *Granada Cancer Registry*, set up in 1985, is run by the Escuela Andaluza de Salud Publica and funded by the Consejeria de Salud de Andalucia. It covers the province of Granada in Andalucia, southern Spain, having a surface area of 12 531 km^2 (density: 62.5 per km^2) and a population of about 800 000 inhabitants. The area is predominantly rural and the active population is mostly employed in agriculture (18%), services (49%) and industry (12%).

There are five public hospitals, one of which is a university hospital, and three private clinics. In two of the public hospitals there are radiotherapeutic facilities.

The index date for computing incidence and survival is the date of diagnosis.

Survival studies are only carried out for some specific tumours. Follow-up in these cases is active, and registry personnel collect information about vital status through hospital records and the municipalities' population files.

The *Tarragona Cancer Registry* is run by the Asociacion Española Contra el Cancer and partially funded by the Department of Health of the Generalitat de Catalunya and the Diputacion de Tarragona. It was set up in 1979 and full population coverage was achieved in 1980. It covers the province of Tarragona in Catalonia, in north-eastern Spain, with a surface area of 6283 km^2 and a population of about 500 000 inhabitants (density: 83 per km^2). The active population is mainly employed in agriculture (21%), industry (21%) and services (48%).

There are five public hospitals, one of which is a university hospital, which has the only radiotherapeutic equipment available in the province, and twelve private clinics.

The index date for computing incidence and survival is the date of diagnosis. Follow-up is mixed active and passive.

The *Girona Cancer Registry*, established in 1980, is run by the Asociacion Española Contra el Cancer and also supported by the Health Department of the Generalitat de Catalunya and the Diputacion de Girona. It is a specific registry for female breast and gynaecological sites, covering the Region of Girona in Catalonia, in the north-east of Spain, with a surface area of 4643 km^2 and 509 000 inhabitants (density: 102 per km^2). The active population is employed mainly in services (52%) and industry (28%).

There are five public hospitals and ten private clinics. One public hospital has radiotherapeutic facilities.

The index date for computing incidence and survival is the date of diagnostic confirmation.

Follow-up is active, and registry personnel collect information about vital status through hospital records and the municipalities' population files.

The *Mallorca Cancer Registry* is run by a cancer epidemiology unit and was created by a collaborative research agreement between the following institutions: Consell Insular de Mallorca, Conselleria de Sanitat i Seguretat Social del Govern Balear, Asociacion Española Contra el Cancer, Universitat de les Illes Balears, INSALUD and the Colorectal Cancer Study Group.

This registry began as a specialized colorectal cancer registry in 1982 and became generalized in 1989. It covers the island of Mallorca in the Balearics, eastern Spain, with a surface area of 3625 km^2 and a population of approximately 600 000 inhabitants (density: 152 inhabitants per km^2). The active population is mostly employed in services (66%) and industry (28%).

There are five public hospitals and seven private clinics. In one public and one private hospital there are radiotherapeutic facilities.

The index date for computing incidence and survival is the date of anatomopathological diagnosis or, if this is not available, the date of the first hospital admission.

Follow-up is mixed active and passive. Passive follow-up is carried out by reviewing death certificates and active follow-up is made regularly, either by interviewing the attending physician or reviewing clinical records.

CHAPTER 14

Health-care system, cancer registration and follow-up of cancer patients in Switzerland

Luc Raymond and Joachim Torhorst

The Swiss health system is characterized by a strong degree of decentralization. The 26 cantons have independence on all health matters except those limited by the Federal Constitution, such as communicable diseases and health insurance. On the whole, medicine is managed on liberal principles, but differences are considerable from one canton to another, especially in hospital care. Certain cantons provide most care within their own establishments, while others subsidize private hospitals.

Health insurance is provided mainly by non-profit-making organizations and is not compulsory in all cantons. Although subsidized by the Confederation and the cantons, a large proportion of the resources comes from insurance premiums, paid by individuals and not from social security taxes. Medical expenses that are not covered are borne by the social services when those involved are in need. In principle, preventive services (check-ups and screening) are not reimbursed, but there are many exceptions.

Swiss cancer registries

Six regional epidemiological registries have been functioning for more than 10 years, the oldest having been founded in 1970. They are: Basel, Geneva, Neuchâtel, St. Gallen and Appenzell, Vaud and Zurich. Although these registries include four out of the five major Swiss cities, the population covered by the registries is less than 50% of the total population; thus those from non-urban areas are underrepresented. The coverage in the French-speaking areas (58%) is higher than the German-speaking ones (43%), while the Italian-speaking region does not, as yet, have any cancer registration. Recently, two new registries were created in Valais (1990) and Grisons (1991). The creation of the six registries was due to local interest rather than part of a concerted action. Registries are supported partially by public and partially by private funds and subsidies are given by the Confederation.

The Swiss cancer registries have formed an Association, the main goals of which are to define and harmonize the data to be recorded and the presentation of the results. The Association has a central office, which keeps an inter-registry incidence data bank and performs statistical epidemiological analyses. The registries keep their autonomy as far as data collection is concerned and, if applicable, follow-up procedures. Population data are provided by the Swiss Central Statistical Office or in some cases by the regional statistical offices. In any event, the population figures are available annually by quinquennia of age.

Two of the Swiss registries participated in the EUROCARE project: Basel and Geneva.

The Basel Registry was established in 1969 and reliable data are available from 1970 onwards. It covers a region situated in the north-west of Switzerland and bordered to the north by France and Germany. The surface area of 450 km^2 has a generally German-speaking population numbering about 450 000, of whom 16% are foreigners. The service sector is preponderant, although industry (mainly chemical) is relatively large. Hospital facilities include approximately 5000 beds, grouped mainly in seven public hospitals, one of them being the central university hospital. No specific cancer beds exist.

Incidence data are obtained on a voluntary basis and then supplemented with surveys done by registry personnel. The index date for incidence and survival calculations is that of histological confirmation or, in its absence, the most conclusive examination. Follow-up is carried out on a set day for all cases. The cases are followed as long as they are residents of the canton. In addition, citizens of the canton are followed up throughout the whole country. Follow-up is, in part, passive (deaths announced by the community offices) and partly active (those presumed still alive).

The Geneva Registry has at its disposal incidence data from 1970 onwards. It is the most western canton of Switzerland, with an area of 250 km^2 and is bordered by France. The essentially urban French-speaking population numbers approximately 400 000, of whom 35% are foreign. The service sector is predominant since production workers make up less than 20% of the working population. Hospital facilities for short-term care comprise one university hospital (2000 beds) and seven private clinics.

Incidence and survival data-collection procedures are more or less the same as in Basel, but death certificates are automatically accessible. The definition of the incidence date index is, however, slightly different, in that it refers to the hospital admission date if this precedes diagnostic confirmation and hospitalization is related to the tumour. Follow-up takes place every fifth year (counted from the index date) rather than at a set date for all cases. Thus the cases are followed exactly at 5, 10, 15 years etc. Cases are removed from the follow-up as soon as they leave the canton.

Emigration effect in survival rate calculation

In Switzerland, foreigners account for a variable and in some places major proportion of residents. In Basel and Geneva, this proportion is 16.0 and 34.7%, respectively (1985 data). Some of these foreigners live in Switzerland only temporarily since their residence authorization is conditional on their working permit.

Analyses of Geneva data showed better cancer survival rates for foreigners than for Swiss nationals. They also revealed that rates of loss-to-follow-up during potential time of observation was higher for foreigners. These results could likely be interpreted as a selection effect in censored observations, the most advanced cases (with bad prognosis) leaving the population under observation to spend the end of their life in another region or country. This selection effect causes an overestimation of survival rates in foreigners.

Depending on the proportion of foreigners in the studied population, this phenomenon can, to a lesser extent, affect the global estimation of the survival rates. According to the Geneva data used in the EUROCARE project, the overall survival overestimation could be about 5% in men (in terms of relative bias). In contrast, this bias is negligible in women, probably for socio-cultural reasons. In Basel, the data available do not allow separate analysis for foreigners, but since the proportion of these is lower than in Geneva, the degree of overestimation of overall survival rates is likely to be smaller.

CHAPTER 15

Health care system, cancer registration and follow-up of cancer patients in the United Kingdom

Sue Wilson, Janine Bell, Roger Black, Michel Coleman, Carole Cummins, Gill Lawrence, Marjorie Page, Lesley Rider, Jennifer Smith and Judith Youngson

All residents of the United Kingdom have access to free health services from general practitioners and hospitals within the National Health Service (NHS). The NHS is funded by taxation, and administered by the Department of Health in England and by the Welsh Common Services Agency in Wales. Hospital services for the 50 million people in England and Wales are provided by District Health Authorities (DHA), each District serving about half a million people and containing at least one acute hospital which is the first point of referral for the majority of cancer patients resident in that District.

Radiotherapy services and specialist oncology services are more centralized, and patterns of referral for such services may vary according to patients' precise diagnosis, age, mobility and distance from the centre. Specialists from these centres generally hold clinics at the district hospitals to which they relate, giving wider access for patients to specialist cancer services. A very small percentage of cancer patients received cancer treatment wholly within private hospitals during the study period 1978–84, although the private health care sector has grown since then.

English and Welsh cancer registries

In England and Wales there has been a voluntary scheme for the registration of cancer patients since 1945, the whole of England and Wales being covered since 1962. There are 12 regional cancer registries, each of which provides a core data-set to the Office of Population, Censuses and Surveys (OPCS) (Ainsworth *et al.*, 1993; Anon., 1993). The data are aggregated by OPCS to provide a national data-set for England and Wales. The registries operate independently and obtain data from a variety of sources including hospitals (NHS and private), general practitioners (GPs) and histopathology labora- tories. OPCS provides the registries with copies of death certificates which mention cancer and the National Health Service Central Register (NHSCR) provides notifications of deaths, for cases registered with OPCS, irrespective of place or cause of death (Woodman *et al.*, 1993).

The cancer registration system in England and Wales has been subject to considerable change in recent years. In 1989, a Working Group of the Registrar General's Medical Advisory Committee was set up to review the operation of the registration system, regional and national data collection methods, quality and timeliness, the uses made of the data and the implications of the growing tendency to treat cancer patients in outpatient departments and the private sector.

Six of the 12 regional registries have contributed data to this volume.

The *East Anglian Cancer Registry* covers an area of approximately 12 800 km^2 with a population of 2.0 million. It is mainly an agricultural community but with industrial centres in Peterborough and Ipswich, light industry in Norwich and Cambridge and seaports in King's Lynn, Great Yarmouth and Lowestoft.

There are three Oncology Centres and eight District Hospitals, one of which is a teaching hospital.

The index date for the computation of incidence and survival rates, during the period of this study, was the date of first treatment. Current policy is to use the date of diagnosis.

Active follow-up is carried out at three years, five years and thereafter five-yearly intervals through hospitals and general practitioners. Where necessary the patient's current GP is traced through the NHSCR.

In addition to data relating to the primary cancer, recurrence, subsequent treatment, subsequent malignancies and date and cause of death are recorded.

The *Thames Cancer Registry* is part of the Public Health Directorate of the Thames Regional Health Authorities (RHA). It was founded in 1956 and since 1985, when it expanded to cover North Thames RHA, has had a population base of 14 million (Thames Cancer Registry, 1993). The data in this volume relate only to the 6.7 million population of South Thames, resident between the river Thames and the south coast, mainly within the counties of Kent, Sussex, Surrey and south London. The region includes some of the most affluent and most deprived areas of England. There is little heavy industry and the most common occupations are in local and national government, finance and industry.

The great majority of cancer patients are treated at NHS hospitals, although the number of private hospitals is increasing. Registrations are mainly drawn from the 120 general acute hospitals, three university hospitals and one specialist cancer hospital. These include nine radiotherapy centres. Substantial numbers of patients are referred to other oncology centres, mainly in North Thames. Cases are actively sought by registry personnel in collaboration with the staff in the hospitals. Ascertainment is supported by routine notification of cancer deaths from OPCS to the Registry, and increasingly by notifications from hospitals on magnetic media.

The index date for computing incidence and survival in this analysis was the date of first attendance at hospital for cancer diagnosis and treatment.

The *Mersey Regional Cancer Registry* was formed in 1944 and registers all cases of cancer occurring in residents covered by the Mersey Regional Health Authority. Data are also collected on patients receiving therapy in the region's hospitals. The Mersey Region lies on the north-west seaboard of England. More than a third of the population of 2.4 million lives in the Liverpool conurbation (Youngson *et al.*, 1992; Williams *et al.*, 1993). Although shipbuilding has almost ceased, industry still centres around the estuary of the river Mersey with a petrochemical complex and a major car factory. Some salt and coal mining still continues, but the east and south of the Region are mainly agricultural.

There are approximately 25 major hospitals in the Region, one of which is a university hospital. There is one specialist oncology centre which includes radiotherapy services in the Region and another in the adjoining North-western Region where some Mersey residents receive their treatment.

The index date is the date of first definitive treatment or the date seen by the diagnosing clinician if the patient received no treatment.

Follow-up is passive, through the NHSCR, which notifies the registry of death in any person registered with cancer.

The *Wessex Cancer Intelligence Unit* has been responsible for collecting data on cancer incidence and mortality for the residents of Wessex Regional Health Authority since 1974. The cancer registry covers a population of approximately 3 million people, of whom 8% are over 75 years of age, resident within the southern counties of Dorset, Hampshire, Wiltshire, Isle of Wight and parts of Avon and Somerset (10 700 km^2) (Wessex Cancer Intelligence Unit, 1993). Compared to the British Isles as a whole, the region is relatively affluent, with less than 21% of the gross domestic product generated by manufacturing industry. The region contains both urban centres and large rural areas.

Primary care services are provided by approximately 1300 GPs; there are 13 major acute hospitals within the region, 4 radiotherapy centres and 2 specialist oncology units (one for children).

The index date for computing incidence and survival is the date of histological verification, or, if this is not available, the date of the first hospital admission where a mention of cancer is recorded.

Data are collected from hospital discharge summaries, pathology laboratories, OPCS, NHSCR and other cancer registries. Today this process is highly computerized, but for the period of this study it included manual collection through hospital coding departments. A passive follow-up system is in operation which relies on OPCS to forward details of Wessex residents dying, with or without cancer, to be combined with the Registry files.

The *West Midlands Regional Cancer Registry* was established in 1936 and has been population-based since 1957. The Registry covers the areas of Birmingham and a large proportion of the Midlands (the central area of England), with a population of 5.2 million (10.4% of the total population of England and Wales).

The Region includes a relatively large proportion of members of ethnic groups other than the indigenous English and Irish, due to immigration from the Indian subcontinent, Africa and the Caribbean. It includes some of the most industrialized sections of England but also large areas of farmland.

There are five radiotherapy and oncology centres within the region, and 22 DHAs, each of which has at least one general hospital that treats cancer patients. There are several specialist units including one for the treatment of children's tumours and one specializing in orthopaedic cases.

Cases are registered from data supplied by clerical staff at individual hospitals who abstract information from hospital inpatient and outpatient records, radiotherapy notes and histopathology reports. Registrations are also made on the basis of data obtained from GPs, domiciliary visits and coroners. This multiple-source system of registration, to-gether with a variety of systems for cross- checking, ensures a high degree of registration efficiency.

A combination of active and passive follow-up procedures are in operation. Copies of all death certificates are sent to the registry by OPCS for linkage to the registry's files. Where a death certificate is the only information received, the case is followed up further through letters to hospitals, GPs and Family Health Service Authorities (FHSAs), as appropriate.

The index date for computing survival is the date of first active treatment or, if the patient was not treated, the date of diagnosis with precedence being given to the date of histological diagnosis.

The *Yorkshire Cancer Registry* was established in 1957 and is now part of the Yorkshire Regional Cancer Organisation located at the Cookridge Hospital site in Leeds.

Covering the Yorkshire Health Region, which spans an area of approximately 13 700 km^2 covering 17 DHAs, the cancer registry serves a population of 3.6 million (density: 265 per km^2) (Yorkshire Cancer Registry, 1992; Yorkshire Regional Cancer Organisation, 1993). The resident population constitutes 7.2% of the total population of England and Wales. There are marked differences in population density, with some 60% of the population living in 15% of the area, which includes the densely populated urban areas of Leeds and Bradford, the remaining areas being relatively sparsely populated rural areas of North and East Yorkshire. 58% of the active population works in industry.

There are 60 hospitals where cancer patients are treated in the region, 14 of which are independent. Two teaching hospitals exist in the region and radiotherapeutic services are provided by the two major radiotherapy hospitals.

The index date for computing incidence and survival is the date of first definitive treatment or first hospital visit. If the patient does not attend hospital, the index date is that of diagnosis by the GP.

Follow-up is mixed; copies of all death certificates are sent to the Registry by OPCS for linkage to the Registry's files. Active follow-up is performed by contacting the GPs of patients for whom no death certificate has been received.

Scottish National Cancer Registry

The Scottish National Cancer Registry attained national coverage in 1959 (Black *et al.*, 1993). There are five constituent regional registries located in hospitals in Glasgow, Edinburgh, Aberdeen, Dundee and Inverness. These submit a minimum core data set to the national Registry.

Registrations are mainly derived from hospital in-patient episodes; other sources include outpatient and pathology departments, histopathology and cytology laboratories and GPs.

The population of Scotland slightly exceeds five million and the national registry encompasses an area of 77 000 km^2. The majority of the population is concentrated in the conurbations of central Scotland surrounding the cities of Glasgow and Edinburgh. Within the central belt, in particular, lie some of the most deprived areas in Britain. The border areas to the south and the highlands to the north are, in the main, rural and sparsely populated. Approximately one third of the employed population works in public administration and other services, with 21% in distribution, hotels and catering and 23% in manufacturing, engineering and construction.

Almost all cancer patients are treated at the National Health Service hospitals. Four specialist cancer centres consisting of integrated units of radiation and medical oncology are based in the teaching hospitals in Glasgow, Edinburgh, Aberdeen and Dundee. A fifth specialist centre in Inverness covers the populations of the Highlands and Western Isles. Each centre has established outpatient clinics in district hospitals nearby and peripheral areas. In addition to these five centres, surgery is carried out at district general and other hospitals.

Follow-up of cancer cases is achieved through the NHS Central Register in Scotland which notifies the registry of death of any person registered with cancer. To attain maximum ascertainment of death, this system is augmented each year by computerized medical records of the Registrar General for Scotland.

The index date for computing incidence and survival in this analysis was the date of first treatment, which represents the date on which the diagnosis of cancer was first confirmed.

References

Ainsworth, I., Gravestock, S., Linklater, K.M. & Page, M. (1993) *Information and Training Manual for Cancer Registration in England and Wales*, London, Cancer Registries Consultative Group

Anon. (1993) *Cancer Statistics: Registrations. England & Wales, 1987* (Series MB1 No. 20), London, HMSO

Black, R.J., Sharp L. & Kendrick, S.W. (1993) *Trends in Cancer Survival in Scotland 1968–1990*, Edinburgh, Information and Statistics Division

Thames Cancer Registry (1993) *Cancer in South-East England, 1990: Cancer Incidence, Prevalence and Survival in Residents of the District Health Authorities in the Thames RHAs,* Sutton, Thames Cancer Registry

Wessex Cancer Intelligence Unit (1993) *Fifth Report*, (1993)

Williams, E.M.I., Youngson, J., Ashby, D. & Donnelly, R.J. (1993) *Lung Cancer Bulletin: a Framework for Action,* Mersey, Mersey Regional Health Authority

Woodman, C., Wilson, S., Moran, T., Donnelly, B. & Hare, L. (1993) *Cancer in the North West Region 1985–89,* Manchester, Centre for Cancer Epidemiology

Yorkshire Cancer Registry (1992) *Report for the Year 1991,* Leeds, Yorkshire Regional Cancer Organisation

Yorkshire Regional Cancer Organisation (1993) *Cancer in Yorkshire — Lung Cancer* (Cancer Registry Special Report Series), Leeds,

Youngson, J., Ashby, D. & Williams, E.M.I. (1992) *Cancer in Mersey: Incidence of Cancer in Mersey Region and its Constituent Health Districts 1986–1990.* Liverpool, Mersey Regional Health Authority

CHAPTER 16

Guide to tables

Gemma Gatta and Milena Sant

The cancer survival results presented in the tables are organized into sections, each of which deals with a single tumour site. Tumour sites are defined by the first three digits of the ICD−9 code. Within each section, data are given by country, followed by a summary page for Europe. Results for children and adults are presented separately. The data for a given country are either those from a single cancer registry or pooled from several, as detailed in Chapter 2 (Table 2.1).

Because the number of patients studied varied greatly according to both cancer site and country, the survival data could not be presented intelligibly in a uniform manner. Five different page layouts (designated A, B, W, NW and R) were therefore chosen to display the data. Page layout A presents country-specific data for the frequent tumour sites; layout B presents country-specific data for infrequent tumour sites; layout W shows weighted pooled European data for frequent sites; layout NW shows unweighted pooled European data (for infrequent tumour sites); and layout R presents pooled data for rare sites. The countries and tumour sites treated, together with the layouts used, are listed in Table 16.1. The following paragraphs explain in detail how the data are presented in each layout.

Layout A: Country-specific information on frequent tumour sites

This layout is used whenever, for a given site, the total number of cases in the EUROCARE database exceeds 10 000. If the total number of cases is less than 10 000, this layout is also used to present the data from countries contributing at least 100 male cases or at least 100 female cases.

Layout A dedicates a whole page to each country, as shown in the example (Figure 16.1). Each page contains two tables and three figures presenting the following information.

(*a*) The main table, in the centre of the page, shows observed and relative survival (as percentages), at 1, 3, 5, 8 and 10 years from diagnosis, according to age and according to period in which diagnosis was made (1978−80, 1981−82 or 1983−85); data are given for each sex and for both sexes combined. The age groups are: 15−44 (20−44 for bone tumours only), 45−54, 55−64, 65−74 and 75+ for adults; and 0−1, 2−4, 5−9, 10−14 (10−19 for bone tumours only) for children. The table also gives (in parentheses) the number of cases in each age class and each diagnosis period at the start of follow-up.

(*b*) The table at the top left of the page lists the cancer registries that provided data, together with the number of cases each registry contributed, by sex and data contribution period. The table also gives the country-specific mean age of all cases.

(*c*) The basic data from the main table are also presented in graphic form. Relative survival, by sex and year up to five years from diagnosis, is shown in the graph in the upper right of the page. Relative survival figures are ratios and not probabilities and cannot strictly be represented by a cumulative survival curve. However, because such curves are readily appreciated, this formalism has been disregarded. At the bottom of the page, two bar charts show relative survival one and five years after diagnosis, by age and period in which diagnosis was made. The aim of these is to facilitate comparison of the effects of age and diagnosis period on short- and long-term prognoses. Also included on the bar charts are error bars representing 95% confidence limits.

For pancreatic and oesophageal cancers, the total number of cases exceeds 10 000, but Spain does not have enough cases for a presentation according to layout A. Therefore the Spain page for these sites reports only the number of cases contributed.

Table 16.1. Page layouts(*) for presentation of survival information according to tumour site and country

ICD–9 code	Adult cancers	DK	NL	ENG	EST	FIN	F	D	I	PL	SCO	E	CH	EUR
		Country												
141	Tongue	A	B	A	B	A	A	A	A	B	A	–	B	NW
143–145	Oral cavity	A	B	A	B	A	A	A	A	B	A	B	A	NW
146	Oropharynx	A	B	A	B	B	A	B	A	B	B	B	B	NW
147	Nasopharynx	A	B	A	B	B	B	B	B	B	B	B	B	NW
148	Hypopharynx	A	B	A	B	B	A	B	A	B	A	B	B	NW
141,143–148	Head & neck	A	A	A	A	A	A	A	A	A	A	A	A	W
150	Oesophagus	A	A	A	A	A	A	A	A	A	A	–	A	W
151	Stomach	A	A	A	A	A	A	A	A	A	A	A	A	W
153	Colon	A	A	A	A	A	A	A	A	A	A	A	A	W
154	Rectum	A	A	A	A	A	A	A	A	A	A	A	A	W
157	Pancreas	A	A	A	A	A	A	A	A	A	A	–	A	W
161	Larynx	A	A	A	A	A	A	A	A	A	A	A	A	W
162	Lung	A	A	A	A	A	A	A	A	A	A	A	A	W
170	Bone	A	B	A	B	A	B	B	B	B	B	–	B	NW
174	Breast	A	A	A	A	A	A	A	A	A	A	A	A	W
180	Cervix uteri	A	A	A	A	A	A	A	A	A	A	A	A	W
182	Corpus uteri	A	A	A	A	A	A	A	A	A	A	A	A	W
183	Ovary	A	A	A	A	A	A	A	A	A	A	A	A	W
184	Vagina & vulva	A	B	A	A	A	B	A	A	B	A	B	B	NW
186	Testis	A	A	A	B	A	A	A	A	B	A	–	A	NW
187	Penis	A	B	A	B	B	B	B	B	B	A	B	B	NW
189	Kidney	A	A	A	A	A	A	A	A	A	A	A	A	W
191	Brain	A	A	A	A	A	A	A	A	A	A	A	A	W
201	Hodgkin's disease	A	B	A	A	A	B	B	A	B	A	B	B	NW
204.0	Acute lymphatic leukaemia	A	B	A	B	A	B	B	B	B	B	B	B	NW
204.1	Chronic lymphatic leukaemia	A	B	A	A	A	B	B	A	B	A	B	B	NW
205.0	Acute myeloid leukaemia	A	B	A	B	A	B	B	B	B	A	B	B	NW
205.1	Chronic myeloid leukaemia	A	B	A	B	A	B	B	B	B	A	B	B	NW
204–208	Leukaemia	A	A	A	A	A	A	A	A	A	A	A	A	W
	Childhood cancers													
147	Nasopharynx	–	–	–	–	–	–	–	–	–	–	–	–	R
170	Bone	–	–	–	–	–	–	–	–	–	–	–	–	R
183	Ovary	–	–	–	–	–	–	–	–	–	–	–	–	R
186	Testis	–	–	–	–	–	–	–	–	–	–	–	–	R
189	Kidney	–	–	–	–	–	–	–	–	–	–	–	–	R
191	Brain	B	B	A	B	A	B	A	B	B	B	–	B	NW
201	Hodgkin's disease	–	–	–	–	–	–	–	–	–	–	–	–	R
204–208	Leukaemia	A	B	A	B	A	B	A	A	B	A	B	B	NW

(*) The page layouts are designated A, B, W, NW or R, presenting, respectively, country-specific data for frequent tumour sites, country-specific data for infrequent tumour sites,weighted pooled European data for frequent sites, unweighted pooled European data for infrequent tumour sites, and pooled data for rare sites.

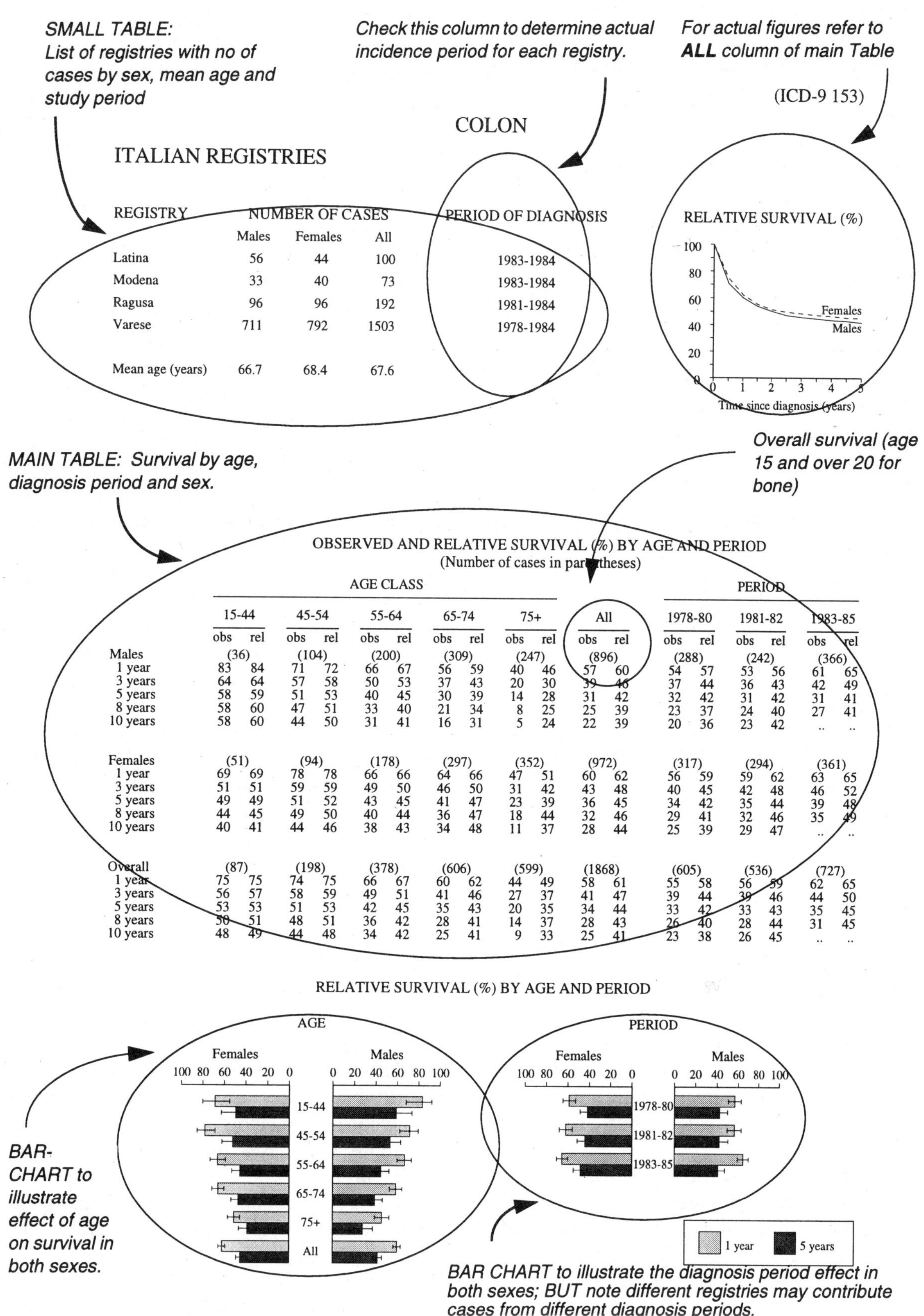

REGISTRY	NUMBER OF CASES Males	Females	All	PERIOD OF DIAGNOSIS
Latina	56	44	100	1983-1984
Modena	33	40	73	1983-1984
Ragusa	96	96	192	1981-1984
Varese	711	792	1503	1978-1984
Mean age (years)	66.7	68.4	67.6	

OBSERVED AND RELATIVE SURVIVAL (%) BY AGE AND PERIOD
(Number of cases in parentheses)

	AGE CLASS 15-44 obs	rel	45-54 obs	rel	55-64 obs	rel	65-74 obs	rel	75+ obs	rel	All obs	rel	PERIOD 1978-80 obs	rel	1981-82 obs	rel	1983-85 obs	rel
Males	(36)		(104)		(200)		(309)		(247)		(896)		(288)		(242)		(366)	
1 year	83	84	71	72	66	67	56	59	40	46	57	60	54	57	53	56	61	65
3 years	64	64	57	58	50	53	37	43	20	30	39	46	37	44	36	43	42	49
5 years	58	59	51	53	40	45	30	39	14	28	31	42	32	42	31	42	31	41
8 years	58	60	47	51	33	40	21	34	8	25	25	39	23	37	24	40	27	41
10 years	58	60	44	50	31	41	16	31	5	24	22	39	20	36	23	42	..	..
Females	(51)		(94)		(178)		(297)		(352)		(972)		(317)		(294)		(361)	
1 year	69	69	78	78	66	66	64	66	47	51	60	62	56	59	59	62	63	65
3 years	51	51	59	59	49	50	46	50	31	42	43	48	40	45	42	48	46	52
5 years	49	49	51	52	43	45	41	47	23	39	36	45	34	42	35	44	39	48
8 years	44	45	49	50	40	44	36	47	18	44	32	46	29	41	32	46	35	49
10 years	40	41	44	46	38	43	34	48	11	37	28	44	25	39	29	47	..	..
Overall	(87)		(198)		(378)		(606)		(599)		(1868)		(605)		(536)		(727)	
1 year	75	75	74	75	66	67	60	62	44	49	58	61	55	58	56	59	62	65
3 years	56	57	58	59	49	51	41	46	27	37	41	47	39	44	39	46	44	50
5 years	53	53	51	53	42	45	35	43	20	35	34	44	33	42	33	43	35	45
8 years	50	51	48	51	36	42	28	41	14	37	28	43	26	40	28	44	31	45
10 years	48	49	44	48	34	42	25	41	9	33	25	41	23	38	26	45	..	..

Figure 16.1. Explanation of presentation of data according to layout A (frequent cancer sites)

Layout B: Country-specific information on infrequent tumour sites

When the total site-specific number of cases in the EUROCARE database is less than 10 000 and the country-specific number less than 100 cases in males and in females, age-specific survival figures are not given, but survival according to sex and diagnosis period is presented. Each page (Figure 16.2) contains the data from two countries arranged as follows:

(*a*) The main table shows observed and relative survival 1, 3, 5, 8 and 10 years from diagnosis, broken down by sex and period in which diagnosis was made.

(*b*) Information on participating registries is presented as in layout A.

(*c*) Overall relative survival in each country is plotted as a curve, and one- and five-year relative survival figures, broken down by diagnosis period, are compared in a bar chart.

Layout W: Weighted pooled European data on frequent tumour sites

At the end of each site-specific section, there is a page presenting European survival information calculated from the pool of all cases contributed by the participating cancer registries.

For frequent cancer sites (more than 10 000 EUROCARE cases), it was assumed that the relative survival, calculated from all the cases provided by the registries of a given country, was a reasonable estimate of survival across that entire country. The European estimates were then obtained by weighting the available relative survival figures for each country with the estimated national average (number of cases per year) (see Chapter 3).

Other details of data presentation (Figure 16.3) are similar to those of layout A:

(*a*) The main table in the middle of the page, and the bar charts at the bottom, give the pooled and weighted age-specific and period-specific relative survival for both sexes and overall.

(*b*) In the table at the top of the page, the contributing countries are listed together with their estimated number of cases yearly.

(*c*) For between-country comparison and country-European pool comparison, the country-specific, age-standardized, relative survival figures (at one and five years from diagnosis) were computed. This information is presented in a bar chart at the top right of the page. To avoid cluttering and obscuring this display, only the one-year survival bars are provided with 95% confidence limits; however, the confidence limit differences between survival at one and five years are usually small. (That the standard errors for one- and five-year relative survival are in fact similar can be appreciated by inspection of the bar chart at the bottom of the page).

Layout NW: Unweighted pooled European data on infrequent tumour sites

For less frequent cancer sites (less than 10 000 total cases), survival for the European pool was computed by simply summing all the cases provided by the participating cancer registries. In most countries the number of cases was insufficient to yield reliable weighted national survival estimates. For this reason, unweighted estimates of European survival are strongly influenced by the large cancer registries of northern Europe. Layout NW is similar to layout W (for an annotated example, see Figure 16.4); differences are: (i) the table at the top left of the page lists participating registries together with the number of cases they contributed to EUROCARE, by sex; (ii) the bar chart at the top right, which compares age-standardized relative survival by country, shows only countries qualifying for layout A presentation (frequent sites), and the bar representing European survival is computed on the basis of the unweighted European pool.

Childhood cancer survival

Childhood cancer survival information is presented in a separate section. The following tumours are considered: leukaemia, Hodgkin's disease and malignant tumours of bone, kidney, brain, ovary, testis and nasopharynx. Only for leukaemia and brain tumours is there a sufficient number of cases to make a country-by-country presentation worthwhile (i.e. according to layout A or B, depending on the number of cases, and layout NW for the European pool).

For rare cancer sites, such as nasopharynx, bone, kidney, ovary, testis and Hodgkin's disease, pooled European survival data only are presented, according to layout R (see Table 16.1 and the annotated example, Figure 16.5). Layout R has a central table showing observed and relative percentage survival by sex and age. This information is also presented

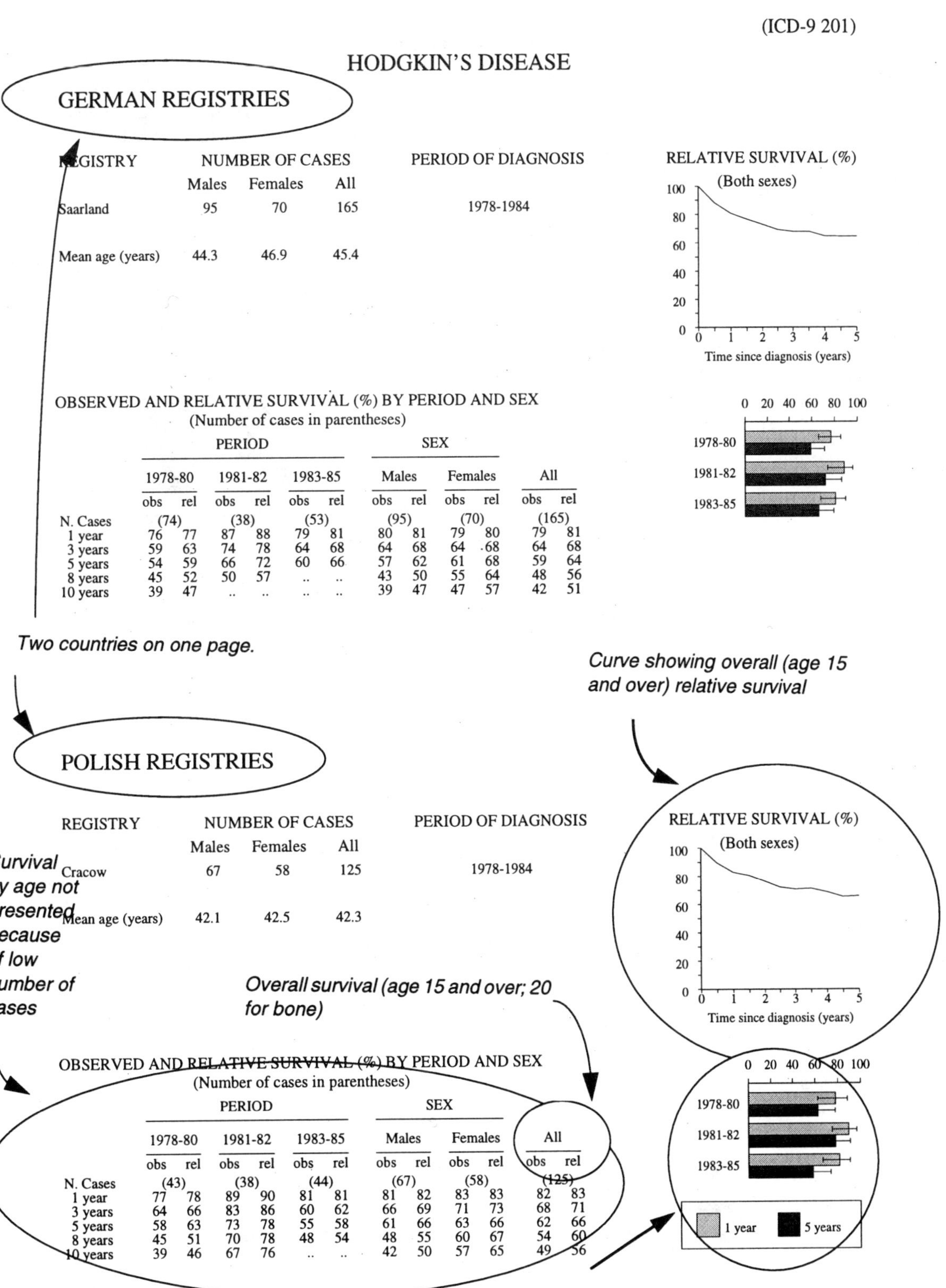

(ICD-9 201)

HODGKIN'S DISEASE

GERMAN REGISTRIES

REGISTRY	NUMBER OF CASES			PERIOD OF DIAGNOSIS
	Males	Females	All	
Saarland	95	70	165	1978-1984
Mean age (years)	44.3	46.9	45.4	

OBSERVED AND RELATIVE SURVIVAL (%) BY PERIOD AND SEX
(Number of cases in parentheses)

	PERIOD						SEX					
	1978-80		1981-82		1983-85		Males		Females		All	
	obs	rel	obs	rel	obs	rel	obs	rel	obs	rel	obs	rel
N. Cases	(74)		(38)		(53)		(95)		(70)		(165)	
1 year	76	77	87	88	79	81	80	81	79	80	79	81
3 years	59	63	74	78	64	68	64	68	64	68	64	68
5 years	54	59	66	72	60	66	57	62	61	68	59	64
8 years	45	52	50	57	..	..	43	50	55	64	48	56
10 years	39	47	..	..	..	..	39	47	47	57	42	51

POLISH REGISTRIES

REGISTRY	NUMBER OF CASES			PERIOD OF DIAGNOSIS
	Males	Females	All	
Cracow	67	58	125	1978-1984
Mean age (years)	42.1	42.5	42.3	

OBSERVED AND RELATIVE SURVIVAL (%) BY PERIOD AND SEX
(Number of cases in parentheses)

	PERIOD						SEX					
	1978-80		1981-82		1983-85		Males		Females		All	
	obs	rel	obs	rel	obs	rel	obs	rel	obs	rel	obs	rel
N. Cases	(43)		(38)		(44)		(67)		(58)		(125)	
1 year	77	78	89	90	81	81	81	82	83	83	82	83
3 years	64	66	83	86	60	62	66	69	71	73	68	71
5 years	58	63	73	78	55	58	61	66	63	66	62	66
8 years	45	51	70	78	48	54	48	55	60	67	54	60
10 years	39	46	67	76	..	..	42	50	57	65	49	56

Figure 16.2. Explanation of presentation of data according to layout B (infrequent cancer sites).

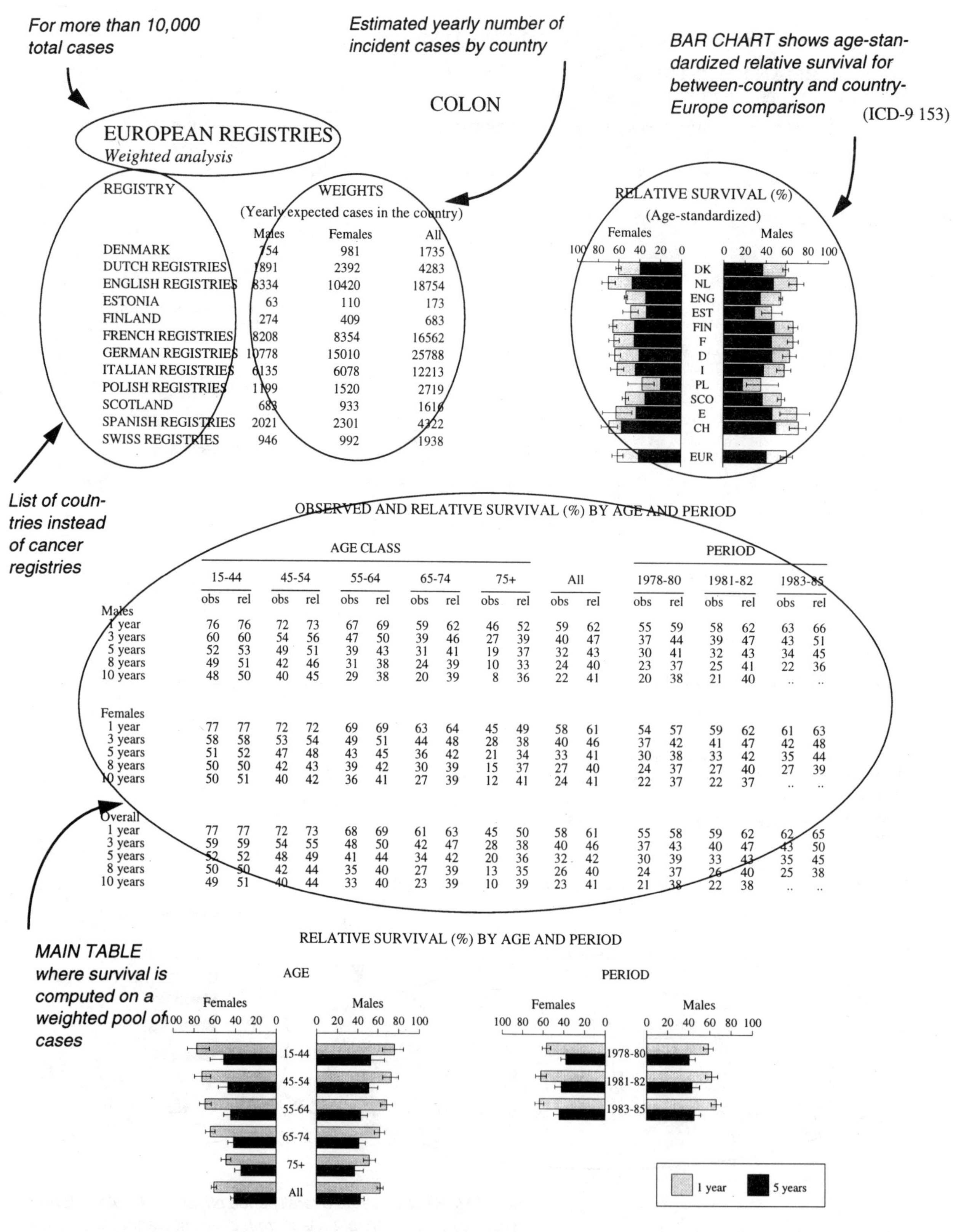

REGISTRY	WEIGHTS (Yearly expected cases in the country) Males	Females	All
DENMARK	754	981	1735
DUTCH REGISTRIES	1891	2392	4283
ENGLISH REGISTRIES	8334	10420	18754
ESTONIA	63	110	173
FINLAND	274	409	683
FRENCH REGISTRIES	8208	8354	16562
GERMAN REGISTRIES	10778	15010	25788
ITALIAN REGISTRIES	6135	6078	12213
POLISH REGISTRIES	1199	1520	2719
SCOTLAND	683	933	1616
SPANISH REGISTRIES	2021	2301	4322
SWISS REGISTRIES	946	992	1938

OBSERVED AND RELATIVE SURVIVAL (%) BY AGE AND PERIOD

	AGE CLASS												PERIOD					
	15-44		45-54		55-64		65-74		75+		All		1978-80		1981-82		1983-85	
	obs	rel	obs	rel	obs	rel	obs	rel	obs	rel	obs	rel	obs	rel	obs	rel	obs	rel
Males																		
1 year	76	76	72	73	67	69	59	62	46	52	59	62	55	59	58	62	63	66
3 years	60	60	54	56	47	50	39	46	27	39	40	47	37	44	39	47	43	51
5 years	52	53	49	51	39	43	31	41	19	37	32	43	30	41	32	43	34	45
8 years	49	51	42	46	31	38	24	39	10	33	24	40	23	37	25	41	22	36
10 years	48	50	40	45	29	38	20	39	8	36	22	41	20	38	21	40	..	..
Females																		
1 year	77	77	72	72	69	69	63	64	45	49	58	61	54	57	59	62	61	63
3 years	58	58	53	54	49	51	44	48	28	38	40	46	37	42	41	47	42	48
5 years	51	52	47	48	43	45	36	42	21	34	33	41	30	38	33	42	35	44
8 years	50	50	42	43	39	42	30	39	15	37	27	40	24	37	27	40	27	39
10 years	50	51	40	42	36	41	27	39	12	41	24	41	22	37	22	37	..	..
Overall																		
1 year	77	77	72	73	68	69	61	63	45	50	58	61	55	58	59	62	62	65
3 years	59	59	54	55	48	50	42	47	28	38	40	46	37	43	40	47	43	50
5 years	52	52	48	49	41	44	34	42	20	36	32	42	30	39	33	43	35	45
8 years	50	50	42	44	35	40	27	39	13	35	26	40	24	37	26	40	25	38
10 years	49	51	40	44	33	40	23	39	10	39	23	41	21	38	22	38	..	..

Figure 16.3. Explanation of presentation of data according to layout W (weighted European pool).

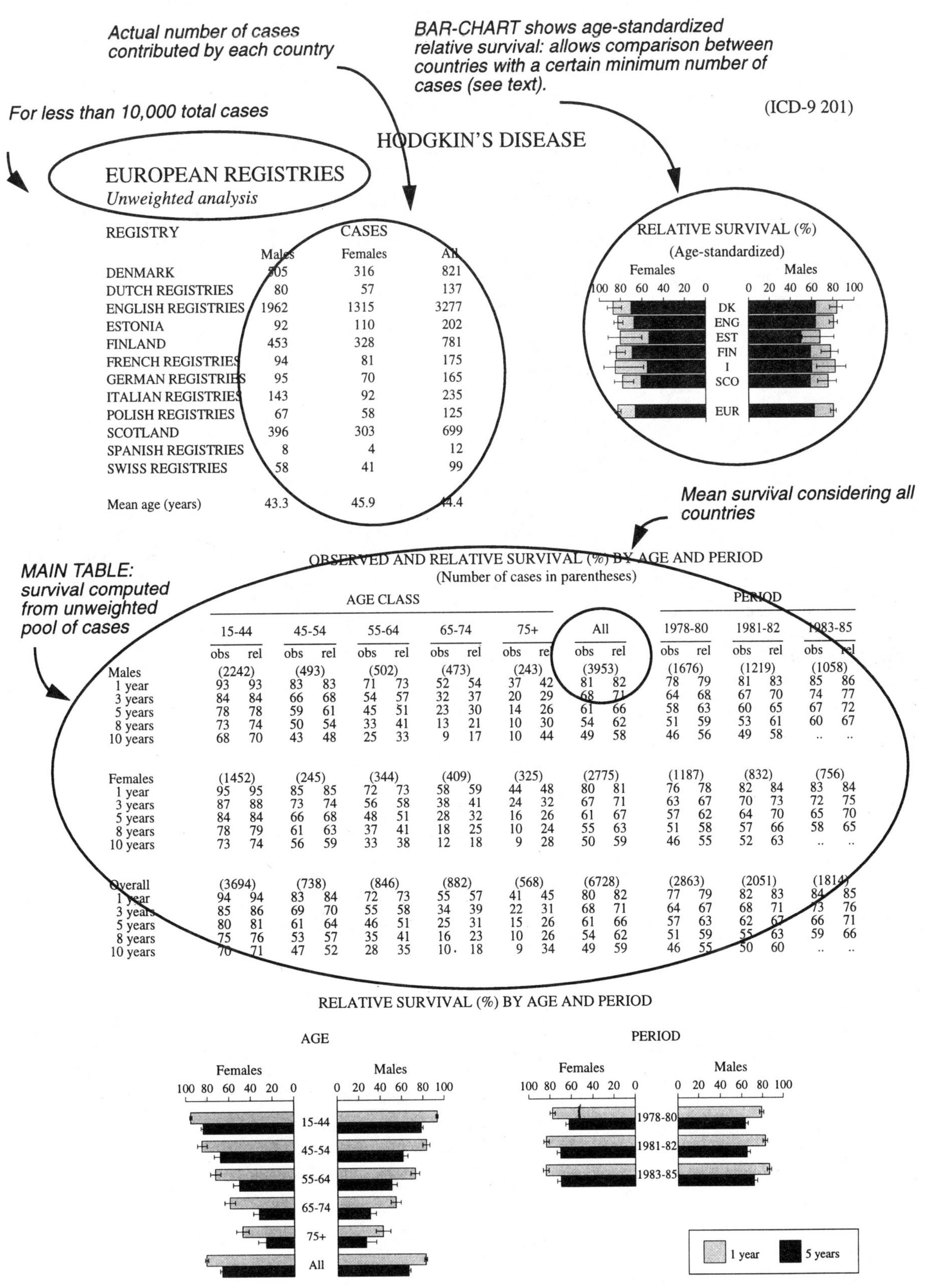

REGISTRY	CASES Males	Females	All
DENMARK	505	316	821
DUTCH REGISTRIES	80	57	137
ENGLISH REGISTRIES	1962	1315	3277
ESTONIA	92	110	202
FINLAND	453	328	781
FRENCH REGISTRIES	94	81	175
GERMAN REGISTRIES	95	70	165
ITALIAN REGISTRIES	143	92	235
POLISH REGISTRIES	67	58	125
SCOTLAND	396	303	699
SPANISH REGISTRIES	8	4	12
SWISS REGISTRIES	58	41	99
Mean age (years)	43.3	45.9	44.4

OBSERVED AND RELATIVE SURVIVAL (%) BY AGE AND PERIOD
(Number of cases in parentheses)

	AGE CLASS 15-44		45-54		55-64		65-74		75+		All	
	obs	rel	obs	rel	obs	rel	obs	rel	obs	rel	obs	rel
Males	(2242)		(493)		(502)		(473)		(243)		(3953)	
1 year	93	93	83	83	71	73	52	54	37	42	81	82
3 years	84	84	66	68	54	57	32	37	20	29	68	71
5 years	78	78	59	61	45	51	23	30	14	26	61	66
8 years	73	74	50	54	33	41	13	21	10	30	54	62
10 years	68	70	43	48	25	33	9	17	10	44	49	58
Females	(1452)		(245)		(344)		(409)		(325)		(2775)	
1 year	95	95	85	85	72	73	58	59	44	48	80	81
3 years	87	88	73	74	56	58	38	41	24	32	67	71
5 years	84	84	66	68	48	51	28	32	16	26	61	67
8 years	78	79	61	63	37	41	18	25	10	24	55	63
10 years	73	74	56	59	33	38	12	18	9	28	50	59
Overall	(3694)		(738)		(846)		(882)		(568)		(6728)	
1 year	94	94	83	84	72	73	55	57	41	45	80	82
3 years	85	86	69	70	55	58	34	39	22	31	68	71
5 years	80	81	61	64	46	51	25	31	15	26	61	66
8 years	75	76	53	57	35	41	16	23	10	26	54	62
10 years	70	71	47	52	28	35	10	18	9	34	49	59

	PERIOD 1978-80		1981-82		1983-85	
	obs	rel	obs	rel	obs	rel
Males	(1676)		(1219)		(1058)	
1 year	78	79	81	83	85	86
3 years	64	68	67	70	74	77
5 years	58	63	60	65	67	72
8 years	51	59	53	61	60	67
10 years	46	56	49	58	..	..
Females	(1187)		(832)		(756)	
1 year	76	78	82	84	83	84
3 years	63	67	70	73	72	75
5 years	57	62	64	70	65	70
8 years	51	58	57	66	58	65
10 years	46	55	52	63	..	..
Overall	(2863)		(2051)		(1814)	
1 year	77	79	82	83	84	85
3 years	64	67	68	71	73	76
5 years	57	63	62	67	66	71
8 years	51	59	55	63	59	66
10 years	46	55	50	60	..	..

Figure 16.4. Explanation of presentation of data according to layout NW (unweighted European pool).

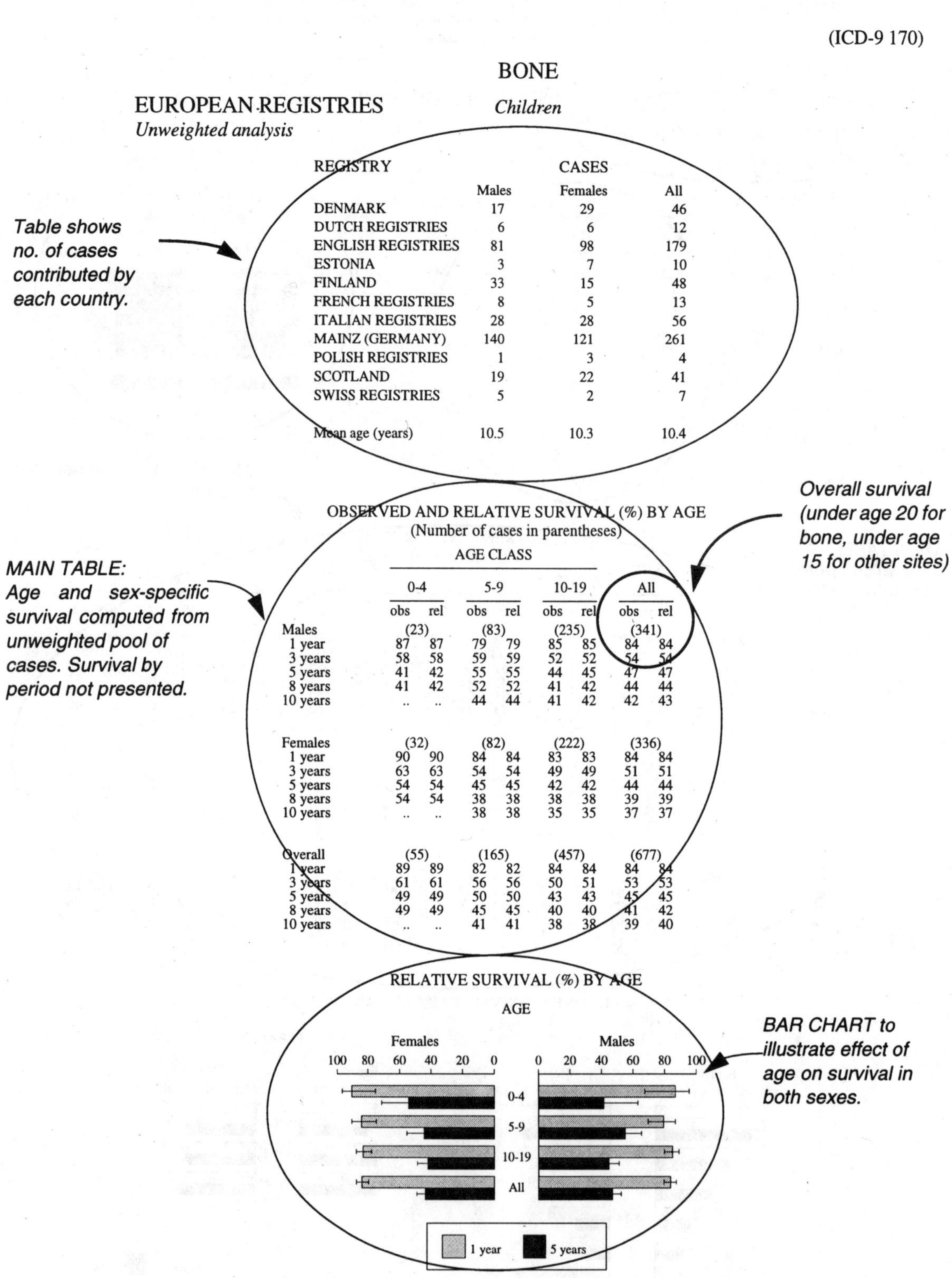

(ICD-9 170)

BONE

EUROPEAN REGISTRIES — *Children*

Unweighted analysis

REGISTRY	CASES Males	Females	All
DENMARK	17	29	46
DUTCH REGISTRIES	6	6	12
ENGLISH REGISTRIES	81	98	179
ESTONIA	3	7	10
FINLAND	33	15	48
FRENCH REGISTRIES	8	5	13
ITALIAN REGISTRIES	28	28	56
MAINZ (GERMANY)	140	121	261
POLISH REGISTRIES	1	3	4
SCOTLAND	19	22	41
SWISS REGISTRIES	5	2	7
Mean age (years)	10.5	10.3	10.4

OBSERVED AND RELATIVE SURVIVAL (%) BY AGE
(Number of cases in parentheses)

AGE CLASS

	0-4 obs	0-4 rel	5-9 obs	5-9 rel	10-19 obs	10-19 rel	All obs	All rel
Males	(23)		(83)		(235)		(341)	
1 year	87	87	79	79	85	85	84	84
3 years	58	58	59	59	52	52	54	54
5 years	41	42	55	55	44	45	47	47
8 years	41	42	52	52	41	42	44	44
10 years	..	..	44	44	41	42	42	43
Females	(32)		(82)		(222)		(336)	
1 year	90	90	84	84	83	83	84	84
3 years	63	63	54	54	49	49	51	51
5 years	54	54	45	45	42	42	44	44
8 years	54	54	38	38	38	38	39	39
10 years	..	..	38	38	35	35	37	37
Overall	(55)		(165)		(457)		(677)	
1 year	89	89	82	82	84	84	84	84
3 years	61	61	56	56	50	51	53	53
5 years	49	49	50	50	43	43	45	45
8 years	49	49	45	45	40	40	41	42
10 years	..	..	41	41	38	38	39	40

Figure 16.5. Explanation of presentation of data according to layout R (rare cancer sites in childhood).

in bar chart form at the bottom of the page. For these rare tumours the age classes are: 0–4, 5–9 and 10–14 (10–19 for bone tumours). As usual, the number of cases by sex and registry is given in the table at the top of the page. For childhood tumours only, the Mainz registry (German Registry of Childhood Malignancies) is in fact a national registry covering West Germany, and, since 1991 also the area of the former GDR. The Piedmont (Italy) Childhood Cancer Registry also contributes data to this section.

Notes and warnings

Increase in relative survival with time

In a few cases relative survival rates increase in the last years of follow-up. This may occur, for example, when the observed survival in these patients is higher than the expected survival in the general population (Hakulinen, 1977; Estève *et al.*, 1990).

Standardized survival

Valid comparison of survival among countries depends on several factors, as discussed in the introductory chapter, and age distribution is one of the most important of these. The reader should therefore also refer to age-specific survival rates when seeking to interpret survival differences.

As described in Chapter 3 on methods of data analysis, survival for each sex was standardized using the entire data set (i.e. both sexes); standardized survival figures in males and females are therefore directly comparable. Note, however, that each cancer site has a different standard age distribution (see Chapter 3, Appendix 1), and survival figures between different sites are thus not directly comparable.

In the bar charts showing standardized survival, a bar may be lacking for one or both sexes in a country, because there were no cases at that site in one or more age groups, and it was therefore not possible to calculate standardized survival.

In a few cases (e.g. testis cancer in Germany and a few head and neck sites in females), standardized survival could be computed but the figure is not very reliable because of the small number of cases in one or more age groups.

Tables 16.2a, b, c and d give the figures for age-standardized one- and five-year survival by cancer site and country, corresponding to the bar charts in the European pooled pages.

Changes in survival with diagnosis period

Survival differences correlating with period in which diagnosis was made should be interpreted with caution, since some countries (specifically England, Spain, Italy, Switzerland and France) include data from registries covering different periods; and in a few cases the apparent variation in survival by diagnosis period may be simply a geographic effect (see Chapter 1 for more detailed discussion).

Survival figures equal to zero

When all the cases entered during a given time interval have died, the corresponding survival figures (both observed and relative) are zero.

In a few cases, especially for older age groups and in the last years of follow-up, observed survival figures were zero and the corresponding relative survival rates were equal to 1% or 2%; this is because the observed survival figures equal to or less than 0.50% were approximated to zero.

Survival figures given as 'blank'

When all the cases entering a given time interval were censored, no survival figure can be computed and none is given.

Table headers

The period of the study was 1978–85; it was decided to divide this into three intervals: 1978–80, 1981–82 and 1983–85, and these intervals form subheadings of the heading PERIOD; however not all registries contributed data for all these periods. The specific periods for which each registry did contribute are specified in the top left table for each country.

The heading ALL in the main table refers to overall survival in patients over 14 years old for adults (over 19 for those with bone tumours), and less than 15 years old for children (less than 20 for those with bone tumours).

References

Estève, J., Benhamou, E., Croasdale, M. & Raymond, L. (1990) Relative survival and the estimation of net survival: elements for further discussion. *Stat. Med.*, **9**, 529–538

Hakulinen T. (1977) On long-term relative survival rates. *J. Chronic Dis.*, **30**, 431–443

Table 16.2a. Age-standardized relative survival; males, one-year survival*

	Denmark	Netherlands	England	Estonia	Finland	France
Tongue	61.4 45.7–75.0	–	63.3 55.8–70.2	–	68.8 51.5–82.1	63.6 46.5–77.8
Oral cavity	70.3 59.4–79.3	–	67.2 60.7–73.0	–	73.4 54.8–86.2	69.9 50.4–84.2
Oropharynx	61.7 49.2–72.8	–	62.1 53.2–70.2	–	–	60.3 46.1–73.0
Nasopharynx	75.5 56.5–87.9	–	64.3 51.5–75.4	–	–	–
Hypopharynx	45.8 29.0–63.6	–	45.3 36.3–54.7	–	–	64.0 48.0–77.5
Head & neck	64.2 58.0–70.1	71.3 53.6–84.3	61.5 57.9–65.1	67.0 50.4–80.2	68.5 59.1–76.6	64.1 56.0–71.4
Oesophagus	17.7 12.7–24.3	–	19.0 16.9–21.3	21.2 10.2–39.0	25.2 18.5–33.4	29.7 24.5–35.4
Stomach	29.7 26.7–32.9	39.5 32.2–47.4	21.7 20.4–23.1	31.2 26.6–36.2	35.8 32.8–38.9	37.2 31.9–42.8
Colon	58.7 55.8–61.6	69.6 61.9–76.3	54.0 52.4–55.7	45.3 35.7–55.3	66.0 61.2–70.5	65.8 60.3–70.8
Rectum	66.2 63.4–69.0	71.9 62.6–79.5	62.7 61.0–64.5	56.9 46.6–66.5	75.7 71.1–79.8	68.8 63.0–73.9
Pancreas	9.6 7.3–12.5	17.4 9.4–29.9	10.6 9.2–12.2	7.1 3.3–14.8	15.2 11.9–19.3	12.8 7.9–20.2
Larynx	84.1 79.0–88.1	89.6 74.6–96.2	83.3 80.4–85.9	75.4 63.2–84.6	88.4 81.8–92.8	79.6 68.0–87.7
Lung	24.2 22.7–25.7	38.9 35.3–42.5	21.2 20.6–21.9	29.2 25.5–33.1	40.4 38.6–42.3	38.6 33.5–44.0
Bone	67.1 47.6–82.0	–	60.6 49.9–70.4	–	72.5 51.6–86.7	–
Testis	94.4 91.5–96.3	95.5 83.2–98.9	92.3 89.8–94.2	–	87.4 78.0–93.1	90.7 74.1–97.1
Penis	86.0 75.2–92.6	–	80.6 74.0–85.9	–	–	–
Kidney	53.2 48.2–58.1	60.5 47.1–72.5	52.8 49.6–56.0	42.0 29.9–55.2	59.8 53.9–65.4	64.5 48.0–78.1
Brain	29.4 25.0–34.2	33.3 20.2–49.7	28.0 25.5–30.8	20.7 10.8–36.1	48.8 41.8–55.9	–
Hodgkin's disease	84.0 77.2–89.1	–	81.0 76.9–84.5	68.1 51.2–81.2	78.1 69.0–85.1	–
ALL	42.9 26.3–61.2	–	44.4 35.7–53.5	–	48.6 32.7–64.9	–
CLL	70.7 64.7–76.1	–	70.2 65.5–74.5	78.0 61.9–88.5	77.9 69.1–84.7	–
AML	24.3 17.8–32.4	–	22.7 18.3–27.7	–	30.0 20.8–41.0	–
CML	55.3 42.2–67.7	–	58.6 50.6–66.1	–	66.7 49.1–80.6	–
Leukaemia	49.9 45.1–54.7	54.2 39.6–68.1	45.7 42.9–48.7	56.8 45.0–68.0	56.8 50.4–62.9	67.9 57.0–77.2
Childhood cancers						
Brain	–	–	69.7 58.7–78.8	–	79.7 61.5–90.6	–
Leukaemia	84.7 71.1–92.6	–	76.3 68.2–82.9	–	79.8 65.2–89.3	–

*Data are given with 95% confidence intervals

– : Data missing or inadequate

Germany	Italy	Poland	Scotland	Spain	Switzerland	EUROPE	ICD-9
61.7 38.4–80.6	59.1 38.3–77.1	–	60.9 45.7–74.2	–	–	63.0 58.2–67.6	**141**
72.8 46.8–89.0	69.0 49.7–83.4	–	70.2 58.0–80.1	–	62.6 40.5–80.4	68.1 64.0–71.9	**143-5**
–	64.8 46.0–79.9	–	–	–	–	62.1 56.9–67.0	**146**
–	–	–	–	–	–	68.7 60.3–75.9	**147**
–	49.6 29.0–70.4	–	47.6 26.7–69.4	–	–	51.1 45.5–56.8	**148**
64.6 51.8–75.6	63.0 53.2–71.9	53.3 33.2–72.4	62.5 54.4–70.1	45.3 20.5–72.7	62.6 50.0–73.8	60.3 46.6–72.6	**141,3-8**
19.8 11.3–32.3	17.5 9.9–29.2	– –	17.5 13.5–22.4	– –	25.6 13.7–42.8	22.9 14.9–33.5	**150**
38.5 32.4–45.0	38.4 33.8–43.2	19.8 13.9–27.3	22.0 19.1–25.2	37.4 17.4–63.0	45.7 35.3–56.5	33.1 26.5–40.5	**151**
62.5 55.7–68.8	57.2 50.2–63.8	35.3 21.7–51.9	54.7 51.0–58.2	70.0 53.8–82.4	71.7 63.0–79.1	60.5 54.4–66.3	**153**
69.9 63.0–76.0	63.2 54.9–70.7	38.2 25.3–53.1	58.8 54.2–63.2	75.2 58.9–86.5	74.2 64.6–81.9	65.4 58.5–71.6	**154**
13.0 6.4–24.6	16.5 9.5–27.0	11.5 4.6–26.1	12.5 9.2–16.8	–	13.2 6.1–26.5	13.1 7.0–23.0	**157**
83.3 71.2–90.9	87.3 79.8–92.2	76.9 61.4–87.5	83.6 76.1–89.0	– –	82.9 67.4–92.0	84.3 73.1–91.4	**161**
27.4 24.1–31.0	30.9 27.8–34.2	20.8 16.8–25.4	21.2 19.8–22.6	25.6 16.7–37.2	36.5 31.8–41.5	28.3 25.0–31.9	**162**
–	–	–	–	–	–	62.8 55.7–69.4	**170**
90.2 82.4–94.7	92.8 79.2–97.7	–	91.5 85.6–95.1	–	91.0 84.7–94.9	92.0 90.4–93.3	**186**
–	–	–	84.0 68.0–92.8	–	–	82.3 77.7–86.1	**187**
66.3 55.0–76.0	64.8 52.5–75.4	39.0 23.0–57.8	49.1 42.5–55.9	– –	66.1 50.8–78.6	61.3 49.5–71.9	**189**
37.4 26.4–49.9	34.2 22.0–48.9	27.1 15.1–43.8	21.5 16.3–27.8	20.3 4.0–61.0	39.1 25.2–55.1	30.5 17.9–46.9	**191**
–	82.4 64.7–92.3	–	75.5 65.6–83.2	–	–	80.3 77.5–82.8	**201**
–	–	–	–	–	–	44.0 37.5–50.8	**204.0**
–	81.8 60.9–92.8	–	71.5 62.0–79.4	–	–	72.6 69.7–75.3	**204.1**
–	–	–	24.2 15.3–36.1	–	–	24.1 21.0–27.5	**205.0**
–	–	–	57.2 38.0–74.5	–	–	59.0 53.6–64.3	**205.1**
52.3 38.5–65.9	49.0 37.8–60.2	29.1 14.0–50.9	46.5 39.6–53.5	48.1 9.6–89.0	67.0 51.6–79.4	52.0 37.8–65.9	**204-8**

Germany	Italy	Poland	Scotland	Spain	Switzerland	EUROPE	ICD-9
75.1 61.5–85.0	–	–	–	–	–	72.3 66.2–77.6	**191**
87.7 82.7–91.5	86.1 72.9–93.5	–	80.6 61.8–91.4	–	–	82.1 78.6–85.1	**204-8**

Table 16.2b. Age-standardized relative survival; males, five-year survival*

	Denmark	Netherlands	England	Estonia	Finland	France
Tongue	30.7 16.8–49.4	–	38.7 30.6–47.4	–	37.0 20.6–57.0	20.2 9.5–37.9
Oral cavity	42.0 29.8–55.2	–	43.6 36.1–51.4	–	42.4 24.4–62.6	43.6 22.5–67.3
Oropharynx	29.2 18.3–43.2	–	33.2 24.3–43.3	–	–	22.8 12.2–38.4
Nasopharynx	44.4 26.7–63.7	–	31.2 20.8–44.0	–	–	–
Hypopharynx	14.0 4.7–34.9	–	19.6 12.6–29.3	–	–	20.3 10.1–36.7
Head & neck	33.8 27.2–41.0	39.0 19.6–62.6	35.8 31.8–40.0	26.6 13.0–46.9	35.8 26.2–46.6	25.9 18.6–34.7
Oesophagus	5.0 2.4–10.1	– –	5.0 3.7–6.5	2.8 0.6–11.7	6.4 3.0–13.3	4.9 2.7–8.7
Stomach	11.6 9.4–14.4	18.1 11.8–26.7	8.1 7.2–9.2	15.1 11.0–20.2	15.9 13.3–18.8	17.2 12.8–22.8
Colon	36.7 33.3–40.2	47.0 37.0–57.3	34.5 32.6–36.4	29.2 19.8–40.9	47.8 41.7–54.1	45.0 38.2–51.9
Rectum	35.4 32.1–38.8	39.4 28.1–51.9	35.4 33.3–37.5	28.0 18.3–40.2	40.7 35.0–46.6	37.7 31.2–44.7
Pancreas	2.6 1.4–4.7	3.9 0.9–16.2	2.1 1.4–3.1	1.7 0.3–9.6	2.0 0.9–4.5	3.0 1.1–8.4
Larynx	58.0 50.8–64.8	71.9 52.1–85.8	64.6 60.2–68.7	44.8 30.7–59.8	61.4 51.9–70.1	45.9 33.0–59.4
Lung	6.2 5.4–7.2	10.5 8.2–13.4	5.8 5.4–6.2	5.6 3.9–8.1	9.1 8.0–10.4	8.7 6.0–12.6
Bone	42.1 22.8–64.3	–	39.2 28.1–51.5	–	42.8 30.1–56.5	–
Testis	88.1 84.2–91.2	89.5 73.8–96.2	85.2 81.8–88.1	–	78.3 66.8–86.6	79.8 59.7–91.3
Penis	72.0 55.4–84.2	–	63.0 53.6–71.5	–	–	–
Kidney	31.4 26.5–36.9	38.7 24.8–54.8	35.9 32.4–39.5	19.5 10.5–33.5	35.9 29.7–42.6	41.0 24.7–59.7
Brain	11.4 8.5–15.2	16.5 8.6–29.5	12.0 10.2–14.2	10.8 3.9–26.6	22.9 17.5–29.5	–
Hodgkin's disease	63.8 54.6–72.1	–	63.8 58.6–68.7	50.1 32.0–68.2	59.0 49.2–68.0	–
ALL	17.8 9.1–31.9	–	14.2 9.1–21.5	–	9.1 4.5–17.5	–
CLL	36.2 29.2–43.8	–	42.5 36.5–48.7	51.1 31.0–70.8	41.0 29.9–53.2	–
AML	4.9 2.5–9.4	–	6.2 3.9–9.8	–	4.6 1.9–10.8	–
CML	16.2 7.6–31.0	–	16.2 10.4–24.3	–	19.9 9.0–38.3	–
Leukaemia	21.2 17.1–26.0	30.6 16.2–50.1	20.3 17.7–23.2	33.5 21.4–48.1	23.7 18.0–30.5	40.1 28.0–53.6
Childhood cancers						
Brain	–	–	48.0 37.4–58.9	–	66.2 48.0–80.6	–
Leukaemia	50.4 36.2–64.5	–	49.7 41.4–58.1	–	50.7 36.3–64.9	–

*Data are given with 95% confidence intervals

– : Data missing or inadequate

Germany	Italy	Poland	Scotland	Spain	Switzerland	EUROPE	ICD-9
34.5	24.1	–	42.9	–	–	34.2	**141**
13.5–64.0	9.4–49.3		23.6–64.6			29.0–39.8	
30.8	31.3	–	41.1	–	39.3	41.0	**143-5**
18.3–46.9	19.2–46.8		28.1–55.5		17.8–66.0	36.2–46.0	
–	20.5	–	–	–	–	28.4	**146**
	8.7–41.0					23.4–34.0	
–	–	–	–	–	–	36.1	**147**
						27.8–45.2	
–	14.3	–	22.2	–	–	18.4	**148**
	4.3–38.1		7.7–49.4			13.9–24.0	
33.5	25.2	19.8	34.6	30.1	31.6	29.2	**141,3-8**
21.6–48.1	17.1–35.5	6.9–45.1	26.2–44.1	9.2–64.7	19.9–46.1	17.4–44.7	
7.3	4.0	–	4.5	–	6.3	4.4	**150**
2.1–22.4	0.9–15.5	–	2.4–8.3	–	1.3–25.3	1.6–11.4	
19.3	16.3	7.3	6.9	11.1	23.3	14.1	**151**
14.0–26.2	12.6–20.8	3.4–14.8	5.0–9.3	4.1–26.7	14.4–35.3	9.5–20.5	
45.5	37.6	18.0	36.8	46.3	49.8	41.1	**153**
37.0–54.2	29.9–46.1	7.5–37.2	32.5–41.3	27.7–65.9	39.2–60.5	33.8–48.8	
37.6	31.9	11.6	29.6	33.4	48.5	34.4	**154**
29.9–46.0	23.4–41.8	4.5–26.6	24.8–34.9	18.6–52.3	36.1–61.0	27.2–42.5	
6.2	2.4	4.5	4.4	–	2.8	3.4	**157**
1.8–19.1	0.6–8.9	1.4–13.2	2.3–8.3		0.9–8.9	0.9–12.6	
61.3	59.9	54.8	65.8	–	59.9	55.8	**161**
45.5–75.1	49.9–69.1	36.3–72.1	55.2–75.0	–	39.5–77.4	39.1–71.2	
8.1	6.0	5.1	6.3	5.0	11.8	7.0	**162**
6.0–10.8	4.6–7.8	3.0–8.5	5.5–7.3	1.6–14.7	8.7–15.9	5.1–9.4	
–	–	–	–	–	–	38.5	**170**
						31.1–46.5	
75.4	87.3	–	80.5	–	83.2	84.3	**186**
65.1–83.4	71.7–94.9		73.4–86.1		74.1–89.5	82.2–86.2	
–	–	–	66.0	–	–	65.9	**187**
			42.7–83.5			59.0–72.2	
52.7	46.7	18.9	32.1	–	46.9	42.2	**189**
38.8–66.2	32.9–61.0	9.7–33.5	25.1–39.9	–	30.0–64.5	29.3–56.4	
17.2	12.6	17.4	10.0	12.3	13.1	13.7	**191**
9.8–28.6	6.3–23.5	7.8–34.4	6.3–15.5	3.0–38.8	7.8–21.1	6.4–27.0	
–	60.1	–	58.6	–	–	62.3	**201**
	46.8–72.1		47.7–68.8			58.8–65.7	
–	–	–	–	–	–	15.1	**204.0**
						11.0–20.2	
–	55.0	–	40.6	–	–	42.6	**204.1**
	30.0–77.6		28.5–53.9			38.8–46.5	
–	–	–	6.7	–	–	5.9	**205.0**
			2.3–18.1			4.2–8.1	
–	–	–	14.8	–	–	17.1	**205.1**
			5.1–36.2			12.9–22.4	
27.7	23.7	9.7	20.3	10.6	39.2	25.6	**204-8**
15.5–44.3	14.5–36.2	1.9–36.9	14.5–27.7	3.0–31.1	24.2–56.6	15.4–39.3	
47.6	–	–	–	–	–	49.8	**191**
34.3–61.2						43.4–56.1	
67.9	54.7	–	43.2	–	–	55.8	**204-8**
61.4–73.8	40.0–68.6		26.6–61.4			51.7–59.9	

Table 16.2c. Age-standardized relative survival; females, one-year survival*

	Denmark	Netherlands	England	Estonia	Finland	France
Tongue	66.8 47.9–81.5	–	68.0 59.2–75.7	–	71.4 55.5–83.3	46.5 26.9–67.3
Oral cavity	76.9 65.6–85.3	–	75.8 68.1–82.1	–	78.9 63.6–88.9	65.8 28.3–90.4
Oropharynx	76.4 56.8–88.8	–	65.7 52.9–76.6	–	–	79.4 34.3–96.6
Nasopharynx	78.7 61.4–89.5	–	58.5 42.7–72.7	–	–	–
Hypopharynx	–	–	45.0 35.6–54.7	–	–	–
Head & neck	74.2 66.5–80.6	64.9 37.3–85.2	64.5 59.9–68.8	60.1 36.4–79.9	72.7 63.6–80.3	70.6 41.5–89.1
Oesophagus	27.2 18.6–37.9	–	23.8 21.1–26.7	26.4 8.5–58.1	39.3 31.0–48.3	–
Stomach	30.6 26.7–34.8	43.9 34.6–53.6	23.5 21.7–25.4	32.1 27.8–36.7	37.8 34.5–41.3	44.9 37.7–52.4
Colon	60.4 57.9–62.9	70.3 63.4–76.4	53.2 51.8–54.6	48.6 41.3–56.0	65.6 61.8–69.2	64.5 59.3–69.4
Rectum	69.3 66.3–72.1	74.3 63.8–82.6	61.6 59.8–63.5	64.4 56.7–71.3	74.9 70.7–78.8	73.5 67.3–78.9
Pancreas	10.4 8.0–13.4	12.0 5.4–24.7	12.3 10.6–14.1	11.7 6.5–20.0	14.0 10.8–17.8	18.8 11.6–28.9
Larynx	87.6 75.8–94.1	–	76.1 69.0–82.0	68.0 30.7–91.0	84.7 65.1–94.2	–
Lung	23.9 21.5–26.4	–	19.5 18.4–20.6	29.8 22.1–38.8	41.1 36.4–45.9	34.8 19.6–54.0
Bone	67.7 42.6–85.6	–	62.8 50.9–73.4	–	72.5 51.2–86.9	–
Breast	91.2 90.2–92.1	93.8 91.0–95.7	86.9 86.3–87.5	87.6 83.8–90.5	94.0 92.7–95.0	94.0 91.2–96.0
Cervix uteri	82.8 80.1–85.2	89.1 76.4–95.4	78.5 76.7–80.1	80.0 73.9–85.1	87.7 83.0–91.2	87.7 79.0–93.1
Corpus uteri	87.6 85.3–89.6	90.0 81.2–95.0	82.9 81.2–84.4	81.1 74.6–86.3	89.6 87.1–91.7	85.5 63.6–95.2
Ovary	56.4 53.2–59.6	60.2 50.2–69.4	51.2 49.3–53.1	49.1 42.3–55.9	64.0 59.8–68.1	65.7 53.6–76.1
Vagina & vulva	76.7 70.3–82.1	–	69.0 65.1–72.6	66.2 50.8–78.7	72.7 64.1–79.9	–
Kidney	51.1 45.6–56.5	57.8 42.4–71.9	50.2 46.1–54.3	45.9 33.5–58.9	63.5 57.4–69.2	66.8 45.8–82.8
Brain	27.8 22.7–33.5	31.8 15.7–53.8	29.1 26.1–32.4	33.0 18.0–52.3	53.9 47.0–60.6	35.7 21.0–53.7
Hodgkin's disease	86.9 78.7–92.3	–	82.3 77.6–86.1	80.2 60.0–91.6	83.9 75.4–89.9	–
ALL	52.6 30.3–74.0	–	50.9 40.0–61.8	–	52.1 29.6–73.8	–
CLL	76.5 69.7–82.1	–	73.7 68.5–78.2	72.7 57.5–83.9	86.9 78.2–92.5	–
AML	27.7 20.6–36.3	–	24.9 20.1–30.4	–	30.0 21.2–40.6	–
CML	66.5 53.2–77.6	–	59.1 50.6–67.2	–	75.9 60.1–86.9	–
Leukaemia	51.2 45.7–56.6	53.0 36.2–69.1	45.9 42.7–49.2	52.4 41.0–63.5	59.5 53.0–65.8	64.5 51.0–76.1
Childhood cancers						
Brain	–	–	68.5 56.1–78.7	–	77.9 61.4–88.7	–
Leukaemia	87.2 72.8–94.6	–	78.5 69.3–85.5	–	83.0 67.5–92.0	–

*Data are given with 95% confidence intervals
– : Data missing or inadequate

Germany	Italy	Poland	Scotland	Spain	Switzerland	EUROPE	ICD-9
76.1 33.7–95.2	76.4 42.2–93.5	–	71.8 54.9–84.2	–	–	69.1 63.1–74.6	**141**
74.3 41.5–92.2	64.3 47.2–78.4	–	75.2 59.0–86.5	–	64 28.1–89.0	75.6 70.6–80.0	**143-5**
–	–	–	–	–	–	68.9 60.5–76.2	**146**
–	–	–	–	–	–	65.6 54.6–75.2	**147**
–	–	–	47.7 27.9–68.2	–	–	47.7 39.8–55.7	**148**
70.4 47.0–86.4	76.5 53.9–90.1	70.1 38.8–89.7	65.3 55.3–74.2	–	61.7 38.0–81.0	69.6 50.0–83.9	**141,3-8**
17.2 4.4–48.3	32 12.7–60.4	–	23.2 18.1–29.4	–	21.2 7.4–47.4	25.0 14.3–39.9	**150**
42.3 35.5–49.5	41.3 35.6–47.2	26.6 18.5–36.7	23.5 19.9–27.5	26.4 12.8–46.8	48 35.3–60.8	36.2 29.0–44.1	**151**
63.6 57.9–69.0	61.2 54.7–67.4	37.3 25.6–50.7	53.2 50.1–56.2	62.1 46.9–75.2	68.9 60.4–76.4	60.6 55.1–65.7	**153**
64.7 58.1–70.8	69 59.9–76.8	45.4 32.7–58.8	61.1 56.6–65.5	66.5 47.9–81.1	80 70.2–87.2	65.8 58.5–72.4	**154**
11.9 5.4–24.2	18 10.2–29.8	11.3 4.5–25.8	12.8 9.5–17.0	–	17.9 8.3–34.3	15.1 8.4–25.5	**157**
–	94.5 65.2–99.4	69 31.0–91.7	77.8 63.8–87.4	–	93.5 58.4–99.3	74.3 45.8–90.8	**161**
29.5 21.1–39.5	29.3 21.6–38.4	23.4 15.9–33.0	20.6 18.5–22.9	–	36.2 26.4–47.3	26.1 19.1–34.6	**162**
–	–	–	–	–	–	64.7 57.1–71.7	**170**
90.4 87.6–92.5	93.7 91.5–95.4	77.5 71.0–82.9	86.9 85.4–88.3	90.8 85.7–94.2	95.4 92.8–97.1	90.4 88.0–92.3	**174**
85.8 78.9–90.7	89.5 81.4–94.4	71.7 63.2–78.9	76.4 72.0–80.3	74.9 54.8–88.0	86.1 73.5–93.3	82.2 74.6–87.9	**180**
90.1 85.1–93.6	88.2 81.3–92.7	71.7 59.8–81.1	82.1 77.6–85.9	82.3 67.8–91.1	88.6 81.2–93.4	85.7 77.2–91.3	**182**
60 50.9–68.6	58.1 48.9–66.8	41.7 29.9–54.5	51.6 47.1–56.1	68.9 50.2–83.0	63.4 52.8–72.9	57.1 48.8–65.1	**183**
64.1 46.7–78.4	65 48.5–78.5	–	69.4 60.3–77.2	–	–	70.4 67.7–72.9	**184**
73.1 60.0–83.1	69.6 52.3–82.6	47.4 27.9–67.7	44.8 36.7–53.2	–	61.8 43.1–77.5	65.6 52.2–77.0	**189**
39.1 25.3–54.8	38.1 25.2–53.0	32.5 17.1–52.8	24.4 18.2–32.0	30.5 18.3–46.1	34.9 20.1–53.3	34.6 22.1–49.6	**191**
–	84.8 58.5–95.7	–	78 67.7–85.7	–	–	82.7 79.6–85.3	**201**
–	–	–	–	–	–	51.5 43.5–59.5	**204.0**
–	80.9 58.8–92.6	–	72.5 58.6–83.1	–	–	76.6 73.4–79.5	**204.1**
–	–	–	23.6 14.7–35.8	–	–	25.3 22.0–28.9	**205.0**
–	–	–	71 50.9–85.2	–	–	64.4 58.9–69.5	**205.1**
44.4 30.2–59.5	53.7 41.3–65.6	34.7 18.9–54.8	45.4 37.9–53.1	–	62.5 46.4–76.2	49.5 37.2–61.8	**204-8**
74.7 59.1–85.8	–	–	–	–	–	71.1 64.3–77.1	**191**
87.7 81.7–91.9	77 61.7–87.4	–	79.5 58.3–91.5	–	–	82.8 78.9–86.1	**204-8**

Table 16.2d. Age–standardized relative survival; females, five–year survival*

	Denmark	Netherlands	England	Estonia	Finland	France
Tongue	41.8 24.0–62.0	–	42.7 33.2–52.8	–	47.4 29.4–66.1	42.8 12.5–79.7
Oral cavity	52.4 39.5–65.1	–	54.1 44.8–63.2	–	55.1 34.4–74.2	39.7 8.3–82.7
Oropharynx	47.1 29.7–65.3	–	40.2 27.3–54.5	–	–	74.1 27.7–95.5
Nasopharynx	41.5 18.0–69.7	–	30.1 16.2–48.8	–	–	–
Hypopharynx	– –	–	18.9 11.9–28.6	–	–	–
Head & neck	46.7 38.1–55.6	54.9 26.7–80.3	39.7 34.8–44.9	40.4 17.1–69.2	43.4 32.4–55.2	49.7 20.8–78.8
Oesophagus	6.7 2.9–14.8	–	7.5 5.8–9.7	14.4 2.4–53.7	10.1 5.4–18.2	–
Stomach	15.0 11.9–18.9	20.1 12.4–30.9	9.3 8.0–10.8	14.6 11.1–18.9	16.9 14.1–20.0	21.2 15.1–29.0
Colon	39.8 36.9–42.7	47.3 38.9–55.9	34.2 32.6–35.8	33.4 25.7–42.0	44.8 40.3–49.3	45.1 39.0–51.5
Rectum	40.1 36.6–43.7	45.8 33.7–58.5	35.8 33.7–38.0	34.9 27.1–43.6	44.6 39.4–49.9	44.7 37.3–52.3
Pancreas	1.2 0.5–2.9	5.3 1.4–17.7	2.4 1.7–3.5	1.3 0.3–5.1	1.6 0.7–3.8	4.9 1.6–14.3
Larynx	67.1 51.6–79.5	–	58.0 49.3–66.1	46.4 12.8–83.6	62.0 40.7–79.5	–
Lung	6.4 5.0–8.0	–	5.4 4.7–6.1	8.2 4.0–16.0	10.3 7.6–13.7	13.0 4.4–32.6
Bone	44.9 20.8–71.6	–	44.9 32.2–58.2	–	51.0 29.1–72.6	–
Breast	68.1 66.2–69.9	69.9 64.5–74.8	62.5 61.5–63.5	58.8 53.1–64.3	73.5 71.2–75.7	71.4 66.1–76.1
Cervix uteri	61.0 57.5–64.5	62.9 46.8–76.6	54.5 52.3–56.8	55.0 47.7–62.0	62.3 55.8–68.5	64.0 51.7–74.7
Corpus uteri	75.7 72.4–78.8	77.5 64.9–86.5	69.7 67.4–71.8	63.5 55.0–71.4	76.8 72.7–80.5	66.1 41.2–84.4
Ovary	26.0 23.0–29.3	32.3 22.9–43.4	26.1 24.3–28.0	21.8 16.2–28.7	34.0 29.7–38.6	31.4 20.5–45.0
Vagina & vulva	56.1 47.8–64.2	–	51.2 46.3–56.1	41.5 25.2–59.8	52.3 42.0–62.5	–
Kidney	31.1 25.9–36.8	43.0 26.8–60.8	33.4 29.3–37.8	24.7 14.6–38.6	40.5 34.0–47.3	42.4 20.9–67.2
Brain	11.0 7.8–15.4	10.0 5.4–17.8	13.9 11.6–16.6	13.3 5.9–27.5	29.8 23.7–36.7	20.0 9.5–37.4
Hodgkin's disease	69.9 59.3–78.7	–	67.3 61.9–72.4	53.3 33.3–72.2	68.9 58.7–77.6	–
ALL	14.6 4.9–36.4	–	23.8 15.1–35.6	–	12.7 6.6–22.9	–
CLL	50.7 41.5–60.0	–	46.8 40.0–53.7	59.5 39.9–76.6	49.8 38.0–61.6	–
AML	6.5 3.5–11.6	–	6.3 4.3–9.3	–	4.6 1.6–12.5	–
CML	17.9 9.5–31.3	–	16.5 10.2–25.5	–	23.8 12.0–41.7	–
Leukaemia	24.6 19.7–30.1	37.8 19.8–59.9	20.8 18.0–24.0	36.3 24.6–49.8	25.0 19.2–31.8	40.0 26.1–55.7
Childhood cancers						
Brain	–	–	56.1 43.7–67.7	–	56.4 35.8–75.1	–
Leukaemia	62.0 44.6–76.8	–	57.9 48.3–66.9	–	64.8 48.5–78.2	–

*Data are given with 95% confidence intervals
– : Data missing or inadequate

Germany	Italy	Poland	Scotland	Spain	Switzerland	EUROPE	**ICD-9**
46 14.6–80.9	53.5 16.8–86.7	–	51.1 30.2–71.7	–	–	43.7 36.8–50.8	**141**
68.8 35.3–90.0	33.9 12.6–64.6	–	54 36.7–70.4	–	51.9 24.4–78.2	53.4 47.2–59.5	**143-5**
–	–	–	–	–	–	43.0 34.1–52.3	**146**
–	–	–	–	–	–	37.0 26.1–49.4	**147**
–	–	–	27.1 11.3–51.9	–	–	19.6 13.6–27.5	**148**
40.7 20.8–64.2	53 30.5–74.3	42.3 15.0–75.2	42.5 32.1–53.7	–	40.6 20.2–64.9	45.4 24.8–67.7	**141,3-8**
3.4 0.6–16.8	1.1 0.7–1.9	–	7.1 4.2–11.7	–	6.2 1.6–20.9	5.4 1.8–15.2	**150**
22 16.1–29.2	21.1 16.1–27.0	15.6 8.9–26.1	9.4 6.9–12.8	14.2 3.9–39.8	23.5 13.5–37.8	18.1 12.1–26.3	**151**
40.5 34.1–47.2	44 36.6–51.6	19.6 10.6–33.3	34.4 31.1–37.8	42.9 27.1–60.4	56.9 46.5–66.7	40.4 34.3–46.8	**153**
40 32.6–47.7	34.3 25.4–44.6	24.5 13.5–40.4	34.1 29.3–39.2	34.1 18.0–55.1	56.7 44.1–68.4	38.1 30.3–46.7	**154**
3.9 1.0–14.2	6.9 2.4–18.2	5.7 1.4–21.3	4.3 2.4–7.5	–	1.8 0.7–4.5	5.1 1.9–12.9	**157**
–	64.7 29.4–89.0	63.3 20.7–91.9	56.4 40.0–71.5	–	66 21.0–93.4	56.0 27.1–81.4	**161**
10 5.0–18.9	11.4 6.4–19.4	9.7 4.8–18.7	6.4 5.1–8.1	–	12.3 6.6–21.8	8.8 4.8–15.7	**162**
–	–	–	–	–	–	44.8 36.2–53.6	**170**
68.4 63.9–72.7	70.8 66.6–74.6	43.9 36.3–51.8	61.8 59.3–64.2	62.5 54.3–69.9	75.7 70.5–80.3	66.5 62.4–70.4	**174**
61.3 52.5–69.5	64 53.3–73.4	51.2 41.9–60.4	51.9 46.6–57.0	40.3 23.2–60.0	64.5 49.3–77.2	57.5 48.1–66.4	**180**
76.2 68.9–82.2	75.3 66.0–82.8	57 43.6–69.4	66.5 60.3–72.3	53.4 37.8–68.4	76.3 66.3–84.0	69.8 58.7–79.0	**182**
31.7 23.1–41.7	28.9 20.7–38.8	24.3 14.7–37.4	27.5 23.3–32.2	35.8 18.6–57.5	36.9 26.1–49.2	29.5 21.7–38.7	**183**
36.1 19.8–56.5	42.4 26.0–60.6	–	44.8 34.2–55.9	–	–	50.3 46.9–53.6	**184**
53.1 38.8–66.9	46.9 29.8–64.8	30.4 14.0–53.9	29.7 22.0–38.6	–	43.3 26.1–62.3	44.0 29.6–59.5	**189**
21.2 12.7–33.2	16.3 8.3–29.5	10.7 4.1–25.4	11.6 7.0–18.7	8.1 2.8–21.6	9.2 5.2–15.6	15.4 7.1–30.3	**191**
–	54.9 37.8–71.0	–	60.7 48.9–71.4	–	–	66.3 62.6–69.9	**201**
–	–	–	–	–	–	19.7 13.9–27.0	**204.0**
–	57.6 31.5–80.0	–	53.1 36.7–68.9	–	–	50.4 46.0–54.7	**204.1**
–	–	–	6.6 3.0–14.0	–	–	6.0 4.4–8.2	**205.0**
–	–	–	18 6.8–39.9	–	–	20.3 15.6–26.0	**205.1**
22 11.1–38.8	25.8 15.5–39.7	16 7.0–32.3	21.9 15.6–29.7	–	35 20.9–52.5	25.9 15.1–40.7	**204-8**
47.4 31.8–63.5	–	–	–	–	–	52.5 45.5–59.5	**191**
72.8 65.5–79.1	48.8 34.8–63.0	–	58.3 38.4–75.8	–	–	62.7 58.0–67.1	**204-8**

CHAPTER 17

RESULTS

The layouts used to present the results in this chapter are described in detail in chapter 16, with annotated examples. The results are summarized and discussed in Chapter 18 (page 447).

In this chapter, the results are presented site by site as follows:

Adult cancers

Childhood cancers

TONGUE

DENMARK

REGISTRY	NUMBER OF CASES			PERIOD OF DIAGNOSIS
	Males	Females	All	
Denmark	201	161	362	1978-1984
Mean age (years)	62.5	69.2	65.5	

RELATIVE SURVIVAL (%)

OBSERVED AND RELATIVE SURVIVAL (%) BY AGE AND PERIOD
(Number of cases in parentheses)

AGE CLASS

	15-44		45-54		55-64		65-74		75+	
	obs	rel	obs	rel	obs	rel	obs	rel	obs	rel
Males	(12)		(40)		(56)		(55)		(38)	
1 year	83	84	70	70	59	60	56	59	47	53
3 years	33	34	33	33	32	34	31	35	24	33
5 years	33	34	28	29	27	30	23	30	18	34
8 years	33	34	24	25	27	32	12	19	18	53
10 years	..	..	24	26	19	24	10	17	18	76
Females	(5)		(17)		(34)		(46)		(59)	
1 year	80	80	65	65	74	74	63	65	53	58
3 years	60	60	53	54	56	58	43	47	25	35
5 years	60	60	41	42	47	50	35	40	16	28
8 years	40	40	41	43	47	52	31	41	8	23
10 years	..	..	41	44	47	55	22	33	..	..
Overall	(17)		(57)		(90)		(101)		(97)	
1 year	82	83	68	69	64	65	59	61	51	56
3 years	41	41	39	39	41	43	37	41	25	34
5 years	41	42	32	33	34	37	29	35	17	30
8 years	34	34	28	30	34	40	20	29	13	36
10 years	..	..	28	31	30	37	15	24	13	51

PERIOD

	All		1978-80		1981-82		1983-85	
	obs	rel	obs	rel	obs	rel	obs	rel
Males	(201)		(89)		(49)		(63)	
1 year	60	62	58	61	63	66	59	60
3 years	30	34	31	36	29	33	30	33
5 years	25	30	28	35	22	28	21	25
8 years	20	29	24	34	18	27	..	..
10 years	17	27	20	32	..	..	..	..
Females	(161)		(69)		(41)		(51)	
1 year	62	65	62	65	61	64	63	65
3 years	41	47	41	46	37	43	45	52
5 years	32	41	33	42	34	45	29	37
8 years	28	41	28	40	31	49	..	..
10 years	24	41	24	39	..	..	..	..
Overall	(362)		(158)		(90)		(114)	
1 year	61	63	60	63	62	65	61	63
3 years	35	40	35	40	32	37	37	41
5 years	28	35	30	38	28	36	25	30
8 years	24	34	25	36	24	36	..	..
10 years	20	33	22	35	..	..	..	..

RELATIVE SURVIVAL (%) BY AGE AND PERIOD

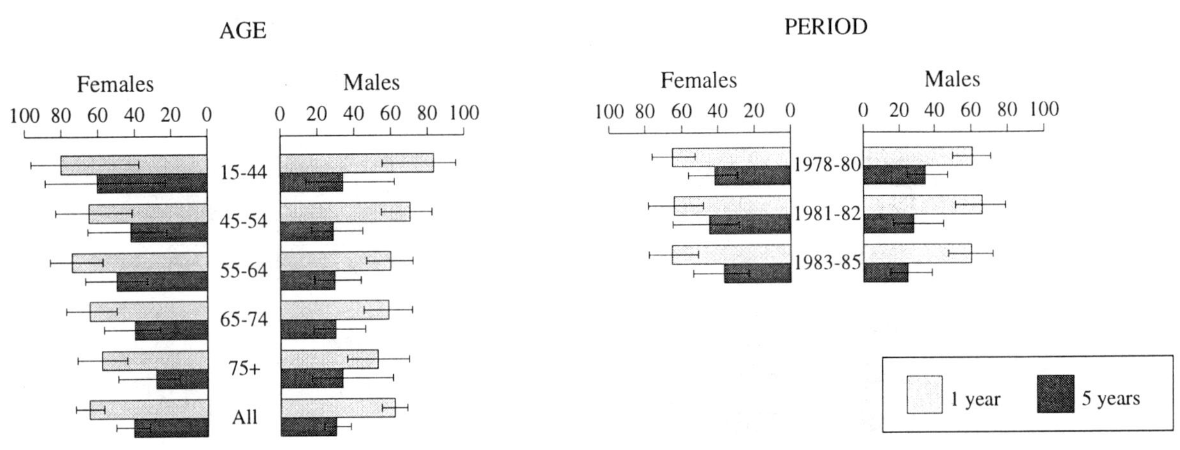

TONGUE

ENGLISH REGISTRIES

REGISTRY	NUMBER OF CASES			PERIOD OF DIAGNOSIS
	Males	Females	All	
East Anglia	59	74	133	1979-1984
Mersey	142	67	209	1978-1984
South Thames	286	242	528	1978-1984
Wessex	41	29	70	1983-1984
West Midlands	183	106	289	1979-1984
Yorkshire	154	127	281	1978-1984
Mean age (years)	63.4	68.1	65.4	

RELATIVE SURVIVAL (%)

100 80 60 40 20 0
Females
Males
0 1 2 3 4 5
Time since diagnosis (years)

OBSERVED AND RELATIVE SURVIVAL (%) BY AGE AND PERIOD
(Number of cases in parentheses)

	AGE CLASS												PERIOD					
	15-44		45-54		55-64		65-74		75+		All		1978-80		1981-82		1983-85	
	obs	rel	obs	rel	obs	rel	obs	rel	obs	rel	obs	rel	obs	rel	obs	rel	obs	rel
Males	(66)		(125)		(259)		(244)		(171)		(865)		(319)		(255)		(291)	
1 year	83	83	66	66	69	70	60	63	41	47	62	65	60	64	61	64	64	66
3 years	70	70	46	47	47	50	33	38	19	30	39	45	39	45	37	43	41	46
5 years	64	64	42	44	39	43	27	35	12	26	33	41	34	44	28	36	35	43
8 years	62	63	34	37	32	39	20	32	9	32	27	39	28	42	25	36	23	33
10 years	62	63	33	36	27	35	16	31	8	42	24	39	25	42	21	35	..	..
Females	(34)		(55)		(136)		(201)		(219)		(645)		(262)		(163)		(220)	
1 year	88	88	69	69	74	74	66	67	49	54	63	66	59	62	63	66	68	71
3 years	65	65	56	57	49	50	41	44	26	37	40	46	36	42	44	50	42	48
5 years	53	53	53	54	45	48	31	36	19	34	33	41	29	37	37	47	35	43
8 years	53	53	46	48	36	40	23	30	15	40	27	39	25	36	28	41	23	33
10 years	23	23	43	45	30	34	19	29	11	41	22	35	20	32	24	40	..	..
Overall	(100)		(180)		(395)		(445)		(390)		(1510)		(581)		(418)		(511)	
1 year	85	85	67	67	70	72	63	65	46	51	62	65	60	63	62	65	65	68
3 years	68	68	49	50	47	50	36	41	23	34	40	45	38	44	40	46	42	47
5 years	60	60	46	47	41	45	29	35	16	31	33	41	32	40	32	40	35	43
8 years	59	60	38	41	33	39	21	31	12	37	27	39	26	39	26	38	23	33
10 years	53	54	36	39	28	35	18	30	10	42	23	37	23	37	22	37	..	..

RELATIVE SURVIVAL (%) BY AGE AND PERIOD

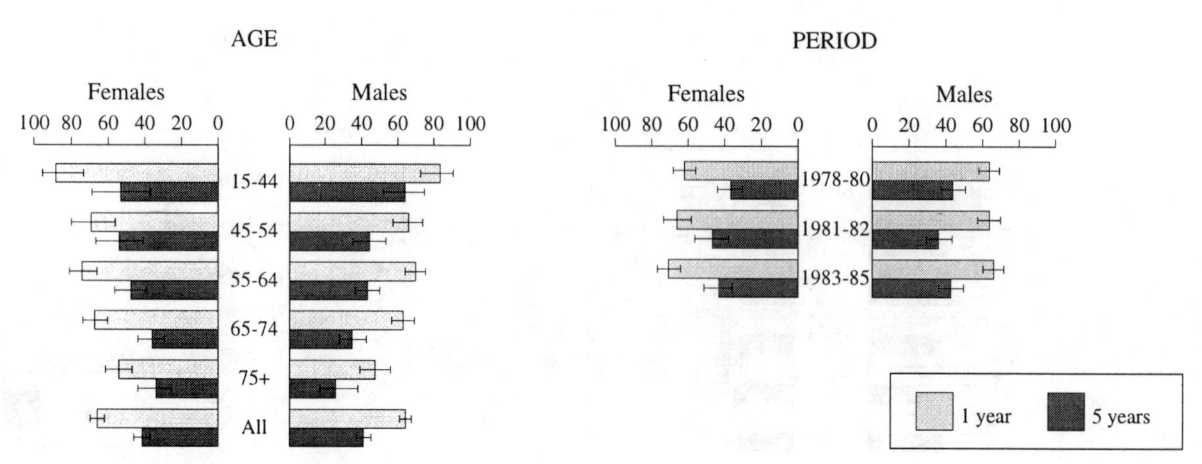

TONGUE

FINLAND

REGISTRY	NUMBER OF CASES			PERIOD OF DIAGNOSIS
	Males	Females	All	
Finland	165	152	317	1978-1984
Mean age (years)	61.0	66.6	63.7	

RELATIVE SURVIVAL (%)

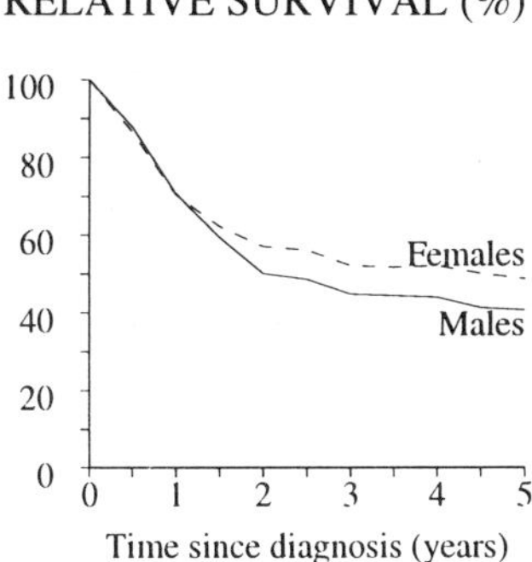

OBSERVED AND RELATIVE SURVIVAL (%) BY AGE AND PERIOD
(Number of cases in parentheses)

	AGE CLASS												PERIOD					
	15-44		45-54		55-64		65-74		75+		All		1978-80		1981-82		1983-85	
	obs	rel	obs	rel	obs	rel	obs	rel	obs	rel	obs	rel	obs	rel	obs	rel	obs	rel
Males	(27)		(21)		(42)		(43)		(32)		(165)		(68)		(51)		(46)	
1 year	81	82	81	82	79	80	63	66	41	46	68	71	71	74	63	65	70	72
3 years	56	56	33	34	55	59	33	38	19	27	39	45	41	47	29	34	48	54
5 years	52	53	29	30	45	51	26	34	13	24	33	41	31	39	25	32	43	53
8 years	48	49	24	26	23	29	15	25	9	29	22	32	22	32	16	23	32	44
10 years	48	50	24	27	23	32	15	30	..	..	21	33	21	33	16	25	..	..
Females	(15)		(15)		(28)		(41)		(53)		(152)		(55)		(45)		(52)	
1 year	100	100	93	94	61	61	68	70	55	60	68	71	67	70	67	69	69	73
3 years	87	87	60	61	50	51	51	56	25	33	46	52	42	47	53	59	44	52
5 years	87	87	53	54	43	45	44	51	17	29	39	49	36	44	47	56	37	47
8 years	87	87	53	55	43	47	34	45	12	30	35	50	33	45	44	61	30	46
10 years	87	88	53	56	43	49	34	51	9	31	34	53	33	49	42	63	..	..
Overall	(42)		(36)		(70)		(84)		(85)		(317)		(123)		(96)		(98)	
1 year	88	88	86	87	71	73	65	68	49	55	68	71	69	72	65	67	69	72
3 years	67	67	44	45	53	56	42	47	22	31	43	48	41	47	41	46	46	53
5 years	64	65	39	40	44	49	35	43	15	27	36	45	33	41	35	43	40	50
8 years	62	63	36	38	31	37	24	36	11	30	28	40	27	38	29	41	30	44
10 years	62	64	36	39	31	39	24	42	7	28	27	43	26	41	28	43	..	..

RELATIVE SURVIVAL (%) BY AGE AND PERIOD

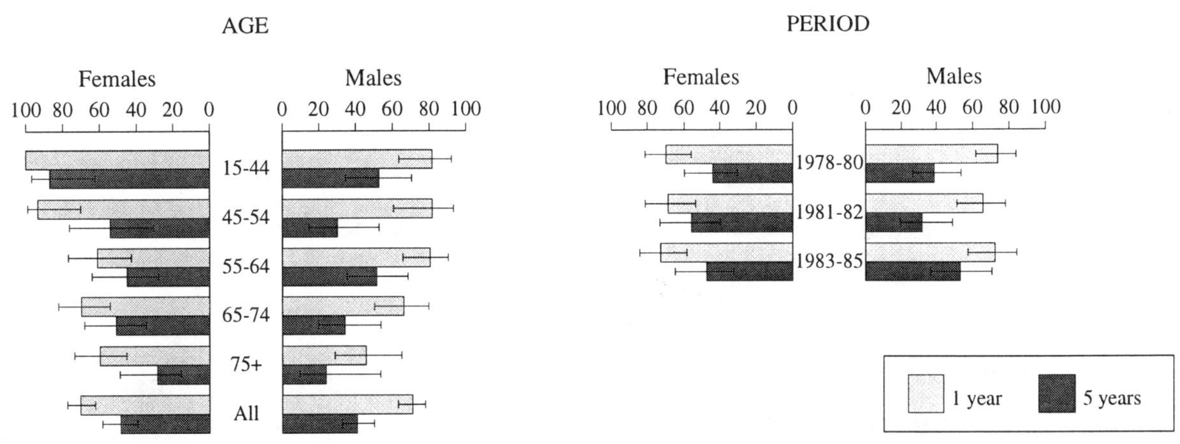

TONGUE

FRENCH REGISTRIES

REGISTRY	NUMBER OF CASES Males	Females	All	PERIOD OF DIAGNOSIS
Amiens	38	5	43	1983-1984
Doubs	165	15	180	1978-1985
Mean age (years)	59.2	64.9	59.8	

RELATIVE SURVIVAL (%)

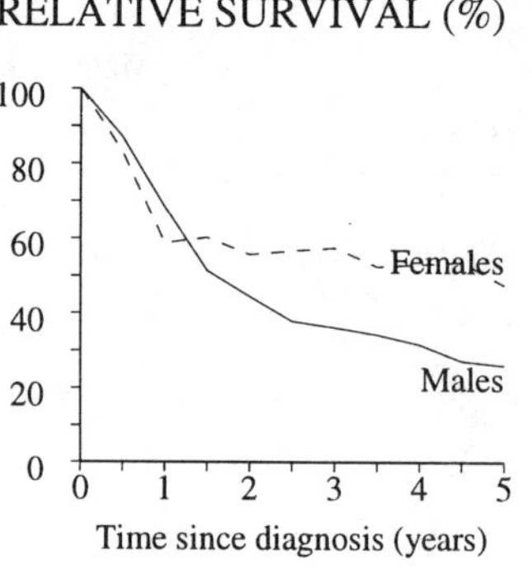

OBSERVED AND RELATIVE SURVIVAL (%) BY AGE AND PERIOD
(Number of cases in parentheses)

	AGE CLASS 15-44 obs	rel	45-54 obs	rel	55-64 obs	rel	65-74 obs	rel	75+ obs	rel	All obs	rel	PERIOD 1978-80 obs	rel	1981-82 obs	rel	1983-85 obs	rel
Males	(14)		(69)		(58)		(38)		(24)		(203)		(59)		(44)		(100)	
1 year	86	86	75	76	69	70	53	55	44	51	66	68	58	60	59	62	75	76
3 years	43	43	40	41	37	39	25	28	9	14	33	36	29	32	23	26	40	43
5 years	35	36	30	31	29	32	6	8	4	9	22	26	18	21	16	19	27	31
8 years	35	36	27	29	16	18	3	5	4	15	17	22	14	19	14	18	..	..
10 years	35	37	9	10	16	19	..	..	..	..	12	16	9	14	..	..	..	..
Females	(1)		(4)		(9)		(1)		(5)		(20)		(4)		(6)		(10)	
1 year	0	0	100	100	44	45	0	0	60	79	55	59	50	50	83	85	40	45
3 years	0	0	100	100	44	45	0	0	40	74	50	57	50	51	83	87	30	39
5 years	0	0	50	51	44	46	0	0	40	96	39	48	50	51	67	73	20	28
8 years	0	0	25	26	33	36	0	0	0	0	21	27	50	53	17	19	..	..
10 years	0	0	0	0	0	0	0	0	0	0	0	0	0	0	..	..	..	..
Overall	(15)		(73)		(67)		(39)		(29)		(223)		(63)		(50)		(110)	
1 year	80	80	77	77	65	66	51	53	47	56	65	68	57	59	62	64	71	74
3 years	40	40	44	45	38	40	24	28	14	23	35	38	30	33	30	34	39	43
5 years	33	33	30	32	31	34	6	8	10	22	24	28	20	24	22	26	27	31
8 years	33	34	26	28	19	22	3	5	5	17	17	22	17	22	13	18	..	..
10 years	33	34	6	7	13	16	..	..	..	..	8	12	8	11	..	..	..	..

RELATIVE SURVIVAL (%) BY AGE AND PERIOD

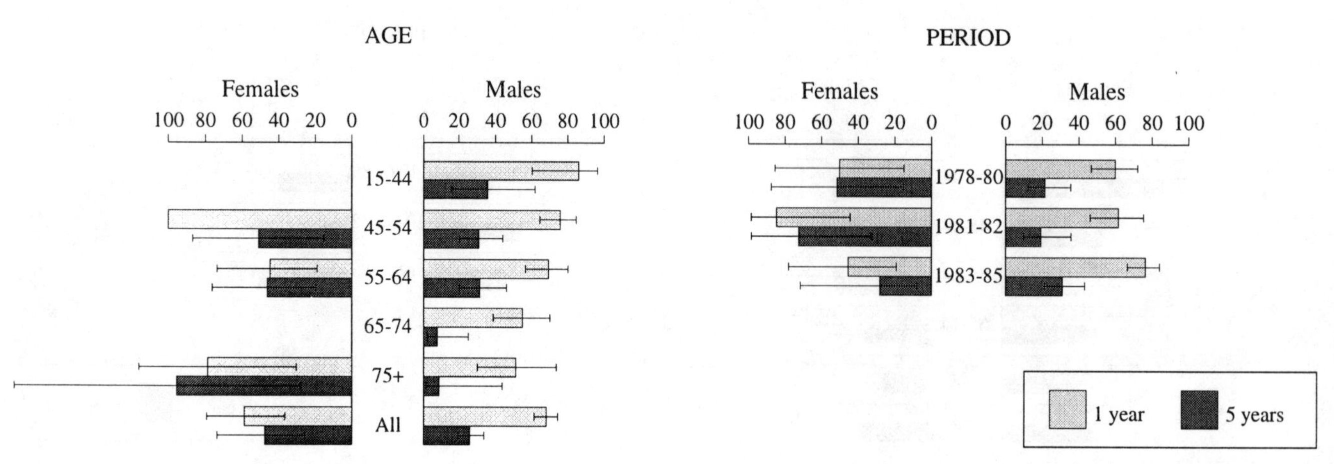

TONGUE

GERMAN REGISTRIES

REGISTRY	NUMBER OF CASES			PERIOD OF DIAGNOSIS
	Males	Females	All	
Saarland	145	34	179	1978-1984
Mean age (years)	55.6	59.9	56.4	

RELATIVE SURVIVAL (%)

100, 80, 60, 40, 20, 0 — Females, Males — 0 1 2 3 4 5 — Time since diagnosis (years)

OBSERVED AND RELATIVE SURVIVAL (%) BY AGE AND PERIOD
(Number of cases in parentheses)

	AGE CLASS												PERIOD					
	15-44		45-54		55-64		65-74		75+		All		1978-80		1981-82		1983-85	
	obs	rel	obs	rel	obs	rel	obs	rel	obs	rel	obs	rel	obs	rel	obs	rel	obs	rel
Males	(21)		(50)		(45)		(23)		(6)		(145)		(58)		(39)		(48)	
1 year	76	76	60	60	67	68	70	74	33	37	65	66	64	65	56	58	73	74
3 years	38	39	26	27	44	47	35	42	33	48	35	38	38	41	33	35	33	35
5 years	24	24	22	23	36	40	30	42	17	32	28	31	36	42	18	20	25	28
8 years	24	25	20	21	21	25	10	18	17	51	19	24	26	33	15	18	..	..
10 years	24	25	20	22	21	27	10	21	0	0	18	24	24	32	..	..	..	..
Females	(3)		(11)		(6)		(8)		(6)		(34)		(18)		(13)		(3)	
1 year	67	67	64	64	83	84	63	64	83	92	71	72	61	63	85	87	67	68
3 years	0	0	45	46	67	68	50	54	50	70	47	51	44	48	46	51	67	70
5 years	0	0	36	37	67	70	25	29	33	59	35	40	33	38	38	45	33	36
8 years	0	0	36	38	67	72	25	33	17	44	32	40	28	34	38	49	..	..
10 years	0	0	36	38	..	..	0	0	..	..	14	18	11	14	..	..	..	..
Overall	(24)		(61)		(51)		(31)		(12)		(179)		(76)		(52)		(51)	
1 year	75	75	61	61	69	70	68	71	58	65	66	67	63	65	63	65	73	74
3 years	33	34	30	30	47	50	39	45	42	59	37	40	39	43	37	39	35	37
5 years	21	21	25	26	39	43	29	38	25	46	29	33	36	41	23	26	25	28
8 years	21	22	23	24	27	32	14	22	17	47	22	27	26	33	21	25	..	..
10 years	21	22	23	25	23	29	5	9	..	..	18	24	22	29	..	..	..	..

RELATIVE SURVIVAL (%) BY AGE AND PERIOD

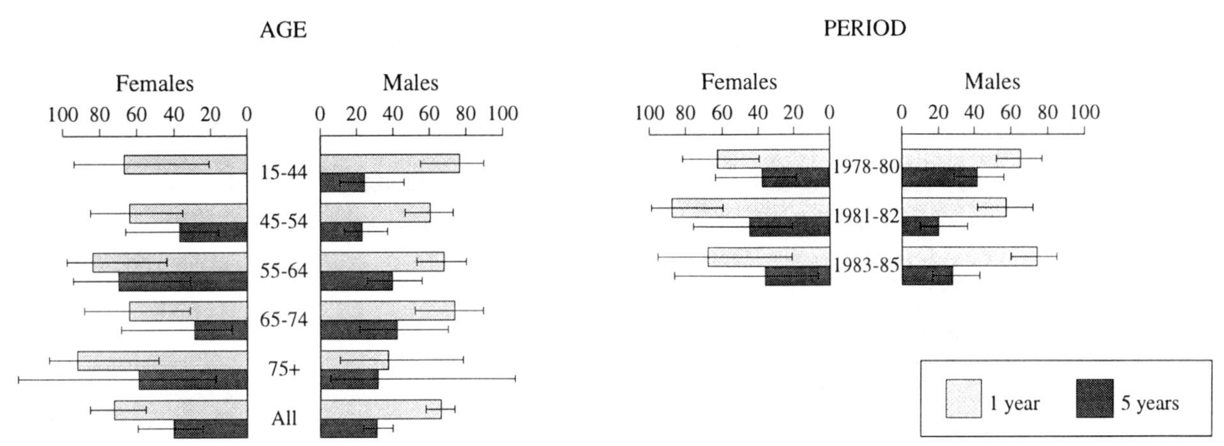

TONGUE

ITALIAN REGISTRIES

REGISTRY	NUMBER OF CASES Males	Females	All	PERIOD OF DIAGNOSIS
Latina	7	2	9	1983-1984
Ragusa	10	3	13	1981-1984
Varese	104	24	128	1978-1985
Mean age (years)	60.8	66.0	61.8	

RELATIVE SURVIVAL (%)

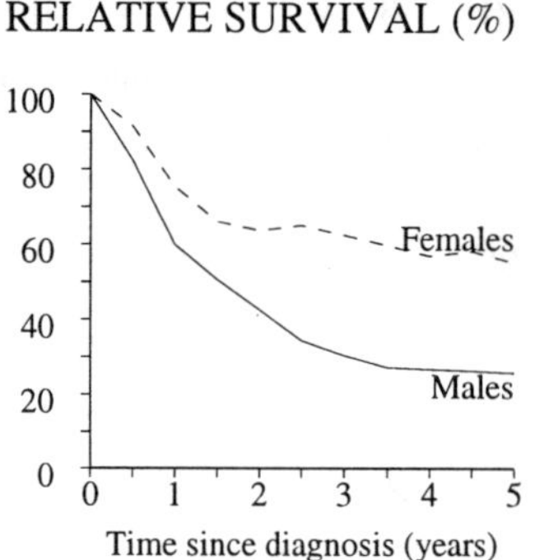

OBSERVED AND RELATIVE SURVIVAL (%) BY AGE AND PERIOD
(Number of cases in parentheses)

AGE CLASS

	15-44 obs	15-44 rel	45-54 obs	45-54 rel	55-64 obs	55-64 rel	65-74 obs	65-74 rel	75+ obs	75+ rel	All obs	All rel
Males	(8)		(28)		(45)		(22)		(18)		(121)	
1 year	88	88	57	58	60	61	50	52	50	56	58	60
3 years	50	50	21	22	38	40	14	16	17	25	27	30
5 years	38	38	21	23	27	30	14	18	11	22	21	26
8 years	38	38	18	19	20	24	9	14	6	18	16	21
10 years	..	..	0	0	20	26	5	9	..	..	8	12
Females	(4)		(3)		(5)		(8)		(9)		(29)	
1 year	100	100	100	100	80	81	63	64	56	62	72	75
3 years	100	100	67	67	60	62	50	55	33	46	55	62
5 years	75	76	67	68	60	63	50	59	11	20	45	55
8 years	75	76	..	..	40	44	33	45	11	31	35	50
10 years	38	38	..	..	40	45	..	..	11	42	28	44
Overall	(12)		(31)		(50)		(30)		(27)		(150)	
1 year	92	92	61	62	62	63	53	56	52	58	61	63
3 years	67	67	26	26	40	43	23	27	22	32	33	36
5 years	50	50	26	27	30	33	23	29	11	21	26	31
8 years	50	51	22	24	22	26	16	24	7	23	19	26
10 years	30	31	0	0	22	28	10	18	7	33	13	20

PERIOD

	1978-80 obs	1978-80 rel	1981-82 obs	1981-82 rel	1983-85 obs	1983-85 rel
Males	(37)		(32)		(52)	
1 year	54	56	50	52	65	67
3 years	19	21	31	35	31	34
5 years	8	10	25	31	29	34
8 years	8	11	19	26	17	23
10 years	3	4	19	29	..	..
Females	(9)		(5)		(15)	
1 year	78	81	80	84	67	69
3 years	67	76	60	70	47	52
5 years	44	56	60	78	40	48
8 years	44	66	40	62	..	..
10 years	33	54	..	..	..	..
Overall	(46)		(37)		(67)	
1 year	59	61	54	56	66	68
3 years	28	32	35	40	34	38
5 years	15	19	30	37	31	37
8 years	15	21	22	31	20	26
10 years	9	13	22	34	..	..

RELATIVE SURVIVAL (%) BY AGE AND PERIOD

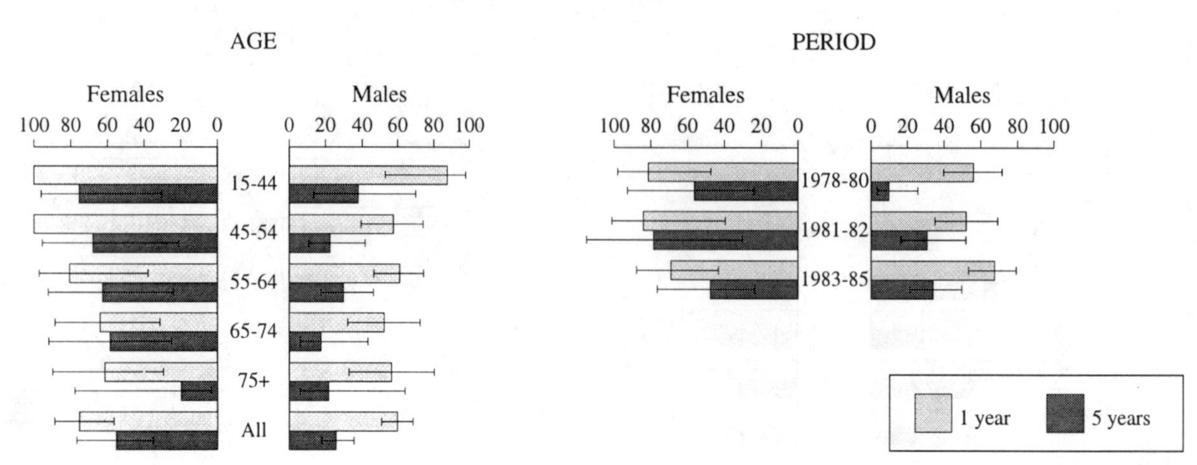

TONGUE

SCOTLAND

REGISTRY	NUMBER OF CASES			PERIOD OF DIAGNOSIS
	Males	Females	All	
Scotland	161	126	287	1978-1982
Mean age (years)	65.1	68.6	66.6	

RELATIVE SURVIVAL (%)

OBSERVED AND RELATIVE SURVIVAL (%) BY AGE AND PERIOD
(Number of cases in parentheses)

	AGE CLASS												PERIOD					
	15-44		45-54		55-64		65-74		75+		All		1978-80		1981-82		1983-85	
	obs	rel	obs	rel	obs	rel	obs	rel	obs	rel	obs	rel	obs	rel	obs	rel	obs	rel
Males	(3)		(29)		(50)		(41)		(38)		(161)		(97)		(64)		(0)	
1 year	100	100	48	49	76	78	54	57	37	43	57	60	51	54	66	68	..	..
3 years	67	67	31	32	52	56	37	44	24	38	38	45	33	40	45	51	..	..
5 years	67	67	24	25	48	55	34	47	13	30	32	43	26	36	42	52	..	..
8 years	67	68	18	20	27	34	31	53	0	0	21	33	17	30	..	..	..	..
10 years	67	69	..	..	..	..	0	0	0	0	10	18	8	16	..	..	..	..
Females	(4)		(17)		(23)		(40)		(42)		(126)		(72)		(54)		(0)	
1 year	100	100	88	89	70	70	78	80	38	43	65	69	61	64	70	74	..	..
3 years	100	100	53	54	61	63	52	58	17	24	44	51	44	52	43	50	..	..
5 years	75	76	41	42	61	65	50	60	12	23	39	51	39	51	39	51	..	..
8 years	..	..	41	43	61	69	37	52	12	36	35	53	35	53	..	..	..	..
10 years	..	..	27	29	..	..	31	49	12	50	27	47	27	46	..	..	..	..
Overall	(7)		(46)		(73)		(81)		(80)		(287)		(169)		(118)		(0)	
1 year	100	100	63	64	74	75	65	68	38	43	60	64	55	58	68	71	..	..
3 years	86	86	39	40	55	58	44	51	20	31	40	48	38	45	44	51	..	..
5 years	71	72	30	32	52	58	42	54	13	26	35	46	31	42	41	52	..	..
8 years	71	73	27	30	38	46	34	53	8	27	27	43	25	40	..	..	..	..
10 years	71	73	18	20	..	..	19	33	8	39	19	34	17	32	..	..	..	..

RELATIVE SURVIVAL (%) BY AGE AND PERIOD

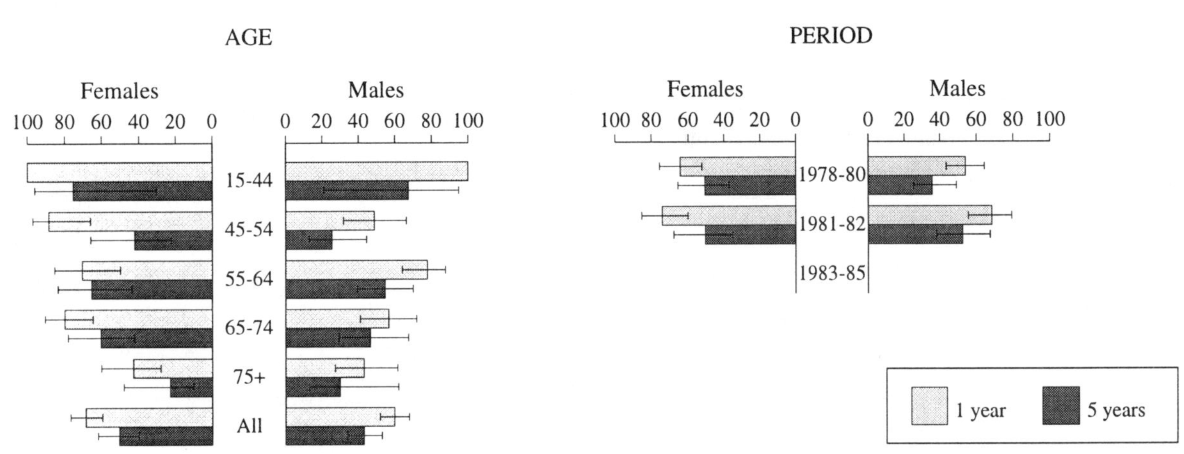

TONGUE

DUTCH REGISTRIES

REGISTRY	NUMBER OF CASES			PERIOD OF DIAGNOSIS
	Males	Females	All	
Eindhoven	36	21	57	1978-1985
Mean age (years)	64.6	71.4	67.1	

RELATIVE SURVIVAL (%)
(Both sexes)

OBSERVED AND RELATIVE SURVIVAL (%) BY PERIOD AND SEX
(Number of cases in parentheses)

	PERIOD						SEX					
	1978-80		1981-82		1983-85		Males		Females		All	
	obs	rel	obs	rel	obs	rel	obs	rel	obs	rel	obs	rel
N. Cases	(17)		(12)		(28)		(36)		(21)		(57)	
1 year	65	68	75	79	68	71	69	72	67	70	68	71
3 years	47	54	17	19	48	56	39	44	46	54	42	48
5 years	35	45	0	0	11	15	17	22	33	45	22	28
8 years	28	43	0	0	..	..	12	17	33	57	17	27
10 years	28	49	0	0	..	..	..	..	33	67	17	31

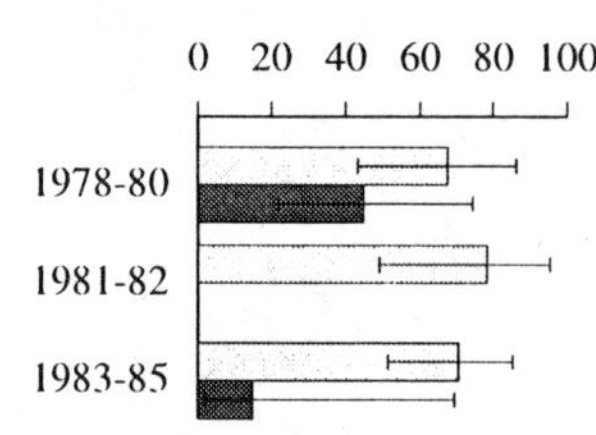

ESTONIA

REGISTRY	NUMBER OF CASES			PERIOD OF DIAGNOSIS
	Males	Females	All	
Estonia	66	22	88	1978-1984
Mean age (years)	60.0	63.0	60.8	

RELATIVE SURVIVAL (%)
(Both sexes)

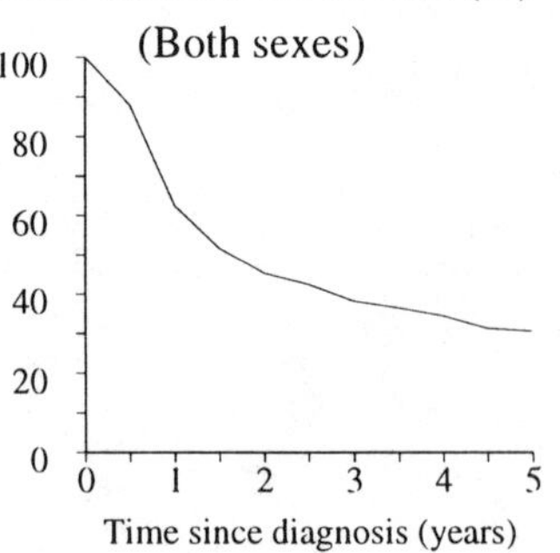

OBSERVED AND RELATIVE SURVIVAL (%) BY PERIOD AND SEX
(Number of cases in parentheses)

	PERIOD						SEX					
	1978-80		1981-82		1983-85		Males		Females		All	
	obs	rel	obs	rel	obs	rel	obs	rel	obs	rel	obs	rel
N. Cases	(43)		(21)		(24)		(66)		(22)		(88)	
1 year	58	61	67	69	58	60	62	65	55	56	60	62
3 years	33	37	38	43	33	37	32	36	41	45	34	38
5 years	23	29	29	35	25	30	23	28	32	38	25	31
8 years	16	23	14	19	..	..	18	25	9	12	16	22
10 years	9	15	..	..	..	..	9	15	9	13	9	14

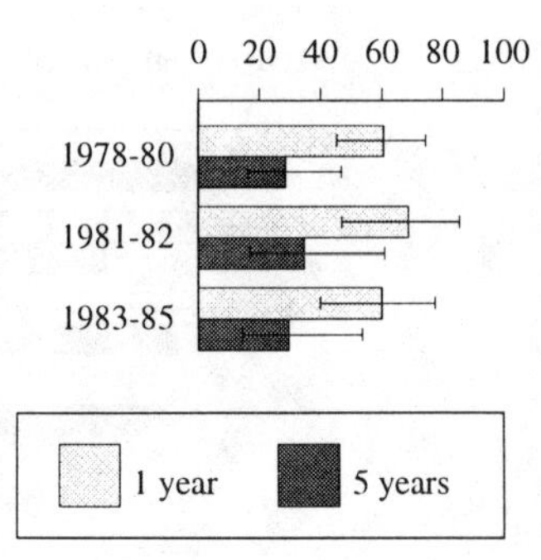

TONGUE

POLISH REGISTRIES

REGISTRY	NUMBER OF CASES			PERIOD OF DIAGNOSIS
	Males	Females	All	
Cracow	29	11	40	1978-1984
Mean age (years)	57.0	59.3	57.7	

RELATIVE SURVIVAL (%)
(Both sexes)

Time since diagnosis (years)

OBSERVED AND RELATIVE SURVIVAL (%) BY PERIOD AND SEX
(Number of cases in parentheses)

	PERIOD						SEX					
	1978-80		1981-82		1983-85		Males		Females		All	
	obs	rel	obs	rel	obs	rel	obs	rel	obs	rel	obs	rel
N. Cases	(16)		(12)		(12)		(29)		(11)		(40)	
1 year	44	45	42	43	42	43	34	36	64	65	43	44
3 years	25	27	17	18	8	9	14	15	27	29	18	19
5 years	13	14	17	19	8	10	10	12	18	21	13	15
8 years	13	16	8	10	..	..	10	14	9	11	10	13
10 years	13	17	8	11	..	..	10	15	9	12	10	14

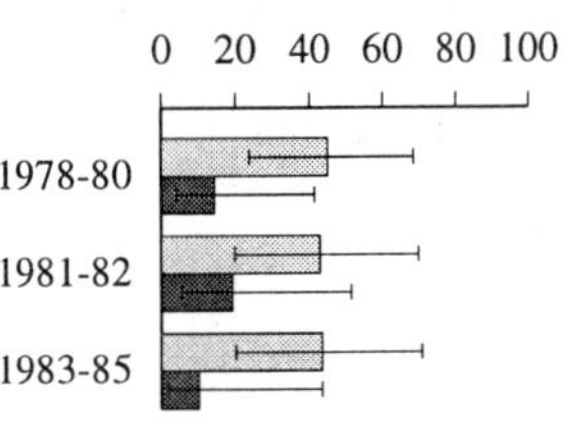

SWISS REGISTRIES

REGISTRY	NUMBER OF CASES			PERIOD OF DIAGNOSIS
	Males	Females	All	
Basel	24	6	30	1981-1984
Geneva	47	9	56	1978-1984
Mean age (years)	60.6	61.8	60.8	

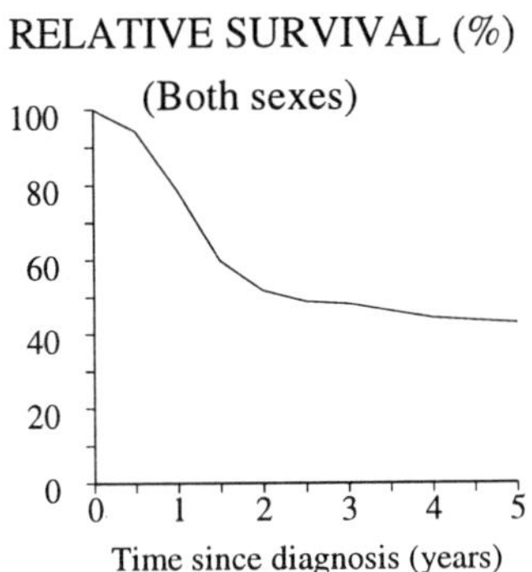

OBSERVED AND RELATIVE SURVIVAL (%) BY PERIOD AND SEX
(Number of cases in parentheses)

	PERIOD						SEX					
	1978-80		1981-82		1983-85		Males		Females		All	
	obs	rel	obs	rel	obs	rel	obs	rel	obs	rel	obs	rel
N. Cases	(21)		(29)		(36)		(71)		(15)		(86)	
1 year	85	87	66	67	80	83	74	76	87	88	76	79
3 years	55	60	34	37	46	51	44	48	47	49	44	48
5 years	55	63	31	35	31	38	39	46	27	29	37	43
8 years	..	..	..	..	..	..	..	..	..	..	..	..
10 years	..	..	..	..	..	..	..	..	..	..	..	..

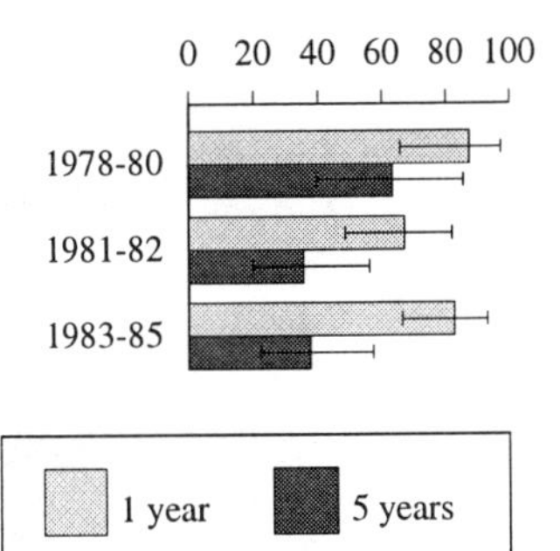

TONGUE

EUROPEAN REGISTRIES

Unweighted analysis

REGISTRY	CASES Males	Females	All
DENMARK	201	161	362
DUTCH REGISTRIES	36	21	57
ENGLISH REGISTRIES	865	645	1510
ESTONIA	66	22	88
FINLAND	165	152	317
FRENCH REGISTRIES	203	20	223
GERMAN REGISTRIES	145	34	179
ITALIAN REGISTRIES	121	29	150
POLISH REGISTRIES	29	11	40
SCOTLAND	161	126	287
SWISS REGISTRIES	71	15	86
Mean age (years)	61.9	67.6	64.0

RELATIVE SURVIVAL (%)

(Age-standardized)

Females 100 80 60 40 20 0 — Males 0 20 40 60 80 100

DK, ENG, FIN, F, D, I, SCO, EUR

OBSERVED AND RELATIVE SURVIVAL (%) BY AGE AND PERIOD

(Number of cases in parentheses)

	AGE CLASS 15-44 obs	rel	45-54 obs	rel	55-64 obs	rel	65-74 obs	rel	75+ obs	rel	All obs	rel	PERIOD 1978-80 obs	rel	1981-82 obs	rel	1983-85 obs	rel
Males	(172)		(406)		(614)		(515)		(356)		(2063)		(804)		(592)		(667)	
1 year	82	83	67	67	67	69	59	62	43	49	62	65	60	63	61	63	66	69
3 years	57	57	38	38	43	45	32	37	20	30	36	41	36	41	34	39	39	43
5 years	50	51	32	33	35	39	24	32	13	26	29	36	29	37	27	33	31	37
8 years	48	49	26	29	26	32	17	27	9	30	23	32	23	34	21	30	21	28
10 years	48	50	23	26	23	30	12	23	7	37	19	30	20	32	19	29	..	..
Females	(72)		(133)		(257)		(362)		(412)		(1236)		(509)		(343)		(384)	
1 year	89	89	77	78	71	72	66	68	50	55	64	67	61	64	66	69	66	69
3 years	67	67	57	58	51	53	43	47	26	36	42	48	39	45	45	51	43	49
5 years	57	57	49	50	47	49	35	41	18	32	34	43	32	41	38	48	34	42
8 years	55	56	44	46	40	45	26	35	13	35	28	41	28	40	30	45	24	34
10 years	40	41	39	42	34	39	21	32	10	38	24	38	23	36	27	45	..	..
Overall	(244)		(539)		(871)		(877)		(768)		(3299)		(1313)		(935)		(1051)	
1 year	84	85	69	70	68	70	62	64	47	52	63	66	60	63	63	65	66	69
3 years	60	60	42	43	45	48	36	41	23	34	38	44	37	43	38	43	40	45
5 years	52	53	36	37	39	43	29	36	16	29	31	39	31	38	31	39	32	39
8 years	50	51	31	33	30	36	21	31	11	33	25	35	25	36	24	35	22	30
10 years	46	48	27	30	26	33	16	27	9	38	21	33	21	34	22	35	..	..

RELATIVE SURVIVAL (%) BY AGE AND PERIOD

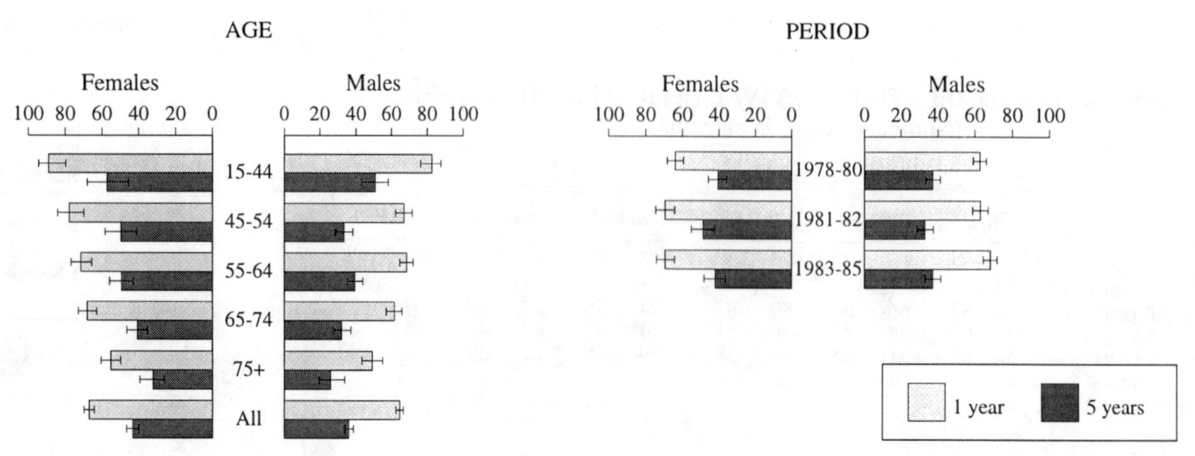

ORAL CAVITY

DENMARK

REGISTRY	NUMBER OF CASES			PERIOD OF DIAGNOSIS
	Males	Females	All	
Denmark	423	375	798	1978-1984
Mean age (years)	65.0	69.6	67.2	

RELATIVE SURVIVAL (%)

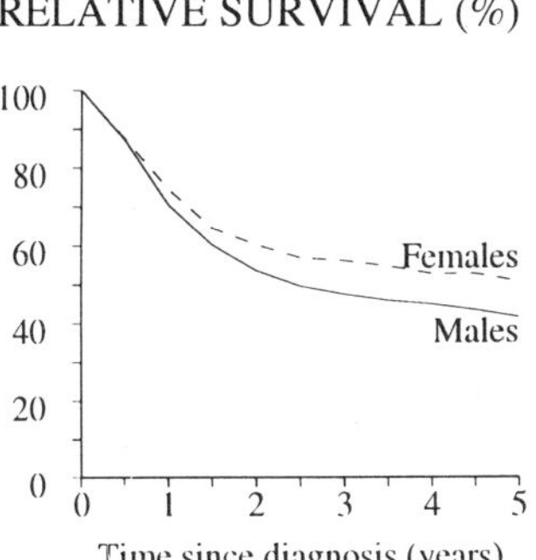

OBSERVED AND RELATIVE SURVIVAL (%) BY AGE AND PERIOD
(Number of cases in parentheses)

	AGE CLASS												PERIOD					
	15-44		45-54		55-64		65-74		75+		All		1978-80		1981-82		1983-85	
	obs	rel	obs	rel	obs	rel	obs	rel	obs	rel	obs	rel	obs	rel	obs	rel	obs	rel
Males	(19)		(61)		(123)		(130)		(90)		(423)		(169)		(119)		(135)	
1 year	84	84	74	74	70	71	68	71	54	62	67	71	69	72	62	65	70	73
3 years	53	53	48	49	46	49	39	45	31	47	41	48	46	53	36	42	40	46
5 years	42	43	44	46	37	41	30	38	22	44	33	42	37	47	28	35	33	42
8 years	34	35	39	43	30	37	18	29	17	57	25	38	30	45	19	29	..	..
10 years	0	0	36	41	24	31	14	27	10	51	19	32	23	39	..	..	..	..
Females	(17)		(33)		(79)		(90)		(156)		(375)		(155)		(115)		(105)	
1 year	88	88	82	82	80	81	76	77	60	66	71	75	70	74	70	72	74	78
3 years	71	71	76	77	58	60	53	58	33	45	49	56	50	57	42	47	55	65
5 years	71	71	66	68	49	52	43	49	25	41	40	51	40	51	37	46	42	55
8 years	71	72	61	65	40	44	30	39	16	40	31	46	30	46	27	38	..	..
10 years	71	72	61	66	40	46	21	30	6	22	26	43	25	43	..	..	..	..
Overall	(36)		(94)		(202)		(220)		(246)		(798)		(324)		(234)		(240)	
1 year	86	86	77	77	74	75	71	74	58	65	69	72	70	73	66	69	72	75
3 years	61	62	57	59	51	54	45	50	33	45	45	52	48	55	39	44	47	54
5 years	56	56	52	54	42	46	35	43	24	42	36	46	38	49	32	41	37	48
8 years	51	53	47	50	34	40	23	33	16	45	28	42	30	45	22	32	..	..
10 years	34	35	44	49	30	38	17	29	8	31	22	37	24	41	..	..	..	..

RELATIVE SURVIVAL (%) BY AGE AND PERIOD

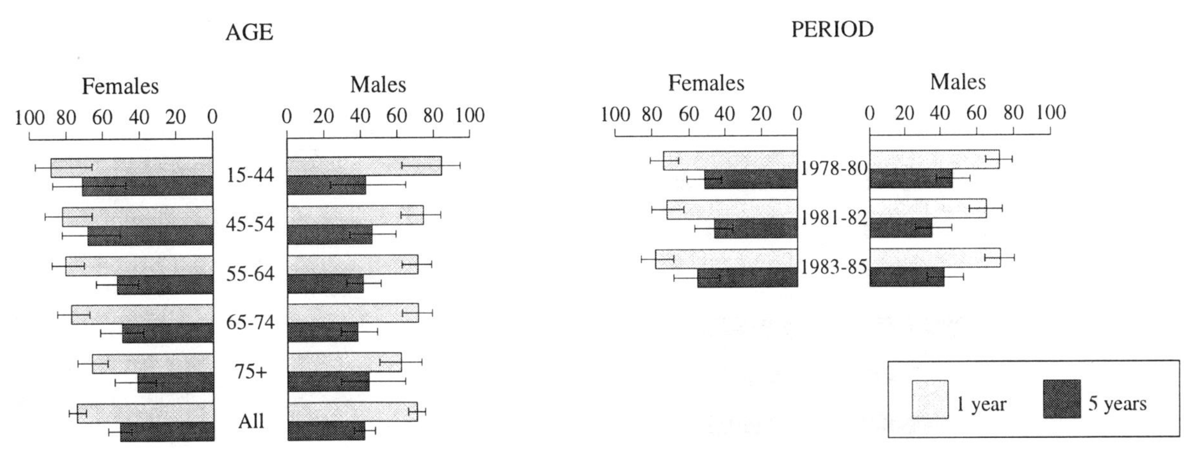

ORAL CAVITY

ENGLISH REGISTRIES

REGISTRY	NUMBER OF CASES			PERIOD OF DIAGNOSIS
	Males	Females	All	
East Anglia	87	62	149	1979-1984
Mersey	200	95	295	1978-1984
South Thames	326	238	564	1978-1984
Wessex	37	24	61	1983-1984
West Midlands	239	118	357	1979-1984
Yorkshire	265	157	422	1978-1984
Mean age (years)	64.5	67.8	65.8	

RELATIVE SURVIVAL (%)

100
80
60
40
20
0
Females
Males
0 1 2 3 4 5
Time since diagnosis (years)

OBSERVED AND RELATIVE SURVIVAL (%) BY AGE AND PERIOD
(Number of cases in parentheses)

	AGE CLASS												PERIOD					
	15-44		45-54		55-64		65-74		75+		All		1978-80		1981-82		1983-85	
	obs	rel	obs	rel	obs	rel	obs	rel	obs	rel	obs	rel	obs	rel	obs	rel	obs	rel
Males	(47)		(164)		(364)		(346)		(233)		(1154)		(426)		(359)		(369)	
1 year	85	85	74	74	67	68	68	71	46	52	65	68	62	65	64	67	69	72
3 years	70	71	52	54	45	48	47	55	21	31	43	49	41	48	40	46	48	54
5 years	64	65	45	47	37	41	38	50	16	32	35	45	33	42	34	43	39	49
8 years	64	65	35	38	32	38	26	43	7	25	27	40	26	39	26	38	29	43
10 years	60	62	30	34	27	35	21	41	5	25	23	38	22	38	21	34	..	..
Females	(34)		(80)		(140)		(194)		(246)		(694)		(252)		(196)		(246)	
1 year	82	82	89	89	81	82	75	77	52	58	70	73	65	68	74	77	72	75
3 years	65	65	79	80	60	62	55	60	32	43	51	58	45	52	55	62	54	61
5 years	56	56	74	76	52	55	45	53	24	40	43	53	39	50	45	57	45	55
8 years	47	47	66	69	44	50	36	48	19	47	35	51	32	47	36	52	40	56
10 years	10	11	66	70	41	47	28	41	15	52	30	49	26	43	36	57	..	..
Overall	(81)		(244)		(504)		(540)		(479)		(1848)		(678)		(555)		(615)	
1 year	84	84	79	79	71	72	71	73	49	55	67	70	63	67	67	70	70	73
3 years	68	68	61	62	49	52	50	57	26	37	46	53	42	49	45	52	50	57
5 years	60	61	55	57	41	45	40	51	20	37	38	48	35	45	38	48	41	51
8 years	57	58	45	48	35	42	30	45	13	38	30	44	28	42	30	43	34	48
10 years	47	49	42	46	31	39	23	41	10	41	25	42	24	40	26	42	..	..

RELATIVE SURVIVAL (%) BY AGE AND PERIOD

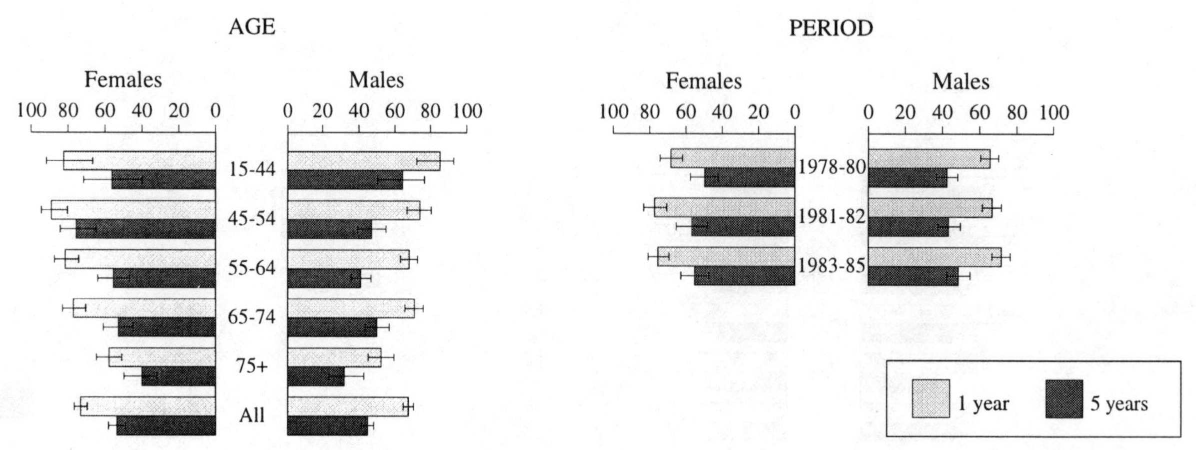

ORAL CAVITY

FINLAND

REGISTRY	NUMBER OF CASES			PERIOD OF DIAGNOSIS
	Males	Females	All	
Finland	151	146	297	1978-1984
Mean age (years)	60.4	67.7	64.0	

RELATIVE SURVIVAL (%)

100
80
60
40
20
0
0 1 2 3 4 5
Females
Males
Time since diagnosis (years)

OBSERVED AND RELATIVE SURVIVAL (%) BY AGE AND PERIOD
(Number of cases in parentheses)

	AGE CLASS												PERIOD					
	15-44		45-54		55-64		65-74		75+		All		1978-80		1981-82		1983-85	
	obs	rel	obs	rel	obs	rel	obs	rel	obs	rel	obs	rel	obs	rel	obs	rel	obs	rel
Males	(16)		(33)		(46)		(28)		(28)		(151)		(65)		(38)		(48)	
1 year	81	81	88	89	78	80	71	75	46	52	74	76	74	77	71	73	75	79
3 years	44	44	70	72	54	58	50	59	18	26	49	55	52	59	42	47	50	58
5 years	44	44	64	67	46	52	29	38	11	21	40	49	42	51	37	44	40	50
8 years	44	45	55	61	30	37	29	48	11	34	33	46	38	53	29	39	23	33
10 years	44	46	44	50	21	28	29	56	11	49	27	41	32	49	24	35	..	..
Females	(4)		(16)		(32)		(54)		(40)		(146)		(66)		(38)		(42)	
1 year	100	100	94	94	81	82	80	82	52	58	75	77	76	79	76	80	71	74
3 years	75	75	81	82	63	64	50	54	33	44	52	58	53	59	53	60	50	55
5 years	75	75	63	64	56	59	43	50	28	47	45	54	47	57	42	53	43	50
8 years	75	76	56	58	50	55	38	51	17	42	38	53	44	61	29	43	38	50
10 years	75	76	56	59	50	57	21	31	13	44	32	49	36	55	29	47	..	..
Overall	(20)		(49)		(78)		(82)		(68)		(297)		(131)		(76)		(90)	
1 year	85	85	90	90	79	81	77	79	50	56	74	77	75	78	74	77	73	76
3 years	50	50	73	75	58	61	50	56	26	37	51	57	53	59	47	53	50	56
5 years	50	51	63	66	50	55	38	46	21	37	42	51	44	54	39	49	41	50
8 years	50	51	56	60	38	45	35	50	14	37	35	49	41	57	29	41	31	43
10 years	50	52	49	54	32	40	24	40	11	42	30	45	34	52	26	40	..	..

RELATIVE SURVIVAL (%) BY AGE AND PERIOD

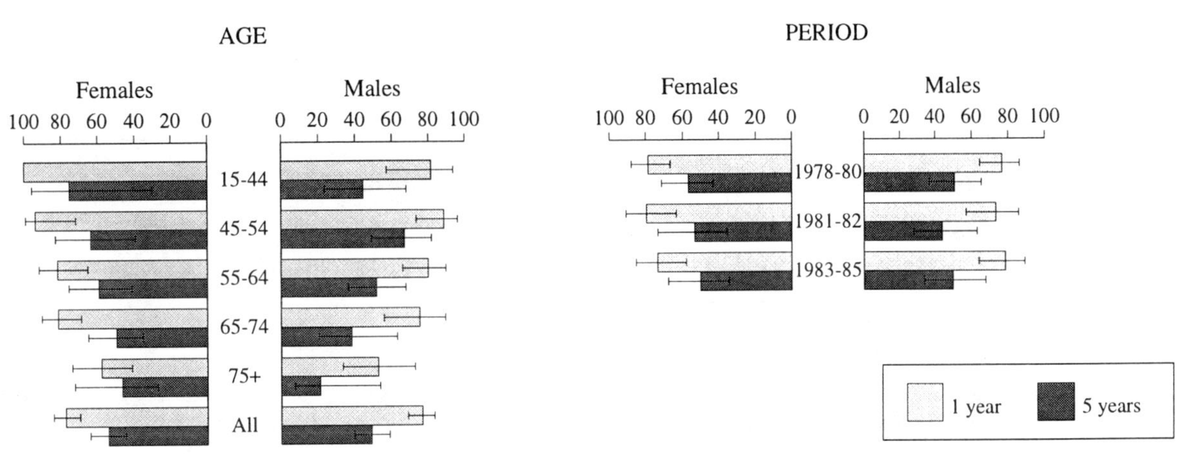

ORAL CAVITY

FRENCH REGISTRIES

REGISTRY	NUMBER OF CASES			PERIOD OF DIAGNOSIS
	Males	Females	All	
Amiens	44	6	50	1983-1984
Doubs	146	14	160	1978-1985
Mean age (years)	58.4	64.8	59.0	

RELATIVE SURVIVAL (%)

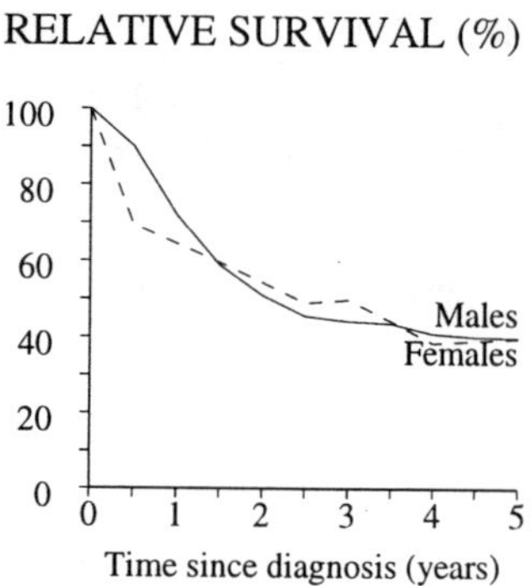

OBSERVED AND RELATIVE SURVIVAL (%) BY AGE AND PERIOD
(Number of cases in parentheses)

	AGE CLASS												PERIOD					
	15-44		45-54		55-64		65-74		75+		All		1978-80		1981-82		1983-85	
	obs	rel	obs	rel	obs	rel	obs	rel	obs	rel	obs	rel	obs	rel	obs	rel	obs	rel
Males	(25)		(44)		(63)		(44)		(14)		(190)		(55)		(45)		(90)	
1 year	76	76	75	75	72	73	64	66	57	66	70	72	73	75	67	68	70	72
3 years	46	47	46	47	41	44	36	41	28	43	41	44	42	45	40	43	41	44
5 years	38	39	39	40	38	41	29	36	28	58	35	40	30	35	35	40	38	44
8 years	38	39	29	32	15	18	14	21	..	..	20	25	15	19	19	24	..	..
10 years	..	..	10	11	10	13	14	25	..	..	11	15	9	12	..	..	..	..
Females	(1)		(4)		(6)		(3)		(6)		(20)		(5)		(2)		(13)	
1 year	100	100	100	100	33	34	67	68	64	69	63	64	78	80	100	100	51	53
3 years	100	100	67	67	17	17	67	71	42	55	46	50	78	85	100	100	26	28
5 years	100	100	67	68	17	17	33	38	21	34	34	40	78	92	100	100	9	10
8 years	..	..	67	69	17	18	33	41	..	..	34	44	78	100	..	..	..	..
10 years	..	..	67	70	0	0	..	..	..	..	23	33	52	76	..	..	..	..
Overall	(26)		(48)		(69)		(47)		(20)		(210)		(60)		(47)		(103)	
1 year	77	77	76	77	69	70	64	66	58	66	69	71	73	75	68	70	68	70
3 years	48	49	48	49	39	41	38	43	31	46	41	45	44	48	42	46	39	42
5 years	40	41	41	42	36	39	29	36	25	49	35	40	33	38	38	43	35	40
8 years	40	42	32	35	16	19	17	25	..	..	22	28	19	24	21	27	..	..
10 years	..	..	16	18	8	10	17	29	..	..	13	18	12	15	..	..	..	..

RELATIVE SURVIVAL (%) BY AGE AND PERIOD

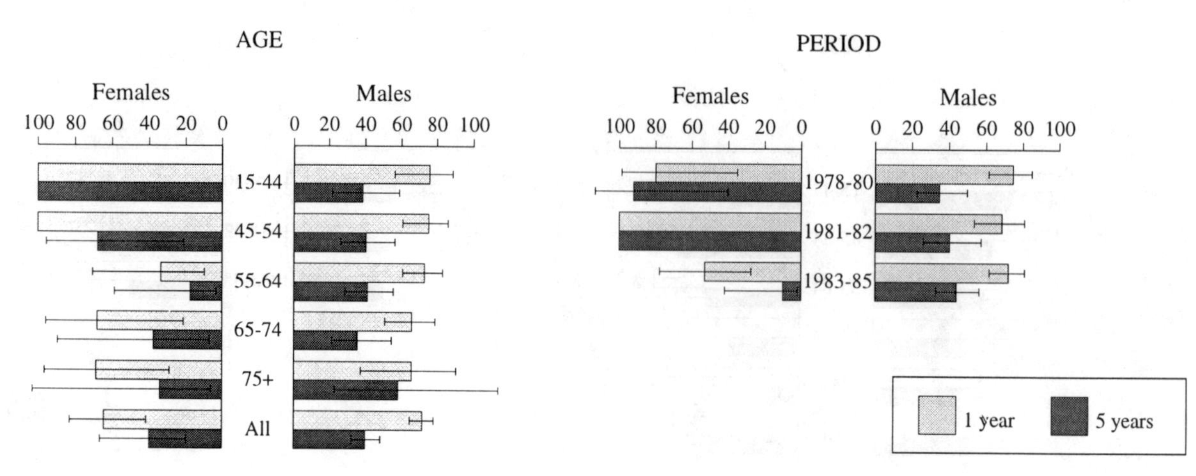

ORAL CAVITY

GERMAN REGISTRIES

REGISTRY	NUMBER OF CASES			PERIOD OF DIAGNOSIS
	Males	Females	All	
Saarland	133	21	154	1978-1984
Mean age (years)	56.7	57.7	56.8	

RELATIVE SURVIVAL (%)

100 80 60 40 20 0

Females

Males

0 1 2 3 4 5

Time since diagnosis (years)

OBSERVED AND RELATIVE SURVIVAL (%) BY AGE AND PERIOD
(Number of cases in parentheses)

	AGE CLASS												PERIOD					
	15-44		45-54		55-64		65-74		75+		All		1978-80		1981-82		1983-85	
	obs	rel	obs	rel	obs	rel	obs	rel	obs	rel	obs	rel	obs	rel	obs	rel	obs	rel
Males	(20)		(48)		(24)		(35)		(6)		(133)		(52)		(37)		(44)	
1 year	80	80	83	84	88	89	60	64	50	56	76	78	71	74	76	77	82	84
3 years	45	45	52	53	46	49	34	41	33	49	44	48	40	45	43	46	50	53
5 years	40	41	46	48	38	42	26	35	0	0	36	42	35	41	35	40	39	43
8 years	33	34	39	43	38	46	22	39	0	0	31	40	33	44	30	37	..	..
10 years	17	17	33	36	25	33	11	24	0	0	20	28	21	31	..	..	..	..
Females	(3)		(7)		(5)		(5)		(1)		(21)		(5)		(11)		(5)	
1 year	100	100	71	72	80	81	40	41	100	100	71	72	80	81	64	65	80	81
3 years	67	67	71	72	80	82	40	45	100	100	67	70	80	84	64	67	60	61
5 years	67	67	71	73	80	84	20	24	100	100	62	67	80	87	55	60	60	62
8 years	67	68	54	56	80	88	..	..	..	..	56	64	60	69	55	64	..	..
10 years	..	..	54	57	80	91	..	..	..	..	56	67	60	72	..	..	..	..
Overall	(23)		(55)		(29)		(40)		(7)		(154)		(57)		(48)		(49)	
1 year	83	83	82	82	86	88	58	61	57	64	75	77	72	74	73	75	82	83
3 years	48	48	55	56	52	55	35	42	43	60	47	51	44	48	48	51	51	54
5 years	43	44	49	51	45	50	25	34	14	26	40	45	39	46	40	45	41	45
8 years	38	39	41	44	45	54	22	37	..	..	35	44	35	47	35	43	..	..
10 years	19	20	36	39	34	43	11	22	..	..	24	33	24	35	..	..	..	..

RELATIVE SURVIVAL (%) BY AGE AND PERIOD

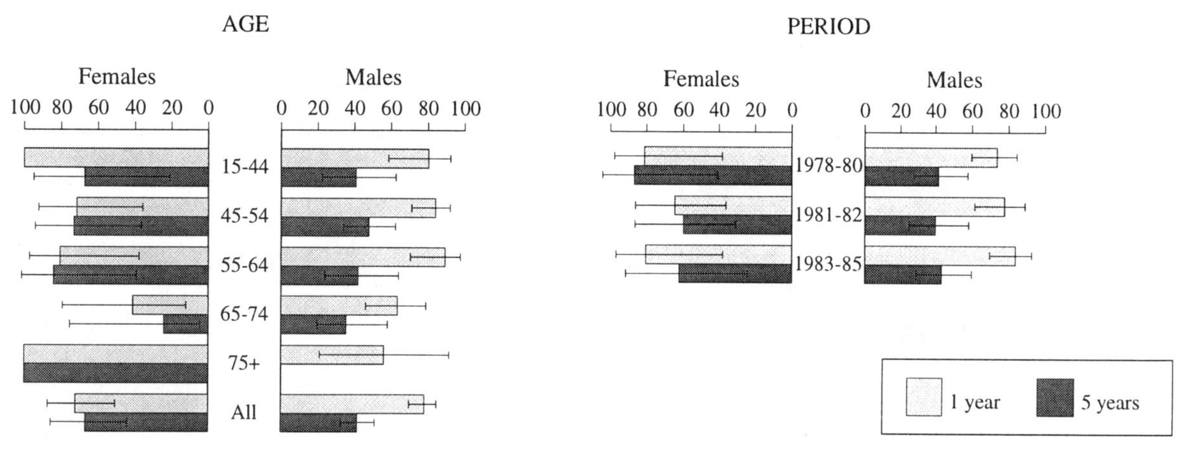

ORAL CAVITY

ITALIAN REGISTRIES

REGISTRY	NUMBER OF CASES			PERIOD OF DIAGNOSIS
	Males	Females	All	
Latina	15	1	16	1983-1984
Ragusa	4	3	7	1981-1984
Varese	118	24	142	1978-1985
Mean age (years)	61.8	67.5	62.7	

RELATIVE SURVIVAL (%)

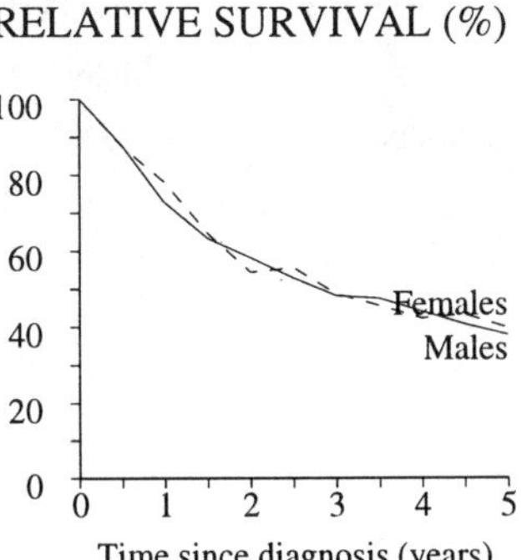

OBSERVED AND RELATIVE SURVIVAL (%) BY AGE AND PERIOD
(Number of cases in parentheses)

	AGE CLASS												PERIOD					
	15-44		45-54		55-64		65-74		75+		All		1978-80		1981-82		1983-85	
	obs	rel	obs	rel	obs	rel	obs	rel	obs	rel	obs	rel	obs	rel	obs	rel	obs	rel
Males	(8)		(30)		(39)		(44)		(16)		(137)		(49)		(27)		(61)	
1 year	75	75	60	60	92	94	68	71	38	43	70	73	67	71	59	61	77	79
3 years	50	50	37	38	51	55	52	61	6	9	43	48	41	48	33	36	49	54
5 years	50	51	33	35	36	40	34	44	0	0	31	38	33	43	26	29	33	38
8 years	50	51	22	24	24	29	21	33	0	0	22	30	18	29	22	28	23	30
10 years	50	52	22	25	18	24	15	29	0	0	18	28	14	25	22	29	..	..
Females	(3)		(1)		(6)		(7)		(11)		(28)		(5)		(8)		(15)	
1 year	100	100	0	0	33	34	100	100	82	90	75	78	40	42	100	100	73	76
3 years	67	67	0	0	17	17	71	75	36	49	43	49	0	0	50	59	53	59
5 years	67	67	0	0	17	17	71	78	9	15	32	40	0	0	25	33	47	55
8 years	..	..	0	0	17	18	26	30	0	0	16	23	0	0	25	38	..	..
10 years	..	..	0	0	17	18	..	..	0	0	16	25	0	0	25	41	..	..
Overall	(11)		(31)		(45)		(51)		(27)		(165)		(54)		(35)		(76)	
1 year	82	82	58	58	84	86	73	76	56	62	71	74	65	68	69	71	76	79
3 years	55	55	35	36	47	49	55	63	19	26	43	48	37	44	37	41	50	55
5 years	55	55	32	34	33	37	39	50	4	7	32	38	30	39	26	30	36	42
8 years	55	56	22	23	23	28	21	32	0	0	21	28	17	26	23	30	19	24
10 years	55	56	22	24	19	24	17	30	0	0	18	27	13	23	23	31	..	..

RELATIVE SURVIVAL (%) BY AGE AND PERIOD

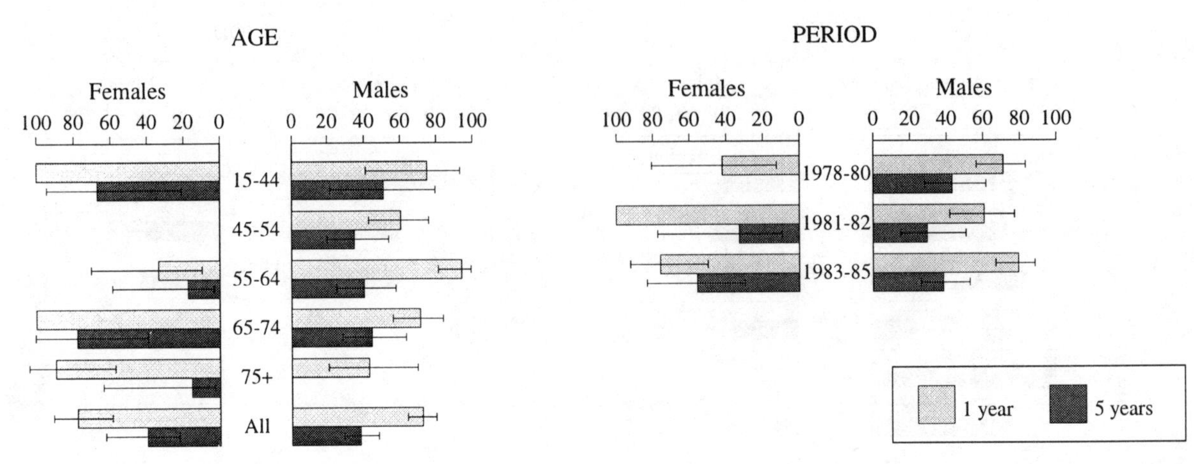

ORAL CAVITY

SCOTLAND

REGISTRY	NUMBER OF CASES			PERIOD OF DIAGNOSIS
	Males	Females	All	
Scotland	323	196	519	1978-1982
Mean age (years)	64.9	69.1	66.5	

RELATIVE SURVIVAL (%)

OBSERVED AND RELATIVE SURVIVAL (%) BY AGE AND PERIOD
(Number of cases in parentheses)

	AGE CLASS												PERIOD					
	15-44		45-54		55-64		65-74		75+		All		1978-80		1981-82		1983-85	
	obs	rel	obs	rel	obs	rel	obs	rel	obs	rel	obs	rel	obs	rel	obs	rel	obs	rel
Males	(18)		(42)		(90)		(96)		(77)		(323)		(177)		(146)		(0)	
1 year	89	89	79	79	74	76	64	67	49	57	67	70	64	68	69	73	..	..
3 years	72	73	50	52	53	57	42	50	19	30	42	50	40	48	45	53	..	..
5 years	67	68	45	48	42	48	27	37	13	28	33	43	33	44	32	42	..	..
8 years	67	68	39	44	30	37	20	34	9	34	25	40	26	42	..	..	..	..
10 years	..	..	30	34	26	35	17	36	0	0	20	36	21	37	..	..	..	..
Females	(7)		(20)		(34)		(59)		(76)		(196)		(110)		(86)		(0)	
1 year	71	72	90	90	76	77	78	80	53	58	69	72	65	69	73	76	..	..
3 years	71	72	80	81	53	55	59	66	33	45	51	59	45	54	57	65	..	..
5 years	71	72	80	82	38	41	51	61	22	38	41	53	38	50	45	57	..	..
8 years	71	73	65	68	33	38	39	53	15	38	32	49	29	45	..	..	..	..
10 years	..	..	..	..	..	..	..	..	15	51	30	53	27	48	..	..	..	..
Overall	(25)		(62)		(124)		(155)		(153)		(519)		(287)		(232)		(0)	
1 year	84	84	82	83	75	76	69	72	51	57	67	71	65	69	71	74	..	..
3 years	72	73	60	61	53	57	48	56	26	38	45	53	42	50	50	58	..	..
5 years	68	69	56	59	41	46	36	47	18	33	36	47	35	47	37	47	..	..
8 years	68	70	48	52	31	37	27	43	12	36	28	44	27	43	..	..	..	..
10 years	..	..	39	44	25	33	25	47	8	33	23	41	23	41	..	..	..	..

RELATIVE SURVIVAL (%) BY AGE AND PERIOD

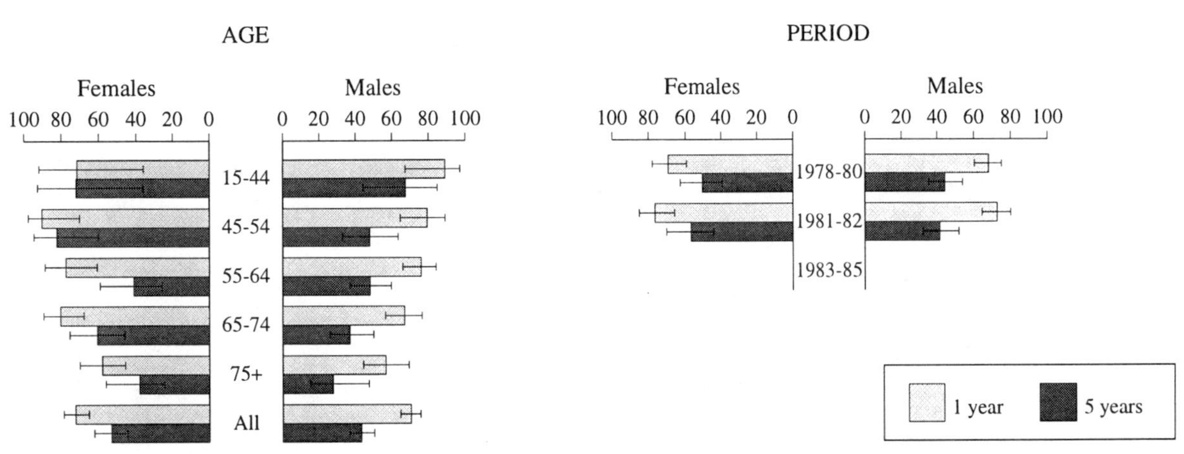

ORAL CAVITY

SWISS REGISTRIES

REGISTRY	NUMBER OF CASES			PERIOD OF DIAGNOSIS
	Males	Females	All	
Basel	20	7	27	1981-1984
Geneva	81	27	108	1978-1984
Mean age (years)	60.6	61.0	60.7	

RELATIVE SURVIVAL (%)

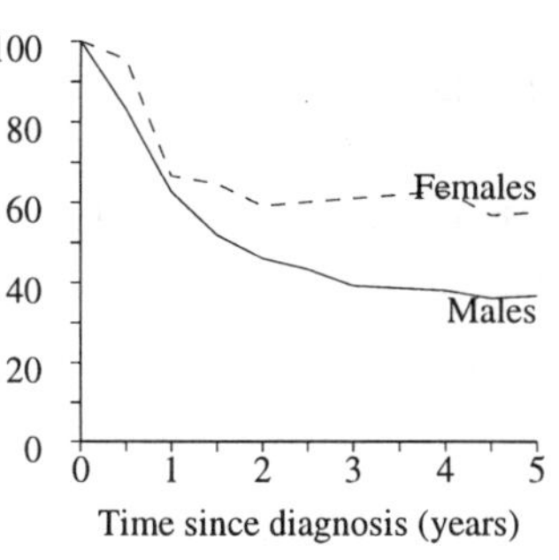

OBSERVED AND RELATIVE SURVIVAL (%) BY AGE AND PERIOD
(Number of cases in parentheses)

	AGE CLASS												PERIOD					
	15-44		45-54		55-64		65-74		75+		All		1978-80		1981-82		1983-85	
	obs	rel	obs	rel	obs	rel	obs	rel	obs	rel	obs	rel	obs	rel	obs	rel	obs	rel
Males	(8)		(21)		(35)		(23)		(14)		(101)		(37)		(37)		(27)	
1 year	25	25	52	53	71	72	78	81	43	47	61	63	64	66	51	52	70	73
3 years	13	13	29	29	43	45	45	51	29	39	36	39	44	48	31	34	32	35
5 years	13	13	29	29	40	43	30	37	29	50	32	37	35	40	28	33	32	38
8 years	..	..	..	..	..	..	..	..	29	77	21	27	..	..	19	24	..	..
10 years	..	..	..	..	..	..	..	..	..	..	..	..	..	..	..	..	..	..
Females	(6)		(9)		(4)		(7)		(8)		(34)		(10)		(19)		(5)	
1 year	83	83	78	78	75	76	71	73	25	28	65	67	80	81	58	60	60	63
3 years	83	84	66	66	75	77	57	61	13	17	56	61	70	74	52	57	40	48
5 years	83	84	53	54	75	78	57	64	0	0	50	58	60	65	47	54	40	55
8 years	..	..	53	54	..	..	..	..	0	0	50	66	..	..	47	60	..	..
10 years	..	..	..	..	..	..	..	..	0	0	..	..	..	..	..	..	..	..
Overall	(14)		(30)		(39)		(30)		(22)		(135)		(47)		(56)		(32)	
1 year	50	50	60	60	71	72	76	79	36	40	62	64	68	69	53	55	69	71
3 years	43	43	40	40	47	49	48	54	23	31	41	45	50	54	38	42	34	37
5 years	43	43	36	37	44	47	37	45	18	32	36	42	40	46	35	40	34	40
8 years	..	..	36	38	..	..	..	..	18	50	26	34	..	..	26	33	..	..
10 years	..	..	..	..	..	..	..	..	..	..	..	..	..	..	..	..	..	..

RELATIVE SURVIVAL (%) BY AGE AND PERIOD

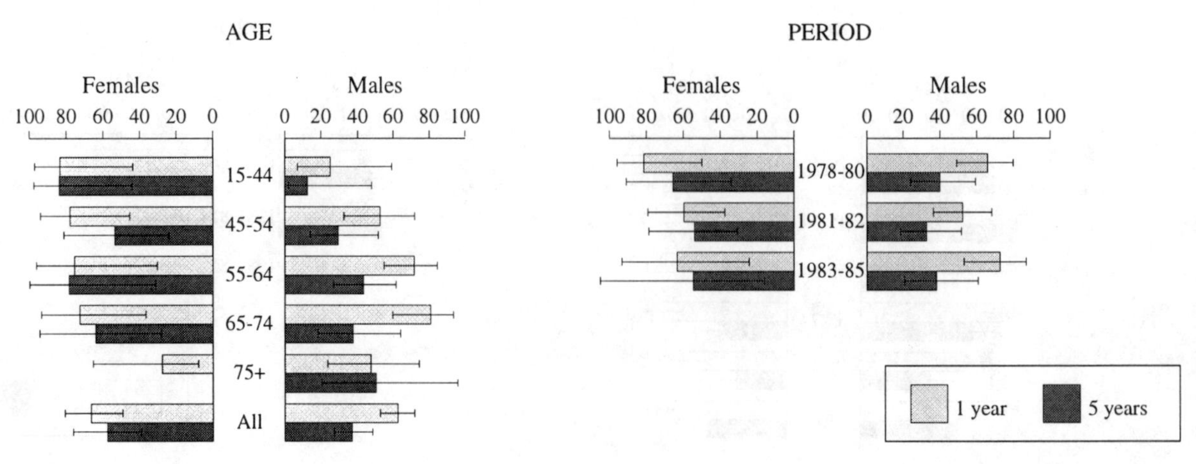

ORAL CAVITY

DUTCH REGISTRIES

REGISTRY	NUMBER OF CASES			PERIOD OF DIAGNOSIS
	Males	Females	All	
Eindhoven	48	24	72	1978-1985
Mean age (years)	63.6	63.7	63.7	

RELATIVE SURVIVAL (%)
(Both sexes)

OBSERVED AND RELATIVE SURVIVAL (%) BY PERIOD AND SEX
(Number of cases in parentheses)

	PERIOD						SEX					
	1978-80		1981-82		1983-85		Males		Females		All	
	obs	rel	obs	rel	obs	rel	obs	rel	obs	rel	obs	rel
N. Cases	(26)		(18)		(28)		(48)		(24)		(72)	
1 year	69	72	56	60	68	70	65	68	67	69	65	68
3 years	54	60	50	63	68	76	54	63	67	75	58	67
5 years	46	56	39	57	61	76	44	58	57	70	49	62
8 years	29	39	..	..	..	..	17	27	57	80	32	49
10 years	29	43	..	..	..	..	..	..	57	87	32	54

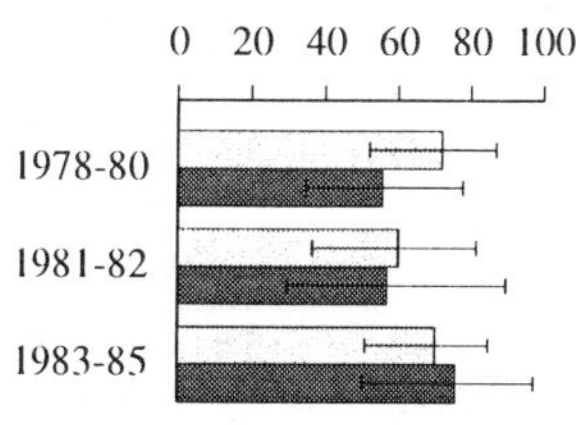

ESTONIA

REGISTRY	NUMBER OF CASES			PERIOD OF DIAGNOSIS
	Males	Females	All	
Estonia	89	19	108	1978-1984
Mean age (years)	56.2	67.0	58.1	

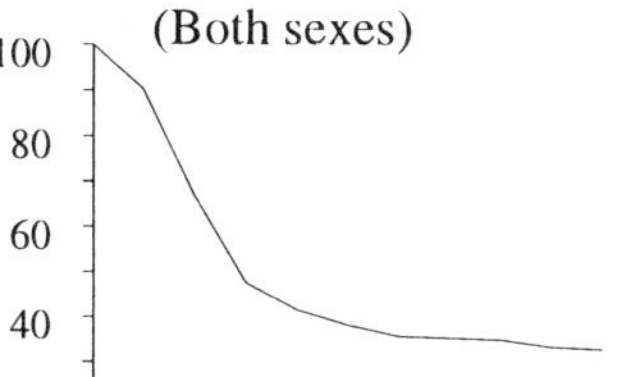

OBSERVED AND RELATIVE SURVIVAL (%) BY PERIOD AND SEX
(Number of cases in parentheses)

	PERIOD						SEX					
	1978-80		1981-82		1983-85		Males		Females		All	
	obs	rel	obs	rel	obs	rel	obs	rel	obs	rel	obs	rel
N. Cases	(51)		(21)		(36)		(89)		(19)		(108)	
1 year	59	61	76	79	67	68	67	69	53	55	65	67
3 years	33	37	33	38	30	33	32	35	32	37	32	36
5 years	24	28	33	42	30	35	28	33	26	34	28	33
8 years	16	21	14	20	..	..	12	16	26	41	15	20
10 years	13	19	..	..	..	..	12	17	13	24	13	19

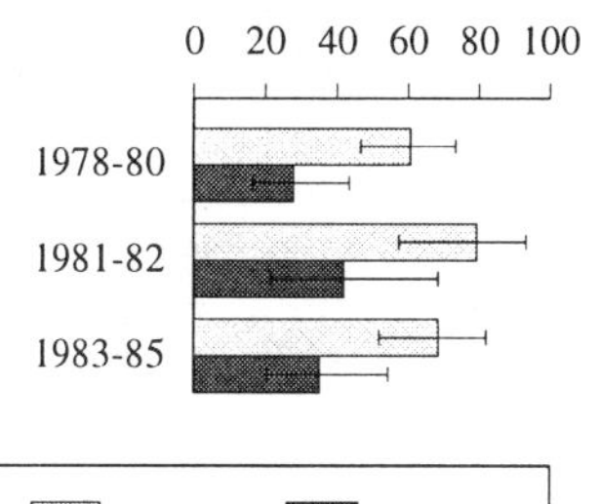

ORAL CAVITY

POLISH REGISTRIES

REGISTRY	NUMBER OF CASES			PERIOD OF DIAGNOSIS
	Males	Females	All	
Cracow	49	14	63	1978-1984
Mean age (years)	57.8	62.6	58.9	

RELATIVE SURVIVAL (%)
(Both sexes)

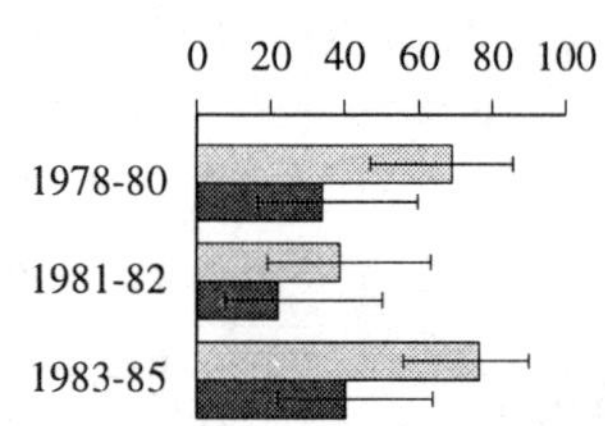

OBSERVED AND RELATIVE SURVIVAL (%) BY PERIOD AND SEX
(Number of cases in parentheses)

	PERIOD						SEX					
	1978-80		1981-82		1983-85		Males		Females		All	
	obs	rel	obs	rel	obs	rel	obs	rel	obs	rel	obs	rel
N. Cases	(21)		(17)		(25)		(49)		(14)		(63)	
1 year	67	69	38	39	75	76	58	60	77	79	62	64
3 years	33	37	25	27	48	52	34	38	46	50	37	40
5 years	29	34	19	22	35	40	24	28	46	53	29	33
8 years	19	25	19	25	27	34	16	21	46	59	23	29
10 years	12	18	..	..	..	..	11	15	46	64	18	26

0 20 40 60 80 100
1978-80
1981-82
1983-85

SPANISH REGISTRIES

REGISTRY	NUMBER OF CASES			PERIOD OF DIAGNOSIS
	Males	Females	All	
Tarragona	13	0	13	1985-1985
Mean age (years)	68.0	..	68.0	

RELATIVE SURVIVAL (%)
(Both sexes)

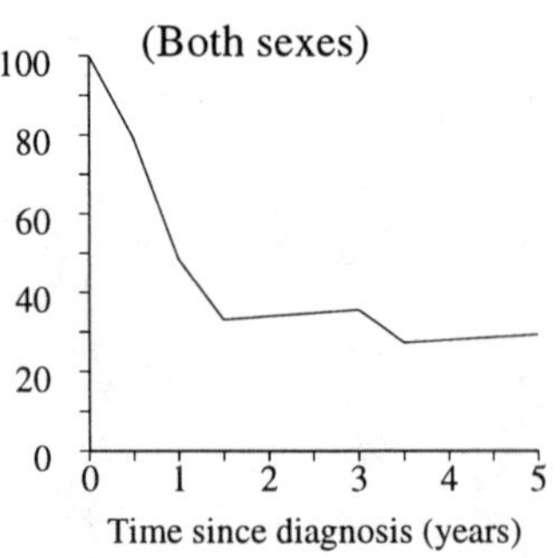

OBSERVED AND RELATIVE SURVIVAL (%) BY PERIOD AND SEX
(Number of cases in parentheses)

	PERIOD						SEX					
	1978-80		1981-82		1983-85		Males		Females		All	
	obs	rel	obs	rel	obs	rel	obs	rel	obs	rel	obs	rel
N. Cases	(0)		(0)		(13)		(13)		(0)		(13)	
1 year	..	..	..	..	46	48	46	48	..	..	46	48
3 years	..	..	..	..	31	36	31	36	..	..	31	36
5 years	..	..	..	..	23	29	23	29	..	..	23	29
8 years	..	..	..	..	..	..	..	..	..	..	..	..
10 years	..	..	..	..	..	..	..	..	..	..	..	..

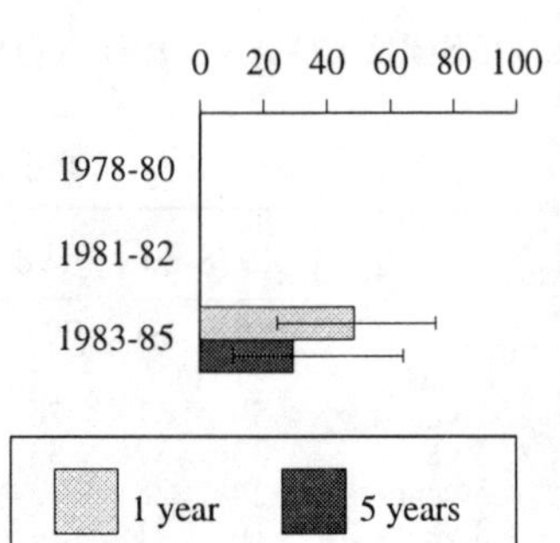

ORAL CAVITY

EUROPEAN REGISTRIES
Unweighted analysis

REGISTRY	CASES Males	Females	All
DENMARK	423	375	798
DUTCH REGISTRIES	48	24	72
ENGLISH REGISTRIES	1154	694	1848
ESTONIA	89	19	108
FINLAND	151	146	297
FRENCH REGISTRIES	190	20	210
GERMAN REGISTRIES	133	21	154
ITALIAN REGISTRIES	137	28	165
POLISH REGISTRIES	49	14	63
SCOTLAND	323	196	519
SPANISH REGISTRIES	13	0	13
SWISS REGISTRIES	101	34	135
Mean age (years)	63.0	68.0	64.8

RELATIVE SURVIVAL (%)
(Age-standardized)

Females: 100 80 60 40 20 0 — Males: 0 20 40 60 80 100

DK, ENG, FIN, F, D, I, SCO, CH, EUR

OBSERVED AND RELATIVE SURVIVAL (%) BY AGE AND PERIOD
(Number of cases in parentheses)

	AGE CLASS 15-44 obs	rel	45-54 obs	rel	55-64 obs	rel	65-74 obs	rel	75+ obs	rel	All obs	rel	PERIOD 1978-80 obs	rel	1981-82 obs	rel	1983-85 obs	rel
Males	(180)		(498)		(851)		(778)		(504)		(2811)		(1103)		(846)		(862)	
1 year	80	80	74	74	71	72	67	70	47	54	67	70	66	69	65	67	70	73
3 years	53	54	49	50	46	49	44	52	22	33	42	48	42	48	40	45	45	51
5 years	47	48	43	45	38	42	33	43	16	32	34	43	34	43	32	40	37	45
8 years	44	45	34	37	29	36	22	37	9	31	26	37	26	38	24	34	26	37
10 years	38	40	28	32	24	31	18	35	5	27	21	33	21	34	19	31	..	..
Females	(81)		(180)		(319)		(428)		(563)		(1571)		(633)		(493)		(445)	
1 year	85	85	87	87	78	79	76	78	54	60	70	73	68	71	72	75	72	75
3 years	69	69	77	78	57	59	55	60	32	43	51	58	48	55	52	59	54	61
5 years	65	66	71	73	50	53	46	53	23	39	42	53	41	51	43	53	44	54
8 years	61	62	63	66	43	47	36	47	16	41	35	50	33	49	34	49	38	53
10 years	44	45	63	67	40	46	25	37	12	43	29	48	27	45	34	54	..	..
Overall	(261)		(678)		(1170)		(1206)		(1067)		(4382)		(1736)		(1339)		(1307)	
1 year	82	82	77	78	73	74	70	73	51	57	68	71	66	70	67	70	71	74
3 years	58	59	56	58	49	52	48	55	27	39	45	52	44	51	44	50	48	54
5 years	53	53	51	53	41	45	37	47	20	36	37	46	36	46	36	45	39	48
8 years	49	50	42	45	33	39	27	41	13	37	29	42	29	42	28	40	30	43
10 years	41	43	37	41	28	36	21	36	9	37	24	38	23	38	25	39	..	..

RELATIVE SURVIVAL (%) BY AGE AND PERIOD

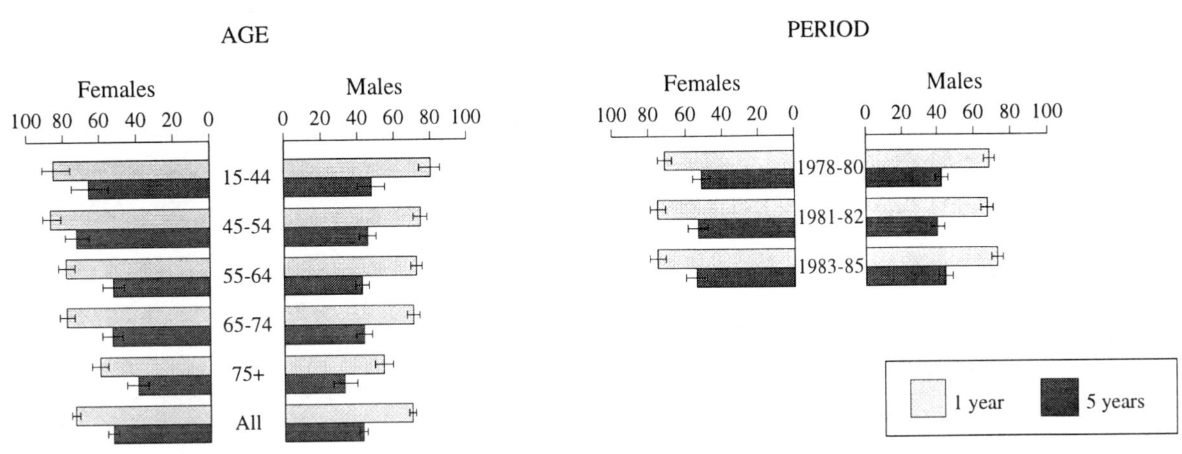

OROPHARYNX

DENMARK

REGISTRY	NUMBER OF CASES			PERIOD OF DIAGNOSIS
	Males	Females	All	
Denmark	310	145	455	1978-1984
Mean age (years)	62.0	65.3	63.1	

RELATIVE SURVIVAL (%)

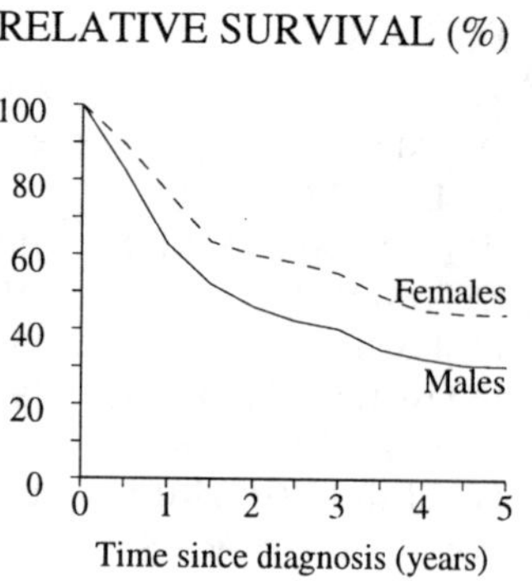

OBSERVED AND RELATIVE SURVIVAL (%) BY AGE AND PERIOD
(Number of cases in parentheses)

	AGE CLASS												PERIOD					
	15-44		45-54		55-64		65-74		75+		All		1978-80		1981-82		1983-85	
	obs	rel	obs	rel	obs	rel	obs	rel	obs	rel	obs	rel	obs	rel	obs	rel	obs	rel
Males	(27)		(55)		(93)		(89)		(46)		(310)		(127)		(88)		(95)	
1 year	85	85	58	59	58	59	66	69	43	49	61	63	60	62	61	63	61	63
3 years	59	60	36	37	29	31	45	51	20	28	36	40	32	36	40	44	38	43
5 years	48	49	29	30	22	25	27	34	10	20	25	31	23	28	31	36	23	28
8 years	44	45	25	27	17	21	19	29	10	32	20	28	19	26	25	34	..	..
10 years	44	45	14	16	17	22	11	21	..	..	16	24	15	22	..	..	..	..
Females	(7)		(20)		(38)		(42)		(38)		(145)		(62)		(38)		(45)	
1 year	71	72	75	75	74	74	79	80	71	77	74	77	71	73	82	85	73	75
3 years	57	57	70	71	66	68	40	44	34	44	50	55	47	51	63	70	44	48
5 years	57	58	70	72	53	56	26	30	16	24	38	44	32	38	50	60	36	41
8 years	57	58	55	58	42	46	26	33	..	..	31	41	27	36	34	46	..	..
10 years	..	..	55	59	42	48	26	36	..	..	31	45	27	39	..	..	..	..
Overall	(34)		(75)		(131)		(131)		(84)		(455)		(189)		(126)		(140)	
1 year	82	83	63	63	63	64	70	73	56	62	65	67	63	66	67	70	65	67
3 years	59	59	45	46	40	42	44	49	26	36	41	45	37	41	47	52	40	44
5 years	50	51	40	42	31	34	26	32	13	22	29	35	26	31	37	44	27	33
8 years	47	48	33	36	24	29	21	30	9	25	24	32	22	29	27	37	..	..
10 years	47	48	26	29	24	30	15	25	..	..	21	31	19	28	..	..	..	..

RELATIVE SURVIVAL (%) BY AGE AND PERIOD

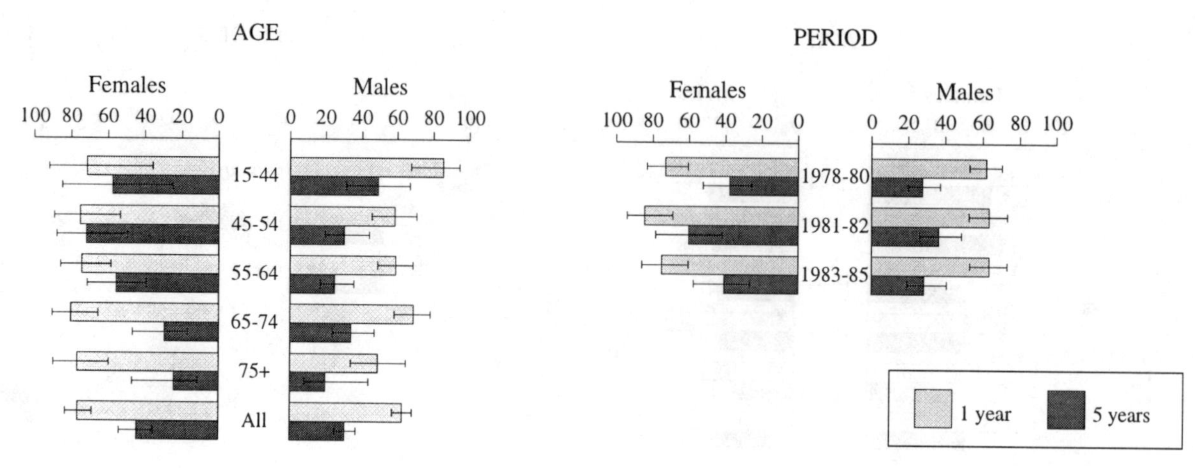

OROPHARYNX

ENGLISH REGISTRIES

REGISTRY	NUMBER OF CASES			PERIOD OF DIAGNOSIS
	Males	Females	All	
East Anglia	47	27	74	1979-1984
Mersey	97	52	149	1978-1984
South Thames	186	81	267	1978-1984
Wessex	13	4	17	1983-1984
West Midlands	159	54	213	1979-1984
Yorkshire	103	65	168	1978-1984
Mean age (years)	63.8	66.3	64.6	

RELATIVE SURVIVAL (%)

100
80
60
40
20
0
Females
Males
0 1 2 3 4 5
Time since diagnosis (years)

OBSERVED AND RELATIVE SURVIVAL (%) BY AGE AND PERIOD
(Number of cases in parentheses)

	AGE CLASS												PERIOD					
	15-44		45-54		55-64		65-74		75+		All		1978-80		1981-82		1983-85	
	obs	rel	obs	rel	obs	rel	obs	rel	obs	rel	obs	rel	obs	rel	obs	rel	obs	rel
Males	(29)		(105)		(168)		(207)		(96)		(605)		(251)		(187)		(167)	
1 year	83	83	70	71	62	63	61	64	32	37	59	62	61	64	57	60	59	62
3 years	59	59	41	42	31	33	37	43	16	24	34	39	36	41	30	34	35	40
5 years	52	52	35	37	27	30	29	37	9	19	27	34	28	35	23	30	31	38
8 years	48	49	30	33	22	27	22	35	2	7	22	31	24	35	17	25	23	32
10 years	48	50	26	29	17	23	17	33	..	..	18	29	20	33	13	20	..	..
Females	(11)		(39)		(71)		(84)		(78)		(283)		(111)		(76)		(96)	
1 year	91	91	72	72	65	65	67	68	40	44	60	63	59	62	54	56	67	69
3 years	82	82	38	39	42	43	49	53	19	26	39	43	38	43	38	43	40	44
5 years	73	73	36	37	36	38	38	44	17	28	33	39	31	37	32	39	35	43
8 years	73	74	33	34	22	24	27	36	7	18	23	32	24	32	23	32	18	24
10 years	73	74	33	35	17	20	23	34	2	8	20	30	20	29	20	29	..	..
Overall	(40)		(144)		(239)		(291)		(174)		(888)		(362)		(263)		(263)	
1 year	85	85	71	71	63	64	63	65	36	40	60	62	61	63	56	59	62	64
3 years	65	65	40	41	35	36	40	46	17	25	35	40	37	41	32	37	37	41
5 years	58	58	35	37	30	33	31	40	13	24	29	36	29	36	26	32	32	40
8 years	55	56	31	33	23	27	24	36	4	12	22	32	24	34	19	27	22	30
10 years	55	56	28	31	17	22	19	33	2	9	19	29	20	32	15	23	..	..

RELATIVE SURVIVAL (%) BY AGE AND PERIOD

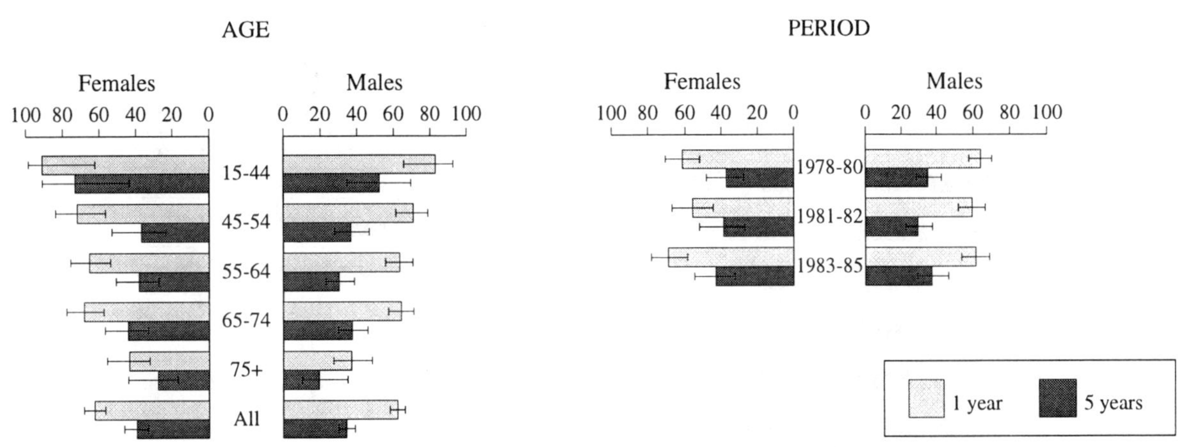

OROPHARYNX

FRENCH REGISTRIES

REGISTRY	NUMBER OF CASES			PERIOD OF DIAGNOSIS
	Males	Females	All	
Amiens	56	8	64	1983-1984
Doubs	216	10	226	1978-1985
Mean age (years)	58.1	58.2	58.1	

RELATIVE SURVIVAL (%)

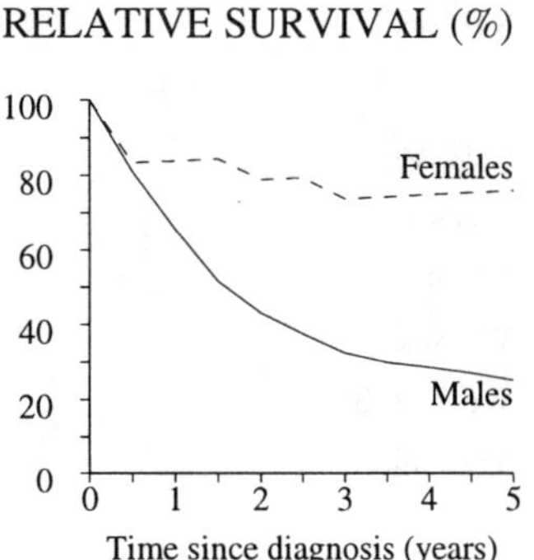

OBSERVED AND RELATIVE SURVIVAL (%) BY AGE AND PERIOD
(Number of cases in parentheses)

	AGE CLASS												PERIOD					
	15-44		45-54		55-64		65-74		75+		All		1978-80		1981-82		1983-85	
	obs	rel	obs	rel	obs	rel	obs	rel	obs	rel	obs	rel	obs	rel	obs	rel	obs	rel
Males	(19)		(89)		(94)		(48)		(22)		(272)		(53)		(60)		(159)	
1 year	58	58	83	84	61	62	46	48	44	48	64	66	75	77	53	54	64	66
3 years	26	27	46	47	25	26	21	24	15	20	30	32	32	34	25	27	32	34
5 years	14	14	34	36	16	18	19	23	10	16	22	25	21	23	13	15	27	31
8 years	..	..	24	26	..	..	0	0	..	..	12	14	8	10	8	9	..	..
10 years	..	..	24	26	..	..	0	0	..	..	12	15	8	11	..	..	..	..
Females	(1)		(5)		(9)		(2)		(1)		(18)		(4)		(2)		(12)	
1 year	100	100	80	80	88	89	50	51	100	100	83	84	50	51	100	100	91	92
3 years	100	100	80	81	63	64	50	53	100	100	71	74	50	55	100	100	73	75
5 years	100	100	80	82	63	65	50	56	100	100	71	76	50	59	100	100	73	77
8 years	..	..	..	..	..	..	..	..	0	0	..	..	0	0	..	..	..	..
10 years	..	..	..	..	..	..	..	..	0	0	..	..	0	0	..	..	..	..
Overall	(20)		(94)		(103)		(50)		(23)		(290)		(57)		(62)		(171)	
1 year	60	60	83	84	64	64	46	48	46	51	65	67	74	75	55	56	66	68
3 years	30	30	47	49	28	29	22	25	19	25	33	35	33	36	27	29	34	37
5 years	19	19	37	39	21	22	20	25	14	24	25	28	22	25	16	18	30	34
8 years	..	..	27	29	..	..	0	0	..	..	15	18	8	10	11	13	..	..
10 years	..	..	27	30	..	..	0	0	..	..	15	19	8	10	..	..	..	..

RELATIVE SURVIVAL (%) BY AGE AND PERIOD

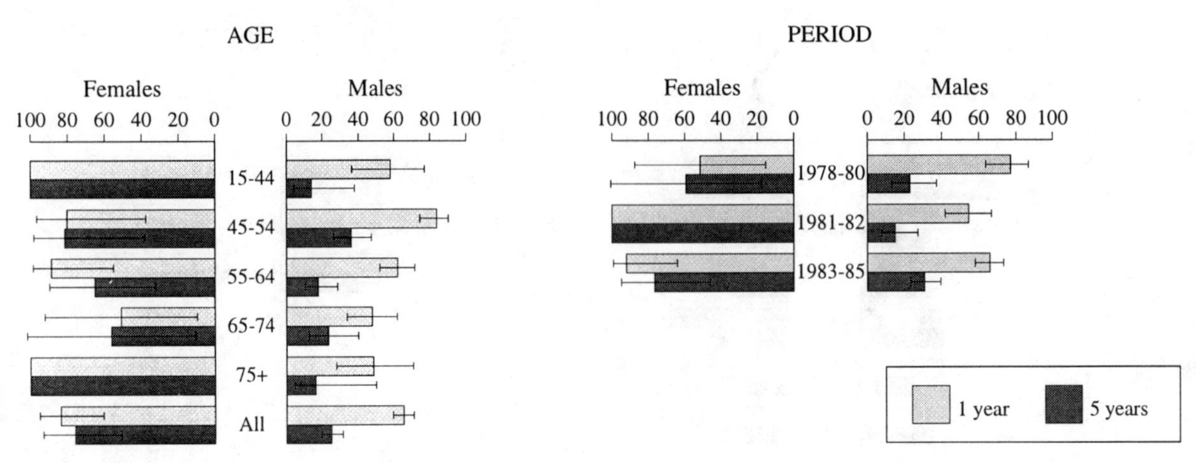

OROPHARYNX

ITALIAN REGISTRIES

REGISTRY	NUMBER OF CASES Males	Females	All	PERIOD OF DIAGNOSIS
Latina	5	0	5	1983-1984
Ragusa	6	0	6	1981-1984
Varese	151	16	167	1978-1985
Mean age (years)	61.0	64.9	61.3	

RELATIVE SURVIVAL (%)

Females
Males
Time since diagnosis (years)

OBSERVED AND RELATIVE SURVIVAL (%) BY AGE AND PERIOD
(Number of cases in parentheses)

	AGE CLASS 15-44 obs	rel	45-54 obs	rel	55-64 obs	rel	65-74 obs	rel	75+ obs	rel	All obs	rel	PERIOD 1978-80 obs	rel	1981-82 obs	rel	1983-85 obs	rel
Males	(7)		(35)		(64)		(37)		(19)		(162)		(55)		(48)		(59)	
1 year	57	57	63	63	58	59	68	71	63	71	62	64	51	53	73	75	63	64
3 years	29	29	26	26	20	22	32	38	21	30	25	27	24	27	25	27	25	28
5 years	14	15	23	24	17	19	16	21	11	20	17	21	15	18	21	24	17	20
8 years	14	15	17	19	12	15	8	13	11	32	12	16	11	16	13	16	13	17
10 years	14	15	..	..	12	16	5	10	0	0	8	12	7	12	..	..	..	..
Females	(0)		(3)		(5)		(4)		(4)		(16)		(5)		(3)		(8)	
1 year	..	..	67	67	80	81	50	51	50	55	63	64	40	41	67	69	75	77
3 years	..	..	67	67	80	82	50	53	0	0	50	55	40	44	33	36	63	69
5 years	..	..	67	68	60	62	50	56	0	0	44	51	40	46	33	39	50	59
8 years	..	..	67	69	20	21	50	60	0	0	27	35	40	50	33	44	0	0
10 years	..	..	67	69	20	22	..	..	0	0	27	37	40	53	..	..	0	0
Overall	(7)		(38)		(69)		(41)		(23)		(178)		(60)		(51)		(67)	
1 year	57	57	63	64	59	61	66	69	61	68	62	64	50	52	73	75	64	66
3 years	29	29	29	30	25	26	34	39	17	25	27	30	25	28	25	28	30	33
5 years	14	15	26	27	20	23	20	25	9	16	20	23	17	21	22	25	21	24
8 years	14	15	21	22	12	15	11	17	9	26	13	18	13	19	14	18	12	16
10 years	14	15	14	15	12	16	8	14	0	0	10	15	10	16	..	..	..	..

RELATIVE SURVIVAL (%) BY AGE AND PERIOD

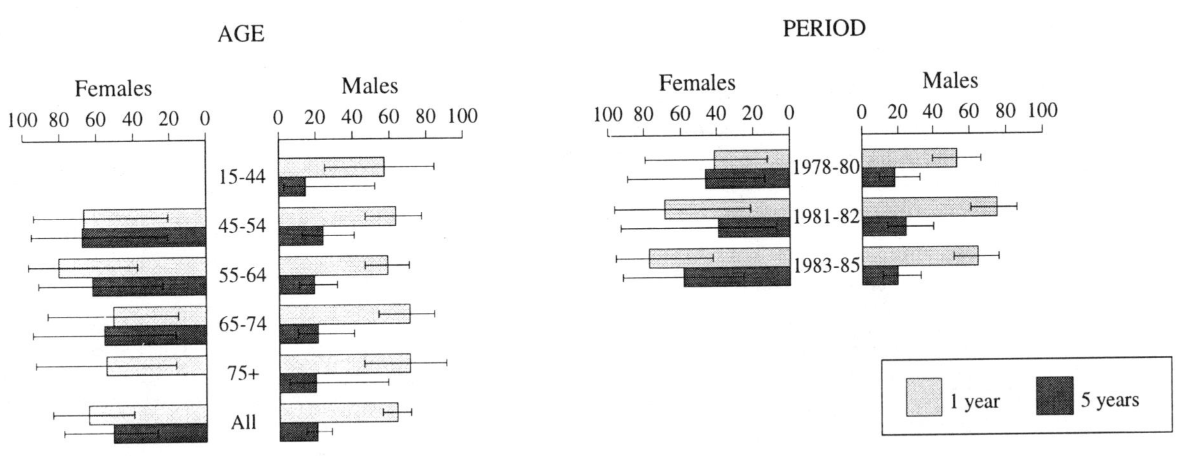

OROPHARYNX

DUTCH REGISTRIES

REGISTRY	NUMBER OF CASES			PERIOD OF DIAGNOSIS
	Males	Females	All	
Eindhoven	24	10	34	1978-1985
Mean age (years)	63.7	56.9	61.7	

RELATIVE SURVIVAL (%)
(Both sexes)

Time since diagnosis (years)

OBSERVED AND RELATIVE SURVIVAL (%) BY PERIOD AND SEX
(Number of cases in parentheses)

	PERIOD						SEX					
	1978-80		1981-82		1983-85		Males		Females		All	
	obs	rel	obs	rel	obs	rel	obs	rel	obs	rel	obs	rel
N. Cases	(10)		(8)		(16)		(24)		(10)		(34)	
1 year	20	21	88	89	69	72	63	65	50	51	59	61
3 years	10	11	63	65	43	49	32	37	50	52	38	42
5 years	10	12	63	68	43	53	32	40	50	55	38	45
8 years	10	14	..	..	..	..	..	..	50	60	28	38
10 years	..	..	..	..	..	..	..	..	..	..	..	..

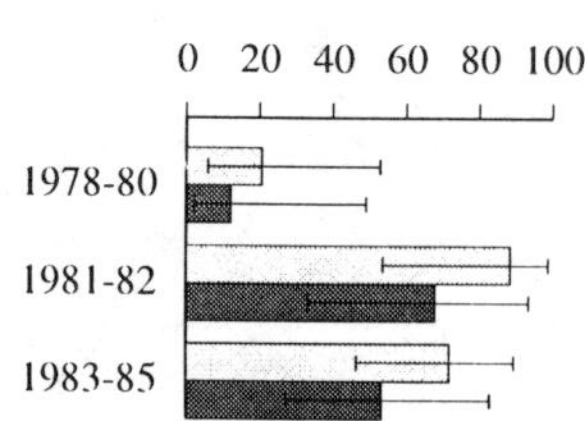

ESTONIA

REGISTRY	NUMBER OF CASES			PERIOD OF DIAGNOSIS
	Males	Females	All	
Estonia	52	13	65	1978-1984
Mean age (years)	55.3	62.8	56.8	

RELATIVE SURVIVAL (%)
(Both sexes)

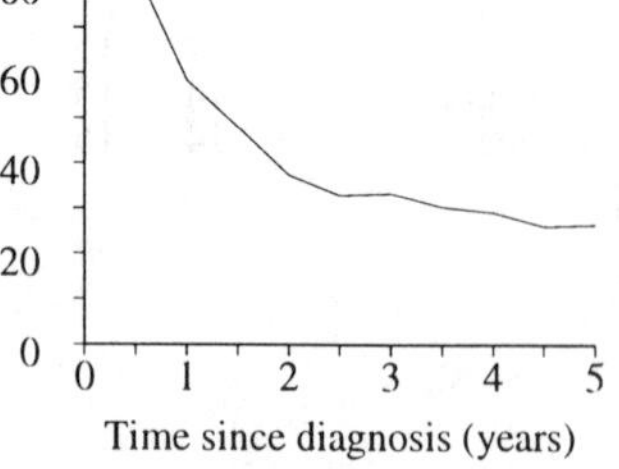

Time since diagnosis (years)

OBSERVED AND RELATIVE SURVIVAL (%) BY PERIOD AND SEX
(Number of cases in parentheses)

	PERIOD						SEX					
	1978-80		1981-82		1983-85		Males		Females		All	
	obs	rel	obs	rel	obs	rel	obs	rel	obs	rel	obs	rel
N. Cases	(18)		(21)		(26)		(52)		(13)		(65)	
1 year	67	68	57	59	50	51	56	57	62	64	57	58
3 years	50	55	33	37	15	16	27	29	46	51	31	33
5 years	39	46	24	28	12	13	17	20	46	54	23	27
8 years	28	37	10	13	..	..	8	10	38	50	14	18
10 years	22	32	..	..	..	..	0	0	38	55	11	16

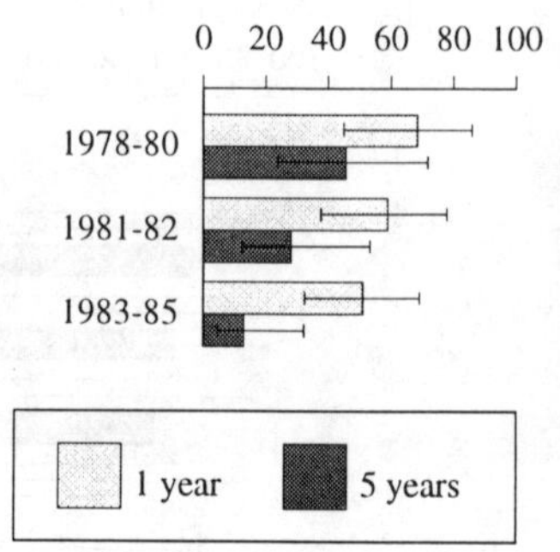

OROPHARYNX

FINLAND

REGISTRY	NUMBER OF CASES			PERIOD OF DIAGNOSIS
	Males	Females	All	
Finland	80	33	113	1978-1984
Mean age (years)	62.2	69.4	64.3	

RELATIVE SURVIVAL (%)

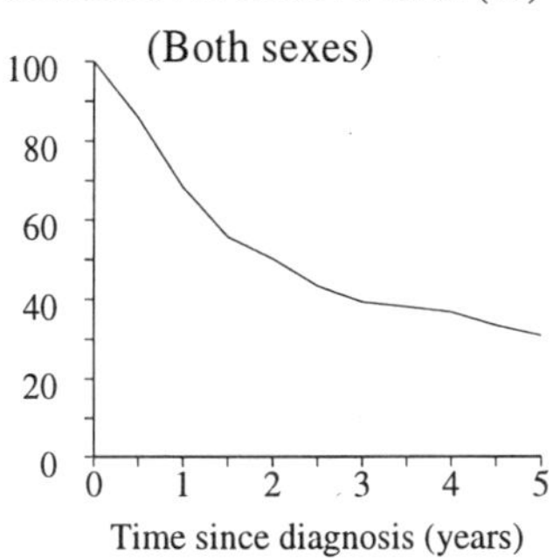

OBSERVED AND RELATIVE SURVIVAL (%) BY PERIOD AND SEX
(Number of cases in parentheses)

	PERIOD						SEX					
	1978-80		1981-82		1983-85		Males		Females		All	
	obs	rel	obs	rel	obs	rel	obs	rel	obs	rel	obs	rel
N. Cases	(47)		(32)		(34)		(80)		(33)		(113)	
1 year	66	69	66	69	65	67	65	68	67	70	65	68
3 years	30	34	31	36	44	49	30	34	45	52	35	39
5 years	19	24	25	32	32	39	24	29	27	35	25	31
8 years	13	19	25	38	29	39	18	26	27	41	21	30
10 years	11	17	21	35	..	..	13	21	22	37	17	27

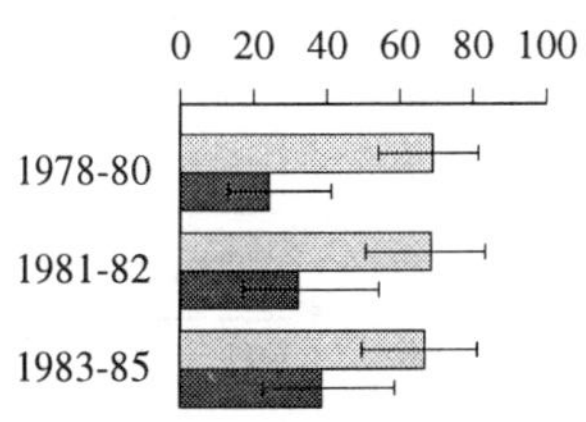

GERMAN REGISTRIES

REGISTRY	NUMBER OF CASES			PERIOD OF DIAGNOSIS
	Males	Females	All	
Saarland	83	34	117	1978-1984
Mean age (years)	54.0	60.1	55.8	

RELATIVE SURVIVAL (%)

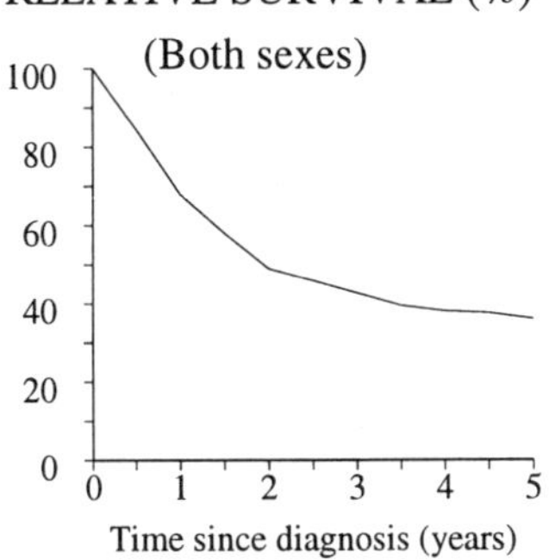

OBSERVED AND RELATIVE SURVIVAL (%) BY PERIOD AND SEX
(Number of cases in parentheses)

	PERIOD						SEX					
	1978-80		1981-82		1983-85		Males		Females		All	
	obs	rel	obs	rel	obs	rel	obs	rel	obs	rel	obs	rel
N. Cases	(48)		(37)		(32)		(83)		(34)		(117)	
1 year	73	74	57	58	69	70	64	65	74	75	67	68
3 years	54	57	24	26	38	40	39	41	44	47	40	43
5 years	48	53	19	21	25	28	31	35	35	40	32	36
8 years	29	34	..	..	..	..	18	22	22	26	19	23
10 years	29	36	..	..	..	..	18	23	22	28	19	24

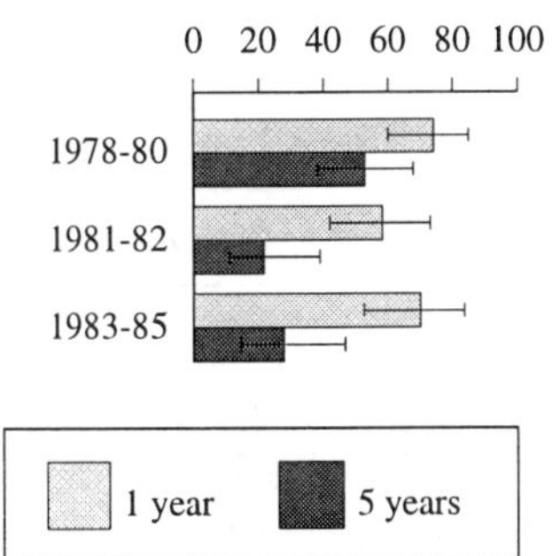

OROPHARYNX

POLISH REGISTRIES

REGISTRY	NUMBER OF CASES			PERIOD OF DIAGNOSIS
	Males	Females	All	
Cracow	27	21	48	1978-1984
Mean age (years)	59.0	57.8	58.5	

RELATIVE SURVIVAL (%)
(Both sexes)

Time since diagnosis (years)

OBSERVED AND RELATIVE SURVIVAL (%) BY PERIOD AND SEX
(Number of cases in parentheses)

	PERIOD						SEX					
	1978-80		1981-82		1983-85		Males		Females		All	
	obs	rel	obs	rel	obs	rel	obs	rel	obs	rel	obs	rel
N. Cases	(17)		(16)		(15)		(27)		(21)		(48)	
1 year	71	72	69	71	65	67	56	57	85	87	68	70
3 years	53	56	38	42	34	37	28	31	60	64	42	46
5 years	53	58	31	37	25	30	20	24	60	66	38	44
8 years	40	48	25	34	25	33	16	22	50	58	30	39
10 years	27	34	25	37	..	..	10	14	37	46	21	29

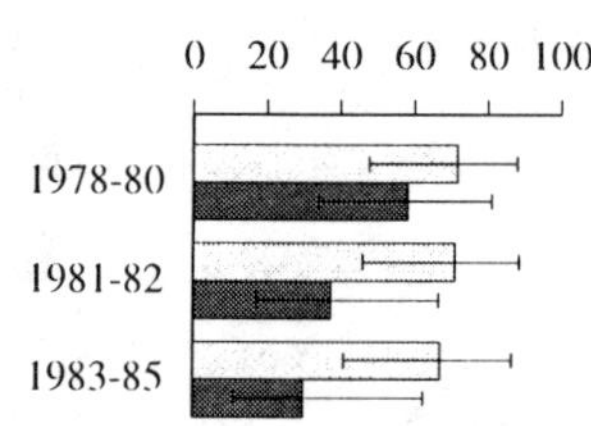

SCOTLAND

REGISTRY	NUMBER OF CASES			PERIOD OF DIAGNOSIS
	Males	Females	All	
Scotland	99	47	146	1978-1982
Mean age (years)	65.4	63.5	64.8	

RELATIVE SURVIVAL (%)
(Both sexes)

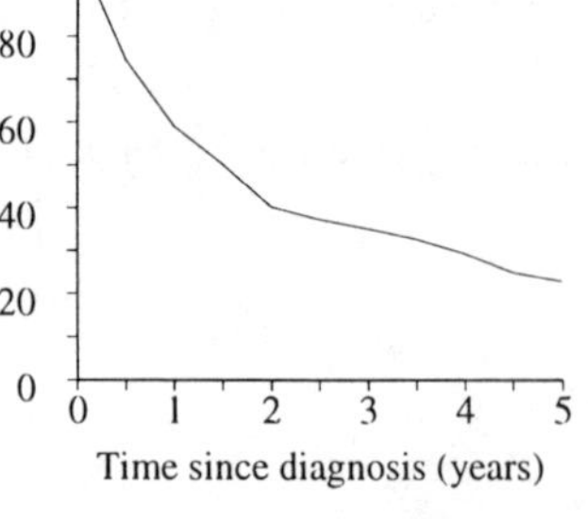

Time since diagnosis (years)

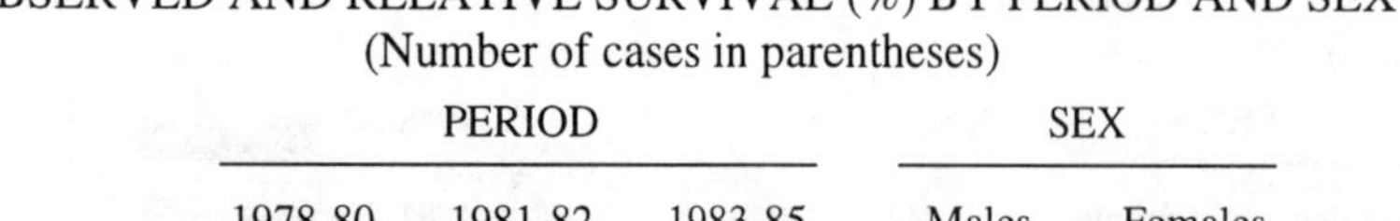

OBSERVED AND RELATIVE SURVIVAL (%) BY PERIOD AND SEX
(Number of cases in parentheses)

	PERIOD						SEX					
	1978-80		1981-82		1983-85		Males		Females		All	
	obs	rel	obs	rel	obs	rel	obs	rel	obs	rel	obs	rel
N. Cases	(91)		(55)		(0)		(99)		(47)		(146)	
1 year	57	60	55	57	..	..	57	60	55	57	56	59
3 years	32	38	27	31	..	..	32	39	26	28	30	35
5 years	21	28	13	16	..	..	16	22	21	25	18	23
8 years	20	31	..	..	..	..	14	23	19	24	16	23
10 years	20	35	..	..	..	..	14	26	..	..	16	26

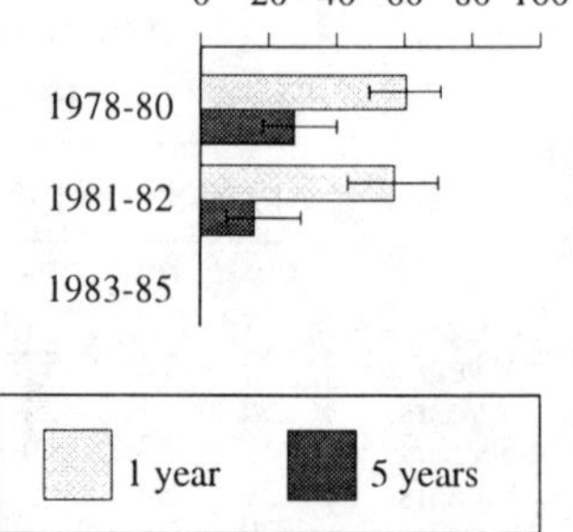

OROPHARYNX

SPANISH REGISTRIES

REGISTRY	NUMBER OF CASES			PERIOD OF DIAGNOSIS
	Males	Females	All	
Tarragona	5	0	5	1985-1985
Mean age (years)	52.0	..	52.0	

RELATIVE SURVIVAL (%)
(Both sexes)

OBSERVED AND RELATIVE SURVIVAL (%) BY PERIOD AND SEX
(Number of cases in parentheses)

	PERIOD						SEX					
	1978-80		1981-82		1983-85		Males		Females		All	
	obs	rel	obs	rel	obs	rel	obs	rel	obs	rel	obs	rel
N. Cases	(0)		(0)		(5)		(5)		(0)		(5)	
1 year	..	..	..	..	60	61	60	61	..	..	60	61
3 years	..	..	..	..	40	41	40	41	..	..	40	41
5 years	..	..	..	..	40	43	40	43	..	..	40	43
8 years	..	..	..	..	..	..	..	..	..	..	..	..
10 years	..	..	..	..	..	..	..	..	..	..	..	..

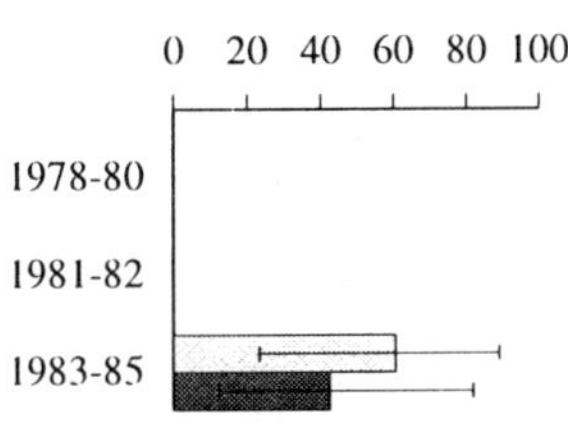

SWISS REGISTRIES

REGISTRY	NUMBER OF CASES			PERIOD OF DIAGNOSIS
	Males	Females	All	
Basel	23	4	27	1981-1984
Geneva	72	19	91	1978-1984
Mean age (years)	59.2	63.6	60.0	

RELATIVE SURVIVAL (%)

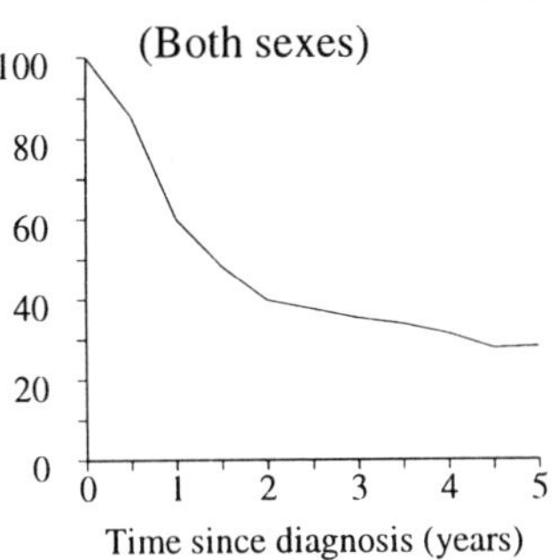

OBSERVED AND RELATIVE SURVIVAL (%) BY PERIOD AND SEX
(Number of cases in parentheses)

	PERIOD						SEX					
	1978-80		1981-82		1983-85		Males		Females		All	
	obs	rel	obs	rel	obs	rel	obs	rel	obs	rel	obs	rel
N. Cases	(45)		(36)		(37)		(95)		(23)		(118)	
1 year	57	58	58	60	61	63	59	61	57	58	59	60
3 years	25	27	33	36	42	45	31	33	39	43	33	35
5 years	20	23	28	31	27	31	21	24	39	45	25	28
8 years	..	..	23	29	..	..	17	21	..	..	20	25
10 years	..	..	..	..	..	..	..	..	..	..	..	..

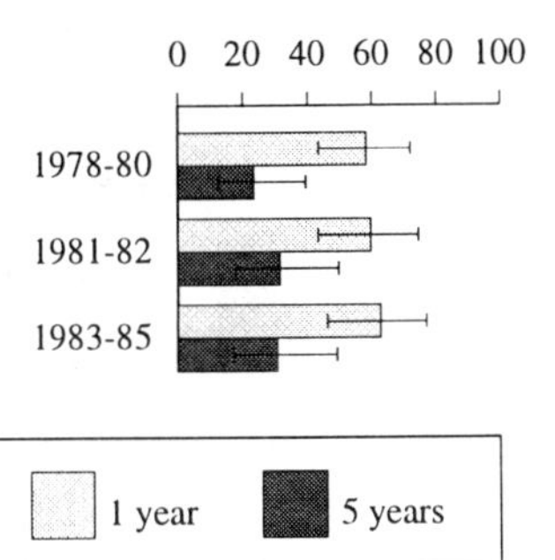

OROPHARYNX

EUROPEAN REGISTRIES

Unweighted analysis

REGISTRY	CASES		
	Males	Females	All
DENMARK	310	145	455
DUTCH REGISTRIES	24	10	34
ENGLISH REGISTRIES	605	283	888
ESTONIA	52	13	65
FINLAND	80	33	113
FRENCH REGISTRIES	272	18	290
GERMAN REGISTRIES	83	34	117
ITALIAN REGISTRIES	162	16	178
POLISH REGISTRIES	27	21	48
SCOTLAND	99	47	146
SPANISH REGISTRIES	5	0	5
SWISS REGISTRIES	95	23	118
Mean age (years)	61.3	64.9	62.3

RELATIVE SURVIVAL (%)
(Age-standardized)

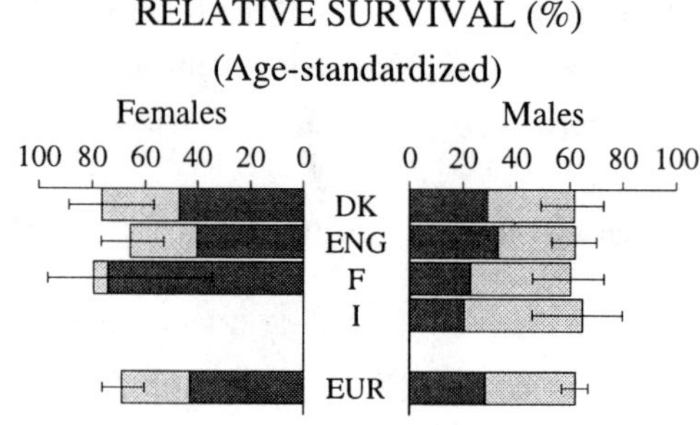

OBSERVED AND RELATIVE SURVIVAL (%) BY AGE AND PERIOD
(Number of cases in parentheses)

	AGE CLASS												PERIOD					
	15-44		45-54		55-64		65-74		75+		All		1978-80		1981-82		1983-85	
	obs	rel	obs	rel	obs	rel	obs	rel	obs	rel	obs	rel	obs	rel	obs	rel	obs	rel
Males	(129)		(402)		(565)		(477)		(241)		(1814)		(684)		(523)		(607)	
1 year	72	72	69	69	60	61	62	65	40	46	61	63	61	64	59	61	61	63
3 years	44	45	38	39	29	31	36	42	18	26	32	36	33	37	31	34	33	37
5 years	34	34	30	32	22	24	25	33	11	21	24	29	24	30	22	27	25	30
8 years	28	29	24	26	18	21	17	27	5	16	18	25	19	27	15	21	20	26
10 years	27	28	19	22	15	19	13	25	..	..	15	22	16	24	12	18	..	..
Females	(29)		(113)		(164)		(180)		(157)		(643)		(260)		(184)		(199)	
1 year	86	86	74	75	70	71	64	66	52	56	65	67	63	65	64	66	71	73
3 years	76	76	50	51	52	53	43	46	24	31	43	48	43	47	42	47	45	49
5 years	66	66	49	50	44	47	32	37	17	27	36	42	34	39	35	43	40	46
8 years	57	58	44	46	33	36	24	32	9	23	27	36	27	34	26	37	23	30
10 years	57	58	44	46	28	32	21	31	4	13	25	35	24	34	22	34	..	..
Overall	(158)		(515)		(729)		(657)		(398)		(2457)		(944)		(707)		(806)	
1 year	75	75	70	71	62	63	63	65	45	50	62	64	62	64	60	62	64	66
3 years	50	51	40	41	34	36	38	43	20	28	35	39	36	40	34	38	36	40
5 years	40	40	34	36	27	30	27	34	13	24	27	33	27	33	26	31	29	34
8 years	34	35	28	30	21	25	19	29	7	19	20	28	21	29	18	25	20	27
10 years	32	34	25	28	18	22	15	27	4	14	17	26	18	27	15	22	..	..

RELATIVE SURVIVAL (%) BY AGE AND PERIOD

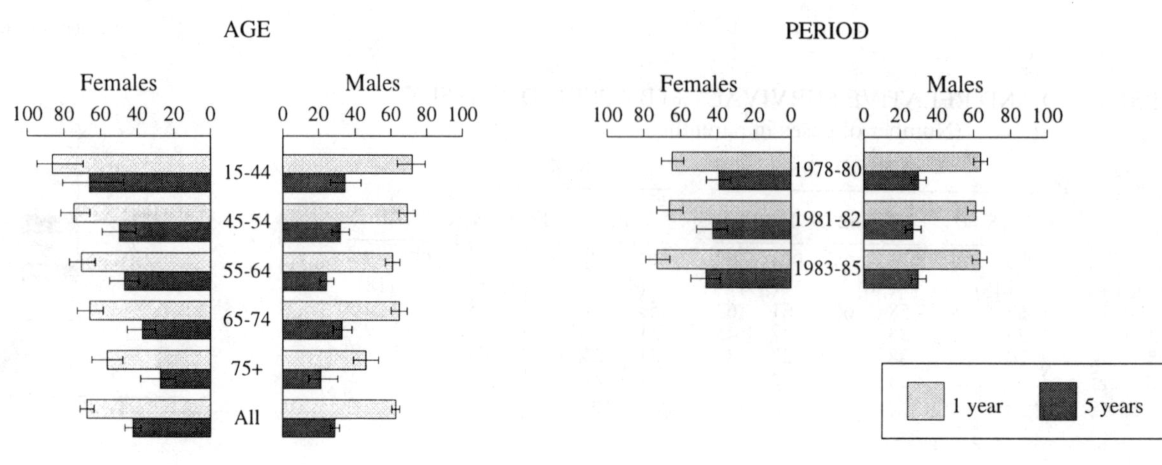

NASOPHARYNX

DENMARK

REGISTRY	NUMBER OF CASES			PERIOD OF DIAGNOSIS
	Males	Females	All	
Denmark	143	63	206	1978-1984
Mean age (years)	58.8	60.8	59.4	

RELATIVE SURVIVAL (%)

OBSERVED AND RELATIVE SURVIVAL (%) BY AGE AND PERIOD
(Number of cases in parentheses)

	AGE CLASS												PERIOD					
	15-44		45-54		55-64		65-74		75+		All		1978-80		1981-82		1983-85	
	obs	rel	obs	rel	obs	rel	obs	rel	obs	rel	obs	rel	obs	rel	obs	rel	obs	rel
Males	(25)		(23)		(35)		(38)		(22)		(143)		(61)		(35)		(47)	
1 year	76	76	78	79	86	87	71	74	45	50	73	75	74	76	77	80	68	71
3 years	64	64	52	53	57	60	37	42	14	19	45	50	49	53	43	48	43	48
5 years	60	61	48	50	51	57	28	36	5	8	39	47	43	49	34	41	40	50
8 years	50	51	48	52	37	45	16	25	..	..	31	41	31	40	31	43	..	..
10 years	42	43	48	53	14	18	5	10	..	..	20	29	20	28	..	..	..	..
Females	(10)		(13)		(11)		(16)		(13)		(63)		(24)		(17)		(22)	
1 year	100	100	77	77	100	100	56	58	46	49	73	75	79	80	65	66	73	75
3 years	60	60	54	55	82	84	44	47	23	29	51	55	58	61	47	50	45	51
5 years	40	40	35	36	64	67	25	29	15	23	34	39	46	50	41	46	15	18
8 years	20	20	35	36	54	60	18	23	15	32	27	34	33	39	35	43	..	..
10 years	20	20	..	..	54	62	18	25	..	..	27	36	33	41	..	..	..	..
Overall	(35)		(36)		(46)		(54)		(35)		(206)		(85)		(52)		(69)	
1 year	83	83	78	78	89	90	67	69	46	50	73	75	75	77	73	75	70	72
3 years	63	63	53	54	63	66	39	44	17	23	47	52	52	56	44	49	43	49
5 years	54	55	43	45	54	59	27	34	10	17	38	44	44	49	37	43	31	38
8 years	41	41	43	47	40	48	17	25	10	26	29	39	32	39	33	43	..	..
10 years	35	36	43	48	27	34	10	17	..	..	22	31	24	32	..	..	..	..

RELATIVE SURVIVAL (%) BY AGE AND PERIOD

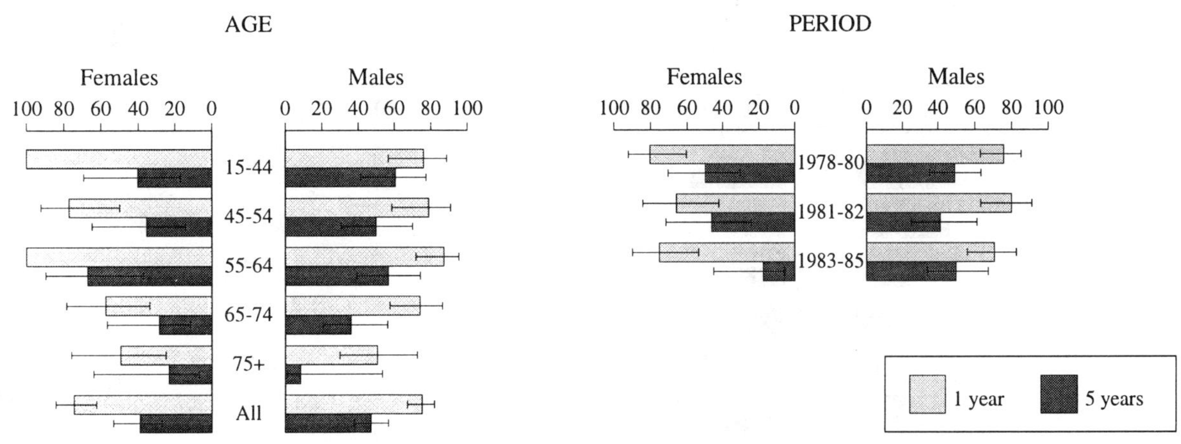

NASOPHARYNX

ENGLISH REGISTRIES

REGISTRY	NUMBER OF CASES			PERIOD OF DIAGNOSIS
	Males	Females	All	
East Anglia	31	22	53	1979-1984
Mersey	37	21	58	1978-1984
South Thames	105	51	156	1978-1984
Wessex	22	3	25	1983-1984
West Midlands	76	28	104	1979-1984
Yorkshire	45	22	67	1978-1984
Mean age (years)	57.5	60.3	58.4	

RELATIVE SURVIVAL (%)

Males
Females
Time since diagnosis (years)

OBSERVED AND RELATIVE SURVIVAL (%) BY AGE AND PERIOD
(Number of cases in parentheses)

	AGE CLASS												PERIOD					
	15-44		45-54		55-64		65-74		75+		All		1978-80		1981-82		1983-85	
	obs	rel	obs	rel	obs	rel	obs	rel	obs	rel	obs	rel	obs	rel	obs	rel	obs	rel
Males	(57)		(56)		(92)		(80)		(31)		(316)		(108)		(97)		(111)	
1 year	82	83	69	70	53	54	59	61	52	59	63	65	69	72	63	65	56	58
3 years	65	65	48	49	27	29	31	35	13	19	37	41	41	45	38	41	32	36
5 years	56	56	40	42	21	24	21	28	3	6	29	34	29	34	29	34	29	34
8 years	48	49	26	28	14	17	15	25	3	11	22	28	21	28	23	30	21	27
10 years	44	45	19	22	9	12	15	29	..	..	18	25	18	24	23	32	..	..
Females	(29)		(14)		(32)		(37)		(35)		(147)		(69)		(46)		(32)	
1 year	83	83	93	93	56	57	27	28	37	41	53	55	55	57	50	51	53	55
3 years	69	69	71	72	31	32	11	12	17	23	34	37	39	43	30	33	28	31
5 years	55	55	50	51	25	26	8	10	9	14	25	29	29	34	20	23	25	30
8 years	51	51	50	52	19	21	3	4	9	20	21	28	25	32	15	18	25	34
10 years	51	51	25	26	19	22	3	4	4	13	19	26	21	30	15	20	..	..
Overall	(86)		(70)		(124)		(117)		(66)		(463)		(177)		(143)		(143)	
1 year	83	83	74	75	54	55	49	51	44	49	60	61	64	66	59	60	55	57
3 years	66	67	52	53	28	30	24	28	15	21	36	40	40	44	35	39	31	35
5 years	56	56	42	44	22	24	17	22	6	11	28	33	29	34	26	30	28	33
8 years	49	50	31	33	15	18	11	17	6	17	22	28	23	30	20	26	22	28
10 years	47	47	21	23	12	16	11	19	3	11	18	26	19	27	20	28	..	..

RELATIVE SURVIVAL (%) BY AGE AND PERIOD

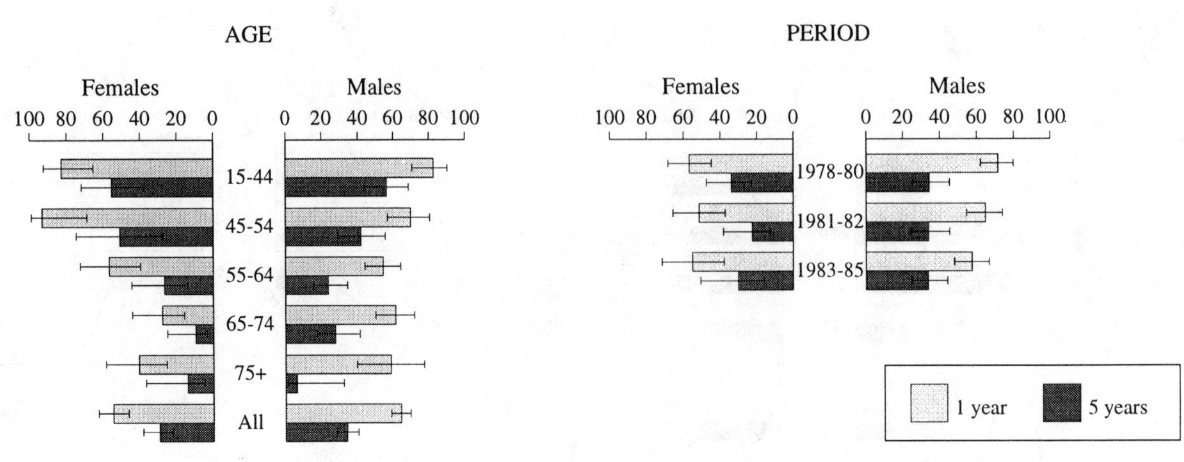

NASOPHARYNX

DUTCH REGISTRIES

REGISTRY	NUMBER OF CASES			PERIOD OF DIAGNOSIS
	Males	Females	All	
Eindhoven	16	5	21	1978-1985
Mean age (years)	58.7	45.4	55.5	

RELATIVE SURVIVAL (%)
(Both sexes)

100
80
60
40
20
0
0 1 2 3 4 5
Time since diagnosis (years)

OBSERVED AND RELATIVE SURVIVAL (%) BY PERIOD AND SEX
(Number of cases in parentheses)

	PERIOD						SEX					
	1978-80		1981-82		1983-85		Males		Females		All	
	obs	rel	obs	rel	obs	rel	obs	rel	obs	rel	obs	rel
N. Cases	(7)		(3)		(11)		(16)		(5)		(21)	
1 year	71	72	100	100	73	75	75	77	80	80	76	78
3 years	57	59	33	35	42	46	32	35	80	81	45	48
5 years	57	60	33	36	..	..	32	36	80	82	45	50
8 years	29	31	..	..	..	..	32	39	27	28	25	29
10 years	..	..	..	..	..	..	..	..	..	..	..	..

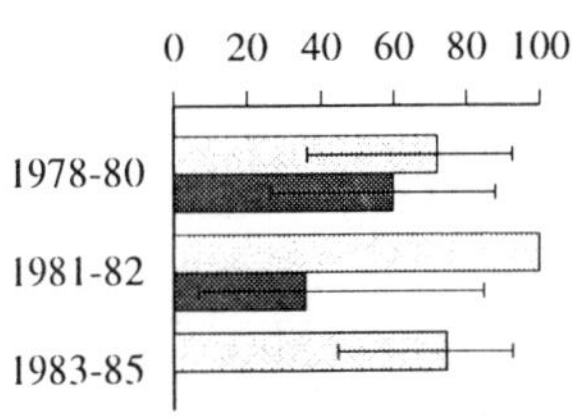

ESTONIA

REGISTRY	NUMBER OF CASES			PERIOD OF DIAGNOSIS
	Males	Females	All	
Estonia	22	11	33	1978-1984
Mean age (years)	56.3	63.3	58.6	

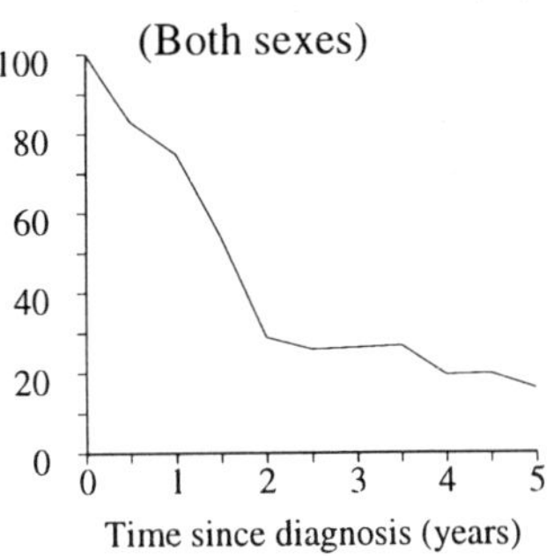

OBSERVED AND RELATIVE SURVIVAL (%) BY PERIOD AND SEX
(Number of cases in parentheses)

	PERIOD						SEX					
	1978-80		1981-82		1983-85		Males		Females		All	
	obs	rel	obs	rel	obs	rel	obs	rel	obs	rel	obs	rel
N. Cases	(13)		(8)		(12)		(22)		(11)		(33)	
1 year	62	63	75	77	83	86	77	79	64	66	73	75
3 years	15	17	38	40	24	26	9	10	55	60	24	26
5 years	8	9	25	28	12	14	5	5	33	39	14	16
8 years	0	0	13	16	..	..	5	6	0	0	5	6
10 years	0	0	..	..	..	..	..	..	0	0	..	..

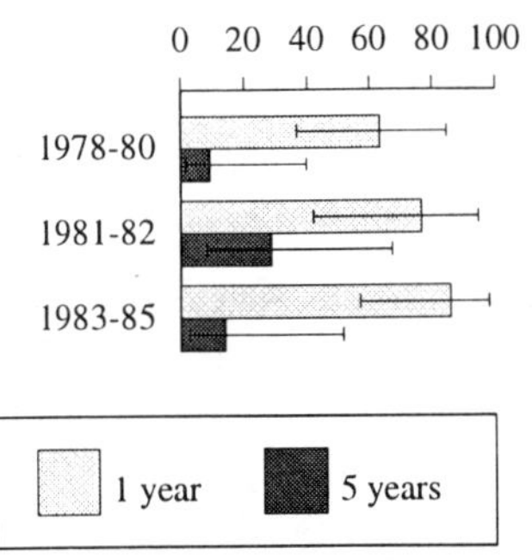

NASOPHARYNX

FINLAND

REGISTRY	NUMBER OF CASES			PERIOD OF DIAGNOSIS
	Males	Females	All	
Finland	55	44	99	1978-1984
Mean age (years)	52.6	58.8	55.3	

RELATIVE SURVIVAL (%)
(Both sexes)

Time since diagnosis (years)

OBSERVED AND RELATIVE SURVIVAL (%) BY PERIOD AND SEX
(Number of cases in parentheses)

	PERIOD						SEX					
	1978-80		1981-82		1983-85		Males		Females		All	
	obs	rel	obs	rel	obs	rel	obs	rel	obs	rel	obs	rel
N. Cases	(40)		(28)		(31)		(55)		(44)		(99)	
1 year	75	76	71	73	77	79	80	82	68	70	75	76
3 years	50	53	54	58	48	52	58	62	41	44	51	54
5 years	43	47	46	53	48	55	51	57	39	44	45	51
8 years	35	42	39	49	39	51	42	51	32	40	37	46
10 years	33	41	39	51	..	..	42	53	28	37	36	46

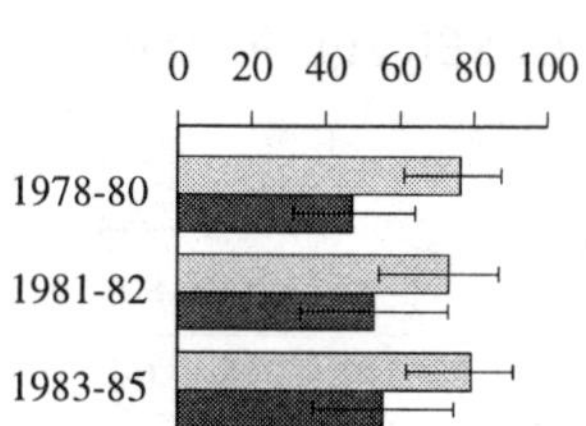

FRENCH REGISTRIES

REGISTRY	NUMBER OF CASES			PERIOD OF DIAGNOSIS
	Males	Females	All	
Amiens	5	2	7	1983-1984
Doubs	18	7	25	1978-1985
Mean age (years)	53.8	60.3	55.7	

RELATIVE SURVIVAL (%)
(Both sexes)

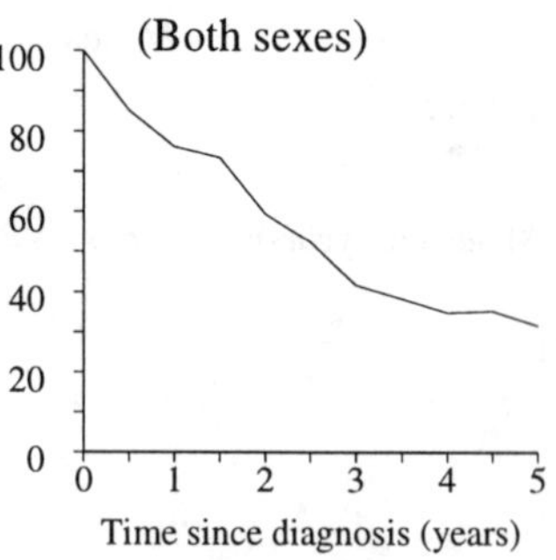

Time since diagnosis (years)

OBSERVED AND RELATIVE SURVIVAL (%) BY PERIOD AND SEX
(Number of cases in parentheses)

	PERIOD						SEX					
	1978-80		1981-82		1983-85		Males		Females		All	
	obs	rel	obs	rel	obs	rel	obs	rel	obs	rel	obs	rel
N. Cases	(13)		(3)		(16)		(23)		(9)		(32)	
1 year	69	71	100	100	75	76	70	71	88	90	75	76
3 years	38	42	50	53	37	39	37	40	44	46	39	42
5 years	31	35	50	55	22	24	28	31	29	32	29	32
8 years	8	10	50	60	..	..	17	20	..	..	15	18
10 years	..	..	..	..	..	..	..	..	..	..	..	..

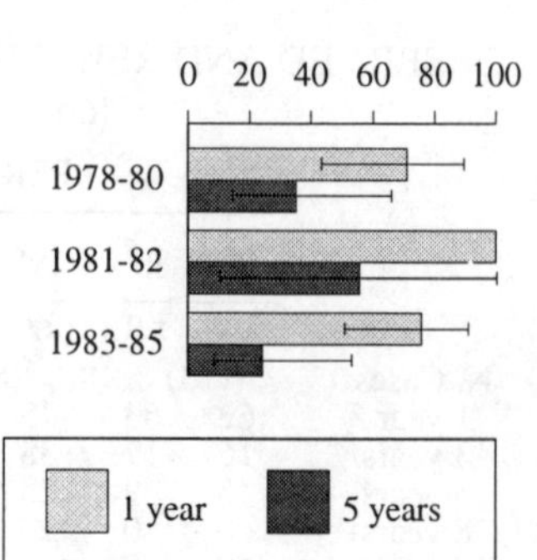

NASOPHARYNX

GERMAN REGISTRIES

REGISTRY	NUMBER OF CASES			PERIOD OF DIAGNOSIS
	Males	Females	All	
Saarland	17	7	24	1978-1984
Mean age (years)	56.4	68.9	60.0	

RELATIVE SURVIVAL (%)

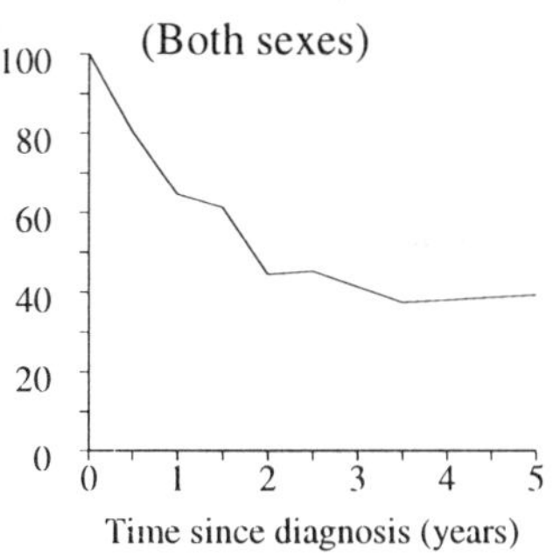

OBSERVED AND RELATIVE SURVIVAL (%) BY PERIOD AND SEX
(Number of cases in parentheses)

	PERIOD						SEX					
	1978-80		1981-82		1983-85		Males		Females		All	
	obs	rel	obs	rel	obs	rel	obs	rel	obs	rel	obs	rel
N. Cases	(5)		(7)		(12)		(17)		(7)		(24)	
1 year	60	62	57	59	67	69	65	67	57	59	63	65
3 years	60	65	29	31	33	37	41	45	29	32	38	41
5 years	60	68	14	17	33	40	41	48	14	17	33	39
8 years	60	73	0	0	..	..	28	36	14	19	24	31
10 years	60	77	0	0	..	..	28	38	..	..	24	33

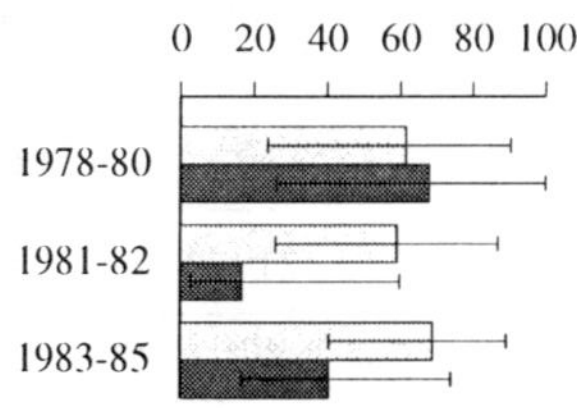

ITALIAN REGISTRIES

REGISTRY	NUMBER OF CASES			PERIOD OF DIAGNOSIS
	Males	Females	All	
Latina	2	1	3	1983-1984
Ragusa	5	1	6	1981-1984
Varese	39	12	51	1978-1985
Mean age (years)	57.8	58.1	57.8	

RELATIVE SURVIVAL (%)

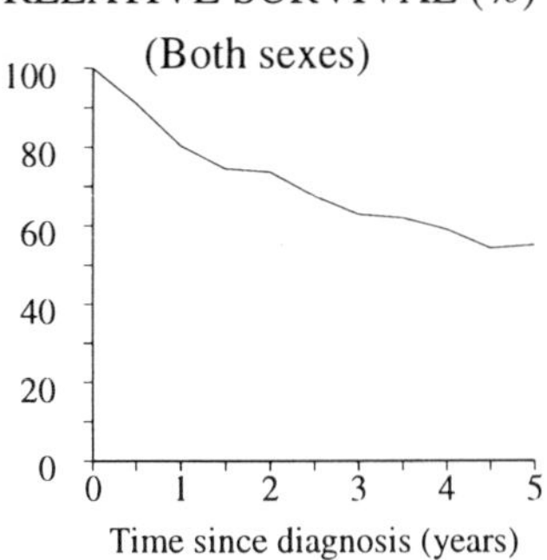

OBSERVED AND RELATIVE SURVIVAL (%) BY PERIOD AND SEX
(Number of cases in parentheses)

	PERIOD						SEX					
	1978-80		1981-82		1983-85		Males		Females		All	
	obs	rel	obs	rel	obs	rel	obs	rel	obs	rel	obs	rel
N. Cases	(25)		(20)		(15)		(46)		(14)		(60)	
1 year	72	74	75	77	93	95	76	78	86	88	78	80
3 years	48	53	55	59	80	85	50	54	86	92	58	63
5 years	48	56	40	45	60	67	39	45	79	89	48	55
8 years	36	47	30	36	46	56	22	27	79	95	35	44
10 years	20	28	30	38	..	..	10	14	61	76	23	30

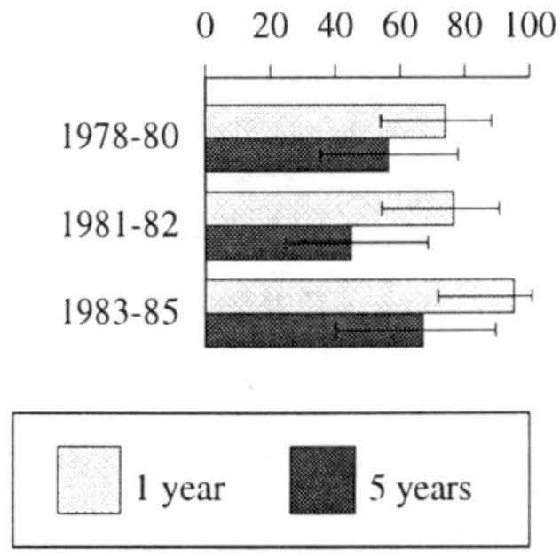

NASOPHARYNX

POLISH REGISTRIES

REGISTRY	NUMBER OF CASES Males	Females	All	PERIOD OF DIAGNOSIS
Cracow	11	9	20	1978-1984
Mean age (years)	54.1	60.0	56.8	

RELATIVE SURVIVAL (%)
(Both sexes)

Time since diagnosis (years)

OBSERVED AND RELATIVE SURVIVAL (%) BY PERIOD AND SEX
(Number of cases in parentheses)

	PERIOD 1978-80 obs	rel	1981-82 obs	rel	1983-85 obs	rel	SEX Males obs	rel	Females obs	rel	All obs	rel
N. Cases	(9)		(4)		(7)		(11)		(9)		(20)	
1 year	56	57	75	76	71	73	73	75	56	57	65	66
3 years	22	24	25	26	43	46	36	39	22	23	30	32
5 years	11	13	25	27	43	49	27	31	22	25	25	28
8 years	11	14	25	28	..	..	18	23	22	27	20	24
10 years	11	15	0	0	..	..	18	24	0	0	10	13

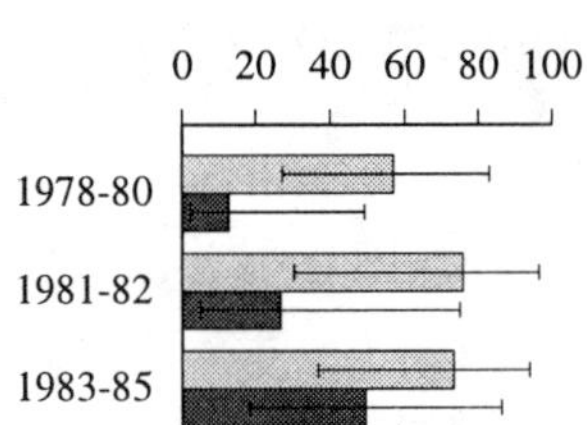

SCOTLAND

REGISTRY	NUMBER OF CASES Males	Females	All	PERIOD OF DIAGNOSIS
Scotland	62	38	100	1978-1982
Mean age (years)	58.8	63.6	60.6	

RELATIVE SURVIVAL (%)
(Both sexes)

Time since diagnosis (years)

OBSERVED AND RELATIVE SURVIVAL (%) BY PERIOD AND SEX
(Number of cases in parentheses)

	PERIOD 1978-80 obs	rel	1981-82 obs	rel	1983-85 obs	rel	SEX Males obs	rel	Females obs	rel	All obs	rel
N. Cases	(64)		(36)		(0)		(62)		(38)		(100)	
1 year	55	57	47	49	..	..	55	57	47	49	52	54
3 years	28	31	31	34	..	..	29	33	29	32	29	32
5 years	20	24	19	24	..	..	19	24	21	25	20	24
8 years	16	21	..	..	..	..	17	24	..	..	15	21
10 years	16	23	..	..	..	..	17	26	..	..	15	23

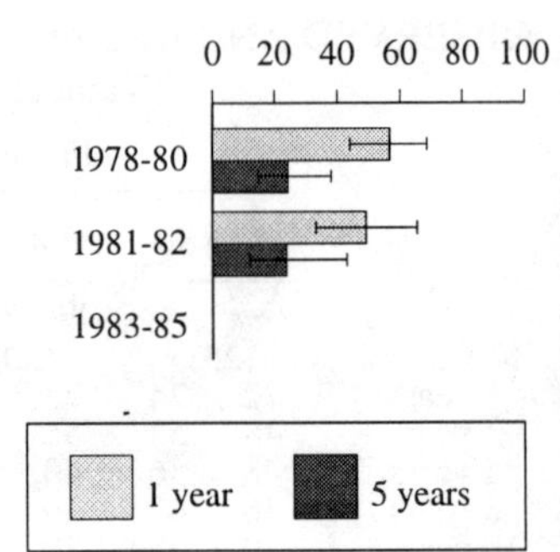

NASOPHARYNX

SPANISH REGISTRIES

REGISTRY	NUMBER OF CASES Males	Females	All	PERIOD OF DIAGNOSIS
Tarragona	6	2	8	1985-1985
Mean age (years)	45.5	56.0	48.1	

RELATIVE SURVIVAL (%)
(Both sexes)

100
80
60
40
20
0
0 1 2 3 4 5
Time since diagnosis (years)

OBSERVED AND RELATIVE SURVIVAL (%) BY PERIOD AND SEX
(Number of cases in parentheses)

	PERIOD 1978-80 obs	rel	1981-82 obs	rel	1983-85 obs	rel	SEX Males obs	rel	Females obs	rel	All obs	rel
N. Cases	(0)		(0)		(8)		(6)		(2)		(8)	
1 year	..	..	..	..	75	76	67	67	100	100	75	76
3 years	..	..	..	..	63	64	50	51	100	100	63	64
5 years	..	..	..	..	50	52	50	53	50	51	50	52
8 years	..	..	..	..	..	..	..	..	..	..	..	..
10 years	..	..	..	..	..	..	..	..	..	..	..	..

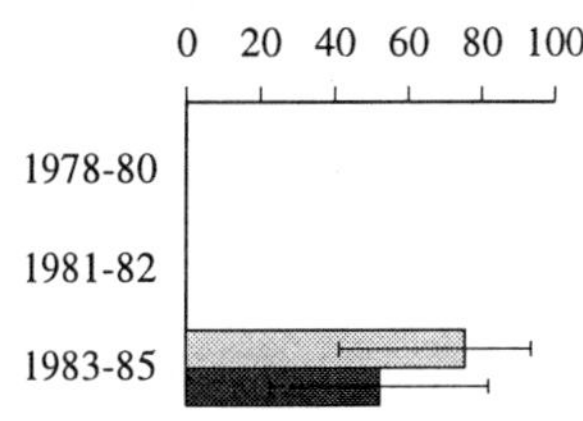

SWISS REGISTRIES

REGISTRY	NUMBER OF CASES Males	Females	All	PERIOD OF DIAGNOSIS
Basel	2	0	2	1984-1984
Geneva	6	4	10	1978-1983
Mean age (years)	57.9	61.3	59.0	

RELATIVE SURVIVAL (%)
(Both sexes)

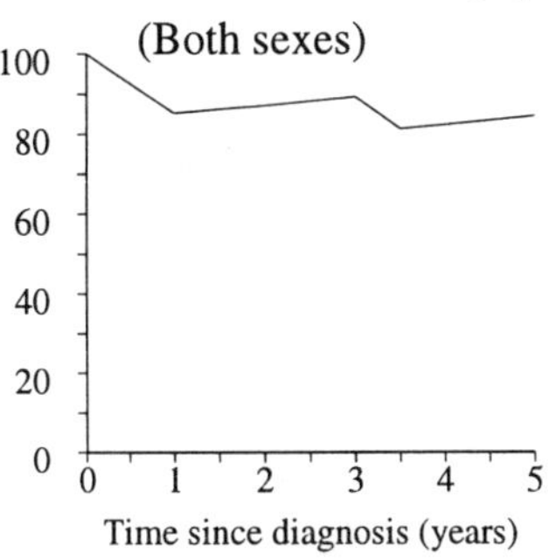

OBSERVED AND RELATIVE SURVIVAL (%) BY PERIOD AND SEX
(Number of cases in parentheses)

	PERIOD 1978-80 obs	rel	1981-82 obs	rel	1983-85 obs	rel	SEX Males obs	rel	Females obs	rel	All obs	rel
N. Cases	(4)		(4)		(4)		(8)		(4)		(12)	
1 year	75	77	75	78	100	100	88	90	75	76	83	85
3 years	75	81	75	84	100	100	88	94	75	80	83	89
5 years	50	57	75	90	100	100	75	85	75	84	75	84
8 years	..	..	..	..	..	..	..	..	..	..	..	..
10 years	..	..	..	..	..	..	..	..	..	..	..	..

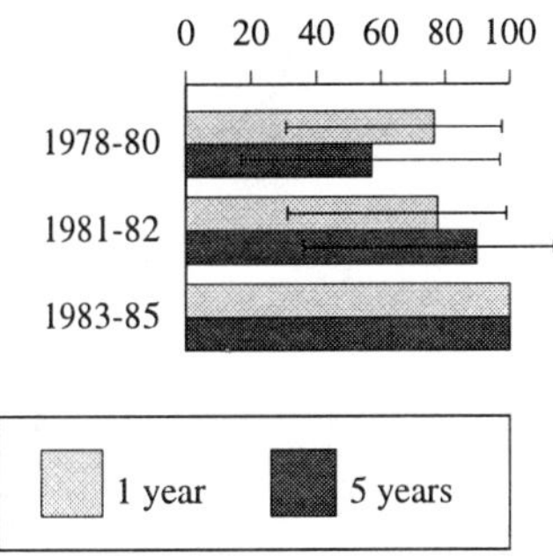

NASOPHARYNX

EUROPEAN REGISTRIES

Unweighted analysis

REGISTRY	CASES		
	Males	Females	All
DENMARK	143	63	206
DUTCH REGISTRIES	16	5	21
ENGLISH REGISTRIES	316	147	463
ESTONIA	22	11	33
FINLAND	55	44	99
FRENCH REGISTRIES	23	9	32
GERMAN REGISTRIES	17	7	24
ITALIAN REGISTRIES	46	14	60
POLISH REGISTRIES	11	9	20
SCOTLAND	62	38	100
SPANISH REGISTRIES	6	2	8
SWISS REGISTRIES	8	4	12
Mean age (years)	57.2	60.5	58.3

RELATIVE SURVIVAL (%)
(Age-standardized)

OBSERVED AND RELATIVE SURVIVAL (%) BY AGE AND PERIOD
(Number of cases in parentheses)

	AGE CLASS												PERIOD					
	15-44		45-54		55-64		65-74		75+		All		1978-80		1981-82		1983-85	
	obs	rel	obs	rel	obs	rel	obs	rel	obs	rel	obs	rel	obs	rel	obs	rel	obs	rel
Males	(128)		(138)		(219)		(167)		(73)		(725)		(280)		(207)		(238)	
1 year	82	82	74	74	67	68	61	64	48	54	68	70	69	71	67	69	66	68
3 years	62	62	48	49	37	39	34	39	15	21	40	44	42	46	39	43	39	43
5 years	53	53	41	43	29	33	26	34	8	16	33	38	32	38	30	35	36	41
8 years	44	45	33	36	20	24	18	28	3	9	25	32	24	32	24	31	26	34
10 years	39	40	27	30	14	19	13	25	..	..	20	28	19	27	24	33	..	..
Females	(62)		(51)		(69)		(94)		(77)		(353)		(162)		(101)		(90)	
1 year	87	87	84	85	67	67	46	47	40	44	61	63	61	63	56	58	68	70
3 years	66	66	62	63	46	48	26	29	21	28	41	45	41	45	41	44	42	47
5 years	56	57	48	49	36	38	20	23	12	19	32	37	34	39	31	35	29	34
8 years	45	46	41	43	27	29	13	18	10	24	25	32	25	31	24	30	27	36
10 years	45	46	35	37	25	28	8	12	5	16	22	29	22	29	21	28	..	..
Overall	(190)		(189)		(288)		(261)		(150)		(1078)		(442)		(308)		(328)	
1 year	84	84	77	77	67	68	56	58	44	49	66	67	66	68	64	65	66	68
3 years	63	63	51	53	39	41	31	35	18	25	41	44	42	45	40	43	40	44
5 years	54	54	43	44	31	34	24	30	10	18	32	38	33	38	30	35	34	40
8 years	44	45	35	38	22	26	16	24	7	19	25	32	25	31	24	31	27	35
10 years	42	43	29	32	17	22	11	19	4	13	21	29	20	28	23	31	..	..

RELATIVE SURVIVAL (%) BY AGE AND PERIOD

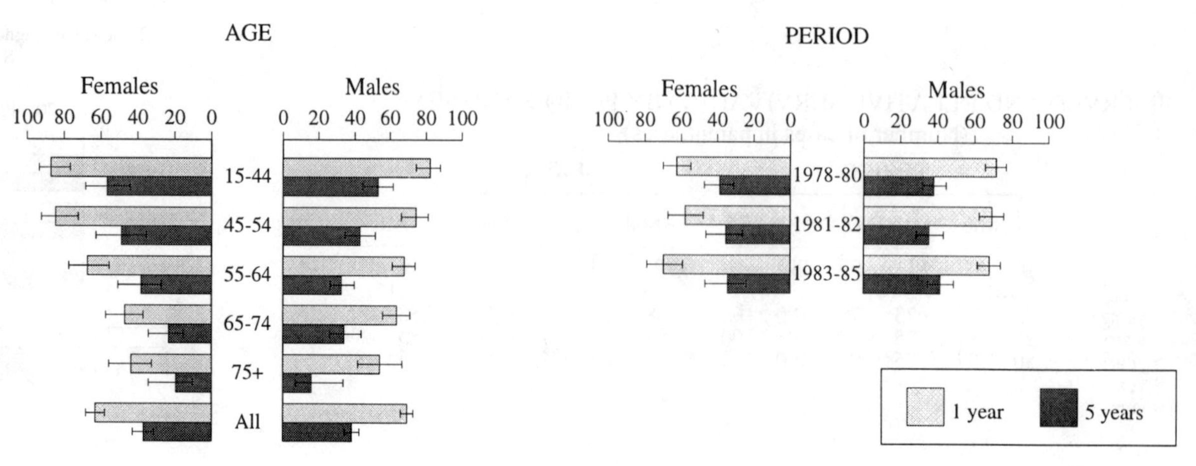

HYPOPHARYNX

DENMARK

REGISTRY	NUMBER OF CASES			PERIOD OF DIAGNOSIS
	Males	Females	All	
Denmark	135	38	173	1978-1984
Mean age (years)	66.1	67.1	66.3	

RELATIVE SURVIVAL (%)

100
80
60
40
20
0
Females
Males
0 1 2 3 4 5
Time since diagnosis (years)

OBSERVED AND RELATIVE SURVIVAL (%) BY AGE AND PERIOD

(Number of cases in parentheses)

	AGE CLASS												PERIOD					
	15-44		45-54		55-64		65-74		75+		All		1978-80		1981-82		1983-85	
	obs	rel	obs	rel	obs	rel	obs	rel	obs	rel	obs	rel	obs	rel	obs	rel	obs	rel
Males	(6)		(16)		(42)		(36)		(35)		(135)		(46)		(43)		(46)	
1 year	83	84	63	63	40	41	44	46	26	30	42	45	50	53	40	42	37	39
3 years	50	50	13	13	19	20	22	25	6	9	17	20	24	28	16	20	11	12
5 years	33	34	13	13	10	11	16	21	3	6	11	14	13	17	16	22	..	..
8 years	33	34	..	..	5	6	13	20	..	..	8	12	9	13	14	23	..	..
10 years	..	..	..	..	5	6	0	0	..	..	4	7	4	7	..	..	..	..
Females	(0)		(2)		(15)		(9)		(12)		(38)		(13)		(11)		(14)	
1 year	..	..	50	50	80	81	56	57	42	44	61	62	54	56	55	56	71	73
3 years	..	..	0	0	40	41	44	48	0	0	26	29	23	26	36	39	21	23
5 years	..	..	0	0	40	43	33	38	0	0	24	27	23	28	27	31	21	24
8 years	..	..	0	0	33	37	33	43	0	0	21	28	15	21	..	..	..	..
10 years	..	..	0	0	..	..	..	..	0	0	..	..	..	..	..	..	..	..
Overall	(6)		(18)		(57)		(45)		(47)		(173)		(59)		(54)		(60)	
1 year	83	84	61	62	51	52	47	48	30	33	46	48	51	53	43	45	45	47
3 years	50	50	11	11	25	26	27	30	4	6	19	22	24	27	20	24	13	15
5 years	33	34	11	12	18	19	20	25	2	4	14	17	15	19	19	24	8	10
8 years	33	34	..	..	10	12	17	26	..	..	10	15	10	15	17	26	..	..
10 years	..	..	..	..	10	12	..	..	..	..	6	10	6	10	..	..	..	..

RELATIVE SURVIVAL (%) BY AGE AND PERIOD

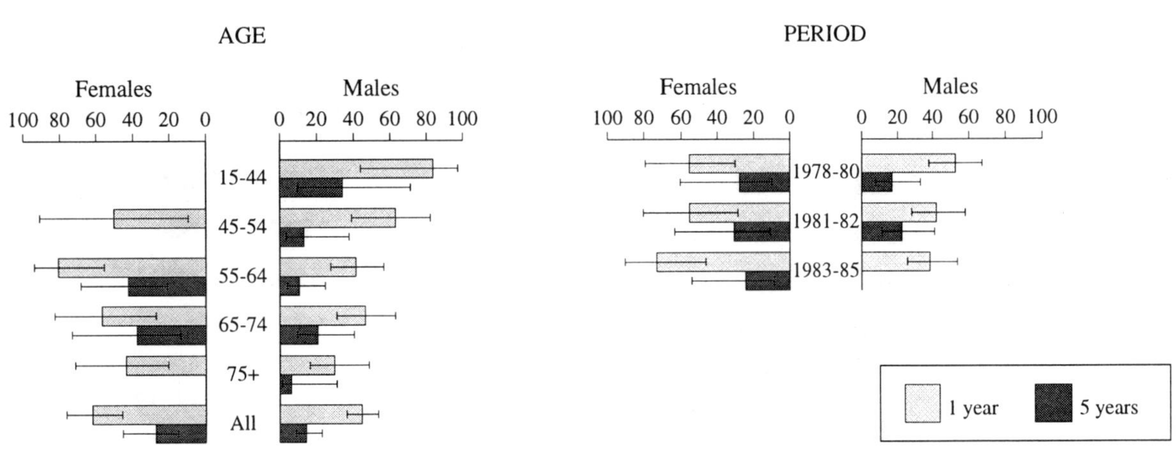

HYPOPHARYNX

ENGLISH REGISTRIES

REGISTRY	NUMBER OF CASES			PERIOD OF DIAGNOSIS
	Males	Females	All	
East Anglia	56	53	109	1979-1984
Mersey	65	71	136	1978-1984
South Thames	178	141	319	1978-1984
Wessex	25	14	39	1983-1984
West Midlands	172	109	281	1979-1984
Yorkshire	93	110	203	1978-1984
Mean age (years)	65.9	66.5	66.2	

RELATIVE SURVIVAL (%)

100
80
60
40
20
0
Males
Females
0 1 2 3 4 5
Time since diagnosis (years)

OBSERVED AND RELATIVE SURVIVAL (%) BY AGE AND PERIOD
(Number of cases in parentheses)

	AGE CLASS												PERIOD					
	15-44		45-54		55-64		65-74		75+		All		1978-80		1981-82		1983-85	
	obs	rel	obs	rel	obs	rel	obs	rel	obs	rel	obs	rel	obs	rel	obs	rel	obs	rel
Males	(16)		(63)		(177)		(198)		(135)		(589)		(215)		(169)		(205)	
1 year	50	50	46	46	45	46	48	50	31	35	43	45	43	46	41	43	44	47
3 years	31	31	24	24	25	27	24	27	12	18	22	25	22	26	20	23	23	27
5 years	25	25	14	15	18	20	17	23	9	18	15	20	15	19	11	15	19	25
8 years	25	26	9	10	12	14	11	18	6	17	10	16	10	15	10	15	8	13
10 years	..	..	9	10	10	14	6	11	4	19	7	13	8	14	3	5	..	..
Females	(16)		(56)		(143)		(154)		(129)		(498)		(215)		(140)		(143)	
1 year	38	38	57	57	54	54	39	40	27	30	42	44	45	47	41	43	38	40
3 years	31	31	28	28	24	25	17	18	10	13	19	21	18	20	21	23	17	19
5 years	31	32	28	28	20	21	13	16	6	10	15	19	14	17	18	21	15	18
8 years	31	32	19	20	16	18	8	10	5	11	12	16	12	16	13	17	5	8
10 years	31	32	16	18	15	17	6	8	2	6	9	14	9	14	12	16	..	..
Overall	(32)		(119)		(320)		(352)		(264)		(1087)		(430)		(309)		(348)	
1 year	44	44	51	51	49	50	44	46	29	33	43	45	44	46	41	43	42	44
3 years	31	31	26	26	25	26	21	23	11	16	20	23	20	23	20	23	21	24
5 years	28	28	20	21	19	20	16	19	8	14	15	19	15	18	14	18	17	22
8 years	28	29	14	15	14	16	10	14	5	14	11	16	11	16	11	16	7	11
10 years	28	29	13	14	12	15	5	9	3	11	8	13	9	14	8	12	..	..

RELATIVE SURVIVAL (%) BY AGE AND PERIOD

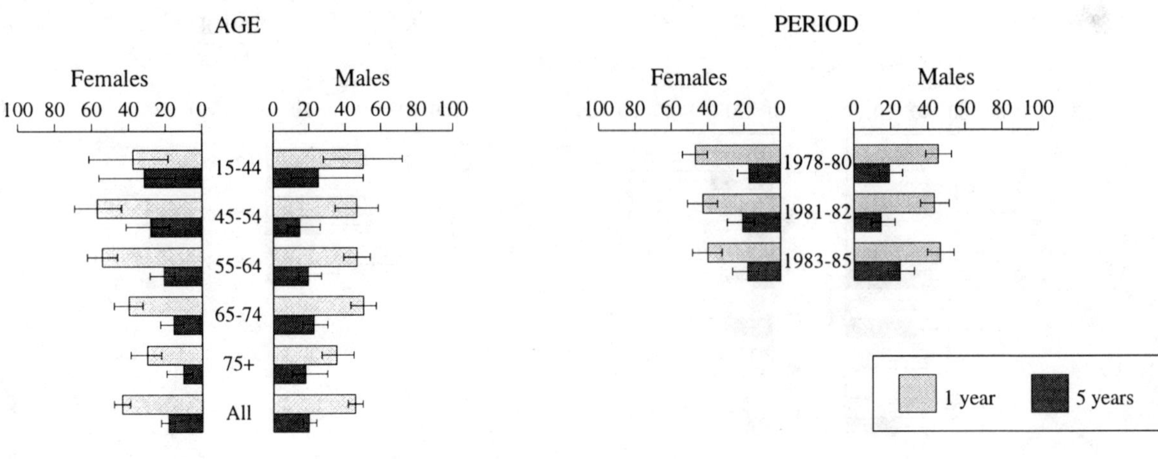

HYPOPHARYNX

FRENCH REGISTRIES

REGISTRY	NUMBER OF CASES			PERIOD OF DIAGNOSIS
	Males	Females	All	
Amiens	59	3	62	1983-1984
Doubs	184	3	187	1978-1985
Mean age (years)	57.7	63.2	57.8	

RELATIVE SURVIVAL (%)

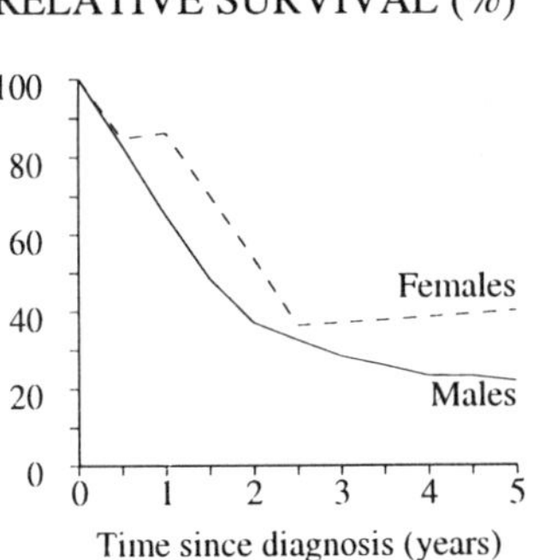

OBSERVED AND RELATIVE SURVIVAL (%) BY AGE AND PERIOD
(Number of cases in parentheses)

	AGE CLASS												PERIOD					
	15-44		45-54		55-64		65-74		75+		All		1978-80		1981-82		1983-85	
	obs	rel	obs	rel	obs	rel	obs	rel	obs	rel	obs	rel	obs	rel	obs	rel	obs	rel
Males	(19)		(85)		(80)		(37)		(22)		(243)		(77)		(43)		(123)	
1 year	78	78	64	65	63	64	62	65	55	60	63	65	69	70	72	74	57	58
3 years	39	39	24	25	29	30	27	31	14	19	26	28	32	35	16	18	26	28
5 years	33	34	21	22	18	19	22	27	5	8	19	22	23	26	9	11	21	23
8 years	26	27	11	11	10	11	11	17	0	0	11	13	14	17	5	6	..	..
10 years	26	27	7	8	10	12	11	20	0	0	10	13	12	16	..	..	..	..
Females	(0)		(3)		(1)		(0)		(2)		(6)		(1)		(1)		(4)	
1 year	..	..	100	100	100	100	..	..	50	55	83	86	100	100	100	100	75	79
3 years	..	..	33	34	100	100	..	..	0	0	33	37	0	0	100	100	25	29
5 years	..	..	..	..	100	100	..	..	0	0	33	40	0	0	100	100	..	..
8 years	..	..	..	..	0	0	..	..	0	0	0	0	0	0	0	0	..	..
10 years	..	..	..	..	0	0	..	..	0	0	0	0	0	0	0	0	..	..
Overall	(19)		(88)		(81)		(37)		(24)		(249)		(78)		(44)		(127)	
1 year	78	78	66	66	63	64	62	65	54	60	64	65	69	71	73	75	57	59
3 years	39	39	25	25	30	31	27	31	13	17	27	29	32	34	18	20	26	28
5 years	33	34	21	22	19	21	22	27	4	7	20	22	23	26	11	13	21	23
8 years	26	27	11	12	8	10	11	17	0	0	10	13	13	17	5	6	..	..
10 years	26	27	7	8	8	10	11	20	0	0	9	12	12	16	..	..	..	..

RELATIVE SURVIVAL (%) BY AGE AND PERIOD

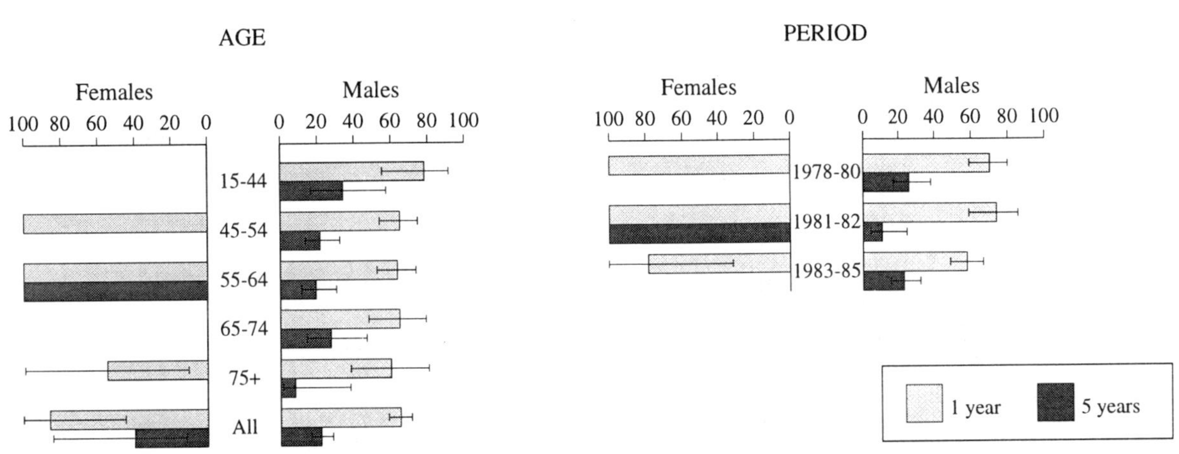

HYPOPHARYNX

ITALIAN REGISTRIES

REGISTRY	NUMBER OF CASES			PERIOD OF DIAGNOSIS
	Males	Females	All	
Varese	104	3	107	1978-1985
Mean age (years)	60.8	61.7	60.8	

RELATIVE SURVIVAL (%)

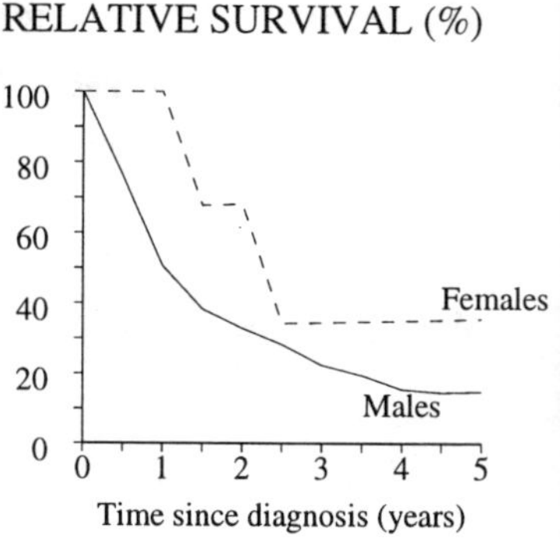

OBSERVED AND RELATIVE SURVIVAL (%) BY AGE AND PERIOD
(Number of cases in parentheses)

	AGE CLASS												PERIOD					
	15-44		45-54		55-64		65-74		75+		All		1978-80		1981-82		1983-85	
	obs	rel	obs	rel	obs	rel	obs	rel	obs	rel	obs	rel	obs	rel	obs	rel	obs	rel
Males	(5)		(28)		(31)		(27)		(13)		(104)		(42)		(21)		(41)	
1 year	60	60	57	58	48	49	41	43	46	51	49	51	52	55	33	35	54	55
3 years	0	0	36	37	16	17	19	22	8	11	20	22	19	22	14	16	24	26
5 years	0	0	18	19	13	14	11	15	8	14	13	15	5	6	10	12	22	25
8 years	0	0	18	19	13	16	6	9	8	21	10	14	5	7	5	7	22	28
10 years	0	0	18	20	..	..	0	0	..	..	7	10	2	4	..	..	..	..
Females	(0)		(1)		(1)		(1)		(0)		(3)		(2)		(0)		(1)	
1 year	..	..	100	100	100	100	100	100	..	..	100	100	100	100	..	..	100	100
3 years	..	..	0	0	0	0	100	100	..	..	33	35	0	0	..	..	100	100
5 years	..	..	0	0	0	0	100	100	..	..	33	36	0	0	..	..	100	100
8 years	..	..	0	0	0	0	..	..	..	..	..	..	0	0	..	..	..	..
10 years	..	..	0	0	0	0	..	..	..	..	..	..	0	0	..	..	..	..
Overall	(5)		(29)		(32)		(28)		(13)		(107)		(44)		(21)		(42)	
1 year	60	60	59	59	50	51	43	45	46	51	50	52	55	57	33	35	55	56
3 years	0	0	34	35	16	17	21	25	8	11	21	23	18	21	14	16	26	28
5 years	0	0	17	18	13	14	14	19	8	14	13	16	5	6	10	12	24	27
8 years	0	0	17	19	13	15	7	12	8	21	10	14	5	6	5	7	24	30
10 years	0	0	17	19	..	..	0	0	..	..	7	10	2	4	..	..	..	..

RELATIVE SURVIVAL (%) BY AGE AND PERIOD

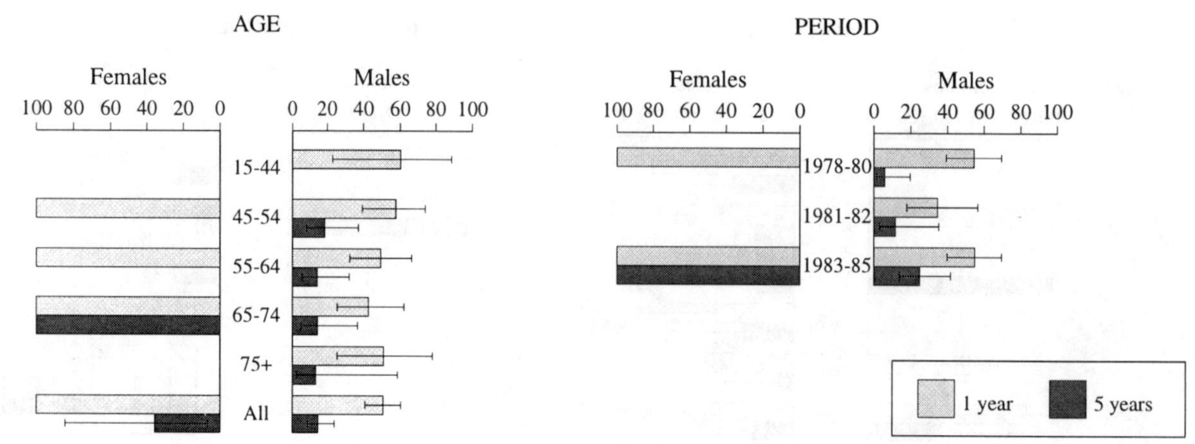

HYPOPHARYNX

SCOTLAND

REGISTRY	NUMBER OF CASES Males	Females	All	PERIOD OF DIAGNOSIS
Scotland	103	98	201	1978-1982
Mean age (years)	65.4	65.2	65.3	

RELATIVE SURVIVAL (%)

Females

Males

Time since diagnosis (years)

OBSERVED AND RELATIVE SURVIVAL (%) BY AGE AND PERIOD
(Number of cases in parentheses)

	AGE CLASS 15-44		45-54		55-64		65-74		75+		All		PERIOD 1978-80		1981-82		1983-85	
	obs	rel	obs	rel	obs	rel	obs	rel	obs	rel	obs	rel	obs	rel	obs	rel	obs	rel
Males	(2)		(12)		(32)		(39)		(18)		(103)		(55)		(48)		(0)	
1 year	50	50	42	42	59	61	41	43	33	38	46	48	45	47	46	49	..	..
3 years	50	51	8	9	34	37	18	21	17	26	22	26	24	27	21	25	..	..
5 years	50	51	8	9	28	32	10	14	11	23	17	22	20	25	13	17	..	..
8 years	..	..	..	..	25	31	10	18	11	40	15	24	18	27	..	..	..	..
10 years	..	..	..	..	..	..	..	..	0	0	..	..	..	..	..	..	..	..
Females	(8)		(11)		(26)		(27)		(26)		(98)		(53)		(45)		(0)	
1 year	63	63	36	37	58	58	52	53	27	29	46	48	40	41	53	55	..	..
3 years	38	38	36	37	38	40	19	20	19	25	28	31	23	25	33	38	..	..
5 years	25	25	27	28	31	33	19	22	15	25	22	27	17	20	29	35	..	..
8 years	25	25	27	29	31	35	19	25	..	..	21	29	17	23	..	..	..	..
10 years	..	..	..	..	31	37	..	..	..	..	21	32	17	25	..	..	..	..
Overall	(10)		(23)		(58)		(66)		(44)		(201)		(108)		(93)		(0)	
1 year	60	60	39	39	59	60	45	48	30	33	46	48	43	44	49	52	..	..
3 years	40	40	22	22	36	38	18	21	18	25	25	28	23	26	27	31	..	..
5 years	30	30	17	18	29	32	14	18	14	24	19	24	19	23	20	26	..	..
8 years	30	31	17	19	27	33	14	21	11	29	18	27	18	25	..	..	..	..
10 years	..	..	..	..	27	35	..	..	0	0	16	26	16	24	..	..	..	..

RELATIVE SURVIVAL (%) BY AGE AND PERIOD

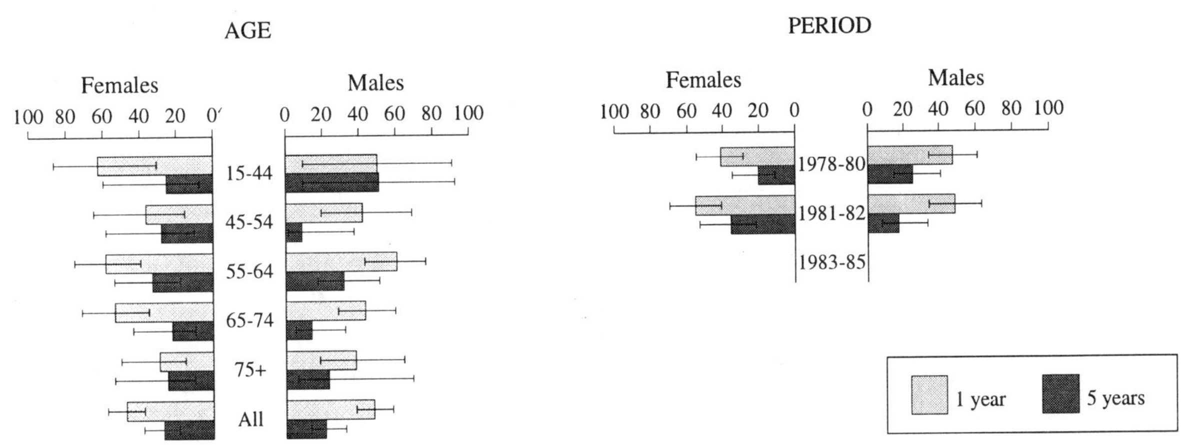

HYPOPHARYNX

DUTCH REGISTRIES

REGISTRY	NUMBER OF CASES			PERIOD OF DIAGNOSIS
	Males	Females	All	
Eindhoven	13	6	19	1978-1985
Mean age (years)	67.2	63.0	65.9	

RELATIVE SURVIVAL (%)
(Both sexes)

Time since diagnosis (years)

OBSERVED AND RELATIVE SURVIVAL (%) BY PERIOD AND SEX
(Number of cases in parentheses)

	PERIOD						SEX					
	1978-80		1981-82		1983-85		Males		Females		All	
	obs	rel	obs	rel	obs	rel	obs	rel	obs	rel	obs	rel
N. Cases	(5)		(3)		(11)		(13)		(6)		(19)	
1 year	60	63	67	67	82	86	85	88	50	53	74	77
3 years	60	68	33	35	55	65	62	70	33	39	53	60
5 years	60	72	0	0	0	0	27	34	33	43	28	36
8 years	40	53	0	0	0	0	14	20	33	48	19	27
10 years	..	..	0	0	0	0	..	..	..	..	..	..

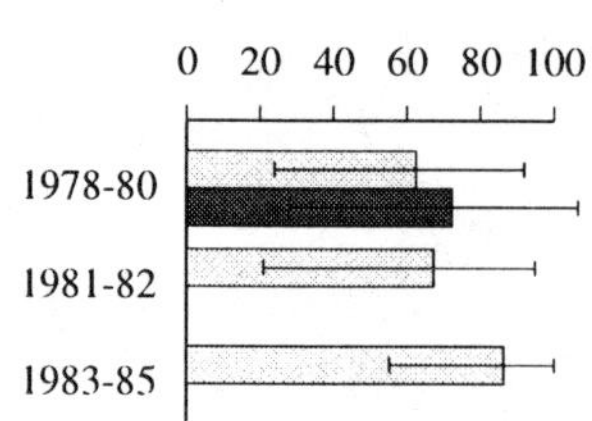

ESTONIA

REGISTRY	NUMBER OF CASES			PERIOD OF DIAGNOSIS
	Males	Females	All	
Estonia	37	3	40	1978-1984
Mean age (years)	57.1	53.0	56.8	

RELATIVE SURVIVAL (%)
(Both sexes)

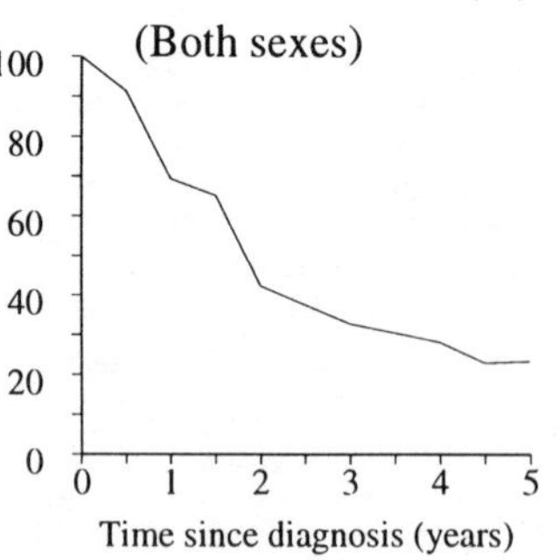

Time since diagnosis (years)

OBSERVED AND RELATIVE SURVIVAL (%) BY PERIOD AND SEX
(Number of cases in parentheses)

	PERIOD						SEX					
	1978-80		1981-82		1983-85		Males		Females		All	
	obs	rel	obs	rel	obs	rel	obs	rel	obs	rel	obs	rel
N. Cases	(9)		(15)		(16)		(37)		(3)		(40)	
1 year	78	80	67	68	63	65	65	67	100	100	68	69
3 years	44	48	20	21	31	35	27	30	67	70	30	33
5 years	33	38	7	8	25	31	16	19	67	73	20	23
8 years	22	28	7	8	..	..	12	16	67	81	16	21
10 years	11	15	..	..	..	..	6	9	..	..	8	11

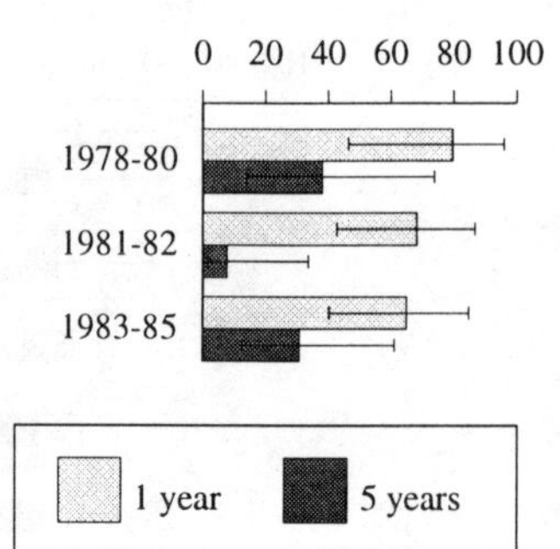

HYPOPHARYNX

FINLAND

REGISTRY	NUMBER OF CASES			PERIOD OF DIAGNOSIS
	Males	Females	All	
Finland	85	50	135	1978-1984
Mean age (years)	67.4	66.9	67.2	

RELATIVE SURVIVAL (%)
(Both sexes)

Time since diagnosis (years)

OBSERVED AND RELATIVE SURVIVAL (%) BY PERIOD AND SEX
(Number of cases in parentheses)

	PERIOD						SEX					
	1978-80		1981-82		1983-85		Males		Females		All	
	obs	rel	obs	rel	obs	rel	obs	rel	obs	rel	obs	rel
N. Cases	(56)		(42)		(37)		(85)		(50)		(135)	
1 year	36	37	64	67	51	54	49	52	48	49	49	51
3 years	7	8	14	16	14	16	12	14	10	11	11	13
5 years	4	5	12	15	5	7	8	11	4	5	7	8
8 years	2	3	10	14	..	..	6	10	4	5	5	8
10 years	2	3	..	..	..	..	6	11	..	..	5	9

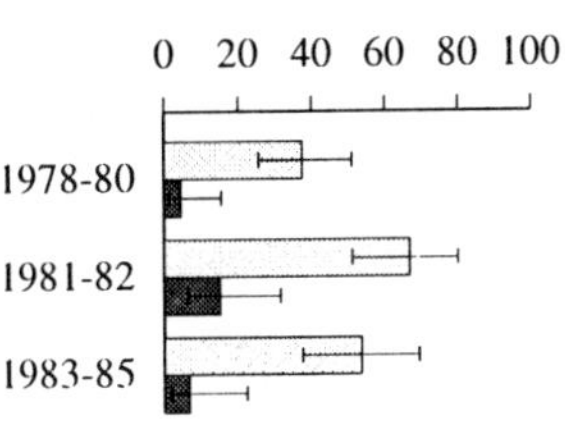

GERMAN REGISTRIES

REGISTRY	NUMBER OF CASES			PERIOD OF DIAGNOSIS
	Males	Females	All	
Saarland	77	7	84	1978-1984
Mean age (years)	54.1	47.9	53.6	

RELATIVE SURVIVAL (%)
(Both sexes)

Time since diagnosis (years)

OBSERVED AND RELATIVE SURVIVAL (%) BY PERIOD AND SEX
(Number of cases in parentheses)

	PERIOD						SEX					
	1978-80		1981-82		1983-85		Males		Females		All	
	obs	rel	obs	rel	obs	rel	obs	rel	obs	rel	obs	rel
N. Cases	(26)		(21)		(37)		(77)		(7)		(84)	
1 year	58	59	52	54	57	58	56	57	57	57	56	57
3 years	15	16	10	10	27	29	21	22	0	0	19	20
5 years	12	13	10	11	22	24	17	19	0	0	15	17
8 years	8	9	10	12	..	..	15	18	0	0	14	16
10 years	8	9	..	..	..	..	15	19	0	0	14	17

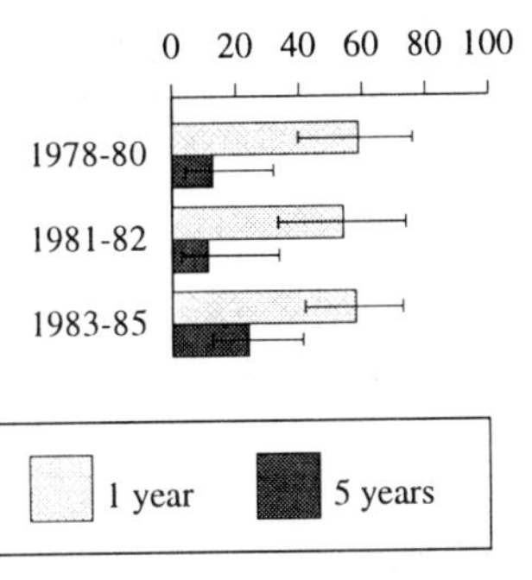

HYPOPHARYNX

POLISH REGISTRIES

REGISTRY	NUMBER OF CASES			PERIOD OF DIAGNOSIS
	Males	Females	All	
Cracow	17	3	20	1979-1984
Mean age (years)	64.4	66.0	64.6	

RELATIVE SURVIVAL (%)
(Both sexes)

Time since diagnosis (years)

OBSERVED AND RELATIVE SURVIVAL (%) BY PERIOD AND SEX
(Number of cases in parentheses)

	PERIOD						SEX					
	1978-80		1981-82		1983-85		Males		Females		All	
	obs	rel	obs	rel	obs	rel	obs	rel	obs	rel	obs	rel
N. Cases	(2)		(11)		(7)		(17)		(3)		(20)	
1 year	50	54	55	57	57	60	59	62	33	35	55	58
3 years	0	0	9	10	14	17	12	14	0	0	10	12
5 years	0	0	9	12	0	0	6	8	0	0	5	7
8 years	0	0	0	0	0	0	0	0	0	0	0	0
10 years	0	0	0	0	0	0	0	0	0	0	0	0

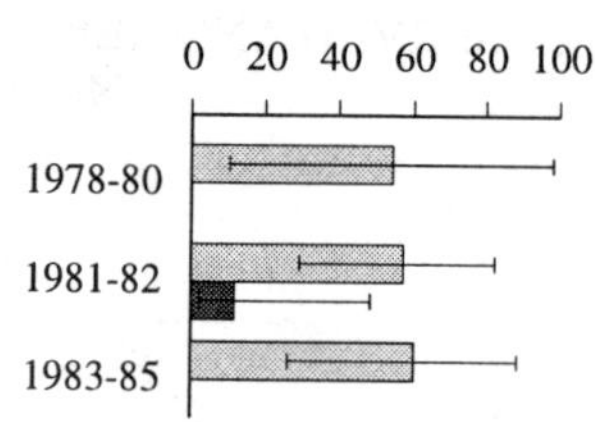

SPANISH REGISTRIES

REGISTRY	NUMBER OF CASES			PERIOD OF DIAGNOSIS
	Males	Females	All	
Tarragona	3	0	3	1985-1985
Mean age (years)	49.7	..	49.7	

RELATIVE SURVIVAL (%)
(Both sexes)

Time since diagnosis (years)

OBSERVED AND RELATIVE SURVIVAL (%) BY PERIOD AND SEX
(Number of cases in parentheses)

	PERIOD						SEX					
	1978-80		1981-82		1983-85		Males		Females		All	
	obs	rel	obs	rel	obs	rel	obs	rel	obs	rel	obs	rel
N. Cases	(0)		(0)		(3)		(3)		(0)		(3)	
1 year	..	..	..	..	33	34	33	34	..	..	33	34
3 years	..	..	..	..	0	0	0	0	..	..	0	0
5 years	..	..	..	..	0	0	0	0	..	..	0	0
8 years	..	..	..	..	0	0	0	0	..	..	0	0
10 years	..	..	..	..	0	0	0	0	..	..	0	0

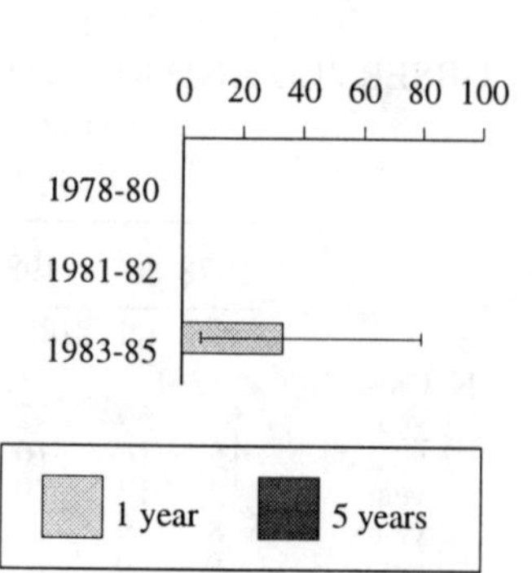

HYPOPHARYNX

SWISS REGISTRIES

REGISTRY	NUMBER OF CASES			PERIOD OF DIAGNOSIS
	Males	Females	All	
Basel	20	2	22	1981-1984
Geneva	55	4	59	1978-1984
Mean age (years)	60.3	66.0	60.7	

RELATIVE SURVIVAL (%)
(Both sexes)

Time since diagnosis (years)

OBSERVED AND RELATIVE SURVIVAL (%) BY PERIOD AND SEX
(Number of cases in parentheses)

	PERIOD						SEX					
	1978-80		1981-82		1983-85		Males		Females		All	
	obs	rel	obs	rel	obs	rel	obs	rel	obs	rel	obs	rel
N. Cases	(26)		(30)		(25)		(75)		(6)		(81)	
1 year	46	47	63	65	50	51	56	57	27	28	54	55
3 years	19	21	23	26	21	22	21	23	27	29	21	23
5 years	15	18	13	15	8	9	12	14	27	30	13	14
8 years	..	..	..	..	..	..	..	..	..	..	..	..
10 years	..	..	..	..	..	..	..	..	..	..	..	..

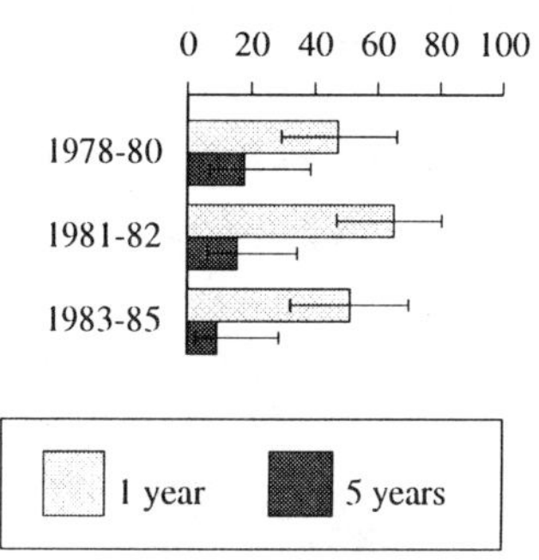

HYPOPHARYNX

EUROPEAN REGISTRIES

Unweighted analysis

REGISTRY	CASES Males	Females	All
DENMARK	135	38	173
DUTCH REGISTRIES	13	6	19
ENGLISH REGISTRIES	589	498	1087
ESTONIA	37	3	40
FINLAND	85	50	135
FRENCH REGISTRIES	243	6	249
GERMAN REGISTRIES	77	7	84
ITALIAN REGISTRIES	104	3	107
POLISH REGISTRIES	17	3	20
SCOTLAND	103	98	201
SPANISH REGISTRIES	3	0	3
SWISS REGISTRIES	75	6	81
Mean age (years)	63.1	66.1	64.1

RELATIVE SURVIVAL (%)
(Age-standardized)

Females Males
100 80 60 40 20 0 0 20 40 60 80 100
DK
ENG
F
I
SCO
EUR

OBSERVED AND RELATIVE SURVIVAL (%) BY AGE AND PERIOD
(Number of cases in parentheses)

	AGE CLASS 15-44 obs	rel	45-54 obs	rel	55-64 obs	rel	65-74 obs	rel	75+ obs	rel	All obs	rel	PERIOD 1978-80 obs	rel	1981-82 obs	rel	1983-85 obs	rel
Males	(74)		(275)		(453)		(415)		(264)		(1481)		(529)		(421)		(531)	
1 year	62	62	58	58	52	53	48	50	37	41	50	52	49	52	49	52	50	52
3 years	29	29	22	23	25	27	22	25	13	19	22	25	23	26	18	21	23	26
5 years	22	22	16	17	17	19	15	20	8	16	15	19	15	19	12	15	17	21
8 years	20	21	11	12	12	14	10	15	5	17	10	15	10	15	8	12	10	13
10 years	20	21	9	10	11	14	4	8	3	15	7	12	8	13	4	6	..	..
Females	(28)		(85)		(208)		(213)		(184)		(718)		(314)		(222)		(182)	
1 year	46	47	59	60	56	57	42	43	28	31	45	46	45	47	46	48	43	45
3 years	32	32	27	27	25	26	19	20	10	14	20	22	18	20	24	26	18	20
5 years	29	29	25	26	21	22	16	18	7	11	16	20	14	17	20	24	15	19
8 years	29	29	19	20	17	19	12	15	5	11	13	17	12	16	15	20	6	8
10 years	29	29	16	17	15	18	10	14	2	6	11	15	10	14	14	19	..	..
Overall	(102)		(360)		(661)		(628)		(448)		(2199)		(843)		(643)		(713)	
1 year	58	58	58	58	53	54	46	48	33	37	48	50	48	50	48	50	48	50
3 years	30	30	23	24	25	27	21	24	12	16	21	24	21	24	20	23	22	24
5 years	24	24	18	19	18	20	15	19	8	14	15	19	15	18	15	18	17	21
8 years	23	23	13	14	13	16	10	15	5	14	11	16	11	16	11	15	8	12
10 years	23	23	10	12	12	15	5	9	3	10	8	13	9	13	8	12	..	..

RELATIVE SURVIVAL (%) BY AGE AND PERIOD

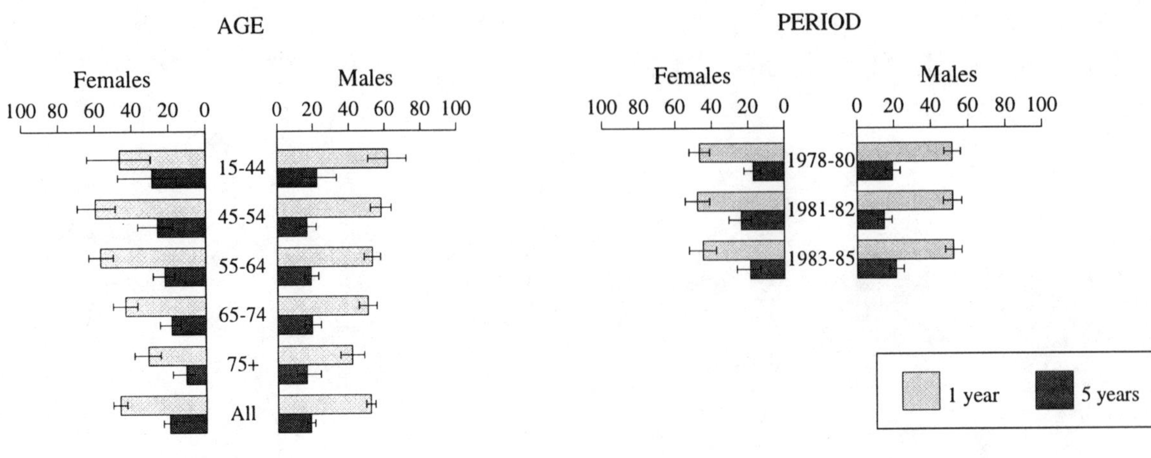

HEAD & NECK

DENMARK

REGISTRY	NUMBER OF CASES			PERIOD OF DIAGNOSIS
	Males	Females	All	
Denmark	1212	782	1994	1978-1984
Mean age (years)	63.2	67.9	65.0	

RELATIVE SURVIVAL (%)

OBSERVED AND RELATIVE SURVIVAL (%) BY AGE AND PERIOD
(Number of cases in parentheses)

	AGE CLASS												PERIOD					
	15-44		45-54		55-64		65-74		75+		All		1978-80		1981-82		1983-85	
	obs	rel	obs	rel	obs	rel	obs	rel	obs	rel	obs	rel	obs	rel	obs	rel	obs	rel
Males	(89)		(195)		(349)		(348)		(231)		(1212)		(492)		(334)		(386)	
1 year	82	82	68	69	63	64	64	66	46	52	62	65	64	66	61	63	62	64
3 years	55	55	39	40	37	39	37	43	22	32	36	41	38	43	34	39	35	39
5 years	47	48	34	36	30	33	26	34	15	29	28	35	30	37	27	34	26	32
8 years	41	42	31	33	23	28	17	26	13	40	22	31	24	34	21	31	..	..
10 years	32	34	27	30	18	23	10	19	10	46	16	26	18	28	..	..	..	..
Females	(39)		(85)		(177)		(203)		(278)		(782)		(323)		(222)		(237)	
1 year	87	87	75	76	79	79	71	73	59	64	70	72	69	72	69	72	71	74
3 years	64	64	65	66	59	61	47	51	30	40	47	53	47	53	45	50	48	55
5 years	59	59	56	58	50	53	36	41	20	33	37	45	37	45	39	47	34	43
8 years	50	51	51	53	42	47	28	37	12	30	29	42	29	41	29	41	..	..
10 years	50	52	51	54	42	48	22	31	5	17	26	42	26	40	..	..	..	..
Overall	(128)		(280)		(526)		(551)		(509)		(1994)		(815)		(556)		(623)	
1 year	84	84	70	71	68	69	66	69	53	59	65	68	66	68	64	67	65	68
3 years	58	58	47	48	45	47	41	46	26	37	40	45	42	47	38	43	40	45
5 years	51	51	41	43	36	40	30	37	18	31	31	39	33	40	32	39	29	36
8 years	44	45	37	39	30	35	21	30	12	34	25	35	26	37	24	34	..	..
10 years	37	38	33	37	26	33	14	24	8	30	20	32	21	33	..	..	..	..

RELATIVE SURVIVAL (%) BY AGE AND PERIOD

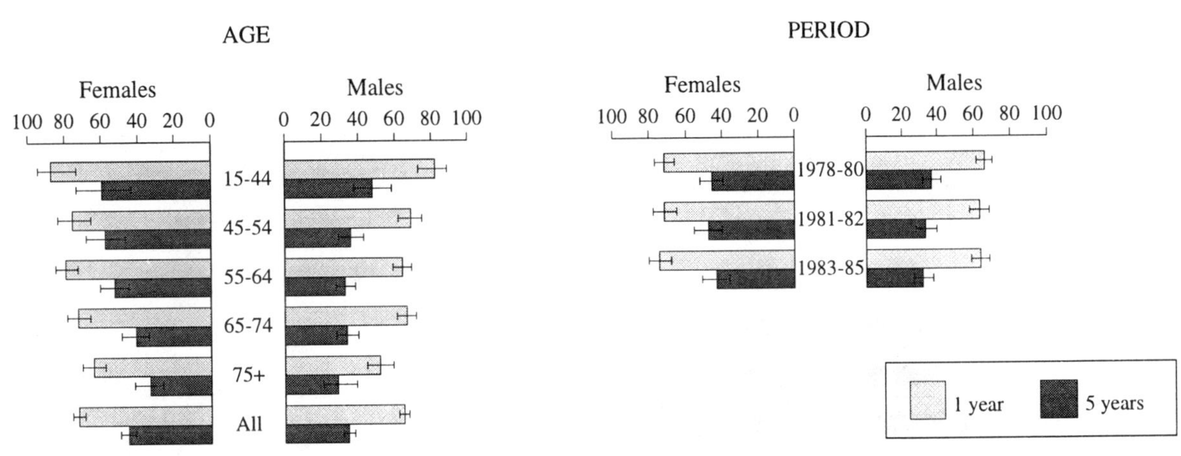

HEAD & NECK

DUTCH REGISTRIES

REGISTRY	NUMBER OF CASES			PERIOD OF DIAGNOSIS
	Males	Females	All	
Eindhoven	137	66	203	1978-1985
Mean age (years)	63.6	63.7	63.7	

RELATIVE SURVIVAL (%)

100
80
60
40
20
0
0 1 2 3 4 5
Females
Males
Time since diagnosis (years)

OBSERVED AND RELATIVE SURVIVAL (%) BY AGE AND PERIOD
(Number of cases in parentheses)

	AGE CLASS												PERIOD					
	15-44		45-54		55-64		65-74		75+		All		1978-80		1981-82		1983-85	
	obs	rel	obs	rel	obs	rel	obs	rel	obs	rel	obs	rel	obs	rel	obs	rel	obs	rel
Males	(9)		(22)		(42)		(39)		(25)		(137)		(45)		(27)		(65)	
1 year	100	100	82	82	67	68	67	70	52	59	69	72	58	60	74	77	74	77
3 years	77	77	59	60	40	42	46	53	28	42	45	51	38	43	37	42	53	61
5 years	77	78	59	61	31	34	19	25	15	32	32	40	31	38	26	32	28	37
8 years	0	0	47	50	19	22	6	11	0	0	16	24	17	23	..	..	..	..
10 years	0	0	..	..	..	..	..	..	0	0	..	..	..	..	..	..	..	..
Females	(7)		(15)		(12)		(9)		(23)		(66)		(20)		(17)		(29)	
1 year	86	86	87	87	67	67	56	57	43	48	64	66	65	67	65	69	62	64
3 years	86	86	80	81	58	60	44	48	35	47	56	63	65	70	47	57	54	60
5 years	86	86	80	81	58	61	30	34	25	43	49	60	60	69	35	49	54	66
8 years	86	86	80	83	35	38	30	38	25	66	43	61	50	62	..	..	..	..
10 years	..	..	80	84	35	39	..	..	..	..	43	67	50	68	..	..	..	..
Overall	(16)		(37)		(54)		(48)		(48)		(203)		(65)		(44)		(94)	
1 year	94	94	84	84	67	68	65	67	48	54	67	70	60	62	70	74	70	73
3 years	81	81	67	68	44	46	45	52	31	45	48	55	46	52	41	47	53	60
5 years	81	81	67	69	37	40	20	26	20	38	38	47	40	48	30	38	36	46
8 years	65	65	58	61	23	27	10	16	16	49	25	37	27	37	..	..	..	..
10 years	..	..	58	63	23	28	..	..	..	..	25	41	27	40	..	..	..	..

RELATIVE SURVIVAL (%) BY AGE AND PERIOD

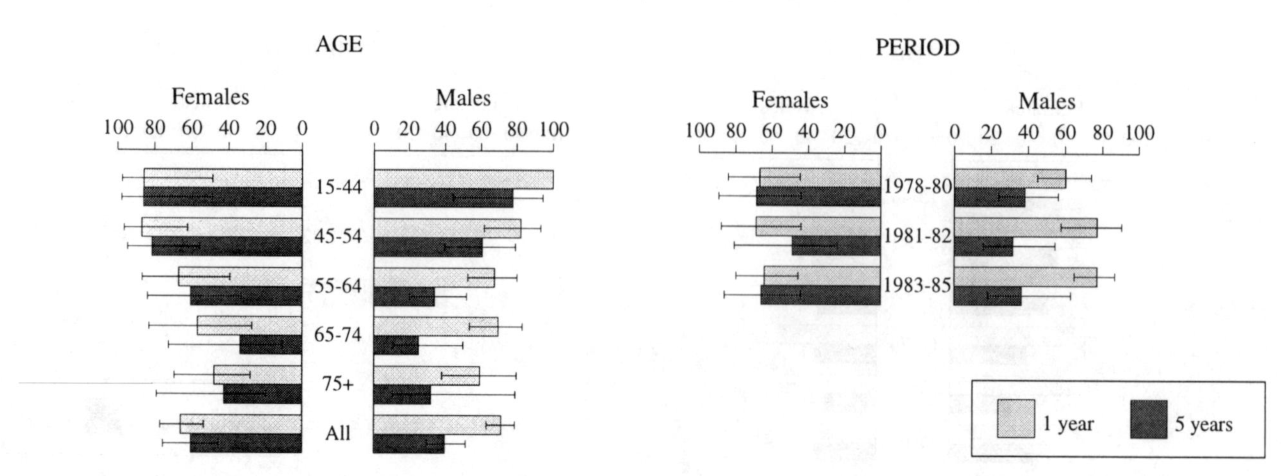

HEAD & NECK

ENGLISH REGISTRIES

REGISTRY	NUMBER OF CASES			PERIOD OF DIAGNOSIS
	Males	Females	All	
East Anglia	280	238	518	1979-1984
Mersey	541	306	847	1978-1984
South Thames	1081	753	1834	1978-1984
Wessex	138	74	212	1983-1984
West Midlands	829	415	1244	1979-1984
Yorkshire	660	481	1141	1978-1984
Mean age (years)	63.7	67.0	65.0	

RELATIVE SURVIVAL (%)

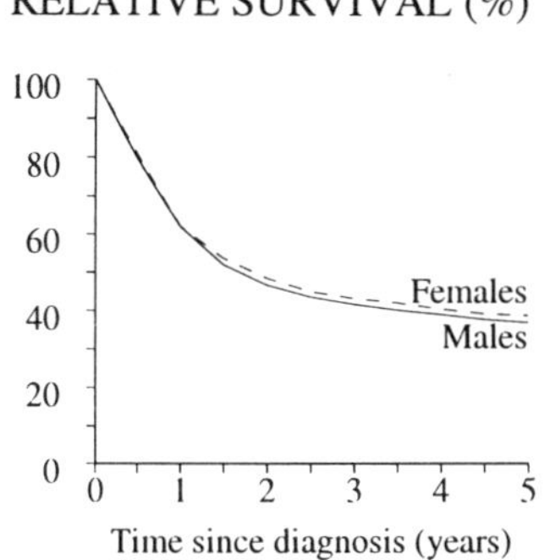

OBSERVED AND RELATIVE SURVIVAL (%) BY AGE AND PERIOD
(Number of cases in parentheses)

	AGE CLASS												PERIOD					
	15-44		45-54		55-64		65-74		75+		All		1978-80		1981-82		1983-85	
	obs	rel	obs	rel	obs	rel	obs	rel	obs	rel	obs	rel	obs	rel	obs	rel	obs	rel
Males	(215)		(513)		(1060)		(1075)		(666)		(3529)		(1319)		(1067)		(1143)	
1 year	81	81	67	68	62	63	60	63	40	46	59	62	59	62	58	61	60	63
3 years	64	65	45	46	38	41	36	42	18	26	36	42	36	42	34	39	38	44
5 years	57	58	38	40	31	35	28	37	12	25	29	37	29	37	27	34	32	40
8 years	54	55	30	32	25	31	20	33	6	22	23	33	23	34	21	31	23	32
10 years	52	54	26	29	21	28	16	30	5	26	19	31	20	33	17	27	..	..
Females	(124)		(244)		(522)		(670)		(707)		(2267)		(909)		(621)		(737)	
1 year	79	79	75	75	68	69	60	62	45	49	60	62	57	60	60	62	63	65
3 years	63	63	55	56	43	44	39	42	24	33	38	43	35	40	40	45	40	46
5 years	53	54	51	52	37	40	31	36	18	30	32	39	29	35	33	41	34	42
8 years	50	51	44	47	30	33	23	30	13	33	25	36	24	33	25	36	25	36
10 years	41	41	42	44	26	31	18	27	9	31	21	33	19	30	24	36	..	..
Overall	(339)		(757)		(1582)		(1745)		(1373)		(5796)		(2228)		(1688)		(1880)	
1 year	80	80	70	70	64	65	60	63	42	47	59	62	58	61	59	61	61	64
3 years	64	64	48	49	40	42	37	42	21	30	37	42	36	41	36	41	39	44
5 years	56	56	42	44	33	37	29	37	15	28	30	38	29	36	29	36	33	41
8 years	53	54	35	37	27	32	21	32	10	28	24	34	23	34	23	33	24	34
10 years	48	49	31	34	23	29	17	29	7	29	20	32	20	32	20	31	..	..

RELATIVE SURVIVAL (%) BY AGE AND PERIOD

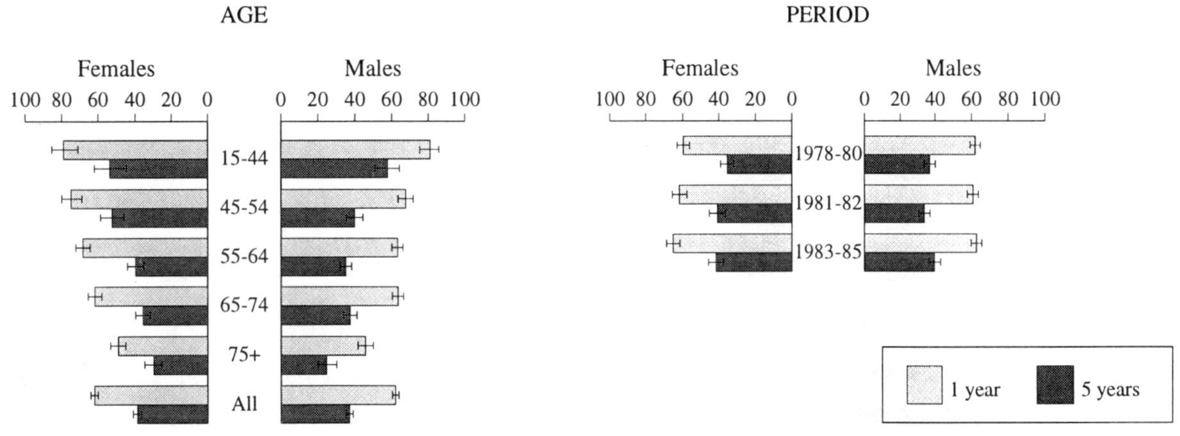

HEAD & NECK

ESTONIA

REGISTRY	NUMBER OF CASES			PERIOD OF DIAGNOSIS
	Males	Females	All	
Estonia	266	68	334	1978-1984
Mean age (years)	57.1	63.7	58.4	

RELATIVE SURVIVAL (%)

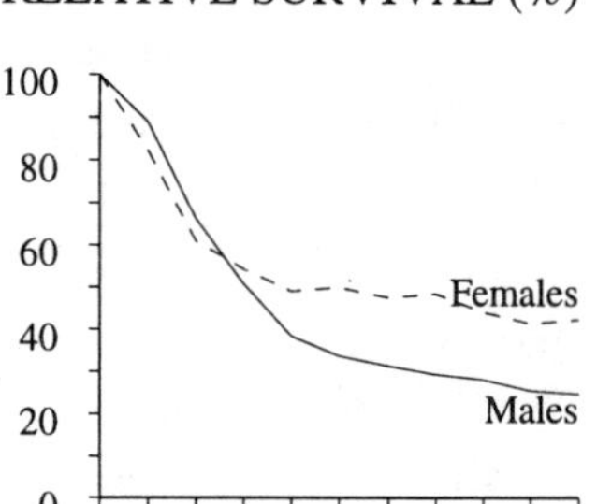

OBSERVED AND RELATIVE SURVIVAL (%) BY AGE AND PERIOD
(Number of cases in parentheses)

	AGE CLASS												PERIOD					
	15-44		45-54		55-64		65-74		75+		All		1978-80		1981-82		1983-85	
	obs	rel	obs	rel	obs	rel	obs	rel	obs	rel	obs	rel	obs	rel	obs	rel	obs	rel
Males	(26)		(91)		(90)		(42)		(17)		(266)		(100)		(68)		(98)	
1 year	77	77	66	67	60	62	62	65	65	73	64	66	64	66	66	68	63	65
3 years	42	43	29	31	23	25	31	37	24	34	29	31	34	38	29	32	22	24
5 years	27	28	23	25	19	22	19	26	18	35	21	25	22	26	24	28	18	21
8 years	18	19	12	14	14	19	12	20	0	0	12	16	14	19	11	15	..	..
10 years	18	20	6	8	14	21	4	8	0	0	8	12	9	13	..	..	..	..
Females	(6)		(11)		(17)		(18)		(16)		(68)		(34)		(18)		(16)	
1 year	100	100	73	73	53	53	56	57	44	48	59	61	53	55	72	75	56	58
3 years	83	84	55	55	41	43	32	36	31	43	43	47	35	39	44	50	56	61
5 years	67	67	55	56	35	37	26	32	19	33	35	42	32	39	28	34	49	57
8 years	50	51	27	29	23	26	19	30	0	0	22	30	24	33	11	16	..	..
10 years	50	51	27	29	23	27	0	0	0	0	18	28	20	31	..	..	..	..
Overall	(32)		(102)		(107)		(60)		(33)		(334)		(134)		(86)		(114)	
1 year	81	82	67	68	59	60	60	63	55	61	63	65	61	63	67	70	62	64
3 years	50	51	32	34	26	28	31	37	27	39	31	35	34	38	33	36	27	29
5 years	34	36	26	28	21	25	21	28	18	34	24	28	25	29	24	29	22	26
8 years	23	25	14	16	16	20	14	23	0	0	14	19	16	22	11	15	..	..
10 years	23	25	8	10	16	22	4	8	0	0	10	15	12	18	..	..	..	..

RELATIVE SURVIVAL (%) BY AGE AND PERIOD

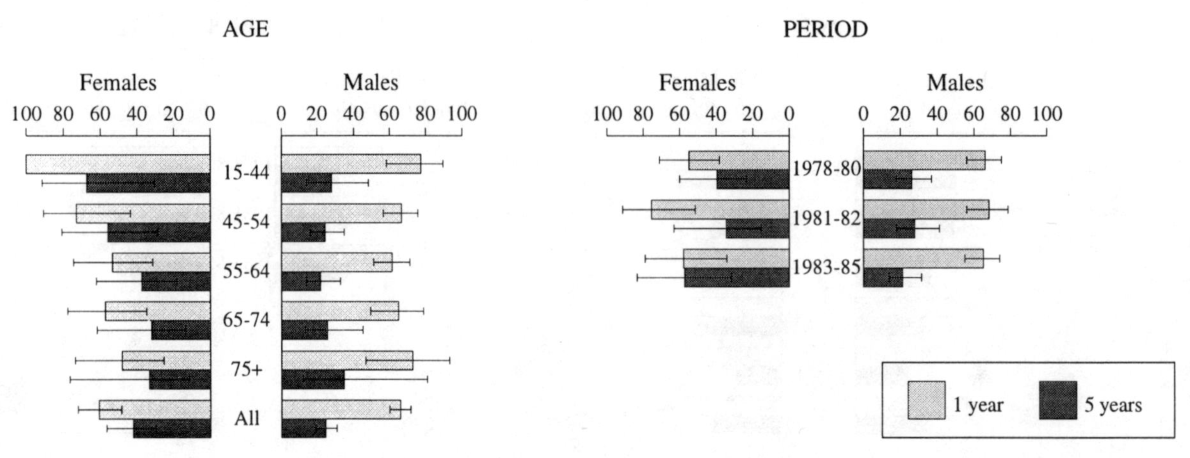

HEAD & NECK

FINLAND

REGISTRY	NUMBER OF CASES			PERIOD OF DIAGNOSIS
	Males	Females	All	
Finland	536	425	961	1978-1984
Mean age (years)	61.1	66.4	63.5	

RELATIVE SURVIVAL (%)

100
80
60
40
20
0
0 1 2 3 4 5
Females
Males
Time since diagnosis (years)

OBSERVED AND RELATIVE SURVIVAL (%) BY AGE AND PERIOD
(Number of cases in parentheses)

	AGE CLASS												PERIOD					
	15-44		45-54		55-64		65-74		75+		All		1978-80		1981-82		1983-85	
	obs	rel	obs	rel	obs	rel	obs	rel	obs	rel	obs	rel	obs	rel	obs	rel	obs	rel
Males	(64)		(89)		(153)		(137)		(93)		(536)		(221)		(154)		(161)	
1 year	81	81	81	82	71	73	63	66	45	51	67	70	67	69	68	71	68	70
3 years	55	55	48	50	44	48	31	37	17	25	38	43	38	43	33	37	43	49
5 years	48	49	43	45	38	43	22	29	12	23	31	39	29	37	29	35	37	45
8 years	44	45	37	41	26	32	15	26	8	25	24	34	24	34	21	30	28	38
10 years	44	45	33	37	22	29	15	31	6	25	21	33	21	33	20	30	..	..
Females	(32)		(43)		(87)		(137)		(126)		(425)		(176)		(120)		(129)	
1 year	97	97	95	96	68	68	69	71	49	54	68	70	66	69	68	70	70	72
3 years	78	78	60	61	47	48	43	47	26	35	43	48	42	47	46	52	43	48
5 years	75	75	49	50	39	41	36	41	20	33	36	44	35	42	38	47	35	43
8 years	75	76	47	48	35	39	30	40	14	34	31	43	32	43	33	48	30	42
10 years	75	76	47	48	35	40	20	30	10	33	28	42	28	42	31	49	..	..
Overall	(96)		(132)		(240)		(274)		(219)		(961)		(397)		(274)		(290)	
1 year	86	87	86	86	70	71	66	69	47	53	68	70	66	69	68	70	69	71
3 years	63	63	52	53	45	48	37	42	22	31	40	46	40	45	39	44	43	49
5 years	57	58	45	47	38	42	29	36	16	29	33	41	32	39	33	40	36	44
8 years	54	55	40	44	29	35	23	34	11	30	27	38	27	38	27	38	28	40
10 years	54	56	38	42	27	34	18	31	8	30	24	38	24	37	25	38	..	..

RELATIVE SURVIVAL (%) BY AGE AND PERIOD

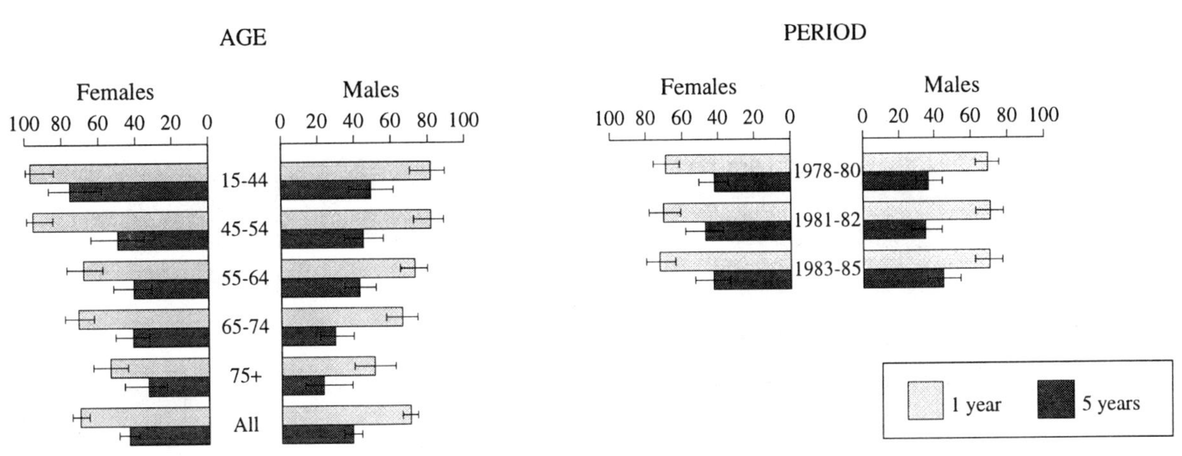

HEAD & NECK

FRENCH REGISTRIES

REGISTRY	NUMBER OF CASES			PERIOD OF DIAGNOSIS
	Males	Females	All	
Amiens	202	24	226	1983-1984
Doubs	729	49	778	1978-1985
Mean age (years)	58.2	62.5	58.5	

RELATIVE SURVIVAL (%)

100 80 60 40 20 0

Females

Males

0 1 2 3 4 5

Time since diagnosis (years)

OBSERVED AND RELATIVE SURVIVAL (%) BY AGE AND PERIOD
(Number of cases in parentheses)

	AGE CLASS												PERIOD					
	15-44		45-54		55-64		65-74		75+		All		1978-80		1981-82		1983-85	
	obs	rel	obs	rel	obs	rel	obs	rel	obs	rel	obs	rel	obs	rel	obs	rel	obs	rel
Males	(81)		(294)		(302)		(170)		(84)		(931)		(253)		(195)		(483)	
1 year	75	75	74	75	65	66	56	58	50	57	66	67	68	70	63	64	66	67
3 years	39	39	38	39	31	33	27	31	17	24	32	35	34	37	26	29	34	36
5 years	29	30	30	31	24	26	20	25	12	22	24	28	23	27	18	21	28	31
8 years	27	28	21	23	12	14	8	13	4	12	15	18	13	16	12	15	..	..
10 years	27	28	12	14	10	12	8	15	..	..	11	15	10	13	..	..	..	..
Females	(4)		(18)		(27)		(8)		(16)		(73)		(18)		(11)		(44)	
1 year	75	75	94	95	62	62	63	64	61	70	70	73	65	67	91	92	67	70
3 years	50	50	69	70	46	47	63	67	38	55	52	57	47	51	91	95	44	49
5 years	50	50	55	56	46	48	38	42	30	56	45	51	47	53	82	88	33	39
8 years	..	..	46	48	33	35	25	31	..	..	30	38	34	41	38	44	..	..
10 years	..	..	23	24	0	0	..	..	..	..	11	14	12	16	..	..	..	..
Overall	(85)		(312)		(329)		(178)		(100)		(1004)		(271)		(206)		(527)	
1 year	75	75	75	76	65	66	56	58	52	59	66	68	68	70	64	66	66	67
3 years	39	40	40	41	32	34	29	33	20	29	34	36	35	38	30	32	34	37
5 years	30	31	31	33	26	28	21	26	14	26	26	29	25	28	22	25	28	32
8 years	28	29	22	24	14	16	9	14	4	11	16	20	14	18	13	16	..	..
10 years	28	30	13	14	9	12	9	16	..	..	11	14	10	13	..	..	..	..

RELATIVE SURVIVAL (%) BY AGE AND PERIOD

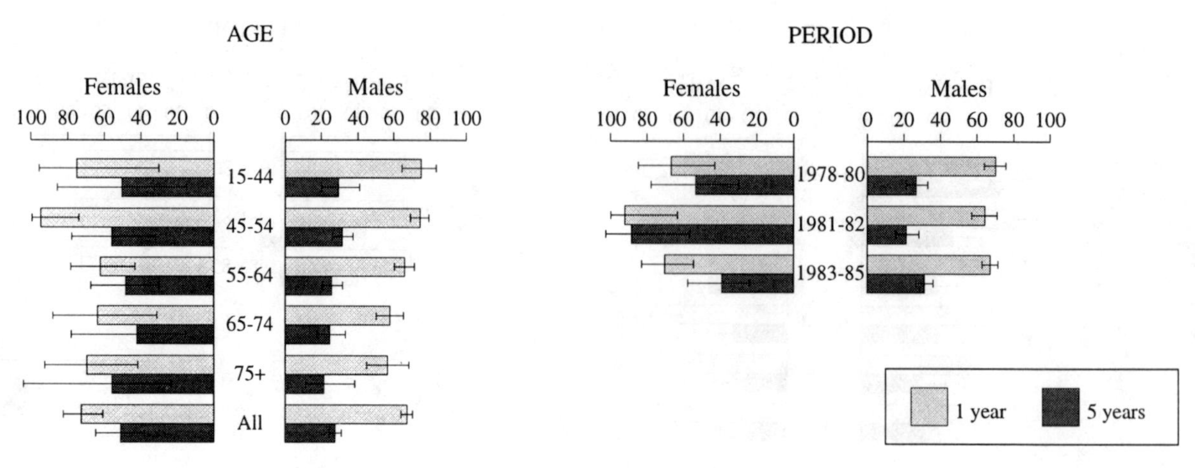

HEAD & NECK

GERMAN REGISTRIES

REGISTRY	NUMBER OF CASES			PERIOD OF DIAGNOSIS
	Males	Females	All	
Saarland	455	103	558	1978-1984
Mean age (years)	55.4	59.3	56.1	

RELATIVE SURVIVAL (%)

OBSERVED AND RELATIVE SURVIVAL (%) BY AGE AND PERIOD
(Number of cases in parentheses)

	AGE CLASS												PERIOD					
	15-44		45-54		55-64		65-74		75+		All		1978-80		1981-82		1983-85	
	obs	rel	obs	rel	obs	rel	obs	rel	obs	rel	obs	rel	obs	rel	obs	rel	obs	rel
Males	(80)		(155)		(113)		(83)		(24)		(455)		(170)		(128)		(157)	
1 year	69	69	69	70	69	70	61	65	46	51	66	68	66	68	59	61	72	73
3 years	36	37	35	36	40	42	36	43	29	42	36	39	39	42	30	32	39	41
5 years	28	28	30	32	33	36	30	41	13	23	29	33	35	41	22	25	29	33
8 years	19	20	26	28	25	30	17	30	8	25	22	27	27	34	16	19	..	..
10 years	16	17	24	27	22	29	12	25	0	0	19	25	23	31	..	..	..	..
Females	(12)		(33)		(22)		(20)		(16)		(103)		(42)		(37)		(24)	
1 year	67	67	76	76	77	78	55	57	69	75	70	71	69	70	76	78	63	64
3 years	33	34	48	49	64	65	45	49	25	33	46	49	52	55	46	50	33	35
5 years	25	25	42	43	59	62	25	29	19	30	37	41	43	47	35	41	29	32
8 years	17	17	36	38	54	59	20	27	13	28	30	36	31	36	35	45	..	..
10 years	..	..	36	38	44	50	0	0	..	..	24	30	24	29	..	..	..	..
Overall	(92)		(188)		(135)		(103)		(40)		(558)		(212)		(165)		(181)	
1 year	68	69	70	71	70	72	60	63	55	61	67	69	67	69	63	65	71	72
3 years	36	36	37	38	44	46	38	44	28	38	38	41	42	45	33	36	38	41
5 years	27	28	32	34	37	41	29	39	15	26	31	35	37	42	25	28	29	33
8 years	19	20	28	30	30	36	17	28	10	26	24	29	28	35	20	25	..	..
10 years	15	16	27	29	26	33	9	17	..	..	20	26	23	31	..	..	..	..

RELATIVE SURVIVAL (%) BY AGE AND PERIOD

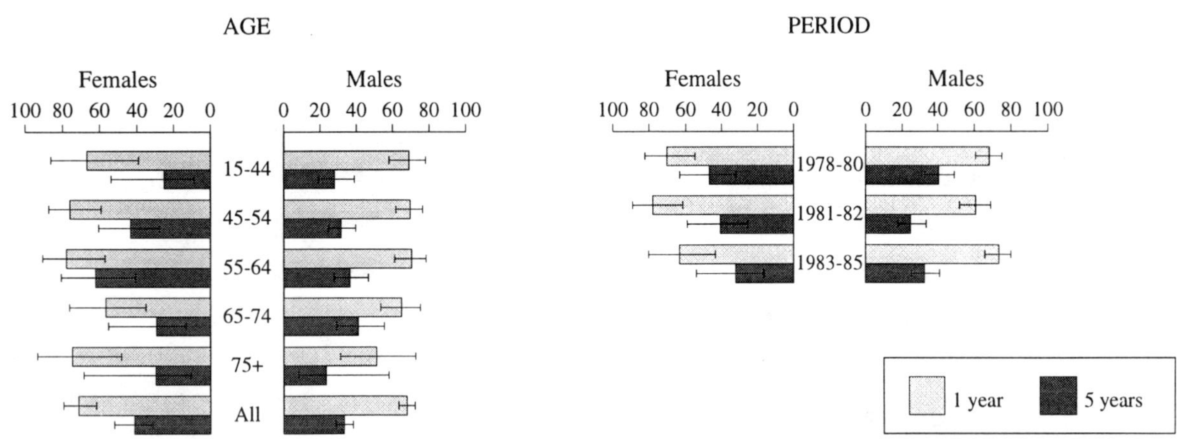

HEAD & NECK

ITALIAN REGISTRIES

REGISTRY	NUMBER OF CASES			PERIOD OF DIAGNOSIS
	Males	Females	All	
Latina	29	4	33	1983-1984
Ragusa	25	7	32	1981-1984
Varese	516	79	595	1978-1985
Mean age (years)	60.8	64.9	61.4	

RELATIVE SURVIVAL (%)

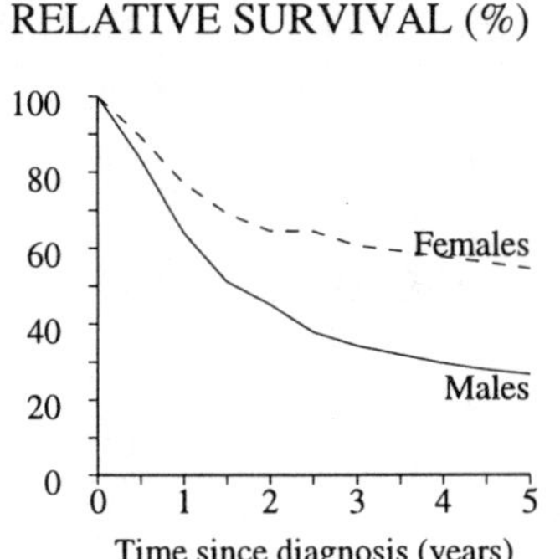

OBSERVED AND RELATIVE SURVIVAL (%) BY AGE AND PERIOD
(Number of cases in parentheses)

	AGE CLASS												PERIOD					
	15-44		45-54		55-64		65-74		75+		All		1978-80		1981-82		1983-85	
	obs	rel	obs	rel	obs	rel	obs	rel	obs	rel	obs	rel	obs	rel	obs	rel	obs	rel
Males	(34)		(130)		(195)		(144)		(67)		(570)		(204)		(142)		(224)	
1 year	76	77	61	61	66	67	60	63	49	55	62	64	57	60	60	62	67	69
3 years	41	41	32	32	32	34	35	40	13	19	31	34	27	31	29	32	35	38
5 years	32	33	25	27	24	27	22	29	7	14	22	27	18	23	22	26	27	31
8 years	32	33	20	22	16	19	13	20	6	17	16	21	12	18	15	19	19	25
10 years	32	33	9	10	14	18	7	14	..	..	11	16	7	12	14	19	..	..
Females	(9)		(12)		(20)		(23)		(26)		(90)		(25)		(22)		(43)	
1 year	100	100	83	84	70	70	74	75	65	72	74	77	68	70	82	85	74	77
3 years	89	89	67	67	55	56	61	65	31	42	54	61	48	53	55	62	58	64
5 years	78	78	67	68	45	47	61	69	12	20	46	55	40	48	45	56	49	58
8 years	78	79	67	69	30	32	38	48	7	18	35	47	40	53	41	57	25	32
10 years	58	59	67	69	30	33	0	0	7	25	30	42	32	46	41	60	..	..
Overall	(43)		(142)		(215)		(167)		(93)		(660)		(229)		(164)		(267)	
1 year	81	82	63	63	66	67	62	64	54	60	63	66	59	61	63	65	68	70
3 years	51	51	35	35	34	36	38	44	18	26	34	38	30	34	32	36	39	42
5 years	42	42	29	30	26	29	28	35	9	16	26	31	21	26	25	30	30	35
8 years	42	43	24	26	17	21	16	25	6	18	18	25	15	22	18	24	20	25
10 years	37	39	15	17	16	20	9	16	4	17	13	20	10	16	17	24	..	..

RELATIVE SURVIVAL (%) BY AGE AND PERIOD

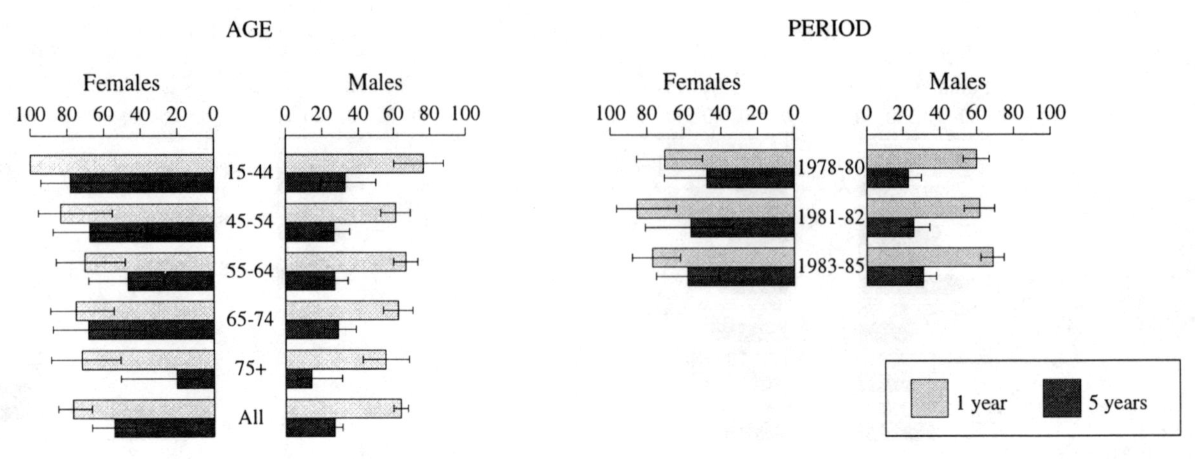

HEAD & NECK

POLISH REGISTRIES

REGISTRY	NUMBER OF CASES			PERIOD OF DIAGNOSIS
	Males	Females	All	
Cracow	133	58	191	1978-1984
Mean age (years)	58.4	60.0	58.9	

RELATIVE SURVIVAL (%)

100
80
60
40
20
0
Females
Males
0 1 2 3 4 5
Time since diagnosis (years)

OBSERVED AND RELATIVE SURVIVAL (%) BY AGE AND PERIOD
(Number of cases in parentheses)

	AGE CLASS												PERIOD					
	15-44		45-54		55-64		65-74		75+		All		1978-80		1981-82		1983-85	
	obs	rel	obs	rel	obs	rel	obs	rel	obs	rel	obs	rel	obs	rel	obs	rel	obs	rel
Males	(13)		(37)		(45)		(25)		(13)		(133)		(41)		(42)		(50)	
1 year	69	69	62	63	47	48	53	56	38	43	54	55	49	50	52	54	59	61
3 years	27	27	27	28	31	33	22	27	8	11	26	28	29	32	19	21	28	32
5 years	18	18	22	23	20	23	13	19	8	15	18	21	22	26	14	17	17	21
8 years	18	19	16	18	15	19	4	8	8	26	13	17	17	22	10	13	11	15
10 years	9	9	16	18	11	16	4	10	..	..	10	14	12	17	10	14	..	..
Females	(6)		(15)		(17)		(14)		(6)		(58)		(24)		(18)		(16)	
1 year	83	83	73	74	88	88	55	57	50	56	72	73	79	81	53	54	80	82
3 years	33	34	47	47	50	52	39	43	17	24	41	44	42	45	36	38	47	51
5 years	33	34	47	48	50	54	31	37	17	32	39	45	38	42	36	40	47	53
8 years	17	17	47	49	43	49	22	31	17	55	34	41	28	34	30	37	47	58
10 years	..	..	47	50	21	25	22	34	..	..	25	32	22	29	23	30	..	..
Overall	(19)		(52)		(62)		(39)		(19)		(191)		(65)		(60)		(66)	
1 year	74	74	65	66	57	59	54	57	42	47	59	61	60	62	53	54	64	66
3 years	29	29	33	34	36	39	28	33	11	15	30	33	34	37	24	26	33	36
5 years	23	24	29	30	28	31	20	26	11	21	24	29	28	32	20	24	25	29
8 years	17	18	25	27	22	28	10	17	11	35	19	25	21	27	15	20	20	27
10 years	9	9	25	28	13	17	10	20	..	..	14	20	16	22	13	18	..	..

RELATIVE SURVIVAL (%) BY AGE AND PERIOD

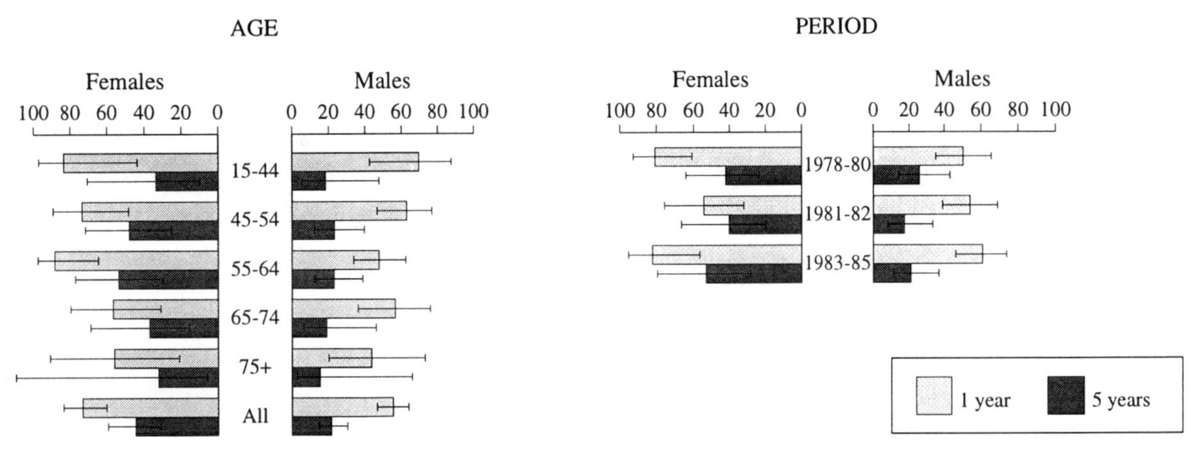

HEAD & NECK

SCOTLAND

REGISTRY	NUMBER OF CASES			PERIOD OF DIAGNOSIS
	Males	Females	All	
Scotland	748	505	1253	1978-1982
Mean age (years)	64.6	67.3	65.7	

RELATIVE SURVIVAL (%)

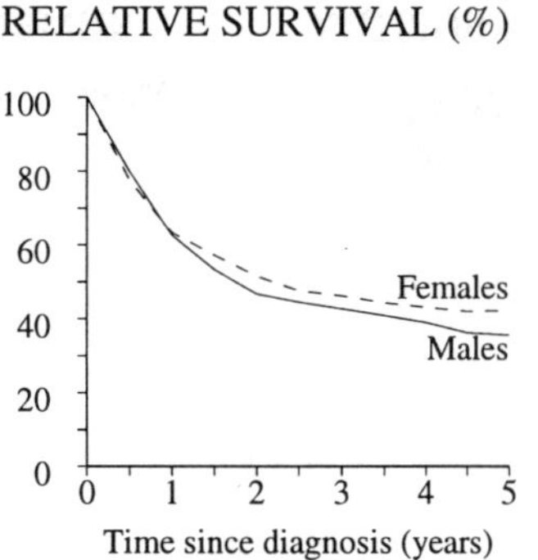

OBSERVED AND RELATIVE SURVIVAL (%) BY AGE AND PERIOD
(Number of cases in parentheses)

	AGE CLASS												PERIOD					
	15-44		45-54		55-64		65-74		75+		All		1978-80		1981-82		1983-85	
	obs	rel	obs	rel	obs	rel	obs	rel	obs	rel	obs	rel	obs	rel	obs	rel	obs	rel
Males	(40)		(107)		(217)		(215)		(169)		(748)		(438)		(310)		(0)	
1 year	78	78	62	62	71	73	56	59	43	49	59	63	58	61	62	65	..	..
3 years	52	53	36	38	47	51	35	42	19	30	36	43	35	41	38	45	..	..
5 years	45	46	31	33	36	41	24	33	12	26	27	36	27	36	27	35	..	..
8 years	41	42	26	28	26	33	20	35	7	27	21	33	22	35	..	..	..	..
10 years	41	42	21	24	25	34	16	33	0	0	17	30	17	31	..	..	..	..
Females	(26)		(61)		(103)		(152)		(163)		(505)		(281)		(224)		(0)	
1 year	73	73	74	74	66	67	66	69	45	50	61	63	57	60	65	68	..	..
3 years	62	62	52	53	48	50	43	48	25	34	40	46	37	43	44	50	..	..
5 years	54	54	46	47	40	43	39	47	17	29	34	42	31	39	37	46	..	..
8 years	44	45	39	41	38	43	31	42	12	31	28	40	25	37	..	..	..	..
10 years	..	..	31	33	31	37	28	43	12	42	24	40	22	36	..	..	..	..
Overall	(66)		(168)		(320)		(367)		(332)		(1253)		(719)		(534)		(0)	
1 year	76	76	66	67	69	71	60	63	44	49	60	63	57	60	63	66	..	..
3 years	56	56	42	43	48	51	39	45	22	32	38	44	36	42	41	47	..	..
5 years	48	49	36	38	38	42	31	39	14	27	30	38	29	37	31	40	..	..
8 years	42	43	30	33	30	37	25	38	10	29	24	36	23	36	..	..	..	..
10 years	42	44	25	27	27	35	20	37	6	27	20	34	19	33	..	..	..	..

RELATIVE SURVIVAL (%) BY AGE AND PERIOD

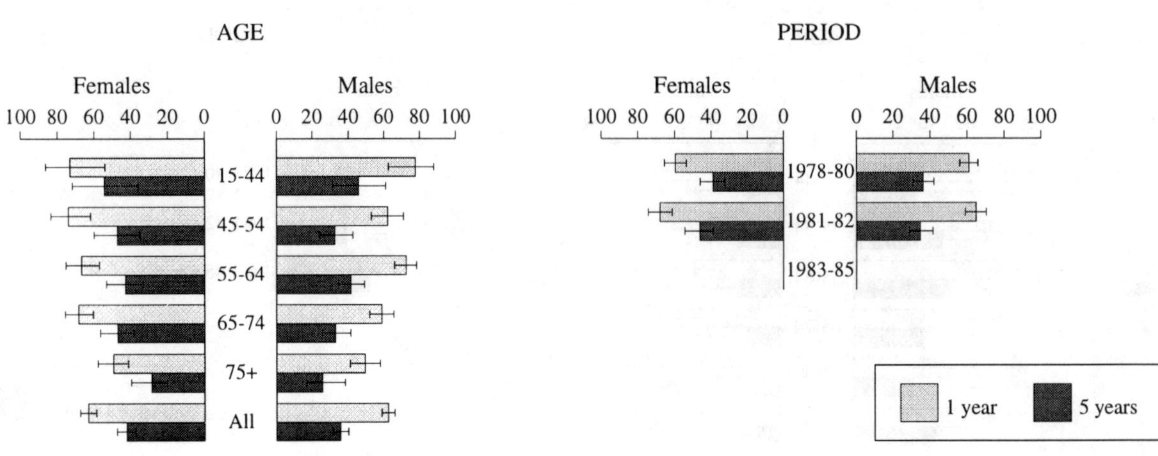

HEAD & NECK

SPANISH REGISTRIES

REGISTRY	NUMBER OF CASES			PERIOD OF DIAGNOSIS
	Males	Females	All	
Tarragona	32	4	36	1985-1985
Mean age (years)	58.6	63.3	59.1	

RELATIVE SURVIVAL (%)

100
80
60
40
20
0
Females
Males
0 1 2 3 4 5
Time since diagnosis (years)

OBSERVED AND RELATIVE SURVIVAL (%) BY AGE AND PERIOD
(Number of cases in parentheses)

	AGE CLASS												PERIOD					
	15-44		45-54		55-64		65-74		75+		All		1978-80		1981-82		1983-85	
	obs	rel	obs	rel	obs	rel	obs	rel	obs	rel	obs	rel	obs	rel	obs	rel	obs	rel
Males	(6)		(6)		(7)		(7)		(6)		(32)		(0)		(0)		(32)	
1 year	83	83	67	67	57	58	43	44	0	0	50	51	..	..	..	..	50	51
3 years	50	50	50	51	29	30	43	47	0	0	34	37	..	..	..	..	34	37
5 years	50	50	50	51	29	31	29	34	0	0	31	36	..	..	..	..	31	36
8 years	..	..	..	..	..	..	..	..	0	0	..	..	..	..	..	..	..	..
10 years	..	..	..	..	..	..	..	..	0	0	..	..	..	..	..	..	..	..
Females	(0)		(1)		(2)		(0)		(1)		(4)		(0)		(0)		(4)	
1 year	..	..	100	100	100	100	..	..	0	0	75	76	..	..	..	..	75	76
3 years	..	..	100	100	100	100	..	..	0	0	75	79	..	..	..	..	75	79
5 years	..	..	100	100	50	52	..	..	0	0	50	55	..	..	..	..	50	55
8 years	..	..	..	..	..	..	..	..	0	0	..	..	..	..	..	..	..	..
10 years	..	..	..	..	..	..	..	..	0	0	..	..	..	..	..	..	..	..
Overall	(6)		(7)		(9)		(7)		(7)		(36)		(0)		(0)		(36)	
1 year	83	83	71	72	67	67	43	44	0	0	53	54	..	..	..	..	53	54
3 years	50	50	57	58	44	46	43	47	0	0	39	42	..	..	..	..	39	42
5 years	50	50	57	59	33	36	29	34	0	0	33	38	..	..	..	..	33	38
8 years	..	..	..	..	..	..	..	..	0	0	..	..	..	..	..	..	..	..
10 years	..	..	..	..	..	..	..	..	0	0	..	..	..	..	..	..	..	..

RELATIVE SURVIVAL (%) BY AGE AND PERIOD

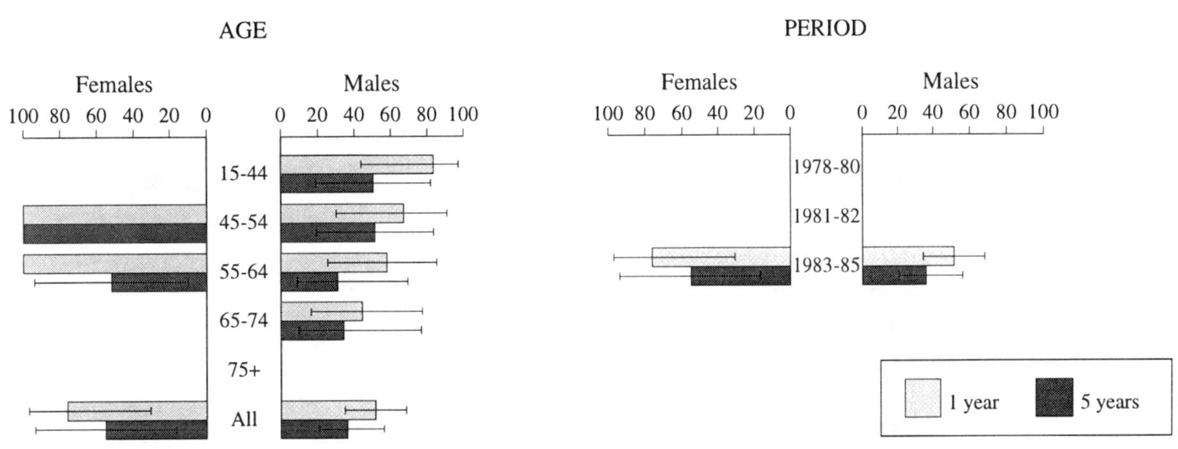

HEAD & NECK

SWISS REGISTRIES

REGISTRY	NUMBER OF CASES			PERIOD OF DIAGNOSIS
	Males	Females	All	
Basel	89	19	108	1981-1984
Geneva	261	63	324	1978-1984
Mean age (years)	60.1	62.3	60.5	

RELATIVE SURVIVAL (%)

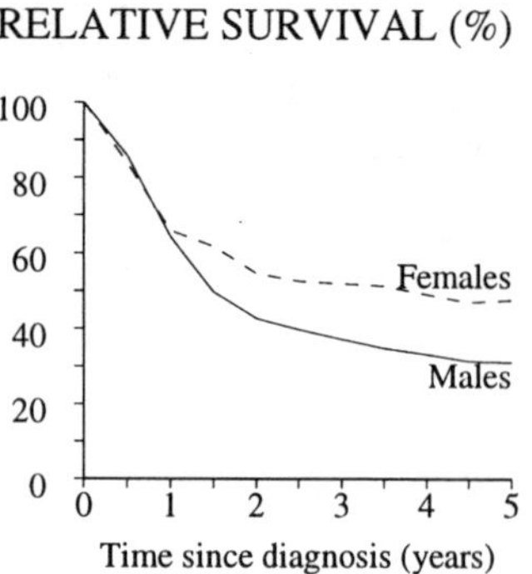

OBSERVED AND RELATIVE SURVIVAL (%) BY AGE AND PERIOD
(Number of cases in parentheses)

	AGE CLASS												PERIOD					
	15-44		45-54		55-64		65-74		75+		All		1978-80		1981-82		1983-85	
	obs	rel	obs	rel	obs	rel	obs	rel	obs	rel	obs	rel	obs	rel	obs	rel	obs	rel
Males	(27)		(81)		(129)		(69)		(44)		(350)		(117)		(122)		(111)	
1 year	56	56	65	65	68	69	64	66	45	50	63	64	62	64	59	60	67	69
3 years	32	32	36	37	38	40	31	35	25	35	34	37	34	37	32	35	37	40
5 years	32	33	30	31	28	31	23	28	20	37	27	31	28	32	27	30	27	31
8 years	..	..	28	30	17	19	..	..	13	37	18	24	..	..	18	22	..	..
10 years	..	..	..	..	..	..	..	..	..	..	..	..	..	..	..	..	..	..
Females	(7)		(24)		(12)		(23)		(16)		(82)		(26)		(33)		(23)	
1 year	86	86	83	83	58	59	65	66	31	34	64	66	65	66	61	63	68	70
3 years	71	72	70	70	42	43	43	46	19	25	48	52	54	56	42	46	50	55
5 years	71	72	60	61	33	35	43	49	6	11	42	48	50	54	39	45	36	43
8 years	..	..	60	62	..	..	..	..	..	..	42	54	..	..	39	51	..	..
10 years	..	..	..	..	..	..	..	..	..	..	..	..	..	..	..	..	..	..
Overall	(34)		(105)		(141)		(92)		(60)		(432)		(143)		(155)		(134)	
1 year	63	63	69	69	67	68	64	66	42	46	63	65	63	65	59	61	67	69
3 years	41	41	44	44	39	40	34	38	23	32	37	40	38	41	34	37	39	42
5 years	41	41	37	38	29	31	28	34	17	29	30	34	32	36	29	33	29	33
8 years	..	..	35	37	17	20	..	..	11	30	21	27	..	..	21	26	..	..
10 years	..	..	..	..	..	..	..	..	..	..	..	..	..	..	..	..	..	..

RELATIVE SURVIVAL (%) BY AGE AND PERIOD

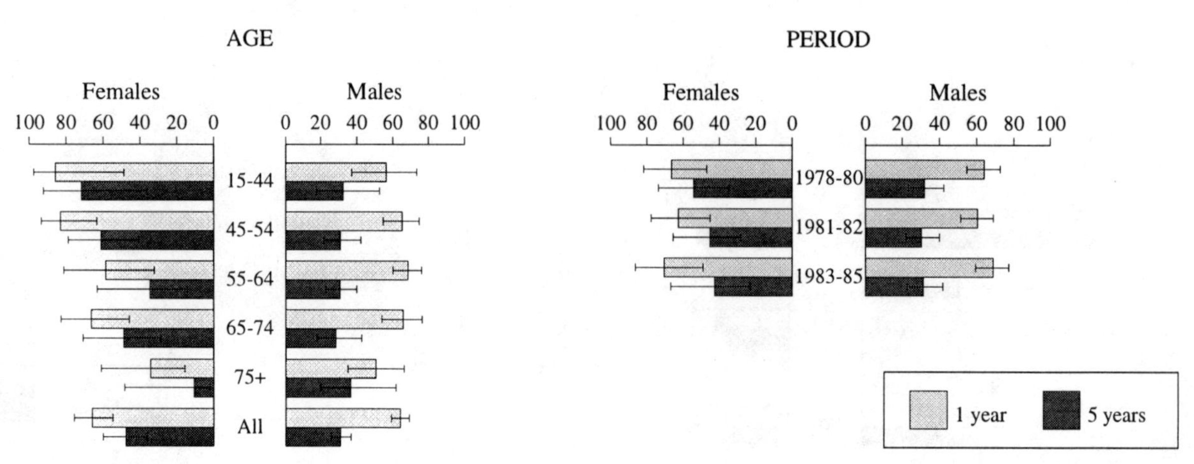

HEAD & NECK

EUROPEAN REGISTRIES

Weighted analysis

REGISTRY	WEIGHTS (Yearly expected cases in the country)		
	Males	Females	All
DENMARK	174	112	286
DUTCH REGISTRIES	459	180	639
ENGLISH REGISTRIES	2370	1079	3449
ESTONIA	38	9	47
FINLAND	85	71	156
FRENCH REGISTRIES	1175	981	2156
GERMAN REGISTRIES	3562	806	4368
ITALIAN REGISTRIES	5099	823	5922
POLISH REGISTRIES	1722	585	2307
SCOTLAND	150	101	251
SPANISH REGISTRIES	2207	350	2557
SWISS REGISTRIES	520	127	647

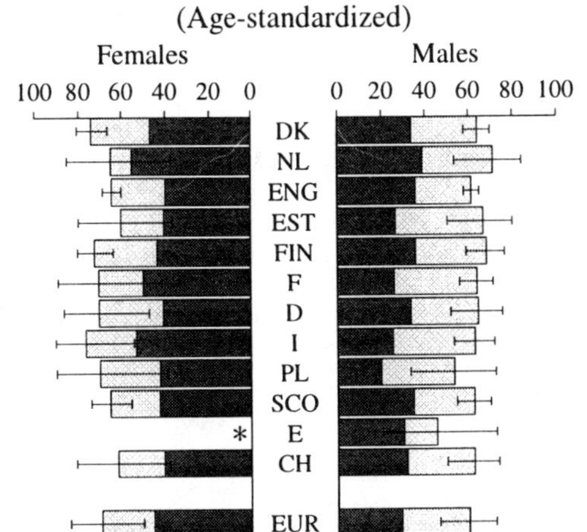

* Not enough cases for reliable estimation

OBSERVED AND RELATIVE SURVIVAL (%) BY AGE AND PERIOD

	AGE CLASS												PERIOD					
	15-44		45-54		55-64		65-74		75+		All		1978-80		1981-82		1983-85	
	obs	rel	obs	rel	obs	rel	obs	rel	obs	rel	obs	rel	obs	rel	obs	rel	obs	rel
Males																		
1 year	76	76	66	66	63	64	57	60	40	45	61	63	60	62	59	61	64	66
3 years	44	44	37	38	34	37	35	40	16	23	33	37	33	37	29	32	36	39
5 years	37	37	32	34	27	31	24	32	9	18	26	31	26	31	22	26	28	32
8 years	30	31	24	26	19	24	14	23	6	18	18	24	19	25	15	20	19	25
10 years	28	28	17	19	17	22	10	19	2	8	14	21	14	21	14	20	..	..
Females																		
1 year	81	81	82	83	73	73	62	63	52	58	69	71	66	68	72	74	69	71
3 years	58	58	62	63	54	56	49	53	26	36	49	53	45	49	54	59	47	51
5 years	52	52	57	58	47	49	37	42	18	32	40	47	40	46	46	54	39	45
8 years	46	46	49	51	37	41	26	34	12	31	31	40	32	40	34	44	30	40
10 years	49	50	43	46	25	28	11	17	7	25	23	32	23	32	29	43	..	..
Overall																		
1 year	77	77	70	70	65	66	59	61	43	48	62	64	61	64	62	64	65	67
3 years	47	47	43	44	39	41	38	43	18	26	37	41	36	40	35	38	39	42
5 years	40	41	38	39	32	35	27	34	11	21	29	35	29	34	27	32	30	35
8 years	34	34	30	32	23	27	17	25	7	21	21	28	22	29	20	26	21	28
10 years	33	33	23	25	19	23	10	19	3	12	16	23	16	24	17	26	..	..

RELATIVE SURVIVAL (%) BY AGE AND PERIOD

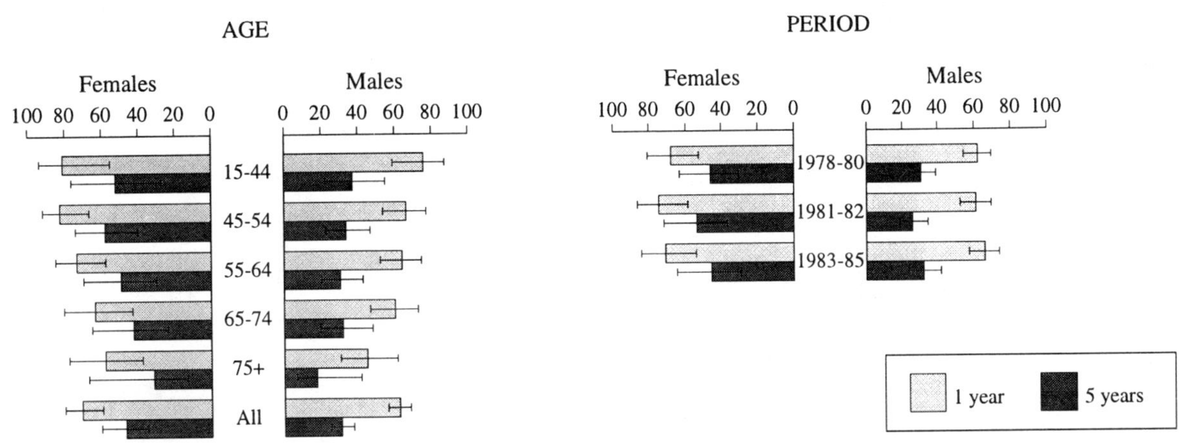

OESOPHAGUS

DENMARK

REGISTRY	NUMBER OF CASES			PERIOD OF DIAGNOSIS
	Males	Females	All	
Denmark	774	405	1179	1978-1984
Mean age (years)	67.1	72.2	68.8	

RELATIVE SURVIVAL (%)

OBSERVED AND RELATIVE SURVIVAL (%) BY AGE AND PERIOD

(Number of cases in parentheses)

	AGE CLASS												PERIOD					
	15-44		45-54		55-64		65-74		75+		All		1978-80		1981-82		1983-85	
	obs	rel	obs	rel	obs	rel	obs	rel	obs	rel	obs	rel	obs	rel	obs	rel	obs	rel
Males	(17)		(77)		(223)		(262)		(195)		(774)		(309)		(210)		(255)	
1 year	29	29	26	26	22	22	16	16	12	13	18	19	19	20	17	18	17	18
3 years	6	6	5	5	6	6	5	6	4	5	5	6	5	6	5	6	5	5
5 years	0	0	4	4	4	4	4	5	3	6	4	5	4	5	4	5	3	4
8 years	0	0	2	2	3	3	3	5	1	4	2	4	3	4	3	4	..	..
10 years	0	0	..	..	..	..	3	5	..	..	2	4	2	4	..	..	..	..
Females	(5)		(28)		(78)		(103)		(191)		(405)		(175)		(117)		(113)	
1 year	60	60	39	39	32	32	22	23	20	22	25	26	22	24	24	25	30	32
3 years	0	0	11	11	14	15	10	10	3	4	7	9	7	8	9	10	7	8
5 years	0	0	11	11	10	10	7	8	2	3	5	7	5	6	6	8	5	7
8 years	0	0	..	..	6	6	5	7	1	3	3	5	3	5	4	6	..	..
10 years	0	0	..	..	..	..	..	..	..	..	..	..	..	..	..	..	..	..
Overall	(22)		(105)		(301)		(365)		(386)		(1179)		(484)		(327)		(368)	
1 year	36	36	30	30	24	25	18	18	16	18	20	21	20	21	20	21	21	22
3 years	5	5	7	7	8	8	6	7	3	5	6	7	6	7	6	7	5	6
5 years	0	0	6	6	5	6	5	6	2	4	4	5	4	5	5	6	4	5
8 years	0	0	3	4	4	4	4	6	1	4	3	4	3	4	3	5	..	..
10 years	0	0	..	..	..	..	3	6	..	..	3	5	2	4	..	..	..	..

RELATIVE SURVIVAL (%) BY AGE AND PERIOD

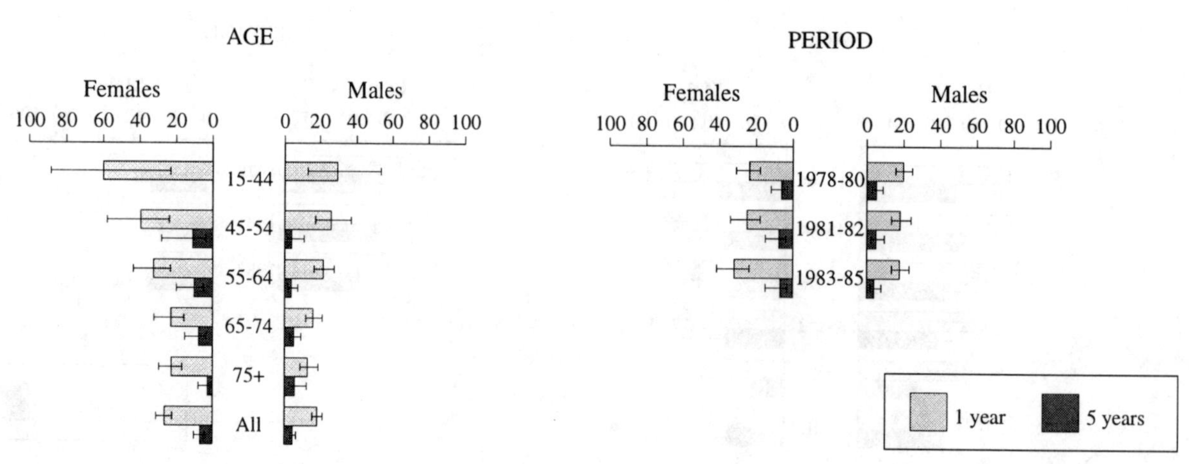

OESOPHAGUS

DUTCH REGISTRIES

REGISTRY	NUMBER OF CASES			PERIOD OF DIAGNOSIS
	Males	Females	All	
Eindhoven	95	36	131	1978-1985
Mean age (years)	64.9	70.3	66.4	

RELATIVE SURVIVAL (%)

OBSERVED AND RELATIVE SURVIVAL (%) BY AGE AND PERIOD
(Number of cases in parentheses)

	AGE CLASS												PERIOD					
	15-44		45-54		55-64		65-74		75+		All		1978-80		1981-82		1983-85	
	obs	rel	obs	rel	obs	rel	obs	rel	obs	rel	obs	rel	obs	rel	obs	rel	obs	rel
Males	(5)		(12)		(27)		(34)		(17)		(95)		(36)		(21)		(38)	
1 year	80	80	67	67	22	23	21	22	12	13	28	30	17	18	33	34	37	39
3 years	40	40	8	8	4	4	15	17	0	0	9	11	8	10	10	10	10	12
5 years	..	..	8	9	0	0	11	14	0	0	5	7	3	4	10	11	5	7
8 years	..	..	0	0	0	0	0	0	0	0	0	0	0	0	..	..	..	..
10 years	..	..	0	0	0	0	0	0	0	0	0	0	0	0	..	..	..	..
Females	(0)		(5)		(4)		(13)		(14)		(36)		(12)		(9)		(15)	
1 year	..	..	40	40	75	75	23	24	7	8	25	26	0	0	33	34	40	41
3 years	..	..	20	20	25	26	0	0	0	0	5	6	0	0	11	12	7	7
5 years	..	..	..	..	25	26	0	0	0	0	5	6	0	0	11	13	..	..
8 years	..	..	..	..	..	..	0	0	0	0	..	..	0	0	..	..	..	..
10 years	..	..	..	..	..	..	0	0	0	0	..	..	0	0	..	..	..	..
Overall	(5)		(17)		(31)		(47)		(31)		(131)		(48)		(30)		(53)	
1 year	80	80	59	59	29	29	21	22	10	11	27	29	13	13	33	34	38	39
3 years	40	40	10	10	6	7	11	12	0	0	8	9	6	7	10	11	9	10
5 years	..	..	10	10	3	4	8	10	0	0	5	7	2	3	10	12	5	6
8 years	..	..	0	0	..	..	0	0	0	0	0	0	0	0	..	..	..	..
10 years	..	..	0	0	..	..	0	0	0	0	0	0	0	0	..	..	..	..

RELATIVE SURVIVAL (%) BY AGE AND PERIOD

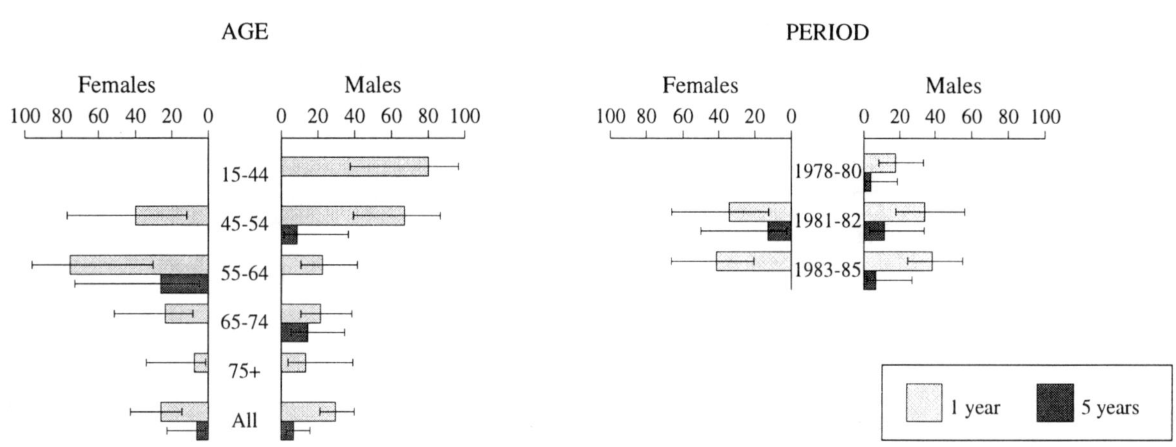

OESOPHAGUS

ENGLISH REGISTRIES

REGISTRY	NUMBER OF CASES			PERIOD OF DIAGNOSIS
	Males	Females	All	
East Anglia	571	390	961	1979-1984
Mersey	877	701	1578	1978-1984
South Thames	1824	1532	3356	1978-1984
Wessex	305	206	511	1983-1984
West Midlands	1044	919	1963	1979-1984
Yorkshire	1103	816	1919	1978-1984
Mean age (years)	67.8	72.3	69.8	

RELATIVE SURVIVAL (%)

100 80 60 40 20 0
Females
Males
0 1 2 3 4 5
Time since diagnosis (years)

OBSERVED AND RELATIVE SURVIVAL (%) BY AGE AND PERIOD
(Number of cases in parentheses)

	AGE CLASS												PERIOD					
	15-44		45-54		55-64		65-74		75+		All		1978-80		1981-82		1983-85	
	obs	rel	obs	rel	obs	rel	obs	rel	obs	rel	obs	rel	obs	rel	obs	rel	obs	rel
Males	(126)		(476)		(1437)		(2088)		(1597)		(5724)		(2101)		(1673)		(1950)	
1 year	32	32	24	24	23	24	19	19	12	13	19	20	17	18	19	20	20	21
3 years	14	14	9	9	8	8	6	7	3	5	6	7	5	6	6	8	7	8
5 years	10	10	5	5	5	6	4	5	2	4	4	5	3	5	4	6	4	6
8 years	9	9	4	5	4	5	3	5	1	3	3	5	3	5	3	4	4	6
10 years	9	9	4	4	4	5	3	5	1	4	3	5	3	5	2	4	..	..
Females	(67)		(246)		(792)		(1313)		(2146)		(4564)		(1726)		(1344)		(1494)	
1 year	33	33	34	34	31	31	24	25	13	14	21	22	19	20	21	22	23	24
3 years	18	18	14	14	14	14	10	11	3	5	8	10	7	8	9	10	9	10
5 years	13	14	11	11	10	10	8	9	2	3	5	7	5	6	6	8	6	8
8 years	12	12	9	9	8	9	5	7	1	3	4	7	3	6	5	8	4	7
10 years	12	12	9	9	7	8	5	7	1	3	4	7	3	5	5	9	..	..
Overall	(193)		(722)		(2229)		(3401)		(3743)		(10288)		(3827)		(3017)		(3444)	
1 year	32	32	27	27	26	26	21	22	12	14	19	21	18	19	20	21	21	22
3 years	16	16	11	11	10	10	8	9	3	5	7	8	6	7	7	9	8	9
5 years	11	12	7	7	7	8	5	7	2	3	5	6	4	5	5	7	5	7
8 years	10	10	6	6	6	7	4	6	1	3	3	6	3	5	4	6	4	6
10 years	10	10	5	6	5	6	3	6	1	4	3	6	3	5	3	6	..	..

RELATIVE SURVIVAL (%) BY AGE AND PERIOD

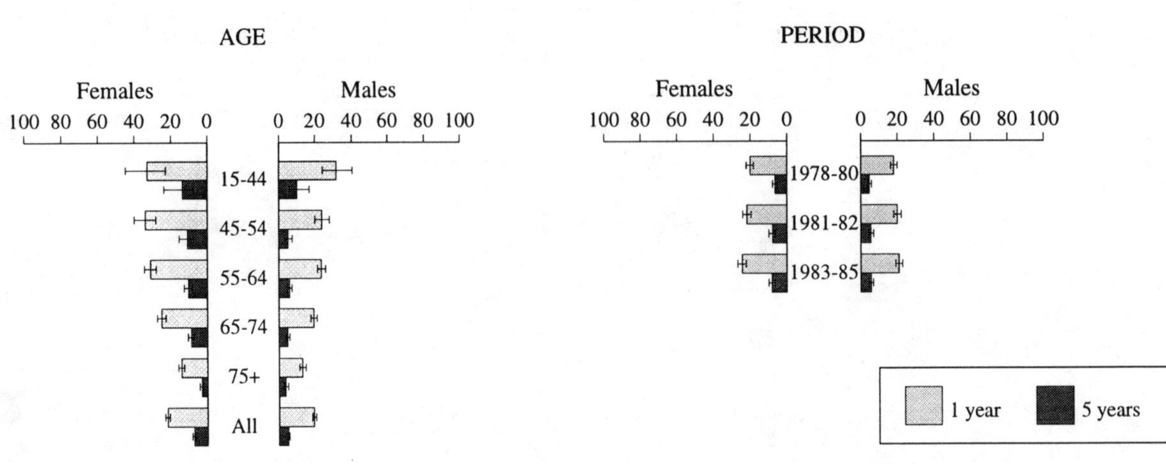

OESOPHAGUS

ESTONIA

REGISTRY	NUMBER OF CASES			PERIOD OF DIAGNOSIS
	Males	Females	All	
Estonia	145	65	210	1978-1984
Mean age (years)	62.2	74.1	65.9	

RELATIVE SURVIVAL (%)

Females
Males
Time since diagnosis (years)

OBSERVED AND RELATIVE SURVIVAL (%) BY AGE AND PERIOD
(Number of cases in parentheses)

	AGE CLASS												PERIOD					
	15-44		45-54		55-64		65-74		75+		All		1978-80		1981-82		1983-85	
	obs	rel	obs	rel	obs	rel	obs	rel	obs	rel	obs	rel	obs	rel	obs	rel	obs	rel
Males	(8)		(33)		(41)		(39)		(24)		(145)		(68)		(25)		(52)	
1 year	13	13	15	15	29	30	23	24	13	14	21	22	21	22	12	12	25	26
3 years	0	0	6	6	7	8	7	8	0	0	5	6	4	4	4	5	8	9
5 years	0	0	0	0	5	6	3	5	0	0	2	3	2	2	0	0	4	5
8 years	0	0	0	0	5	6	..	..	0	0	2	3	2	3	0	0	..	..
10 years	0	0	0	0	..	..	..	..	0	0	..	..	..	..	0	0	..	..
Females	(2)		(3)		(5)		(12)		(43)		(65)		(27)		(16)		(22)	
1 year	0	0	33	33	20	20	33	34	20	23	23	24	19	20	17	18	32	34
3 years	0	0	33	34	20	21	8	9	8	11	10	12	4	5	8	11	18	23
5 years	0	0	33	34	20	21	8	10	5	10	8	13	4	6	8	13	14	21
8 years	0	0	..	..	..	..	0	0	..	..	..	..	0	0	0	0	..	..
10 years	0	0	..	..	..	..	0	0	..	..	..	..	0	0	0	0	..	..
Overall	(10)		(36)		(46)		(51)		(67)		(210)		(95)		(41)		(74)	
1 year	10	10	17	17	28	29	25	27	17	20	21	23	20	21	14	15	27	28
3 years	0	0	8	9	9	9	7	8	5	7	7	8	4	4	6	7	11	13
5 years	0	0	3	3	7	8	5	6	3	6	4	6	2	3	3	4	7	9
8 years	0	0	..	..	7	8	..	..	..	..	3	4	1	2	0	0	..	..
10 years	0	0	..	..	..	..	..	..	..	..	..	..	..	..	0	0	..	..

RELATIVE SURVIVAL (%) BY AGE AND PERIOD

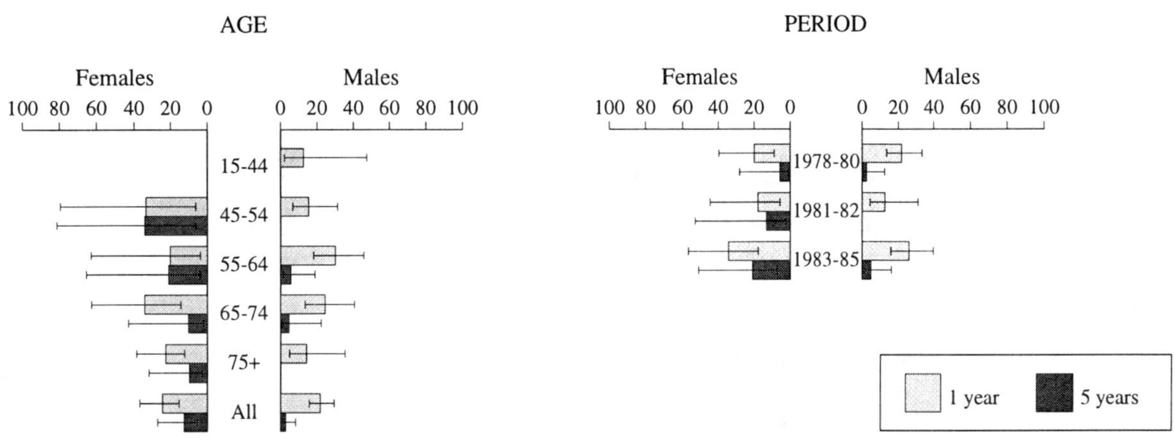

OESOPHAGUS

FINLAND

REGISTRY	NUMBER OF CASES			PERIOD OF DIAGNOSIS
	Males	Females	All	
Finland	609	740	1349	1978-1984
Mean age (years)	68.2	73.4	71.0	

RELATIVE SURVIVAL (%)

100 80 60 40 20 0

0 1 2 3 4 5

Females

Males

Time since diagnosis (years)

OBSERVED AND RELATIVE SURVIVAL (%) BY AGE AND PERIOD
(Number of cases in parentheses)

	AGE CLASS												PERIOD					
	15-44		45-54		55-64		65-74		75+		All		1978-80		1981-82		1983-85	
	obs	rel	obs	rel	obs	rel	obs	rel	obs	rel	obs	rel	obs	rel	obs	rel	obs	rel
Males	(19)		(46)		(133)		(229)		(182)		(609)		(268)		(173)		(168)	
1 year	53	53	33	33	27	28	23	24	18	21	24	26	26	28	25	26	20	21
3 years	32	32	9	9	9	10	6	7	4	6	7	8	6	7	9	10	7	9
5 years	21	21	9	9	8	9	4	5	2	4	5	7	4	5	6	8	7	9
8 years	16	16	2	2	6	8	2	3	2	5	3	6	2	4	3	5	6	10
10 years	16	17	2	3	2	3	..	..	..	..	2	4	1	3	2	3	..	..
Females	(5)		(19)		(103)		(257)		(356)		(740)		(305)		(218)		(217)	
1 year	60	60	53	53	54	55	37	38	22	25	33	35	35	37	31	33	33	35
3 years	20	20	26	27	18	19	12	14	4	5	9	11	9	11	10	12	10	11
5 years	20	20	21	21	15	15	8	10	2	3	6	9	5	7	7	9	8	11
8 years	..	..	21	22	11	12	6	8	2	4	5	8	4	6	6	10	6	11
10 years	..	..	21	22	8	9	6	9	1	4	4	8	3	6	5	11	..	..
Overall	(24)		(65)		(236)		(486)		(538)		(1349)		(573)		(391)		(385)	
1 year	54	54	38	39	39	40	31	32	21	23	29	31	31	33	28	30	27	29
3 years	29	29	14	14	13	14	9	10	4	5	8	10	7	9	9	11	9	10
5 years	21	21	12	13	11	12	6	8	2	4	6	8	5	6	6	9	7	10
8 years	16	17	8	8	8	10	4	6	2	5	4	7	3	5	5	8	6	10
10 years	16	17	8	9	5	6	4	7	1	4	3	6	2	4	4	7	..	..

RELATIVE SURVIVAL (%) BY AGE AND PERIOD

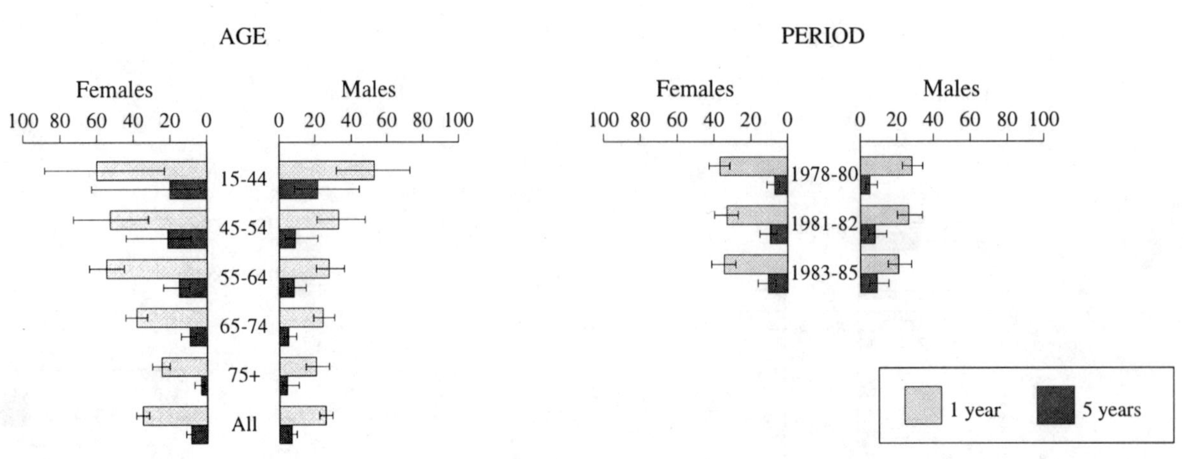

OESOPHAGUS

FRENCH REGISTRIES

REGISTRY	NUMBER OF CASES			PERIOD OF DIAGNOSIS
	Males	Females	All	
Amiens	122	9	131	1983-1984
Calvados	751	47	798	1978-1985
Côte-d'Or	267	25	292	1978-1985
Doubs	288	28	316	1978-1985
Mean age (years)	62.7	70.0	63.2	

RELATIVE SURVIVAL (%)

OBSERVED AND RELATIVE SURVIVAL (%) BY AGE AND PERIOD
(Number of cases in parentheses)

	AGE CLASS												PERIOD					
	15-44		45-54		55-64		65-74		75+		All		1978-80		1981-82		1983-85	
	obs	rel	obs	rel	obs	rel	obs	rel	obs	rel	obs	rel	obs	rel	obs	rel	obs	rel
Males	(53)		(293)		(467)		(400)		(215)		(1428)		(519)		(298)		(611)	
1 year	43	43	31	31	32	33	27	28	24	27	30	31	30	31	28	29	31	32
3 years	20	20	8	8	8	9	7	8	4	6	8	9	7	7	7	7	9	10
5 years	14	14	4	4	5	6	4	5	2	3	4	5	4	4	4	5	5	6
8 years	11	11	3	3	3	3	3	4	1	3	3	4	2	3	2	3	..	..
10 years	11	12	2	2	2	3	2	4	1	4	2	3	2	3	..	..	..	..
Females	(0)		(15)		(21)		(34)		(39)		(109)		(27)		(28)		(54)	
1 year	..	..	27	27	38	38	26	27	21	23	27	28	26	27	18	19	31	33
3 years	..	..	0	0	10	10	0	0	5	7	4	5	4	4	0	0	6	7
5 years	..	..	0	0	10	10	0	0	3	5	3	4	4	5	0	0	4	5
8 years	..	..	0	0	..	..	0	0	3	8	3	4	4	6	0	0	..	..
10 years	..	..	0	0	..	..	0	0	3	12	3	5	4	6	0	0	..	..
Overall	(53)		(308)		(488)		(434)		(254)		(1537)		(546)		(326)		(665)	
1 year	43	43	31	31	33	33	27	28	24	27	30	31	30	31	27	28	31	32
3 years	20	20	8	8	8	9	7	8	4	6	8	8	6	7	6	7	9	10
5 years	14	14	4	4	5	6	4	5	2	4	4	5	4	4	4	4	5	6
8 years	11	11	2	3	3	4	2	4	1	4	3	4	3	3	2	3	..	..
10 years	11	12	1	2	2	3	2	3	1	5	2	3	2	3	..	..	..	..

RELATIVE SURVIVAL (%) BY AGE AND PERIOD

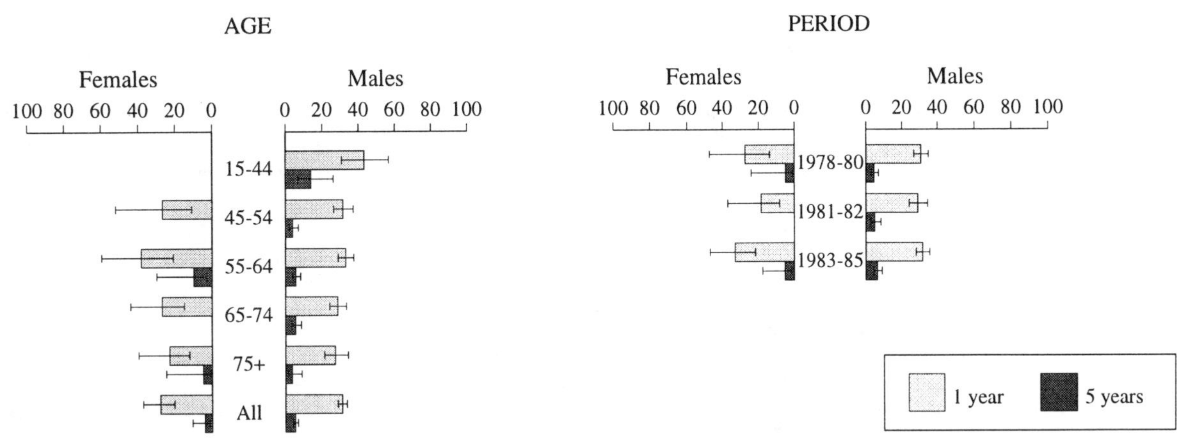

OESOPHAGUS

GERMAN REGISTRIES

REGISTRY	NUMBER OF CASES			PERIOD OF DIAGNOSIS
	Males	Females	All	
Saarland	229	46	275	1978-1984
Mean age (years)	62.3	68.9	63.4	

RELATIVE SURVIVAL (%)

OBSERVED AND RELATIVE SURVIVAL (%) BY AGE AND PERIOD
(Number of cases in parentheses)

	AGE CLASS												PERIOD					
	15-44		45-54		55-64		65-74		75+		All		1978-80		1981-82		1983-85	
	obs	rel	obs	rel	obs	rel	obs	rel	obs	rel	obs	rel	obs	rel	obs	rel	obs	rel
Males	(14)		(50)		(64)		(66)		(35)		(229)		(89)		(49)		(91)	
1 year	29	29	14	14	36	37	21	22	6	7	22	23	22	24	24	26	20	21
3 years	7	7	4	4	6	7	8	9	3	4	6	6	3	4	12	14	4	5
5 years	7	7	2	2	6	7	8	10	3	6	5	7	3	4	10	13	4	5
8 years	7	7	..	..	4	5	6	11	..	..	4	6	3	5	6	9	..	..
10 years	0	0	..	..	..	..	6	13	..	..	3	5	2	4	..	..	..	..
Females	(1)		(7)		(8)		(11)		(19)		(46)		(22)		(12)		(12)	
1 year	0	0	14	14	13	13	27	28	11	12	15	16	9	10	17	17	25	26
3 years	0	0	0	0	0	0	9	10	0	0	2	3	5	5	0	0	0	0
5 years	0	0	0	0	0	0	9	10	0	0	2	3	5	6	0	0	0	0
8 years	0	0	0	0	0	0	9	12	0	0	2	3	5	7	0	0	0	0
10 years	0	0	0	0	0	0	9	13	0	0	2	4	5	8	0	0	0	0
Overall	(15)		(57)		(72)		(77)		(54)		(275)		(111)		(61)		(103)	
1 year	27	27	14	14	33	34	22	23	7	8	21	22	20	21	23	24	20	21
3 years	7	7	4	4	6	6	8	9	2	3	5	6	4	4	10	11	4	4
5 years	7	7	2	2	6	6	8	10	2	4	5	6	4	5	8	10	4	5
8 years	7	7	..	..	4	4	6	11	..	..	4	5	4	6	5	7	..	..
10 years	0	0	..	..	..	..	6	13	..	..	3	5	3	5	..	..	..	..

RELATIVE SURVIVAL (%) BY AGE AND PERIOD

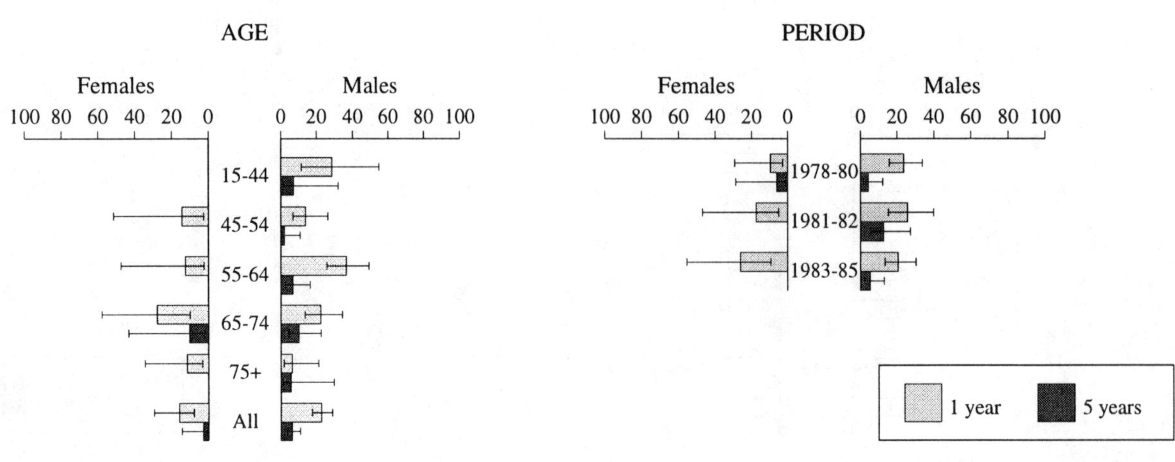

OESOPHAGUS

ITALIAN REGISTRIES

REGISTRY	NUMBER OF CASES			PERIOD OF DIAGNOSIS
	Males	Females	All	
Latina	11	4	15	1983-1984
Ragusa	22	3	25	1981-1984
Varese	209	40	249	1978-1984
Mean age (years)	66.2	70.2	66.9	

RELATIVE SURVIVAL (%)

OBSERVED AND RELATIVE SURVIVAL (%) BY AGE AND PERIOD
(Number of cases in parentheses)

	AGE CLASS												PERIOD					
	15-44		45-54		55-64		65-74		75+		All		1978-80		1981-82		1983-85	
	obs	rel	obs	rel	obs	rel	obs	rel	obs	rel	obs	rel	obs	rel	obs	rel	obs	rel
Males	(4)		(31)		(71)		(82)		(54)		(242)		(88)		(68)		(86)	
1 year	0	0	16	16	21	22	18	19	13	15	17	18	14	14	16	17	22	23
3 years	0	0	10	10	8	9	4	4	2	3	5	6	3	4	6	7	7	8
5 years	0	0	3	3	6	6	2	3	2	4	3	4	1	1	4	6	5	6
8 years	0	0	3	4	3	3	0	0	2	6	2	3	1	2	3	4	..	..
10 years	0	0	..	..	3	4	0	0	..	..	2	3	1	2	..	..	..	..
Females	(2)		(4)		(7)		(16)		(18)		(47)		(12)		(15)		(20)	
1 year	100	100	50	50	29	29	44	45	11	12	32	33	17	18	40	41	35	37
3 years	50	50	25	25	0	0	13	14	0	0	9	10	8	10	7	7	10	12
5 years	50	50	0	0	0	0	0	0	0	0	2	3	0	0	0	0	5	7
8 years	..	..	0	0	0	0	0	0	0	0	..	..	0	0	0	0	..	..
10 years	..	..	0	0	0	0	0	0	0	0	..	..	0	0	0	0	..	..
Overall	(6)		(35)		(78)		(98)		(72)		(289)		(100)		(83)		(106)	
1 year	33	33	20	20	22	22	22	23	13	14	20	21	14	15	20	21	25	26
3 years	17	17	11	12	8	8	5	6	1	2	6	7	4	5	6	7	8	9
5 years	17	17	3	3	5	6	2	3	1	3	3	4	1	1	4	5	5	6
8 years	..	..	3	3	3	3	0	0	1	4	2	3	1	2	2	4	..	..
10 years	..	..	..	..	3	3	0	0	..	..	2	3	1	2	..	..	..	..

RELATIVE SURVIVAL (%) BY AGE AND PERIOD

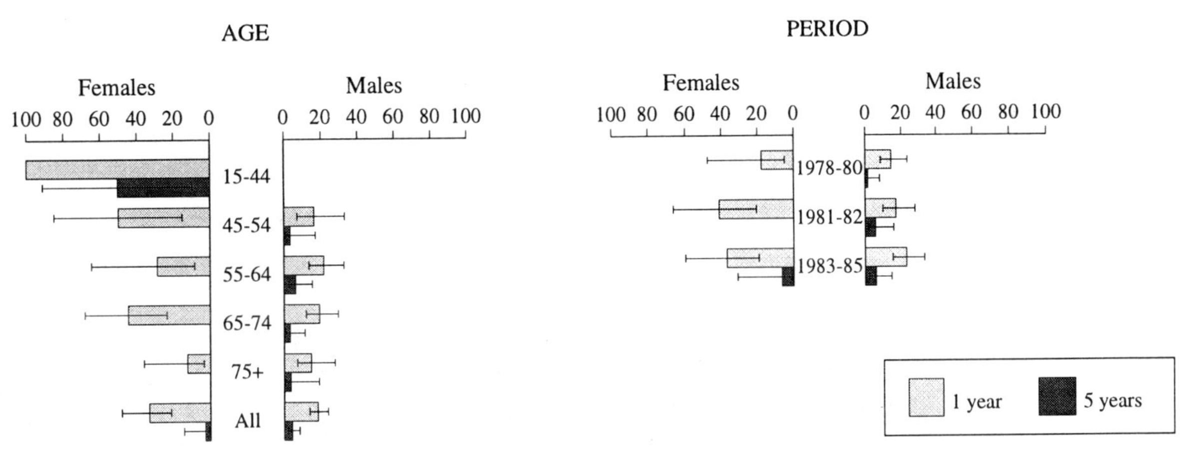

OESOPHAGUS

POLISH REGISTRIES

REGISTRY	NUMBER OF CASES			PERIOD OF DIAGNOSIS
	Males	Females	All	
Cracow	103	29	132	1978-1984
Mean age (years)	62.6	69.2	64.1	

RELATIVE SURVIVAL (%)

100
80
60
40
20
0
Females
Males
0 1 2 3 4 5
Time since diagnosis (years)

OBSERVED AND RELATIVE SURVIVAL (%) BY AGE AND PERIOD
(Number of cases in parentheses)

	AGE CLASS												PERIOD					
	15-44		45-54		55-64		65-74		75+		All		1978-80		1981-82		1983-85	
	obs	rel	obs	rel	obs	rel	obs	rel	obs	rel	obs	rel	obs	rel	obs	rel	obs	rel
Males	(3)		(24)		(30)		(32)		(14)		(103)		(43)		(24)		(36)	
1 year	0	0	13	13	18	18	20	21	17	19	17	17	20	21	13	13	16	17
3 years	0	0	0	0	0	0	0	0	0	0	0	0	0	0	0	0	0	0
5 years	0	0	0	0	0	0	0	0	0	0	0	0	0	0	0	0	0	0
8 years	0	0	0	0	0	0	0	0	0	0	0	0	0	0	0	0	0	0
10 years	0	0	0	0	0	0	0	0	0	0	0	0	0	0	0	0	0	0
Females	(0)		(2)		(8)		(11)		(8)		(29)		(14)		(6)		(9)	
1 year	..	..	50	50	13	13	9	9	25	27	17	18	29	30	17	18	0	0
3 years	..	..	0	0	0	0	0	0	0	0	0	0	0	0	0	0	0	0
5 years	..	..	0	0	0	0	0	0	0	0	0	0	0	0	0	0	0	0
8 years	..	..	0	0	0	0	0	0	0	0	0	0	0	0	0	0	0	0
10 years	..	..	0	0	0	0	0	0	0	0	0	0	0	0	0	0	0	0
Overall	(3)		(26)		(38)		(43)		(22)		(132)		(57)		(30)		(45)	
1 year	0	0	16	16	17	17	17	18	20	22	17	17	22	23	13	14	12	13
3 years	0	0	0	0	0	0	0	0	0	0	0	0	0	0	0	0	0	0
5 years	0	0	0	0	0	0	0	0	0	0	0	0	0	0	0	0	0	0
8 years	0	0	0	0	0	0	0	0	0	0	0	0	0	0	0	0	0	0
10 years	0	0	0	0	0	0	0	0	0	0	0	0	0	0	0	0	0	0

RELATIVE SURVIVAL (%) BY AGE AND PERIOD

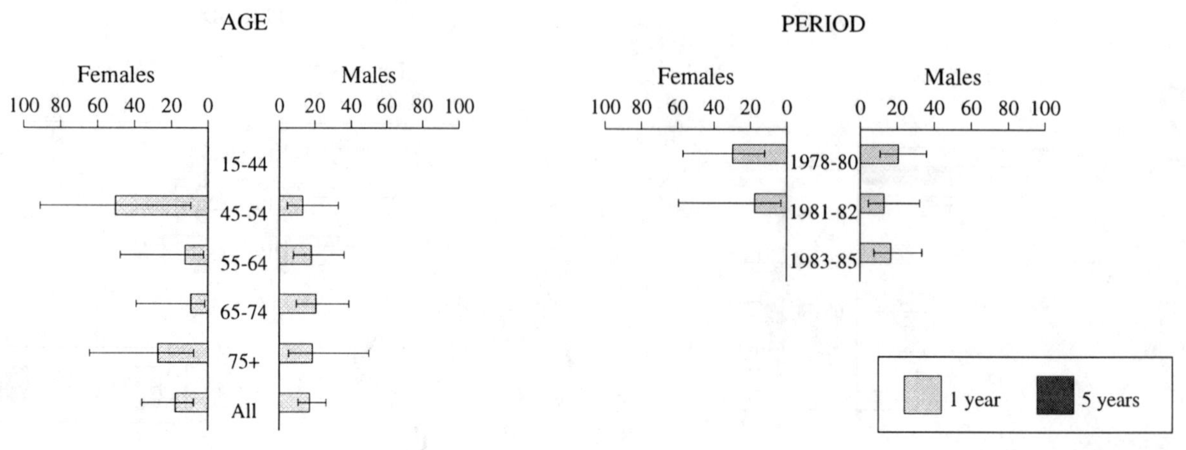

OESOPHAGUS

SCOTLAND

REGISTRY	NUMBER OF CASES			PERIOD OF DIAGNOSIS
	Males	Females	All	
Scotland	1324	1091	2415	1978-1982
Mean age (years)	66.8	71.6	68.9	

RELATIVE SURVIVAL (%)

OBSERVED AND RELATIVE SURVIVAL (%) BY AGE AND PERIOD
(Number of cases in parentheses)

	AGE CLASS												PERIOD					
	15-44		45-54		55-64		65-74		75+		All		1978-80		1981-82		1983-85	
	obs	rel	obs	rel	obs	rel	obs	rel	obs	rel	obs	rel	obs	rel	obs	rel	obs	rel
Males	(47)		(117)		(334)		(507)		(319)		(1324)		(771)		(553)		(0)	
1 year	36	36	32	33	18	18	15	15	12	14	17	18	17	18	18	19	..	..
3 years	11	11	9	9	6	6	4	5	2	2	5	6	5	6	4	5	..	..
5 years	9	9	7	7	4	5	3	4	2	3	4	5	4	5	4	5	..	..
8 years	6	7	2	2	3	4	2	3	1	3	2	3	2	3	..	..	..	..
10 years	..	..	2	2	..	..	..	..	..	..	2	3	2	4	..	..	..	..
Females	(19)		(61)		(188)		(358)		(465)		(1091)		(647)		(444)		(0)	
1 year	37	37	28	28	29	30	23	24	14	16	21	22	21	22	22	23	..	..
3 years	11	11	7	7	10	10	9	10	4	6	7	8	8	9	6	7	..	..
5 years	5	5	5	5	9	9	7	8	3	5	5	7	6	7	5	7	..	..
8 years	..	..	5	5	5	6	5	7	1	4	4	6	4	6	..	..	..	..
10 years	..	..	5	5	5	6	..	..	1	5	3	6	3	6	..	..	..	..
Overall	(66)		(178)		(522)		(865)		(784)		(2415)		(1418)		(997)		(0)	
1 year	36	36	31	31	22	22	18	19	14	15	19	20	18	19	20	21	..	..
3 years	11	11	8	8	7	8	6	7	3	5	6	7	6	7	5	6	..	..
5 years	8	8	6	6	6	7	5	6	2	4	4	6	4	6	4	6	..	..
8 years	6	6	3	3	4	5	3	5	1	3	3	4	3	4	..	..	..	..
10 years	..	..	3	3	4	5	..	..	1	5	2	5	3	5	..	..	..	..

RELATIVE SURVIVAL (%) BY AGE AND PERIOD

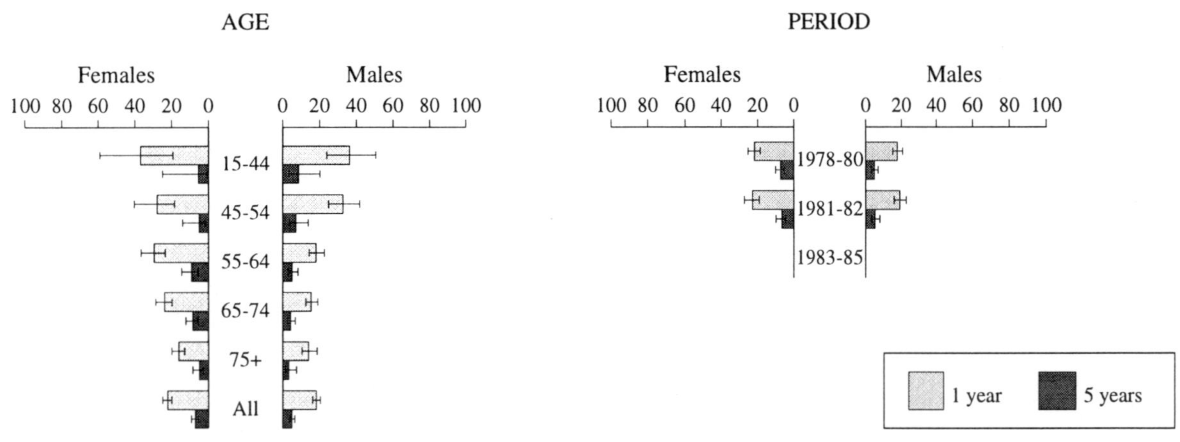

OESOPHAGUS

SPANISH REGISTRIES

REGISTRY	NUMBER OF CASES			PERIOD OF DIAGNOSIS
	Males	Females	All	
Tarragona	23	0	23	1985-1985
Mean age (years)	62.4	..	62.4	

Not enough cases for reliable estimation

OESOPHAGUS

SWISS REGISTRIES

REGISTRY	NUMBER OF CASES Males	Females	All	PERIOD OF DIAGNOSIS
Basel	40	8	48	1981-1984
Geneva	107	25	132	1978-1984
Mean age (years)	63.4	68.4	64.3	

RELATIVE SURVIVAL (%)

100 80 60 40 20 0
Females
Males
0 1 2 3 4 5
Time since diagnosis (years)

OBSERVED AND RELATIVE SURVIVAL (%) BY AGE AND PERIOD
(Number of cases in parentheses)

	AGE CLASS 15-44 obs	rel	45-54 obs	rel	55-64 obs	rel	65-74 obs	rel	75+ obs	rel	All obs	rel	PERIOD 1978-80 obs	rel	1981-82 obs	rel	1983-85 obs	rel
Males	(4)		(25)		(51)		(43)		(24)		(147)		(51)		(49)		(47)	
1 year	0	0	32	32	31	32	23	24	21	23	27	27	27	28	27	27	26	26
3 years	0	0	20	20	6	6	7	8	8	11	9	10	8	9	6	7	13	14
5 years	0	0	12	12	4	4	5	6	4	7	5	6	6	7	2	2	9	10
8 years	0	0	..	..	..	..	..	..	..	..	..	..	..	..	0	0	..	..
10 years	0	0	..	..	..	..	..	..	..	..	..	..	..	..	0	0	..	..
Females	(1)		(5)		(9)		(7)		(11)		(33)		(8)		(13)		(12)	
1 year	0	0	40	40	33	34	0	0	27	30	24	25	25	26	15	16	33	35
3 years	0	0	40	40	11	11	0	0	0	0	9	10	13	15	8	8	8	10
5 years	0	0	40	41	11	12	0	0	0	0	9	11	13	16	8	9	8	11
8 years	0	0	..	..	11	12	0	0	0	0	9	13	..	..	8	10	..	..
10 years	0	0	..	..	..	..	0	0	0	0	..	..	..	..	..	..	..	..
Overall	(5)		(30)		(60)		(50)		(35)		(180)		(59)		(62)		(59)	
1 year	0	0	33	34	32	32	20	21	23	25	26	27	27	28	24	25	27	28
3 years	0	0	23	24	7	7	6	7	6	8	9	10	8	9	6	7	12	13
5 years	0	0	17	17	5	5	4	5	3	5	6	7	7	8	3	4	8	10
8 years	0	0	..	..	5	6	..	..	..	..	5	6	..	..	2	2	..	..
10 years	0	0	..	..	..	..	..	..	..	..	..	..	..	..	..	..	..	..

RELATIVE SURVIVAL (%) BY AGE AND PERIOD

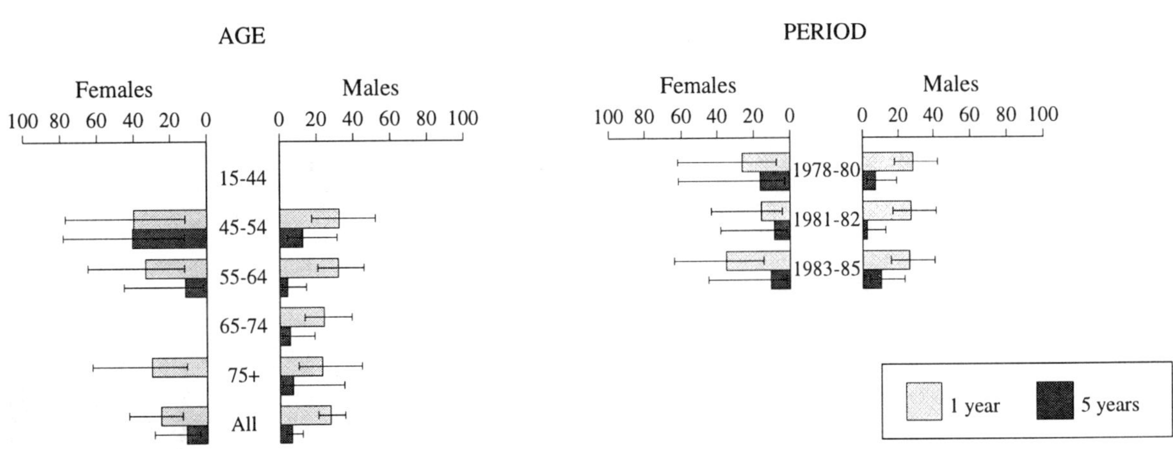

OESOPHAGUS

EUROPEAN REGISTRIES

Weighted analysis

REGISTRY	WEIGHTS (Yearly expected cases in the country) Males	Females	All
DENMARK	110	58	168
DUTCH REGISTRIES	307	170	477
ENGLISH REGISTRIES	2069	1651	3720
ESTONIA	20	9	29
FINLAND	87	105	192
FRENCH REGISTRIES	4005	582	4587
GERMAN REGISTRIES	1558	562	2120
ITALIAN REGISTRIES	1623	447	2070
POLISH REGISTRIES	696	183	879
SCOTLAND	264	218	482
SWISS REGISTRIES	256	73	329

RELATIVE SURVIVAL (%)
(Age-standardized)

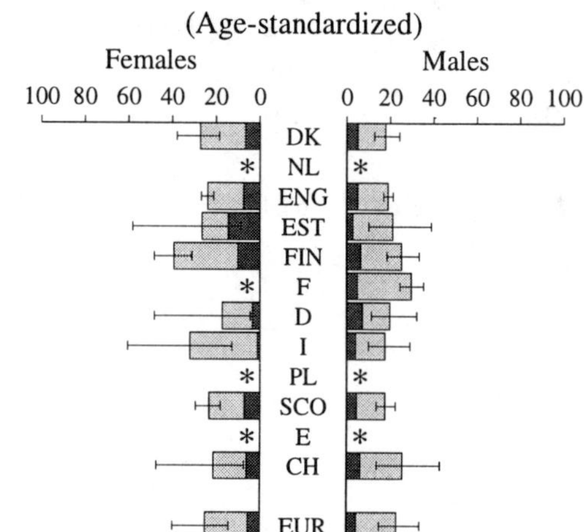

* Not enough cases for reliable estimation

OBSERVED AND RELATIVE SURVIVAL (%) BY AGE AND PERIOD

	AGE CLASS 15-44 obs	15-44 rel	45-54 obs	45-54 rel	55-64 obs	55-64 rel	65-74 obs	65-74 rel	75+ obs	75+ rel	All obs	All rel	PERIOD 1978-80 obs	1978-80 rel	1981-82 obs	1981-82 rel	1983-85 obs	1983-85 rel
Males																		
1 year	27	27	27	27	30	30	22	23	15	17	24	25	22	23	23	24	25	26
3 years	11	12	7	7	7	7	7	8	3	4	6	7	5	6	7	8	7	8
5 years	8	8	4	4	4	5	4	5	2	3	4	5	3	4	5	6	4	5
8 years	6	7	2	3	3	3	2	4	1	3	2	3	2	3	3	4	2	3
10 years	6	6	2	2	2	3	2	4	1	3	2	3	2	3	2	3	..	..
Females																		
1 year	37	37	33	33	31	31	26	27	14	16	23	24	19	20	22	23	26	28
3 years	18	18	11	11	9	10	8	9	3	4	6	7	6	7	6	7	7	8
5 years	15	15	6	6	8	8	5	6	1	2	4	5	4	5	4	5	4	6
8 years	8	8	5	5	5	6	4	5	1	3	3	5	3	5	3	4	3	5
10 years	8	8	5	5	4	5	4	5	1	3	3	5	3	5	2	4	..	..
Overall																		
1 year	30	30	28	28	30	30	23	24	15	16	23	24	21	22	23	24	25	26
3 years	13	13	8	8	7	8	7	8	3	4	6	7	5	6	7	8	7	8
5 years	10	10	4	4	5	6	4	5	2	3	4	5	3	4	4	6	4	5
8 years	7	7	3	3	3	4	3	4	1	3	3	4	2	4	3	4	2	4
10 years	6	6	3	3	3	3	2	4	1	3	2	4	2	3	2	3	..	..

RELATIVE SURVIVAL (%) BY AGE AND PERIOD

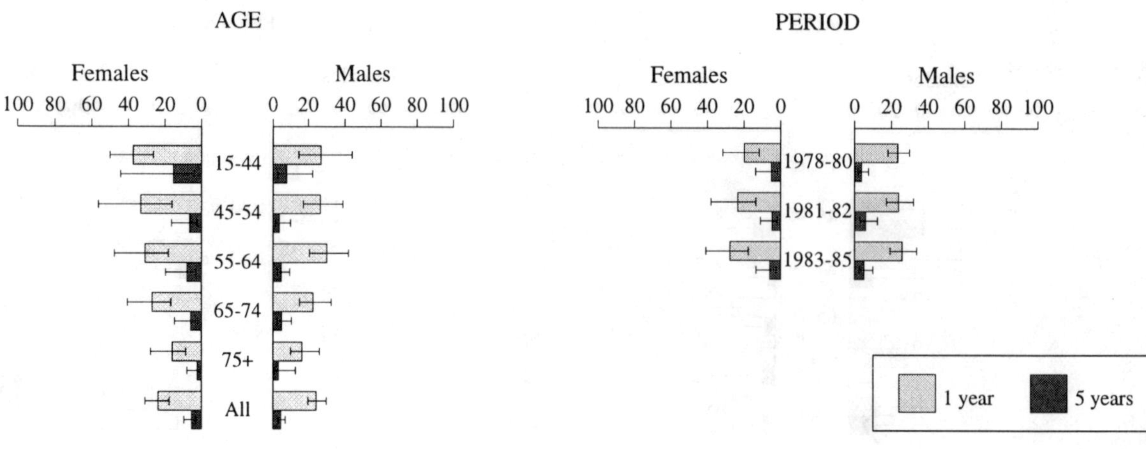

STOMACH

DENMARK

REGISTRY	NUMBER OF CASES			PERIOD OF DIAGNOSIS
	Males	Females	All	
Denmark	3902	2478	6380	1978-1984
Mean age (years)	69.9	72.2	70.8	

RELATIVE SURVIVAL (%)

— Males
- - Females

Time since diagnosis (years)

OBSERVED AND RELATIVE SURVIVAL (%) BY AGE AND PERIOD
(Number of cases in parentheses)

	AGE CLASS												PERIOD					
	15-44		45-54		55-64		65-74		75+		All		1978-80		1981-82		1983-85	
	obs	rel	obs	rel	obs	rel	obs	rel	obs	rel	obs	rel	obs	rel	obs	rel	obs	rel
Males	(105)		(282)		(735)		(1302)		(1478)		(3902)		(1716)		(1085)		(1101)	
1 year	42	42	39	39	38	39	29	30	19	22	28	30	27	28	28	30	30	32
3 years	27	27	19	20	20	21	14	16	7	11	13	16	12	14	14	17	15	18
5 years	23	23	17	17	15	16	9	12	3	7	9	13	8	11	9	13	10	14
8 years	20	21	14	15	11	13	7	11	2	6	7	12	6	11	6	10	..	..
10 years	15	15	13	14	10	14	6	11	1	4	5	11	5	10	..	..	..	..
Females	(90)		(156)		(342)		(620)		(1270)		(2478)		(1106)		(706)		(666)	
1 year	42	42	50	50	40	41	28	29	20	22	28	29	28	29	28	29	27	28
3 years	29	29	31	31	24	25	15	16	10	13	15	18	17	19	15	18	13	15
5 years	26	26	21	22	20	21	12	14	7	11	11	15	12	17	10	14	10	14
8 years	21	22	19	20	18	20	9	12	4	10	9	14	10	16	8	12	..	..
10 years	21	22	19	21	16	18	8	11	3	11	8	15	9	16	..	..	..	..
Overall	(195)		(438)		(1077)		(1922)		(2748)		(6380)		(2822)		(1791)		(1767)	
1 year	42	42	43	43	39	40	29	30	20	22	28	29	27	29	28	30	29	31
3 years	28	28	23	24	21	22	14	16	9	12	14	17	14	16	15	17	14	17
5 years	24	24	18	19	16	18	10	13	5	9	10	14	10	13	10	13	10	14
8 years	21	21	16	17	13	15	8	12	3	8	7	13	8	13	6	11	..	..
10 years	18	19	15	17	12	15	6	11	2	8	6	13	6	13	..	..	..	..

RELATIVE SURVIVAL (%) BY AGE AND PERIOD

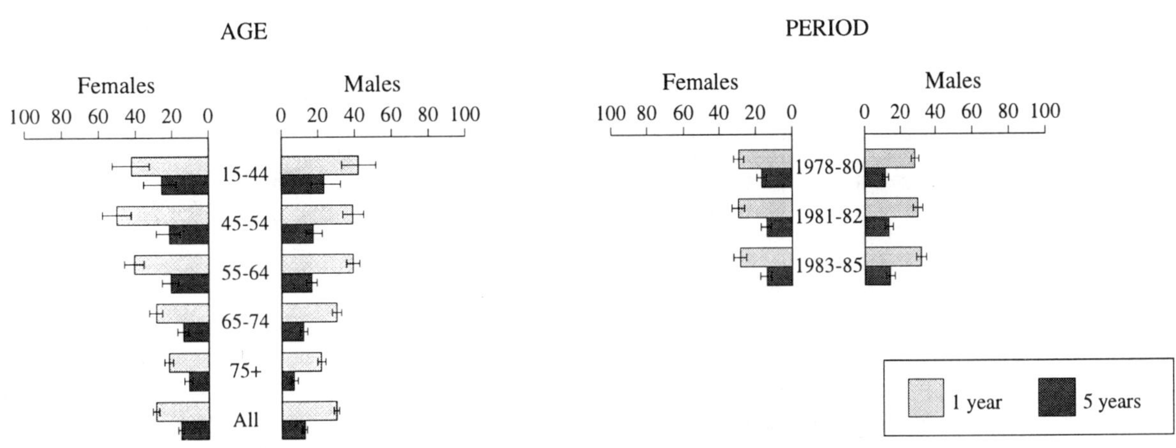

STOMACH

DUTCH REGISTRIES

REGISTRY	NUMBER OF CASES			PERIOD OF DIAGNOSIS
	Males	Females	All	
Eindhoven	717	430	1147	1978-1985
Mean age (years)	66.0	69.9	67.4	

RELATIVE SURVIVAL (%)

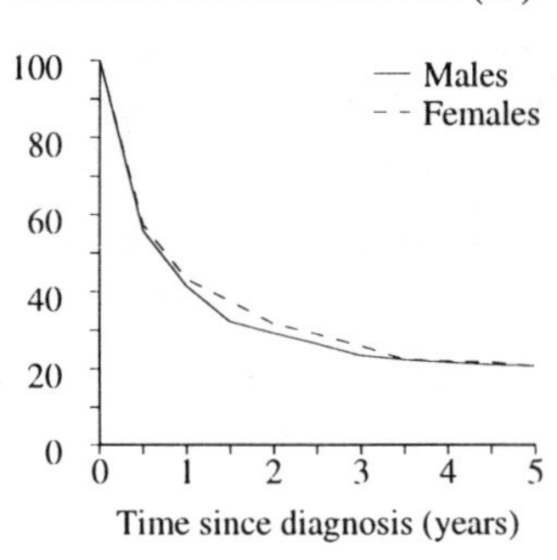

OBSERVED AND RELATIVE SURVIVAL (%) BY AGE AND PERIOD
(Number of cases in parentheses)

	AGE CLASS												PERIOD					
	15-44		45-54		55-64		65-74		75+		All		1978-80		1981-82		1983-85	
	obs	rel	obs	rel	obs	rel	obs	rel	obs	rel	obs	rel	obs	rel	obs	rel	obs	rel
Males	(33)		(88)		(180)		(233)		(183)		(717)		(272)		(167)		(278)	
1 year	64	64	50	50	42	43	37	39	30	34	39	41	37	39	42	44	41	43
3 years	39	40	30	31	22	23	19	22	11	16	20	23	18	21	22	26	21	24
5 years	39	40	29	30	17	19	14	18	7	13	16	21	14	19	19	24	16	20
8 years	32	33	22	24	12	14	9	14	5	16	11	18	9	15	..	..	..	..
10 years	..	..	22	24	12	15	..	..	..	..	10	19	9	15	..	..	..	..
Females	(17)		(34)		(71)		(130)		(178)		(430)		(161)		(105)		(164)	
1 year	41	41	74	74	59	60	42	42	29	31	42	43	40	42	50	52	37	39
3 years	35	35	44	44	35	35	23	24	13	17	23	26	21	24	32	37	18	21
5 years	35	36	25	25	26	27	17	20	9	14	17	21	16	20	24	30	12	16
8 years	35	36	20	21	24	26	11	14	6	15	13	19	12	17	..	..	..	..
10 years	..	..	..	..	24	27	11	16	..	..	13	21	12	20	..	..	..	..
Overall	(50)		(122)		(251)		(363)		(361)		(1147)		(433)		(272)		(442)	
1 year	56	56	57	57	47	48	39	40	29	32	40	42	38	40	45	47	39	41
3 years	38	38	34	35	26	27	20	23	12	17	21	24	19	22	26	30	20	23
5 years	38	38	27	28	20	22	15	19	8	14	16	21	15	19	21	27	14	19
8 years	34	35	22	23	15	18	9	14	6	15	12	18	10	16	..	..	..	..
10 years	..	..	22	23	15	19	9	17	..	..	11	20	10	17	..	..	..	..

RELATIVE SURVIVAL (%) BY AGE AND PERIOD

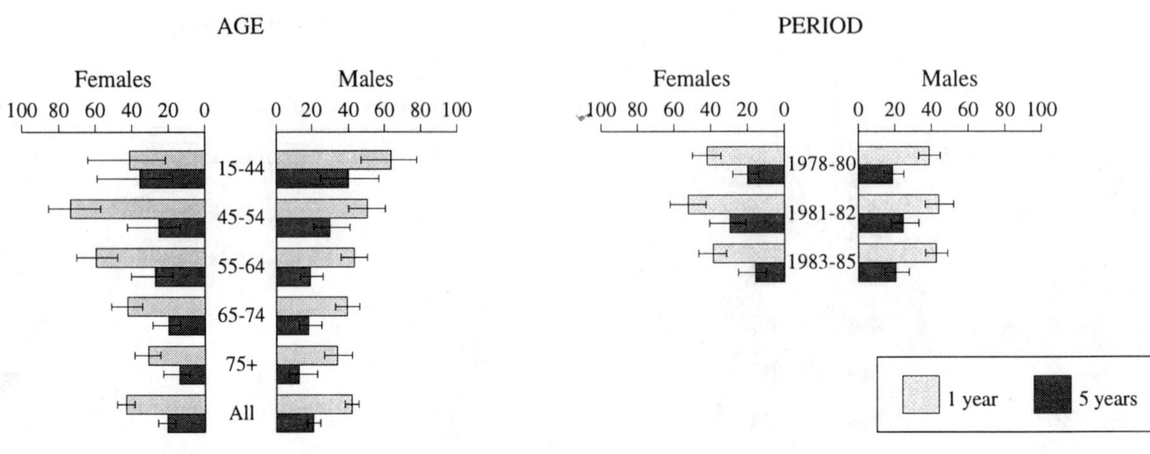

STOMACH

ENGLISH REGISTRIES

REGISTRY	NUMBER OF CASES			PERIOD OF DIAGNOSIS
	Males	Females	All	
East Anglia	1541	898	2439	1979-1984
Mersey	2405	1729	4134	1978-1984
South Thames	5405	3642	9047	1978-1984
Wessex	615	391	1006	1983-1984
West Midlands	4294	2475	6769	1979-1984
Yorkshire	3499	2398	5897	1978-1984
Mean age (years)	68.7	73.5	70.6	

RELATIVE SURVIVAL (%)

— Males
- - Females

Time since diagnosis (years)

OBSERVED AND RELATIVE SURVIVAL (%) BY AGE AND PERIOD
(Number of cases in parentheses)

	AGE CLASS												PERIOD					
	15-44		45-54		55-64		65-74		75+		All		1978-80		1981-82		1983-85	
	obs	rel	obs	rel	obs	rel	obs	rel	obs	rel	obs	rel	obs	rel	obs	rel	obs	rel
Males	(360)		(1251)		(3787)		(7032)		(5329)		(17759)		(7023)		(5260)		(5476)	
1 year	40	40	34	35	29	29	20	21	12	14	21	22	19	20	22	24	23	24
3 years	24	24	17	17	13	13	8	10	4	6	9	11	8	9	9	11	10	12
5 years	20	20	13	14	9	10	6	8	3	5	6	9	5	7	7	9	7	10
8 years	17	18	11	12	7	9	4	7	2	5	5	8	4	7	5	8	5	9
10 years	17	18	10	11	6	8	3	7	1	6	4	8	3	7	4	8	..	..
Females	(182)		(510)		(1445)		(3426)		(5970)		(11533)		(4806)		(3384)		(3343)	
1 year	45	45	36	36	31	31	23	24	13	15	20	21	17	19	19	20	24	26
3 years	24	24	21	21	14	15	11	12	5	7	9	11	7	9	9	10	12	14
5 years	16	16	15	15	11	12	8	10	3	6	6	9	5	7	6	8	9	12
8 years	15	15	13	14	10	11	6	9	2	6	5	9	4	7	5	8	7	12
10 years	15	15	13	13	8	10	6	9	2	6	4	9	3	7	4	8	..	..
Overall	(542)		(1761)		(5232)		(10458)		(11299)		(29292)		(11829)		(8644)		(8819)	
1 year	42	42	35	35	29	30	21	22	13	14	21	22	18	19	21	22	23	25
3 years	24	24	18	19	13	14	9	11	5	6	9	11	8	9	9	11	11	13
5 years	19	19	14	14	10	11	7	8	3	5	6	9	5	7	6	9	8	11
8 years	17	17	12	13	8	9	5	8	2	6	5	8	4	7	5	8	6	10
10 years	17	17	11	12	7	9	4	8	2	6	4	8	3	7	4	8	..	..

RELATIVE SURVIVAL (%) BY AGE AND PERIOD

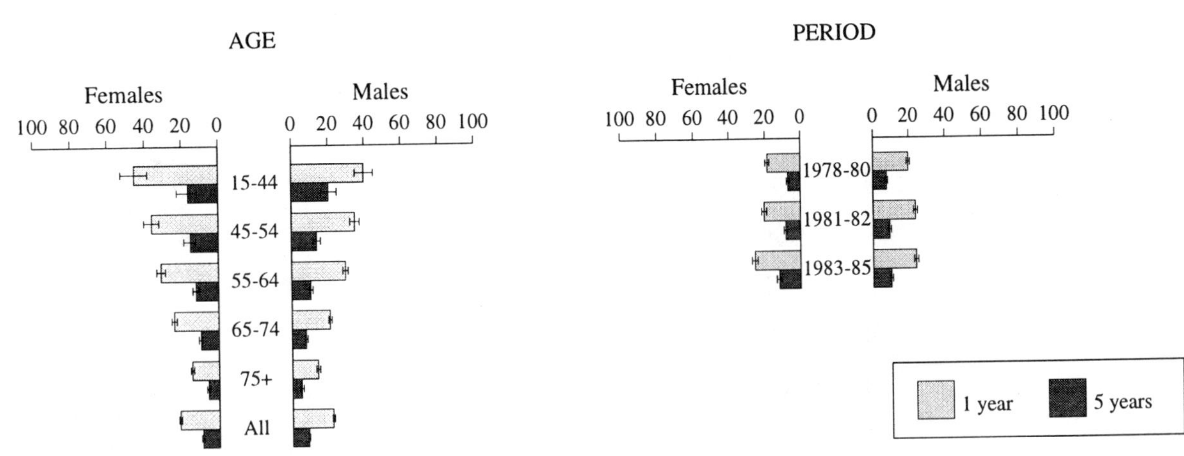

STOMACH

ESTONIA

REGISTRY	NUMBER OF CASES			PERIOD OF DIAGNOSIS
	Males	Females	All	
Estonia	1817	1756	3573	1978-1984
Mean age (years)	61.8	65.8	63.8	

RELATIVE SURVIVAL (%)

100 80 60 40 20 0

— Males
- - Females

0 1 2 3 4 5
Time since diagnosis (years)

OBSERVED AND RELATIVE SURVIVAL (%) BY AGE AND PERIOD
(Number of cases in parentheses)

	AGE CLASS												PERIOD					
	15-44		45-54		55-64		65-74		75+		All		1978-80		1981-82		1983-85	
	obs	rel	obs	rel	obs	rel	obs	rel	obs	rel	obs	rel	obs	rel	obs	rel	obs	rel
Males	(148)		(394)		(442)		(556)		(277)		(1817)		(809)		(488)		(520)	
1 year	42	42	47	48	35	36	30	32	21	23	35	36	35	37	34	35	35	36
3 years	28	28	27	28	21	22	14	17	8	12	19	22	19	21	18	21	20	23
5 years	24	25	21	23	16	18	10	14	6	12	14	18	13	17	14	18	16	21
8 years	21	23	15	17	12	17	7	13	3	12	11	16	10	16	10	15	..	..
10 years	21	24	12	14	11	16	6	12	3	20	9	16	9	15	..	..	..	..
Females	(115)		(214)		(352)		(617)		(458)		(1756)		(764)		(490)		(502)	
1 year	45	45	45	45	47	47	31	32	19	21	34	35	34	36	32	33	34	36
3 years	29	29	28	28	24	25	17	18	7	10	18	20	18	21	17	19	18	20
5 years	22	22	21	22	19	20	13	16	5	9	14	17	14	17	13	16	14	18
8 years	20	20	20	22	17	19	10	14	4	10	12	17	11	16	11	16	..	..
10 years	20	20	20	22	17	20	8	13	3	12	11	17	10	17	..	..	..	..
Overall	(263)		(608)		(794)		(1173)		(735)		(3573)		(1573)		(978)		(1022)	
1 year	43	43	46	47	40	41	31	32	19	22	34	36	35	36	33	34	34	36
3 years	28	29	27	28	22	23	16	18	8	11	18	21	18	21	18	20	19	22
5 years	23	23	21	22	17	19	11	15	5	10	14	18	13	17	13	17	15	19
8 years	21	22	17	19	14	18	9	14	3	11	11	17	11	16	11	16	..	..
10 years	21	22	15	18	13	17	7	13	3	14	10	17	9	16	..	..	..	..

RELATIVE SURVIVAL (%) BY AGE AND PERIOD

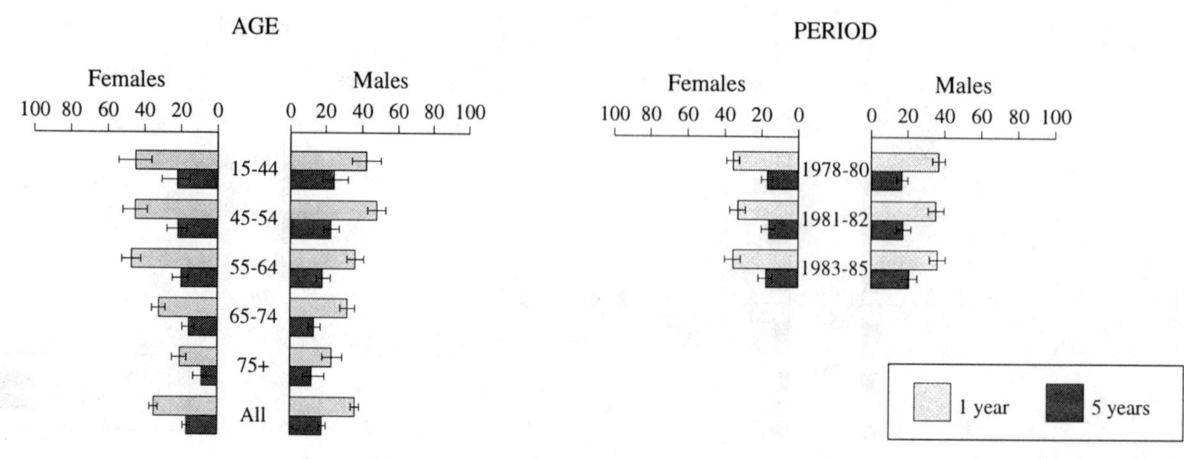

STOMACH

FINLAND

REGISTRY	NUMBER OF CASES			PERIOD OF DIAGNOSIS
	Males	Females	All	
Finland	4048	3498	7546	1978-1984
Mean age (years)	66.5	69.9	68.1	

RELATIVE SURVIVAL (%)

100
80
60
40
20
0
— Males
- - Females
0 1 2 3 4 5
Time since diagnosis (years)

OBSERVED AND RELATIVE SURVIVAL (%) BY AGE AND PERIOD
(Number of cases in parentheses)

	AGE CLASS												PERIOD					
	15-44		45-54		55-64		65-74		75+		All		1978-80		1981-82		1983-85	
	obs	rel	obs	rel	obs	rel	obs	rel	obs	rel	obs	rel	obs	rel	obs	rel	obs	rel
Males	(197)		(446)		(904)		(1412)		(1089)		(4048)		(1798)		(1135)		(1115)	
1 year	43	43	51	52	49	50	34	36	21	24	36	38	37	39	36	38	36	38
3 years	26	27	33	34	26	28	16	19	8	12	19	22	18	21	19	22	20	23
5 years	22	22	27	28	20	23	12	16	5	9	14	19	13	18	14	19	15	21
8 years	21	21	24	26	16	20	8	14	3	8	11	18	10	16	11	18	13	20
10 years	21	22	22	25	15	20	7	14	2	8	10	18	9	16	10	19	..	..
Females	(177)		(252)		(529)		(1107)		(1433)		(3498)		(1512)		(980)		(1006)	
1 year	54	54	51	51	46	46	40	41	24	26	36	38	34	36	37	39	37	38
3 years	31	31	30	30	23	23	22	24	9	12	18	21	17	19	19	22	18	21
5 years	29	29	25	25	18	19	17	19	6	11	14	18	13	16	15	19	14	18
8 years	26	26	23	24	16	18	13	17	4	10	11	17	10	15	12	18	12	18
10 years	25	26	22	23	16	18	10	15	3	9	10	16	9	15	10	17	..	..
Overall	(374)		(698)		(1433)		(2519)		(2522)		(7546)		(3310)		(2115)		(2121)	
1 year	48	49	51	51	48	49	37	38	23	25	36	38	36	38	36	38	36	38
3 years	29	29	32	32	25	26	19	21	9	12	18	21	17	20	19	22	19	22
5 years	25	25	26	27	20	22	14	17	6	10	14	18	13	17	14	19	15	19
8 years	23	24	24	25	16	19	10	16	3	9	11	17	10	16	12	18	12	19
10 years	23	24	22	24	15	19	8	15	2	9	10	17	9	16	10	18	..	..

RELATIVE SURVIVAL (%) BY AGE AND PERIOD

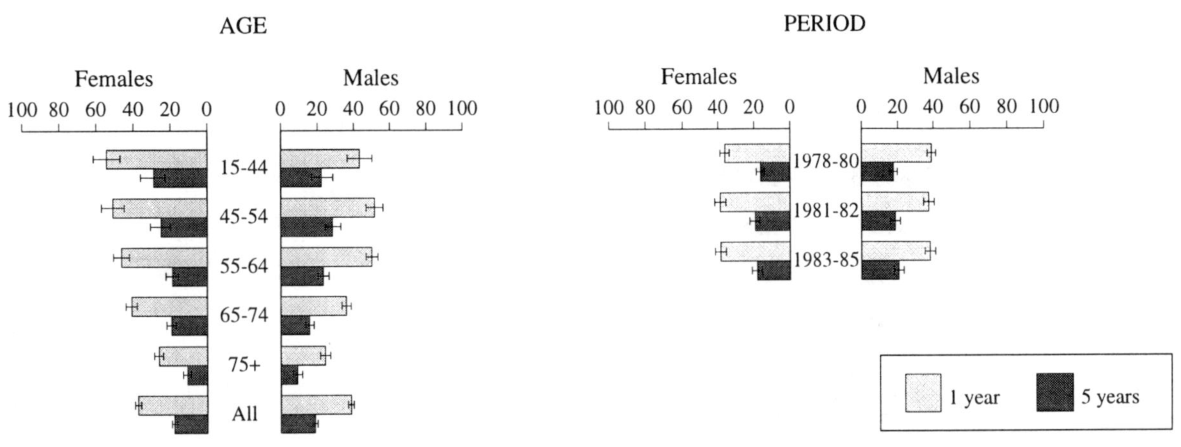

STOMACH

FRENCH REGISTRIES

REGISTRY	NUMBER OF CASES			PERIOD OF DIAGNOSIS
	Males	Females	All	
Amiens	113	82	195	1983-1984
Calvados	455	310	765	1978-1985
Côte-d'Or	381	223	604	1978-1985
Doubs	363	226	589	1978-1985
Mean age (years)	67.6	72.3	69.4	

RELATIVE SURVIVAL (%)

100
80
60
40
20
0
— Males
- - Females
0 1 2 3 4 5
Time since diagnosis (years)

OBSERVED AND RELATIVE SURVIVAL (%) BY AGE AND PERIOD
(Number of cases in parentheses)

	AGE CLASS												PERIOD					
	15-44		45-54		55-64		65-74		75+		All		1978-80		1981-82		1983-85	
	obs	rel	obs	rel	obs	rel	obs	rel	obs	rel	obs	rel	obs	rel	obs	rel	obs	rel
Males	(53)		(130)		(282)		(449)		(398)		(1312)		(438)		(278)		(596)	
1 year	57	58	57	58	44	45	36	38	24	27	37	39	37	38	38	40	37	39
3 years	35	35	43	45	28	29	19	21	8	12	21	24	19	22	21	25	22	26
5 years	33	33	38	40	18	20	14	18	5	9	15	20	14	18	17	23	15	20
8 years	25	25	30	33	16	19	12	18	3	10	12	20	11	16	14	23	13	21
10 years	25	26	30	34	14	18	10	18	2	10	11	20	10	17	12	21	..	..
Females	(24)		(48)		(116)		(242)		(411)		(841)		(282)		(208)		(351)	
1 year	65	66	58	59	59	59	46	46	28	31	40	43	39	41	40	43	42	44
3 years	52	53	41	42	36	37	23	24	11	15	21	24	21	24	18	22	22	26
5 years	40	40	34	35	30	31	18	21	7	12	16	21	16	21	15	20	16	21
8 years	40	41	30	30	26	28	15	19	4	10	13	20	12	19	12	20	14	24
10 years	24	25	30	31	26	28	11	15	2	9	10	19	10	18	12	22	..	..
Overall	(77)		(178)		(398)		(691)		(809)		(2153)		(720)		(486)		(947)	
1 year	60	60	57	58	48	49	40	41	26	29	38	40	37	39	39	41	39	41
3 years	40	41	43	44	30	32	20	22	10	13	21	24	20	23	20	24	22	26
5 years	35	36	37	38	21	23	16	19	6	11	15	20	15	19	16	22	15	21
8 years	29	30	30	32	19	22	13	18	4	10	12	20	11	18	13	22	13	22
10 years	25	26	30	33	18	22	10	16	2	10	11	19	10	17	12	21	..	..

RELATIVE SURVIVAL (%) BY AGE AND PERIOD

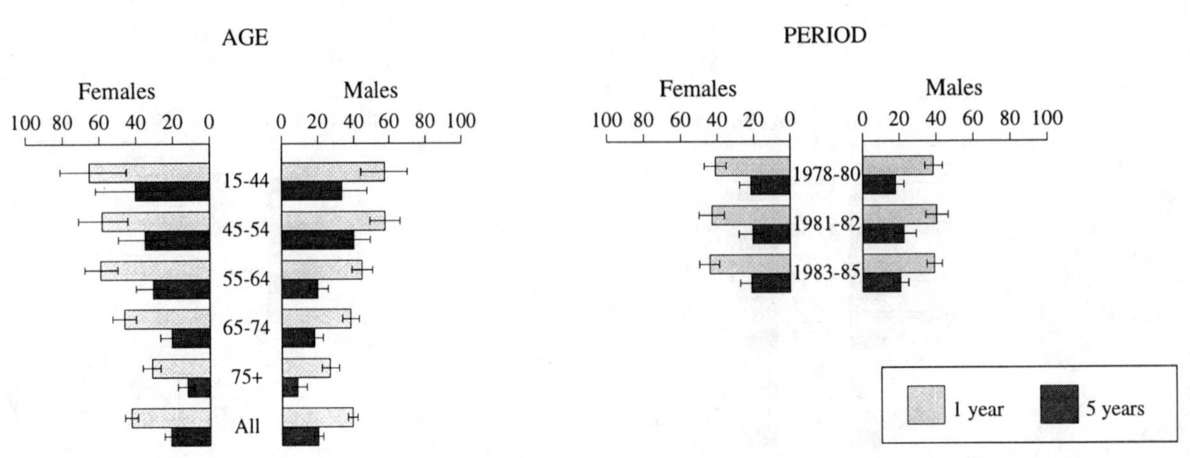

STOMACH

GERMAN REGISTRIES

REGISTRY	NUMBER OF CASES			PERIOD OF DIAGNOSIS
	Males	Females	All	
Saarland	1006	878	1884	1978-1984
Mean age (years)	66.5	70.7	68.4	

RELATIVE SURVIVAL (%)

— Males
- - Females

Time since diagnosis (years)

OBSERVED AND RELATIVE SURVIVAL (%) BY AGE AND PERIOD
(Number of cases in parentheses)

	AGE CLASS												PERIOD					
	15-44		45-54		55-64		65-74		75+		All		1978-80		1981-82		1983-85	
	obs	rel	obs	rel	obs	rel	obs	rel	obs	rel	obs	rel	obs	rel	obs	rel	obs	rel
Males	(50)		(127)		(207)		(342)		(280)		(1006)		(446)		(276)		(284)	
1 year	44	44	57	58	43	44	39	41	25	29	38	41	39	41	35	37	41	43
3 years	34	34	46	47	24	25	18	21	11	16	21	26	21	25	18	22	25	30
5 years	32	33	39	41	18	21	12	17	8	15	17	23	16	21	14	19	21	27
8 years	30	31	36	39	15	18	9	16	7	22	14	23	13	22	11	19	..	..
10 years	26	27	36	40	13	17	9	19	6	28	13	25	13	24	..	..	..	..
Females	(30)		(55)		(126)		(285)		(382)		(878)		(358)		(249)		(271)	
1 year	57	57	62	62	52	53	41	42	29	32	39	41	37	39	35	37	46	49
3 years	37	37	40	41	37	38	23	25	14	18	23	26	22	26	18	21	27	31
5 years	33	34	33	33	29	31	19	22	8	14	17	22	16	21	15	20	20	26
8 years	30	30	23	24	28	30	14	19	7	16	14	22	14	21	12	19	..	..
10 years	30	30	17	18	28	32	12	19	6	20	13	23	13	23	..	..	..	..
Overall	(80)		(182)		(333)		(627)		(662)		(1884)		(804)		(525)		(555)	
1 year	49	49	59	59	47	47	40	41	27	31	39	41	38	40	35	37	44	46
3 years	35	35	44	45	29	30	20	23	12	17	22	26	22	26	18	22	26	30
5 years	33	33	37	39	23	25	15	20	8	14	17	22	16	21	14	20	21	27
8 years	30	31	32	34	20	23	12	18	7	18	14	22	14	22	12	19	..	..
10 years	28	28	30	33	19	24	11	19	6	23	13	24	13	24	..	..	..	..

RELATIVE SURVIVAL (%) BY AGE AND PERIOD

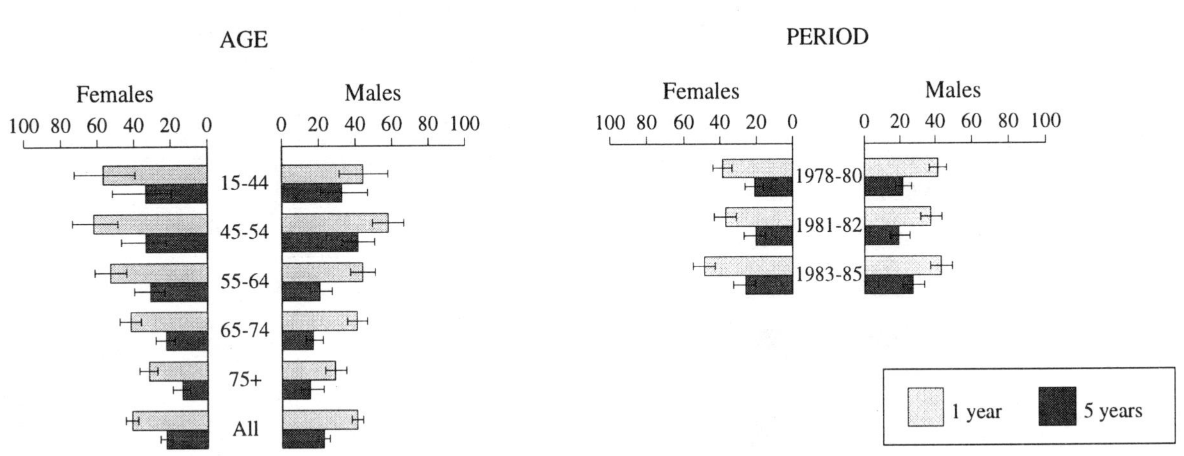

STOMACH

ITALIAN REGISTRIES

REGISTRY	NUMBER OF CASES			PERIOD OF DIAGNOSIS
	Males	Females	All	
Florence	418	275	693	1985-1985
Latina	81	62	143	1983-1984
Ragusa	153	93	246	1981-1984
Varese	1159	833	1992	1978-1984
Mean age (years)	67.3	71.4	69.0	

RELATIVE SURVIVAL (%)

— Males
- - Females

Time since diagnosis (years)

OBSERVED AND RELATIVE SURVIVAL (%) BY AGE AND PERIOD
(Number of cases in parentheses)

	AGE CLASS												PERIOD					
	15-44		45-54		55-64		65-74		75+		All		1978-80		1981-82		1983-85	
	obs	rel	obs	rel	obs	rel	obs	rel	obs	rel	obs	rel	obs	rel	obs	rel	obs	rel
Males	(74)		(174)		(386)		(691)		(486)		(1811)		(488)		(449)		(874)	
1 year	64	64	61	62	43	44	37	38	25	28	38	41	39	41	37	39	39	41
3 years	41	41	44	45	25	26	16	19	8	11	19	23	17	21	21	24	20	23
5 years	35	36	36	37	19	21	12	16	4	8	15	19	13	17	15	20	15	20
8 years	23	24	33	36	16	20	8	13	2	7	11	18	9	15	12	18	13	21
10 years	23	24	29	33	14	19	8	14	1	5	10	18	8	15	11	20	..	..
Females	(38)		(86)		(163)		(406)		(570)		(1263)		(370)		(270)		(623)	
1 year	61	61	59	59	51	51	40	41	28	31	38	40	34	36	38	40	40	42
3 years	47	48	34	34	34	35	25	27	13	17	22	26	17	20	24	28	24	28
5 years	39	40	26	26	28	29	19	22	8	14	16	21	12	16	16	22	19	24
8 years	35	35	24	25	25	27	16	20	7	17	14	22	10	16	14	22	18	26
10 years	35	35	24	25	23	26	12	17	7	22	12	21	9	16	11	19	..	..
Overall	(112)		(260)		(549)		(1097)		(1056)		(3074)		(858)		(719)		(1497)	
1 year	63	63	61	61	45	46	38	39	27	30	38	40	37	39	37	39	39	41
3 years	43	43	40	41	28	29	20	22	10	14	20	24	17	20	22	26	22	25
5 years	37	37	32	33	22	24	15	18	6	11	15	20	13	17	16	21	17	22
8 years	27	28	30	32	19	22	11	16	5	13	12	19	10	15	13	20	15	23
10 years	27	28	27	30	17	21	9	15	4	14	11	19	8	15	11	20	..	..

RELATIVE SURVIVAL (%) BY AGE AND PERIOD

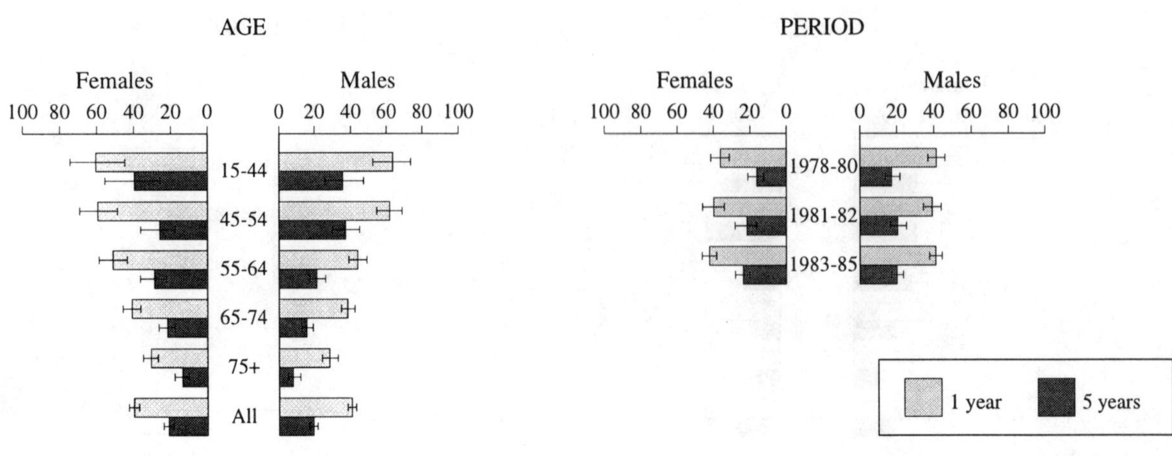

STOMACH

POLISH REGISTRIES

REGISTRY	NUMBER OF CASES			PERIOD OF DIAGNOSIS
	Males	Females	All	
Cracow	659	402	1061	1978-1984
Mean age (years)	64.1	67.5	65.4	

RELATIVE SURVIVAL (%)

— Males
- - Females

Time since diagnosis (years)

OBSERVED AND RELATIVE SURVIVAL (%) BY AGE AND PERIOD

(Number of cases in parentheses)

AGE CLASS

	15-44		45-54		55-64		65-74		75+		All	
	obs	rel	obs	rel	obs	rel	obs	rel	obs	rel	obs	rel
Males	(41)		(82)		(184)		(232)		(120)		(659)	
1 year	28	28	42	42	24	25	18	19	11	12	22	23
3 years	20	21	21	22	11	11	7	8	3	4	10	11
5 years	13	13	17	18	6	7	4	6	3	6	7	9
8 years	10	10	14	16	5	6	2	3	3	9	5	7
10 years	10	10	14	17	3	5	2	4	3	13	4	8
Females	(23)		(33)		(77)		(148)		(121)		(402)	
1 year	35	35	44	44	40	41	27	28	13	14	27	28
3 years	22	22	30	31	23	24	20	22	5	7	17	19
5 years	17	18	30	31	16	17	16	20	5	8	14	17
8 years	17	18	30	32	14	16	12	17	3	7	11	17
10 years	17	18	25	27	14	17	11	18	3	10	11	18
Overall	(64)		(115)		(261)		(380)		(241)		(1061)	
1 year	30	30	42	43	29	29	21	22	12	13	24	25
3 years	21	21	24	24	14	15	11	13	4	6	12	14
5 years	14	15	21	22	9	10	9	11	4	7	9	12
8 years	12	13	19	21	7	9	6	9	3	8	7	11
10 years	12	13	17	20	7	9	5	10	3	11	7	12

PERIOD

	1978-80		1981-82		1983-85	
	obs	rel	obs	rel	obs	rel
Males	(302)		(176)		(181)	
1 year	21	23	23	24	23	24
3 years	11	12	9	10	9	11
5 years	9	11	4	5	7	9
8 years	5	8	4	5	5	8
10 years	5	9	..	..	..	..
Females	(196)		(90)		(116)	
1 year	29	30	23	24	26	27
3 years	20	23	10	12	17	19
5 years	17	21	6	7	16	20
8 years	14	21	5	7	13	18
10 years	13	22	5	8	..	..
Overall	(498)		(266)		(297)	
1 year	24	26	23	24	24	25
3 years	14	16	9	11	12	14
5 years	12	15	4	5	10	13
8 years	9	13	4	6	8	12
10 years	8	14	4	7	..	..

RELATIVE SURVIVAL (%) BY AGE AND PERIOD

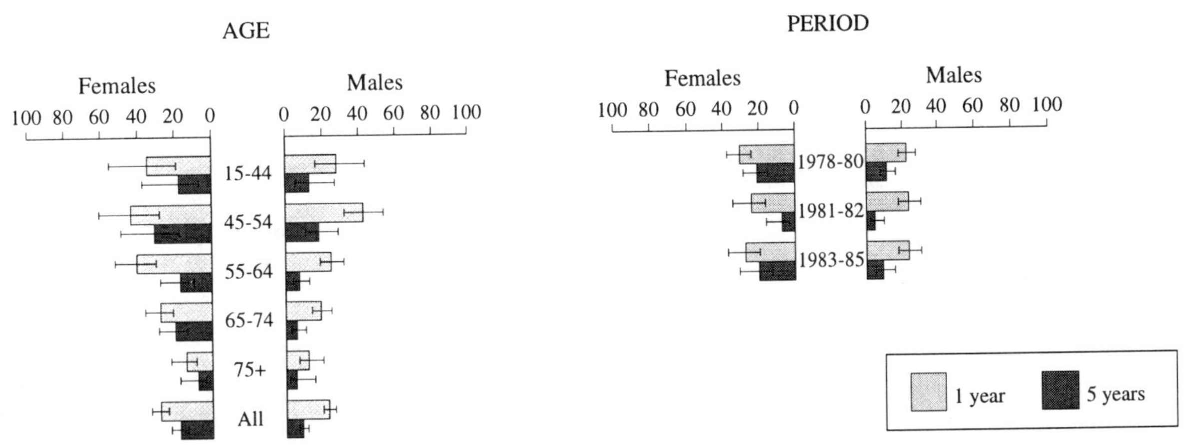

STOMACH

SCOTLAND

REGISTRY	NUMBER OF CASES			PERIOD OF DIAGNOSIS
	Males	Females	All	
Scotland	3333	2428	5761	1978-1982
Mean age (years)	67.1	71.7	69.0	

RELATIVE SURVIVAL (%)

Males / Females

Time since diagnosis (years)

OBSERVED AND RELATIVE SURVIVAL (%) BY AGE AND PERIOD
(Number of cases in parentheses)

	AGE CLASS												PERIOD					
	15-44		45-54		55-64		65-74		75+		All		1978-80		1981-82		1983-85	
	obs	rel	obs	rel	obs	rel	obs	rel	obs	rel	obs	rel	obs	rel	obs	rel	obs	rel
Males	(81)		(334)		(774)		(1302)		(842)		(3333)		(1984)		(1349)		(0)	
1 year	32	32	34	34	28	28	20	21	14	16	22	23	20	22	24	26	..	..
3 years	16	16	16	17	11	12	8	9	4	7	9	10	8	10	10	12	..	..
5 years	10	10	11	11	8	9	5	7	2	4	6	8	6	8	6	8	..	..
8 years	5	5	10	11	7	9	3	6	1	4	4	7	4	8	..	..	..	..
10 years	..	..	7	8	7	10	2	5	1	5	4	7	4	7	..	..	..	..
Females	(51)		(138)		(342)		(846)		(1051)		(2428)		(1424)		(1004)		(0)	
1 year	35	35	36	36	31	32	22	22	15	17	21	23	21	22	22	23	..	..
3 years	20	20	18	18	16	17	9	10	7	10	10	12	10	11	11	13	..	..
5 years	14	14	13	13	13	14	6	7	5	8	7	9	7	9	7	9	..	..
8 years	14	14	12	13	10	11	4	5	3	8	5	8	5	8	..	..	..	..
10 years	..	..	..	..	10	12	3	5	3	11	5	9	5	9	..	..	..	..
Overall	(132)		(472)		(1116)		(2148)		(1893)		(5761)		(3408)		(2353)		(0)	
1 year	33	33	34	35	29	29	20	21	15	17	22	23	20	22	23	25	..	..
3 years	17	18	17	17	12	13	8	10	6	8	9	11	9	10	10	12	..	..
5 years	11	12	11	12	10	11	5	7	4	7	6	9	6	8	6	9	..	..
8 years	8	9	10	11	8	10	4	6	2	6	5	8	5	8	..	..	..	..
10 years	..	..	8	9	8	11	3	5	2	9	4	8	4	8	..	..	..	..

RELATIVE SURVIVAL (%) BY AGE AND PERIOD

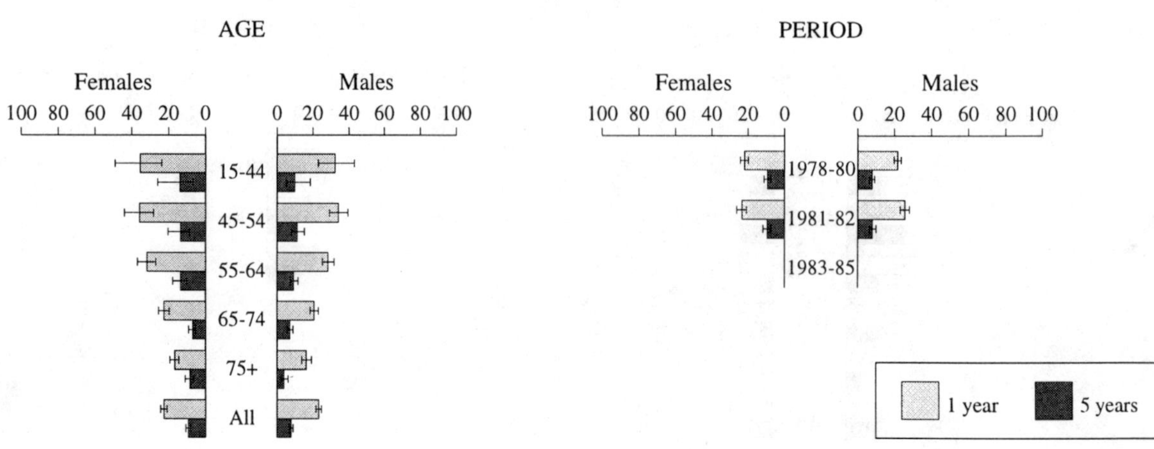

STOMACH

SPANISH REGISTRIES

REGISTRY	NUMBER OF CASES			PERIOD OF DIAGNOSIS
	Males	Females	All	
Tarragona	50	44	94	1985-1985
Mean age (years)	67.5	67.3	67.4	

RELATIVE SURVIVAL (%)

OBSERVED AND RELATIVE SURVIVAL (%) BY AGE AND PERIOD
(Number of cases in parentheses)

	AGE CLASS												PERIOD					
	15-44		45-54		55-64		65-74		75+		All		1978-80		1981-82		1983-85	
	obs	rel	obs	rel	obs	rel	obs	rel	obs	rel	obs	rel	obs	rel	obs	rel	obs	rel
Males	(2)		(8)		(8)		(18)		(14)		(50)		(0)		(0)		(50)	
1 year	100	100	38	38	63	63	39	40	14	16	38	40	..	..	..	..	38	40
3 years	50	50	25	25	50	52	6	6	0	0	16	19	..	..	..	..	16	19
5 years	50	51	25	26	38	40	0	0	0	0	12	15	..	..	..	..	12	15
8 years	..	..	..	..	..	..	0	0	0	0	..	..	..	..	..	..	..	..
10 years	..	..	..	..	..	..	0	0	0	0	..	..	..	..	..	..	..	..
Females	(6)		(3)		(8)		(7)		(20)		(44)		(0)		(0)		(44)	
1 year	67	67	33	33	75	75	0	0	20	22	34	35	..	..	..	..	34	35
3 years	50	50	33	34	38	38	0	0	5	6	18	21	..	..	..	..	18	21
5 years	50	50	33	34	38	39	0	0	5	8	18	22	..	..	..	..	18	22
8 years	..	..	..	..	..	..	0	0	..	..	..	..	..	..	..	..	..	..
10 years	..	..	..	..	..	..	0	0	..	..	..	..	..	..	..	..	..	..
Overall	(8)		(11)		(16)		(25)		(34)		(94)		(0)		(0)		(94)	
1 year	75	75	36	37	69	69	28	29	18	20	36	38	..	..	..	..	36	38
3 years	50	50	27	28	44	45	4	4	3	4	17	19	..	..	..	..	17	19
5 years	50	50	27	28	38	40	0	0	3	5	15	19	..	..	..	..	15	19
8 years	..	..	..	..	..	..	0	0	..	..	..	..	..	..	..	..	..	..
10 years	..	..	..	..	..	..	0	0	..	..	..	..	..	..	..	..	..	..

RELATIVE SURVIVAL (%) BY AGE AND PERIOD

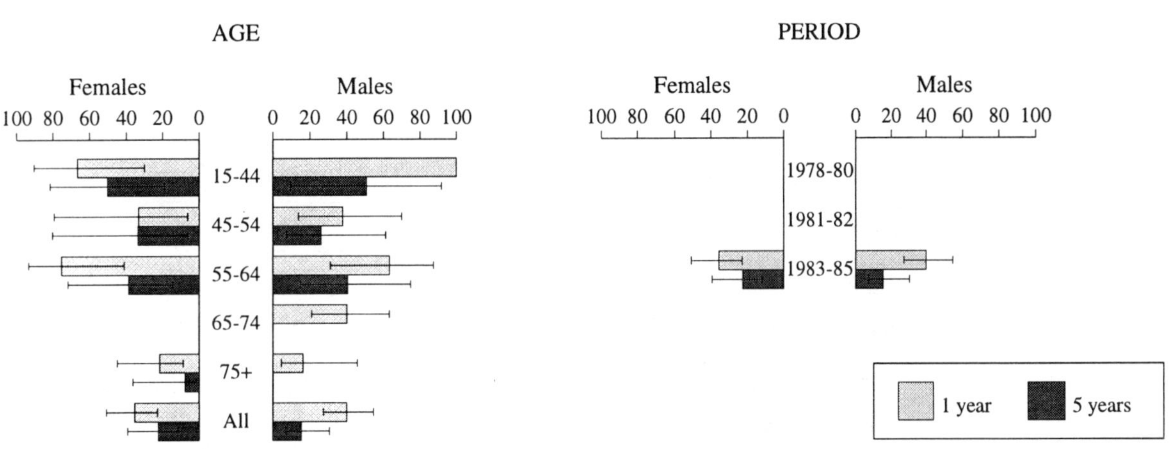

STOMACH

SWISS REGISTRIES

REGISTRY	NUMBER OF CASES			PERIOD OF DIAGNOSIS
	Males	Females	All	
Basel	177	121	298	1981-1984
Geneva	189	148	337	1978-1984
Mean age (years)	68.0	71.7	69.5	

RELATIVE SURVIVAL (%)

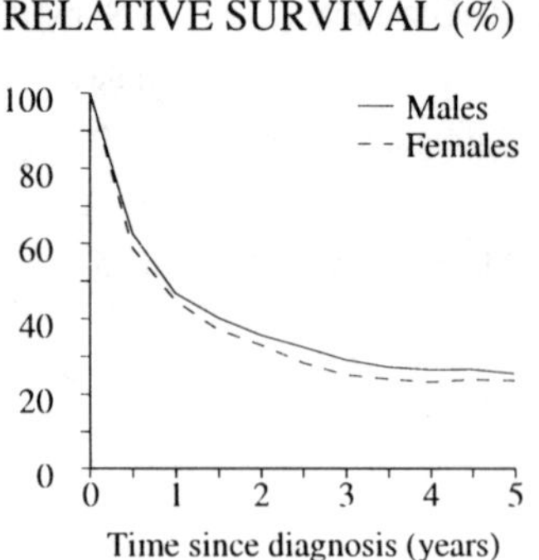

OBSERVED AND RELATIVE SURVIVAL (%) BY AGE AND PERIOD
(Number of cases in parentheses)

	AGE CLASS												PERIOD					
	15-44		45-54		55-64		65-74		75+		All		1978-80		1981-82		1983-85	
	obs	rel	obs	rel	obs	rel	obs	rel	obs	rel	obs	rel	obs	rel	obs	rel	obs	rel
Males	(14)		(41)		(76)		(110)		(125)		(366)		(83)		(147)		(136)	
1 year	64	64	51	51	57	57	41	42	36	40	44	47	46	48	48	50	40	43
3 years	50	50	38	39	36	38	19	22	16	23	25	29	24	28	31	35	19	23
5 years	50	51	35	37	29	32	13	16	11	21	20	26	19	25	24	31	15	19
8 years	50	51	30	32	21	24	8	12	10	30	15	24	..	..	18	27	..	..
10 years	..	..	..	..	..	..	..	..	..	..	..	..	..	..	..	..	..	..
Females	(18)		(19)		(25)		(72)		(135)		(269)		(66)		(114)		(89)	
1 year	61	61	58	58	64	64	51	52	29	32	43	45	37	39	42	44	47	49
3 years	39	39	53	53	24	25	30	32	10	13	22	25	20	24	24	28	20	23
5 years	33	34	42	43	24	25	27	30	7	11	18	24	17	23	19	25	17	22
8 years	26	26	23	24	24	26	20	25	6	14	14	22	..	..	15	23	..	..
10 years	..	..	..	..	..	..	..	..	..	..	..	..	..	..	..	..	..	..
Overall	(32)		(60)		(101)		(182)		(260)		(635)		(149)		(261)		(225)	
1 year	63	63	53	53	58	59	45	46	33	36	44	46	42	44	45	48	43	45
3 years	44	44	43	44	33	34	23	26	13	18	24	27	22	26	28	32	19	23
5 years	41	41	38	39	28	30	18	22	9	16	19	25	18	24	22	29	16	21
8 years	35	36	28	30	21	24	13	18	8	21	15	23	..	..	16	26	..	..
10 years	..	..	..	..	..	..	..	..	..	..	..	..	..	..	..	..	..	..

RELATIVE SURVIVAL (%) BY AGE AND PERIOD

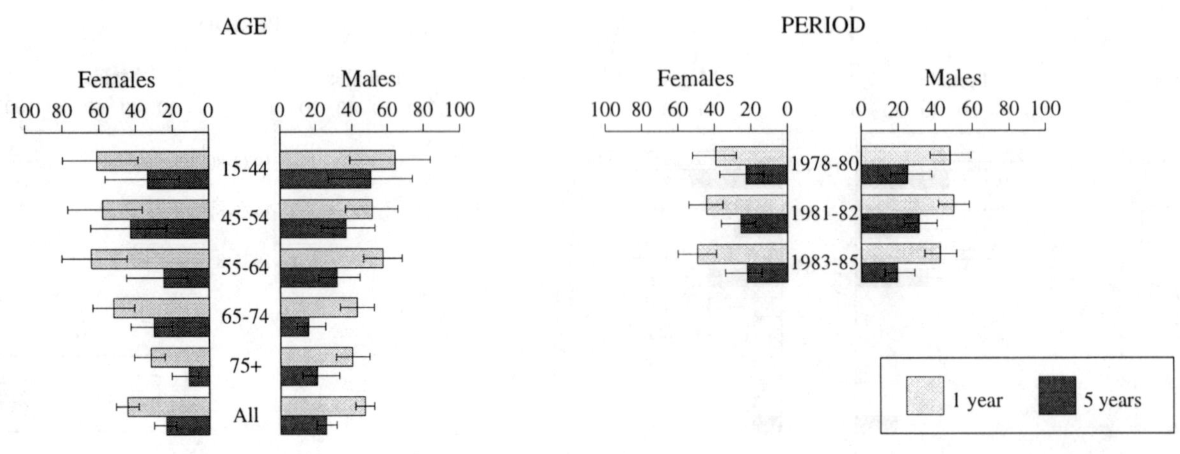

STOMACH

EUROPEAN REGISTRIES

Weighted analysis

REGISTRY	WEIGHTS (Yearly expected cases in the country) Males	Females	All
DENMARK	557	354	911
DUTCH REGISTRIES	2021	1146	3167
ENGLISH REGISTRIES	8946	5586	14532
ESTONIA	259	250	509
FINLAND	592	515	1107
FRENCH REGISTRIES	6407	4278	10685
GERMAN REGISTRIES	12210	10467	22677
ITALIAN REGISTRIES	12872	7991	20863
POLISH REGISTRIES	7172	4061	11233
SCOTLAND	666	485	1151
SPANISH REGISTRIES	6066	3931	9997
SWISS REGISTRIES	734	473	1207

RELATIVE SURVIVAL (%)
(Age-standardized)

OBSERVED AND RELATIVE SURVIVAL (%) BY AGE AND PERIOD

	AGE CLASS 15-44 obs	rel	45-54 obs	rel	55-64 obs	rel	65-74 obs	rel	75+ obs	rel	All obs	rel	PERIOD 1978-80 obs	rel	1981-82 obs	rel	1983-85 obs	rel
Males																		
1 year	54	54	50	50	41	41	32	34	20	23	33	35	32	34	32	34	34	36
3 years	34	34	34	35	24	25	13	16	7	10	17	20	16	19	17	20	18	21
5 years	30	31	29	30	18	20	9	12	4	8	13	17	12	16	12	16	14	18
8 years	23	23	26	28	12	15	6	11	3	10	10	16	9	14	10	16	10	15
10 years	21	22	25	28	11	14	6	11	2	11	9	17	8	15	9	16	..	..
Females																		
1 year	55	55	52	52	51	51	33	34	24	26	34	36	32	34	33	35	37	39
3 years	38	38	34	35	31	32	19	21	10	13	19	22	18	21	18	21	21	24
5 years	33	33	28	29	25	26	15	17	7	11	15	19	13	17	13	17	17	21
8 years	28	28	23	24	22	24	12	15	5	13	12	19	11	17	10	17	13	21
10 years	26	26	21	22	21	24	10	14	5	15	11	19	10	17	8	15	..	..
Overall																		
1 year	54	54	51	51	45	45	32	34	22	24	34	36	32	34	32	34	36	38
3 years	36	36	34	35	27	28	16	18	8	11	18	21	17	20	17	20	19	22
5 years	31	32	29	30	21	22	12	14	5	9	13	18	12	16	13	17	15	19
8 years	25	25	25	27	16	19	9	13	4	11	11	17	10	15	10	16	11	17
10 years	23	24	23	25	15	18	7	13	3	13	10	17	9	16	9	16	..	..

RELATIVE SURVIVAL (%) BY AGE AND PERIOD

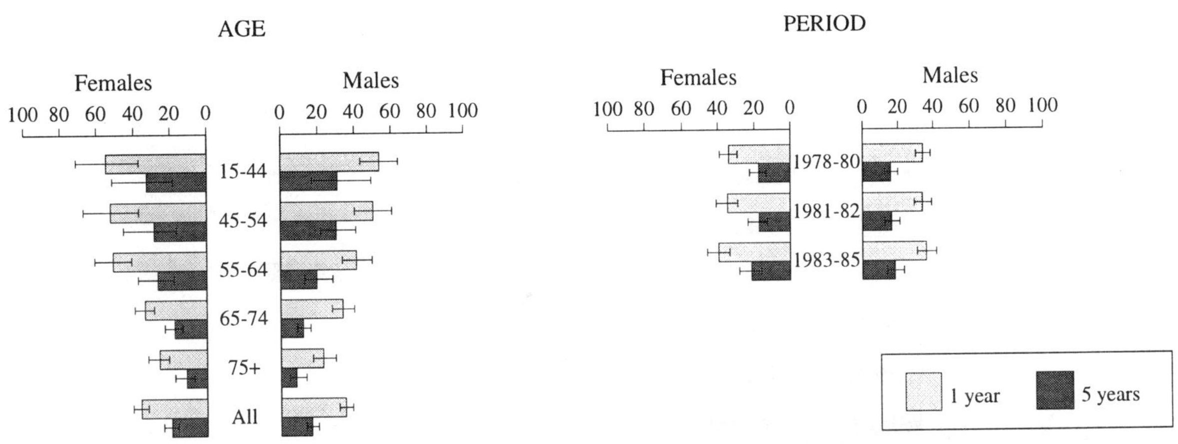

COLON

DENMARK

REGISTRY	NUMBER OF CASES			PERIOD OF DIAGNOSIS
	Males	Females	All	
Denmark	5283	6869	12152	1978-1984
Mean age (years)	69.5	71.3	70.5	

RELATIVE SURVIVAL (%)

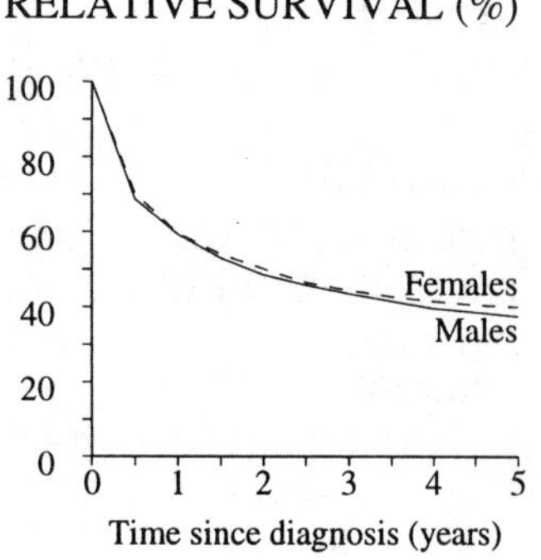

OBSERVED AND RELATIVE SURVIVAL (%) BY AGE AND PERIOD
(Number of cases in parentheses)

	AGE CLASS												PERIOD					
	15-44		45-54		55-64		65-74		75+		All		1978-80		1981-82		1983-85	
	obs	rel	obs	rel	obs	rel	obs	rel	obs	rel	obs	rel	obs	rel	obs	rel	obs	rel
Males	(155)		(386)		(979)		(1854)		(1909)		(5283)		(2203)		(1490)		(1590)	
1 year	65	65	65	65	64	65	60	63	45	50	56	59	54	58	57	61	56	60
3 years	46	46	46	47	43	46	39	46	26	38	36	43	36	44	36	43	36	43
5 years	41	42	38	40	36	40	29	38	17	33	27	38	27	37	28	38	27	37
8 years	37	38	34	37	30	36	21	34	9	28	20	34	20	35	19	33	..	..
10 years	37	38	33	37	26	34	17	33	7	32	17	34	17	35	..	..	..	..
Females	(192)		(416)		(1099)		(2114)		(3048)		(6869)		(2837)		(1984)		(2048)	
1 year	70	70	72	72	67	68	62	64	47	51	57	60	55	57	59	62	58	61
3 years	51	51	50	50	50	51	44	47	28	37	38	44	38	43	40	46	38	44
5 years	44	45	42	43	42	45	36	41	21	35	31	40	30	39	33	43	31	40
8 years	39	40	39	41	37	42	29	38	14	34	25	38	25	38	24	37	..	..
10 years	39	40	38	40	36	42	25	36	10	33	21	38	21	37	..	..	..	..
Overall	(347)		(802)		(2078)		(3968)		(4957)		(12152)		(5040)		(3474)		(3638)	
1 year	68	68	68	69	66	67	61	63	46	51	56	59	55	57	58	61	57	60
3 years	48	49	48	49	47	49	42	46	27	37	37	44	37	44	38	45	37	44
5 years	43	43	40	42	39	43	33	40	20	34	29	39	29	38	31	41	29	39
8 years	38	39	36	39	34	39	25	36	12	32	23	37	23	36	22	35	..	..
10 years	38	39	36	39	31	39	21	35	9	33	19	36	19	36	..	..	..	..

RELATIVE SURVIVAL (%) BY AGE AND PERIOD

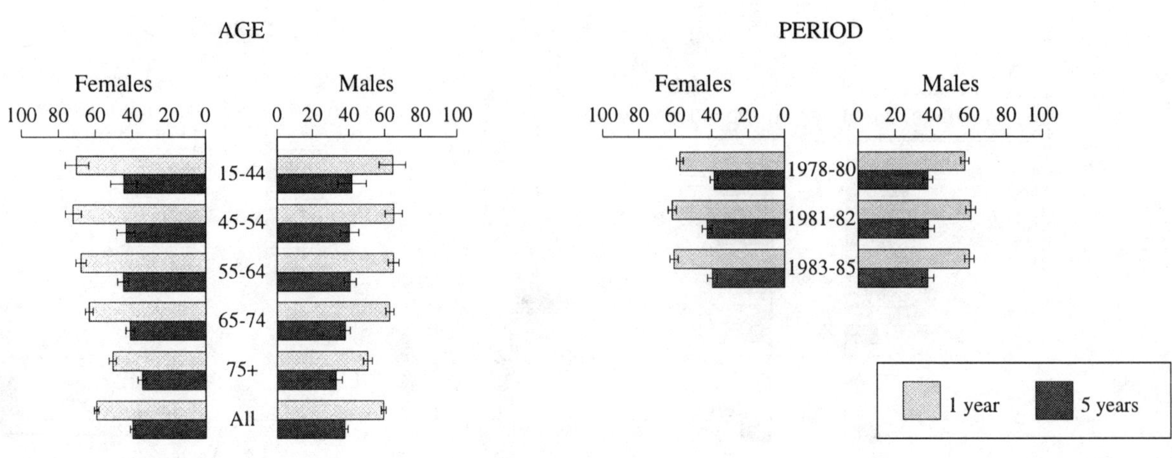

COLON

DUTCH REGISTRIES

REGISTRY	NUMBER OF CASES			PERIOD OF DIAGNOSIS
	Males	Females	All	
Eindhoven	746	857	1603	1978-1985
Mean age (years)	65.6	67.2	66.5	

RELATIVE SURVIVAL (%)

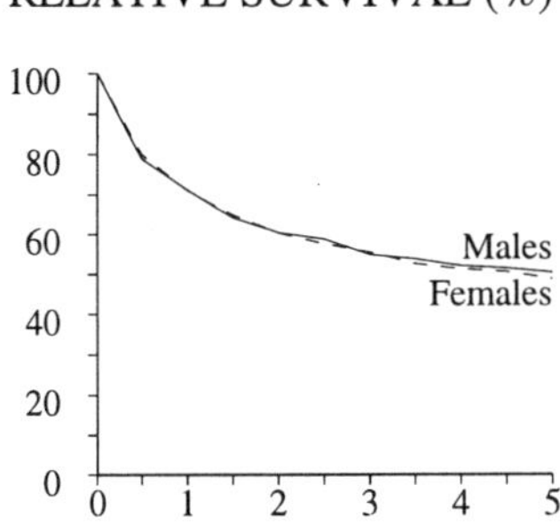

OBSERVED AND RELATIVE SURVIVAL (%) BY AGE AND PERIOD
(Number of cases in parentheses)

	AGE CLASS												PERIOD					
	15-44		45-54		55-64		65-74		75+		All		1978-80		1981-82		1983-85	
	obs	rel	obs	rel	obs	rel	obs	rel	obs	rel	obs	rel	obs	rel	obs	rel	obs	rel
Males	(58)		(82)		(173)		(225)		(208)		(746)		(229)		(194)		(323)	
1 year	72	73	78	78	74	75	69	73	55	62	68	71	66	69	64	68	71	75
3 years	66	66	61	62	53	57	47	55	30	44	47	55	45	52	46	54	49	57
5 years	62	63	51	53	46	51	38	50	20	40	38	50	38	50	37	49	36	47
8 years	58	59	47	50	41	50	30	49	14	47	32	51	32	50	..	..	..	..
10 years	58	60	47	51	41	54	28	55	14	71	32	58	31	57	..	..	..	..
Females	(58)		(79)		(169)		(267)		(284)		(857)		(288)		(236)		(333)	
1 year	79	79	75	75	73	73	70	72	61	66	69	71	67	70	69	71	70	72
3 years	64	64	54	55	52	54	52	56	43	55	50	56	47	52	52	58	51	57
5 years	61	62	46	46	44	46	46	53	27	42	41	49	39	47	41	50	44	54
8 years	58	59	40	41	41	45	38	49	15	34	33	46	32	43	..	..	..	..
10 years	58	59	40	42	39	44	38	55	15	45	32	50	31	47	..	..	..	..
Overall	(116)		(161)		(342)		(492)		(492)		(1603)		(517)		(430)		(656)	
1 year	76	76	76	77	73	74	70	72	59	64	68	71	67	69	67	70	70	73
3 years	65	65	58	58	53	55	50	56	38	51	49	55	46	52	49	56	50	57
5 years	62	62	49	50	45	49	43	52	24	41	40	50	39	48	39	49	40	50
8 years	58	59	43	46	41	47	34	49	15	38	33	48	32	46	..	..	..	..
10 years	58	59	43	47	40	48	33	55	15	53	32	53	31	51	..	..	..	..

RELATIVE SURVIVAL (%) BY AGE AND PERIOD

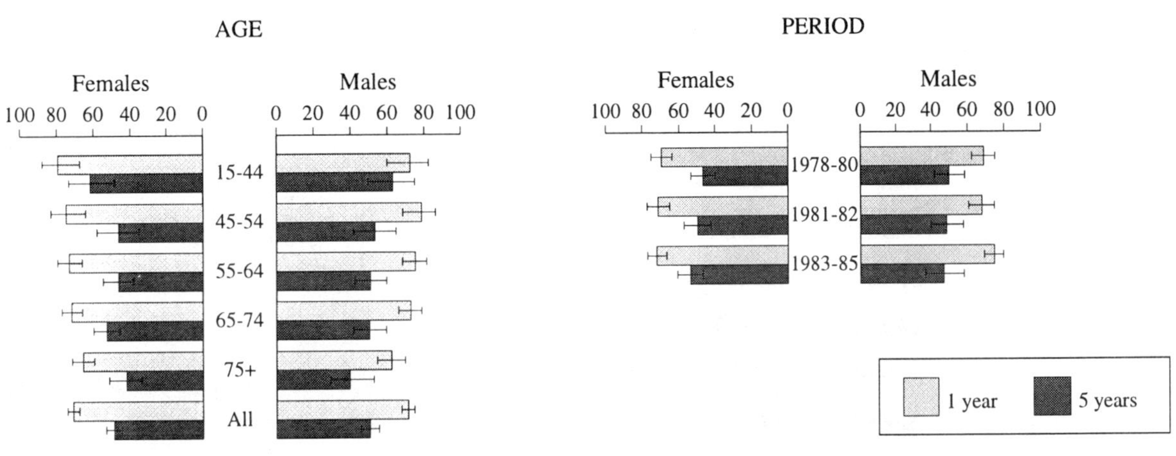

COLON

ENGLISH REGISTRIES

REGISTRY	NUMBER OF CASES			PERIOD OF DIAGNOSIS
	Males	Females	All	
East Anglia	1683	1991	3674	1979-1984
Mersey	1953	2694	4647	1978-1984
South Thames	5326	7607	12933	1978-1984
Wessex	907	1083	1990	1983-1984
West Midlands	3564	4171	7735	1979-1984
Yorkshire	3080	3999	7079	1978-1984
Mean age (years)	68.5	71.6	70.2	

RELATIVE SURVIVAL (%)

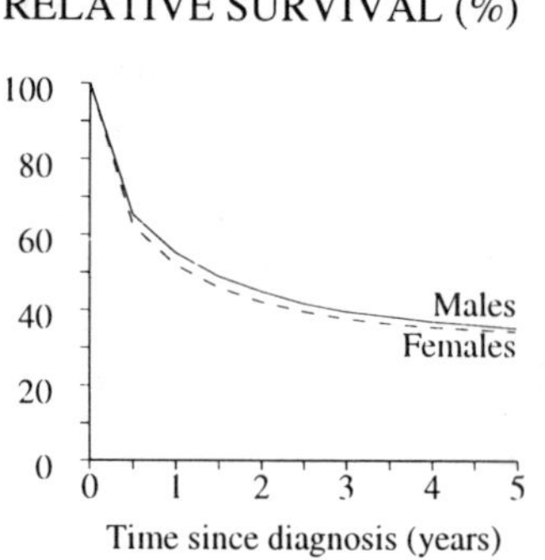

OBSERVED AND RELATIVE SURVIVAL (%) BY AGE AND PERIOD
(Number of cases in parentheses)

	AGE CLASS												PERIOD					
	15-44		45-54		55-64		65-74		75+		All		1978-80		1981-82		1983-85	
	obs	rel	obs	rel	obs	rel	obs	rel	obs	rel	obs	rel	obs	rel	obs	rel	obs	rel
Males	(553)		(1390)		(3335)		(5911)		(5324)		(16513)		(6153)		(4710)		(5650)	
1 year	68	68	65	65	60	61	54	57	39	45	52	55	48	51	53	56	56	59
3 years	48	48	45	46	39	42	35	41	22	33	33	40	30	36	33	40	36	44
5 years	42	43	38	40	31	35	27	36	16	31	26	35	23	32	26	36	28	39
8 years	39	39	33	36	25	31	21	34	10	32	20	33	18	30	20	34	21	35
10 years	38	39	30	34	23	31	17	35	7	34	17	34	16	31	17	33	..	..
Females	(552)		(1374)		(3538)		(6355)		(9726)		(21545)		(8243)		(6308)		(6994)	
1 year	73	73	69	69	64	64	56	57	36	39	49	52	45	48	50	53	53	56
3 years	52	52	47	48	41	42	38	41	22	30	32	38	29	34	33	39	35	42
5 years	46	46	41	42	35	37	31	36	16	29	26	34	23	31	27	35	29	38
8 years	43	43	37	39	30	33	25	34	12	31	21	34	19	30	22	35	24	37
10 years	42	43	36	38	28	33	23	34	9	32	19	35	17	31	19	35	..	..
Overall	(1105)		(2764)		(6873)		(12266)		(15050)		(38058)		(14396)		(11018)		(12644)	
1 year	70	71	67	67	62	63	55	57	37	41	50	53	46	49	51	54	54	57
3 years	50	50	46	47	40	42	36	41	22	31	32	39	29	35	33	39	36	43
5 years	44	44	39	41	33	36	29	36	16	29	26	35	23	31	26	35	28	38
8 years	41	41	35	37	28	32	23	34	11	31	20	34	18	30	21	34	22	36
10 years	40	41	33	36	26	32	20	34	8	33	18	34	16	31	18	34	..	..

RELATIVE SURVIVAL (%) BY AGE AND PERIOD

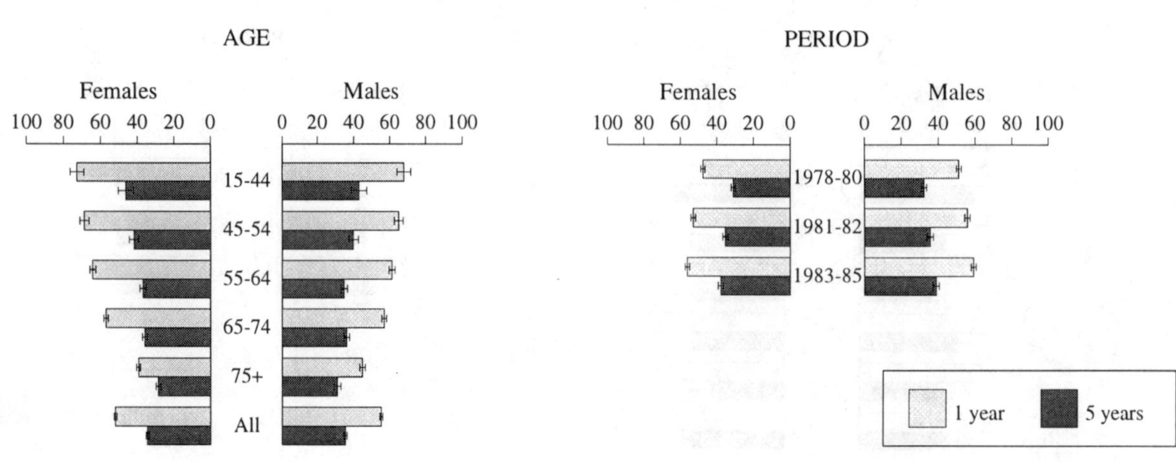

COLON

ESTONIA

REGISTRY	NUMBER OF CASES			PERIOD OF DIAGNOSIS
	Males	Females	All	
Estonia	441	772	1213	1978-1984
Mean age (years)	63.0	65.5	64.6	

RELATIVE SURVIVAL (%)

100
80
60
40
20
0
0 1 2 3 4 5
Males
Females
Time since diagnosis (years)

OBSERVED AND RELATIVE SURVIVAL (%) BY AGE AND PERIOD

(Number of cases in parentheses)

	AGE CLASS												PERIOD					
	15-44		45-54		55-64		65-74		75+		All		1978-80		1981-82		1983-85	
	obs	rel	obs	rel	obs	rel	obs	rel	obs	rel	obs	rel	obs	rel	obs	rel	obs	rel
Males	(39)		(69)		(112)		(134)		(87)		(441)		(168)		(123)		(150)	
1 year	72	72	65	66	59	60	46	48	25	29	50	53	51	53	51	54	49	52
3 years	62	63	58	61	43	47	29	35	10	16	36	42	38	44	33	39	37	44
5 years	56	58	49	53	36	42	24	33	6	12	30	40	32	41	28	37	30	41
8 years	44	47	40	46	34	46	21	38	6	21	26	42	28	42	24	38	..	..
10 years	36	39	36	43	28	41	16	36	..	..	21	39	24	41	..	..	..	..
Females	(44)		(105)		(174)		(254)		(195)		(772)		(325)		(223)		(224)	
1 year	61	61	66	66	57	58	52	53	32	36	50	52	50	52	50	52	51	53
3 years	47	47	48	48	42	43	38	42	17	24	35	40	32	36	39	44	37	42
5 years	42	43	39	40	34	36	32	39	14	25	29	36	26	32	34	42	29	36
8 years	30	31	36	38	32	36	27	40	9	26	25	36	23	33	28	40	..	..
10 years	30	31	36	38	31	36	23	39	4	17	22	35	19	31	..	..	..	..
Overall	(83)		(174)		(286)		(388)		(282)		(1213)		(493)		(346)		(374)	
1 year	66	66	66	66	58	59	49	51	30	34	50	53	50	52	50	52	51	53
3 years	54	55	52	53	42	44	35	40	15	22	36	41	34	38	37	42	37	43
5 years	49	50	43	45	35	39	29	37	11	21	30	38	28	35	32	40	30	38
8 years	37	38	38	41	33	40	25	40	8	25	25	38	24	36	27	39	..	..
10 years	33	35	36	40	29	37	20	38	3	16	22	36	21	34	..	..	..	..

RELATIVE SURVIVAL (%) BY AGE AND PERIOD

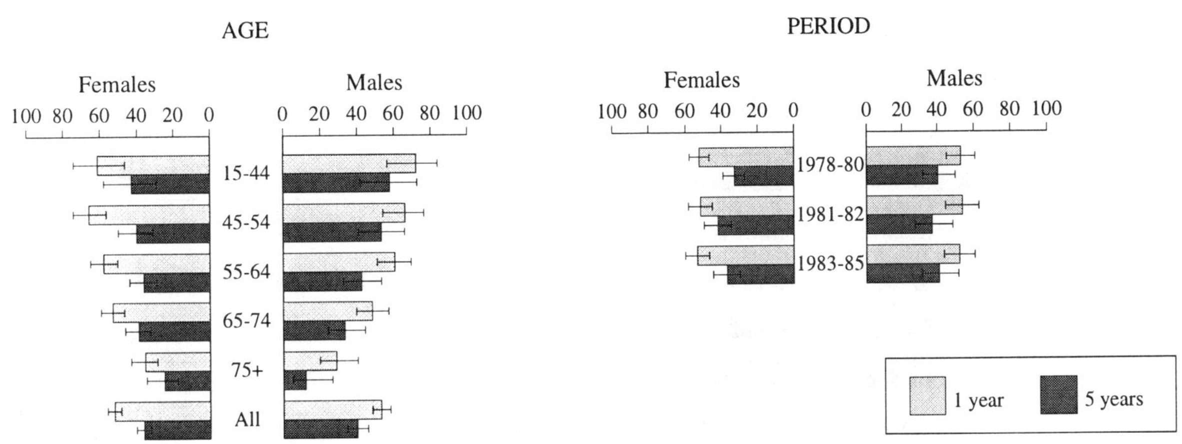

COLON

FINLAND

REGISTRY	NUMBER OF CASES			PERIOD OF DIAGNOSIS
	Males	Females	All	
Finland	1903	2840	4743	1978-1984
Mean age (years)	65.5	68.6	67.4	

RELATIVE SURVIVAL (%)

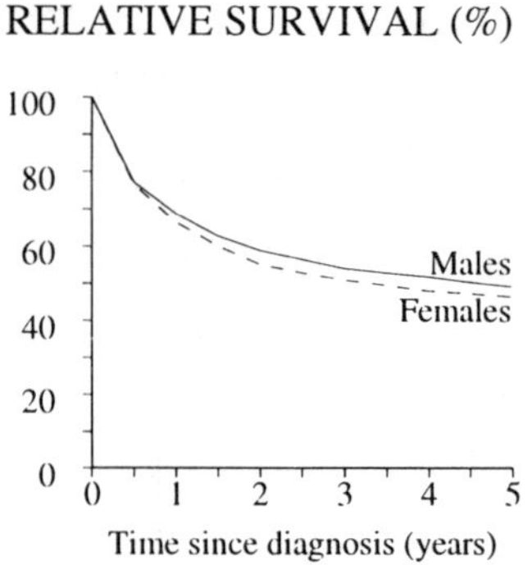

OBSERVED AND RELATIVE SURVIVAL (%) BY AGE AND PERIOD
(Number of cases in parentheses)

	AGE CLASS												PERIOD					
	15-44		45-54		55-64		65-74		75+		All		1978-80		1981-82		1983-85	
	obs	rel	obs	rel	obs	rel	obs	rel	obs	rel	obs	rel	obs	rel	obs	rel	obs	rel
Males	(150)		(189)		(420)		(644)		(500)		(1903)		(704)		(570)		(629)	
1 year	78	78	74	74	73	75	68	71	48	55	65	69	61	65	72	76	64	68
3 years	65	65	56	57	52	56	45	53	32	47	46	54	42	50	52	61	44	53
5 years	59	60	49	51	44	50	34	46	23	46	37	49	35	46	42	56	35	47
8 years	58	59	43	48	37	46	27	45	13	42	29	47	26	42	35	56	28	45
10 years	57	59	41	47	33	45	23	46	8	36	26	46	22	41	30	53	..	..
Females	(209)		(185)		(467)		(905)		(1074)		(2840)		(1109)		(885)		(846)	
1 year	88	88	76	76	71	71	65	67	52	57	64	67	61	64	64	67	66	69
3 years	75	75	59	60	51	53	44	48	33	45	44	51	43	49	44	50	47	54
5 years	72	72	51	52	44	46	36	42	25	42	37	47	35	44	37	46	39	50
8 years	69	69	48	50	38	42	30	40	16	39	30	44	29	42	29	43	31	46
10 years	69	70	47	49	36	41	24	37	11	39	26	43	26	42	22	36	..	..
Overall	(359)		(374)		(887)		(1549)		(1574)		(4743)		(1813)		(1455)		(1475)	
1 year	84	84	75	75	72	73	66	69	51	57	64	67	61	64	67	70	65	68
3 years	71	71	57	59	52	54	45	50	33	45	45	52	43	49	47	54	46	54
5 years	67	67	50	52	44	48	36	44	24	43	37	48	35	45	39	50	37	49
8 years	64	65	46	49	38	44	29	42	15	40	30	45	28	42	32	48	30	45
10 years	64	65	44	48	35	42	24	40	10	38	26	44	24	42	25	42	..	..

RELATIVE SURVIVAL (%) BY AGE AND PERIOD

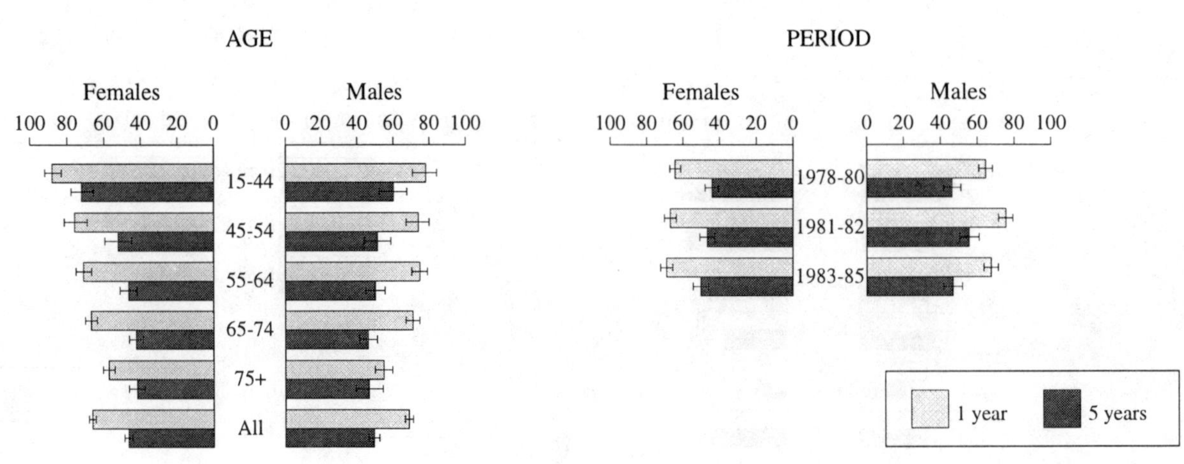

COLON

FRENCH REGISTRIES

REGISTRY	NUMBER OF CASES Males	Females	All	PERIOD OF DIAGNOSIS
Amiens	144	123	267	1983-1984
Calvados	368	426	794	1978-1985
Côte-d'Or	502	535	1037	1978-1985
Doubs	450	436	886	1978-1985
Mean age (years)	68.2	70.4	69.3	

RELATIVE SURVIVAL (%)

Females
Males
Time since diagnosis (years)

OBSERVED AND RELATIVE SURVIVAL (%) BY AGE AND PERIOD
(Number of cases in parentheses)

	AGE CLASS 15-44 obs	rel	45-54 obs	rel	55-64 obs	rel	65-74 obs	rel	75+ obs	rel	All obs	rel	PERIOD 1978-80 obs	rel	1981-82 obs	rel	1983-85 obs	rel
Males	(62)		(135)		(303)		(483)		(481)		(1464)		(462)		(315)		(687)	
1 year	71	71	78	78	71	73	63	66	52	59	63	67	58	62	63	67	66	70
3 years	55	55	54	56	51	54	41	47	33	49	43	51	39	46	44	52	45	53
5 years	43	44	49	51	45	49	32	40	24	46	34	45	31	41	34	45	36	48
8 years	37	38	41	44	36	43	23	35	12	39	24	40	23	36	26	41	22	38
10 years	37	39	37	41	36	45	18	32	9	41	21	39	20	36	25	44	..	..
Females	(53)		(130)		(247)		(434)		(656)		(1520)		(503)		(348)		(669)	
1 year	81	81	72	72	77	78	66	68	47	52	61	64	57	60	59	62	65	68
3 years	59	60	54	55	58	59	48	51	31	42	43	50	42	48	40	47	46	53
5 years	55	55	50	51	48	50	40	45	24	41	36	46	32	41	34	45	40	50
8 years	55	56	44	46	46	49	32	39	18	46	30	45	27	40	28	44	..	..
10 years	55	56	40	42	43	48	29	39	16	59	28	47	25	43	20	34	..	..
Overall	(115)		(265)		(550)		(917)		(1137)		(2984)		(965)		(663)		(1356)	
1 year	76	76	75	75	74	75	65	67	49	55	62	65	58	61	61	64	66	69
3 years	57	57	54	55	54	56	44	49	32	45	43	50	40	47	42	50	45	53
5 years	49	49	49	51	46	50	36	43	24	43	35	46	31	41	34	45	38	49
8 years	45	46	42	45	40	46	27	37	15	43	27	42	25	38	27	43	25	41
10 years	45	47	38	41	39	47	23	36	13	53	24	44	23	40	21	38	..	..

RELATIVE SURVIVAL (%) BY AGE AND PERIOD

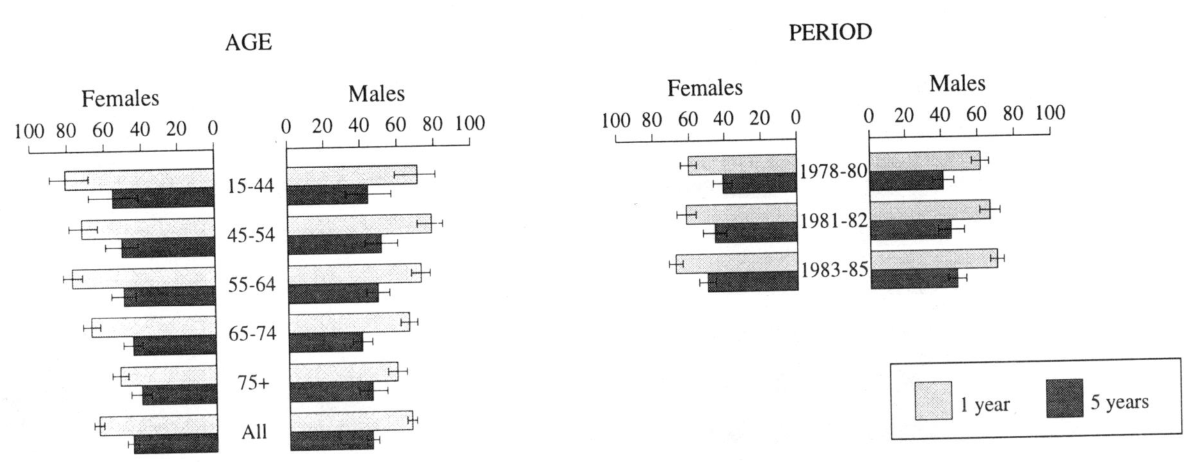

COLON

GERMAN REGISTRIES

REGISTRY	NUMBER OF CASES Males	Females	All	PERIOD OF DIAGNOSIS
Saarland	943	1254	2197	1978-1984
Mean age (years)	66.7	68.9	68.0	

RELATIVE SURVIVAL (%)

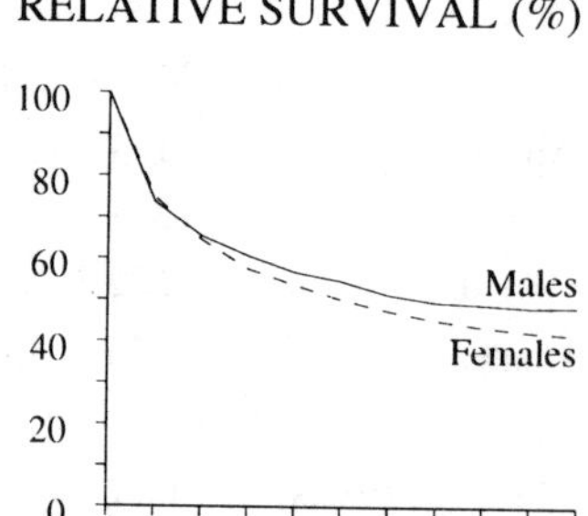

OBSERVED AND RELATIVE SURVIVAL (%) BY AGE AND PERIOD
(Number of cases in parentheses)

	AGE CLASS 15-44 obs	rel	45-54 obs	rel	55-64 obs	rel	65-74 obs	rel	75+ obs	rel	All obs	rel	PERIOD 1978-80 obs	rel	1981-82 obs	rel	1983-85 obs	rel
Males	(37)		(124)		(202)		(318)		(262)		(943)		(368)		(289)		(286)	
1 year	81	81	77	78	73	74	60	63	45	51	62	65	58	61	61	64	67	71
3 years	68	68	63	65	50	53	41	49	27	40	43	51	39	47	42	50	49	59
5 years	62	63	58	61	40	44	35	48	19	39	36	48	32	44	35	48	40	54
8 years	59	61	51	56	33	41	28	50	9	30	28	47	26	43	29	49	..	..
10 years	59	62	49	55	29	38	25	53	8	39	26	49	23	44	..	..	..	..
Females	(41)		(99)		(236)		(444)		(434)		(1254)		(485)		(346)		(423)	
1 year	88	88	73	73	69	69	67	69	48	52	62	64	57	60	66	69	64	66
3 years	66	66	57	57	49	50	45	50	28	37	42	47	38	44	44	50	44	49
5 years	56	57	48	50	44	46	35	42	21	33	33	42	31	39	35	43	36	44
8 years	56	57	44	46	38	42	28	38	16	36	28	40	26	38	27	39	..	..
10 years	56	57	44	47	37	43	25	38	13	38	25	41	24	39	..	..	..	..
Overall	(78)		(223)		(438)		(762)		(696)		(2197)		(853)		(635)		(709)	
1 year	85	85	75	76	71	72	64	67	47	52	62	65	57	60	64	67	65	68
3 years	67	67	60	61	49	51	44	50	28	38	42	49	38	45	43	50	46	53
5 years	59	60	54	56	42	45	35	44	20	35	34	45	31	41	35	45	38	48
8 years	58	59	48	51	36	42	28	42	13	34	28	43	26	40	28	43	..	..
10 years	58	59	47	51	33	41	25	43	11	39	26	44	23	41	..	..	..	..

RELATIVE SURVIVAL (%) BY AGE AND PERIOD

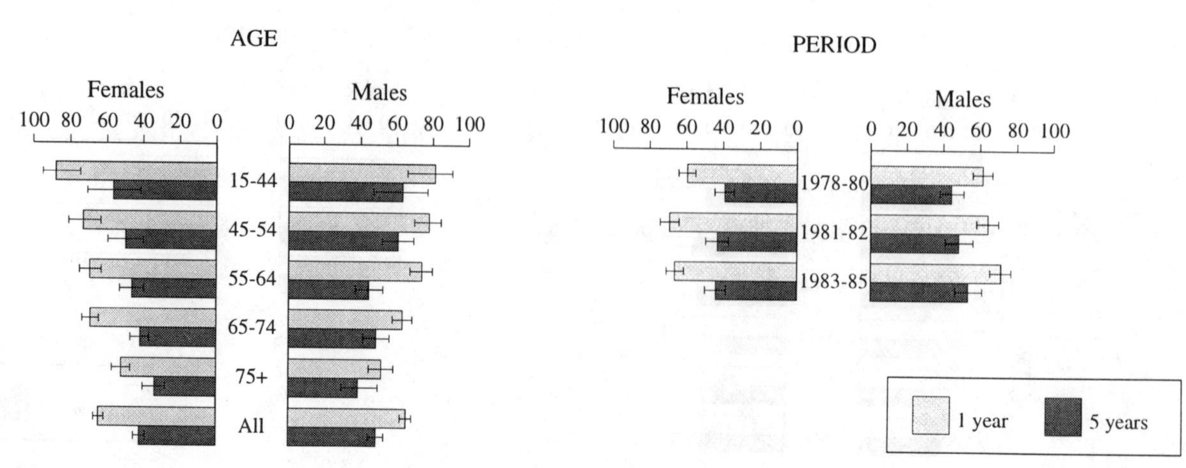

COLON

ITALIAN REGISTRIES

REGISTRY	NUMBER OF CASES			PERIOD OF DIAGNOSIS
	Males	Females	All	
Latina	56	44	100	1983-1984
Modena	33	40	73	1983-1984
Ragusa	96	96	192	1981-1984
Varese	711	792	1503	1978-1984
Mean age (years)	66.7	68.4	67.6	

RELATIVE SURVIVAL (%)

Females
Males
Time since diagnosis (years)

OBSERVED AND RELATIVE SURVIVAL (%) BY AGE AND PERIOD
(Number of cases in parentheses)

	AGE CLASS												PERIOD					
	15-44		45-54		55-64		65-74		75+		All		1978-80		1981-82		1983-85	
	obs	rel	obs	rel	obs	rel	obs	rel	obs	rel	obs	rel	obs	rel	obs	rel	obs	rel
Males	(36)		(104)		(200)		(309)		(247)		(896)		(288)		(242)		(366)	
1 year	83	84	71	72	66	67	56	59	40	46	57	60	54	57	53	56	61	65
3 years	64	64	57	58	50	53	37	43	20	30	39	46	37	44	36	43	42	49
5 years	58	59	51	53	40	45	30	39	14	28	31	42	32	42	31	42	31	41
8 years	58	60	47	51	33	40	21	34	8	25	25	39	23	37	24	40	27	41
10 years	58	60	44	50	31	41	16	31	5	24	22	39	20	36	23	42	..	..
Females	(51)		(94)		(178)		(297)		(352)		(972)		(317)		(294)		(361)	
1 year	69	69	78	78	66	66	64	66	47	51	60	62	56	59	59	62	63	65
3 years	51	51	59	59	49	50	46	50	31	42	43	48	40	45	42	48	46	52
5 years	49	49	51	52	43	45	41	47	23	39	36	45	34	42	35	44	39	48
8 years	44	45	49	50	40	44	36	47	18	44	32	46	29	41	32	46	35	49
10 years	40	41	44	46	38	43	34	48	11	37	28	44	25	39	29	47	..	..
Overall	(87)		(198)		(378)		(606)		(599)		(1868)		(605)		(536)		(727)	
1 year	75	75	74	75	66	67	60	62	44	49	58	61	55	58	56	59	62	65
3 years	56	57	58	59	49	51	41	46	27	37	41	47	39	44	39	46	44	50
5 years	53	53	51	53	42	45	35	43	20	35	34	44	33	42	33	43	35	45
8 years	50	51	48	51	36	42	28	41	14	37	28	43	26	40	28	44	31	45
10 years	48	49	44	48	34	42	25	41	9	33	25	41	23	38	26	45	..	..

RELATIVE SURVIVAL (%) BY AGE AND PERIOD

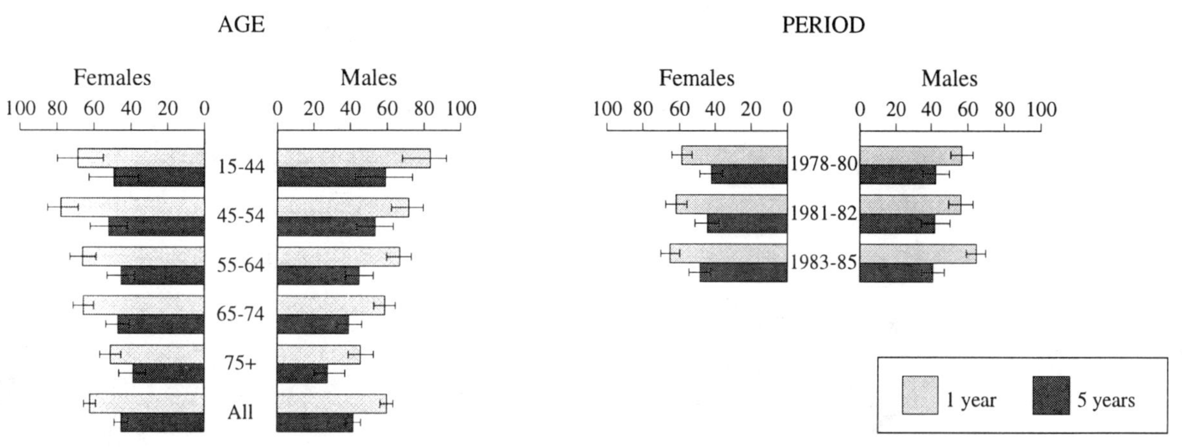

COLON

POLISH REGISTRIES

REGISTRY	NUMBER OF CASES			PERIOD OF DIAGNOSIS
	Males	Females	All	
Cracow	195	246	441	1978-1984
Mean age (years)	63.9	67.1	65.7	

RELATIVE SURVIVAL (%)

100
80
60
40
20
0
Females
Males
0 1 2 3 4 5
Time since diagnosis (years)

OBSERVED AND RELATIVE SURVIVAL (%) BY AGE AND PERIOD
(Number of cases in parentheses)

	AGE CLASS												PERIOD					
	15-44		45-54		55-64		65-74		75+		All		1978-80		1981-82		1983-85	
	obs	rel	obs	rel	obs	rel	obs	rel	obs	rel	obs	rel	obs	rel	obs	rel	obs	rel
Males	(10)		(33)		(49)		(72)		(31)		(195)		(80)		(48)		(67)	
1 year	56	56	45	45	42	43	32	34	26	29	37	38	43	45	34	36	30	32
3 years	42	42	31	32	19	20	21	26	13	19	22	25	26	30	9	11	26	29
5 years	28	28	31	33	11	12	17	23	6	12	16	21	22	28	5	6	18	22
8 years	28	29	23	26	8	11	13	23	0	0	12	18	16	25	5	7	0	0
10 years	28	29	18	22	8	12	13	28	0	0	11	19	15	26	..	..	0	0
Females	(9)		(38)		(42)		(79)		(78)		(246)		(99)		(59)		(88)	
1 year	53	53	54	55	52	53	39	40	21	23	39	40	35	36	43	45	40	41
3 years	53	53	33	33	33	35	27	30	8	11	24	27	17	20	35	39	25	28
5 years	40	40	24	25	29	30	22	27	3	5	19	23	15	19	24	30	19	23
8 years	40	40	16	17	29	32	17	24	..	..	15	22	11	16	19	27	19	26
10 years	..	..	16	17	29	34	12	21	..	..	14	22	8	14	19	30	..	..
Overall	(19)		(71)		(91)		(151)		(109)		(441)		(179)		(107)		(155)	
1 year	54	54	50	50	47	48	36	37	22	24	38	39	39	40	40	41	36	37
3 years	48	48	32	33	26	27	24	28	9	13	23	26	21	24	24	27	25	29
5 years	34	34	27	29	19	21	20	25	4	7	18	22	18	23	16	20	18	23
8 years	34	35	19	20	18	22	15	24	..	..	14	21	13	20	13	19	15	22
10 years	34	35	17	19	18	23	12	23	..	..	12	21	11	19	13	21	..	..

RELATIVE SURVIVAL (%) BY AGE AND PERIOD

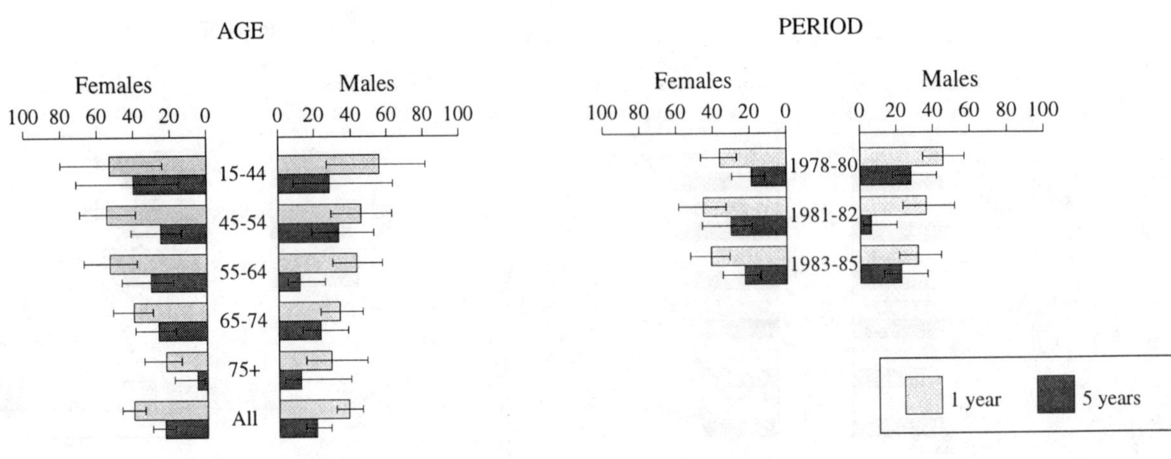

COLON

SCOTLAND

REGISTRY	NUMBER OF CASES			PERIOD OF DIAGNOSIS
	Males	Females	All	
Scotland	3415	4658	8073	1978-1982
Mean age (years)	67.7	70.4	69.3	

RELATIVE SURVIVAL (%)

OBSERVED AND RELATIVE SURVIVAL (%) BY AGE AND PERIOD
(Number of cases in parentheses)

	AGE CLASS												PERIOD					
	15-44		45-54		55-64		65-74		75+		All		1978-80		1981-82		1983-85	
	obs	rel	obs	rel	obs	rel	obs	rel	obs	rel	obs	rel	obs	rel	obs	rel	obs	rel
Males	(121)		(318)		(741)		(1215)		(1020)		(3415)		(2041)		(1374)		(0)	
1 year	69	69	70	71	63	64	52	55	40	45	53	56	53	57	52	56	..	..
3 years	55	55	49	51	44	47	33	39	24	36	35	42	35	42	34	42	..	..
5 years	49	49	43	46	37	43	24	33	17	35	27	38	28	39	26	37	..	..
8 years	46	47	39	43	31	39	16	28	10	36	21	36	21	37	..	..	..	..
10 years	46	47	39	45	28	39	14	30	10	50	19	39	20	40	..	..	..	..
Females	(150)		(321)		(787)		(1483)		(1917)		(4658)		(2795)		(1863)		(0)	
1 year	71	71	70	71	63	64	53	55	37	41	50	53	49	52	51	54	..	..
3 years	53	54	46	47	45	47	36	40	22	31	33	39	32	38	34	40	..	..
5 years	50	50	42	44	37	40	29	34	16	28	27	35	26	34	28	37	..	..
8 years	49	50	39	41	31	36	23	32	12	31	22	35	21	33	..	..	..	..
10 years	49	50	39	42	30	36	20	31	11	39	20	37	20	35	..	..	..	..
Overall	(271)		(639)		(1528)		(2698)		(2937)		(8073)		(4836)		(3237)		(0)	
1 year	70	70	70	71	63	64	53	55	38	42	51	54	51	54	52	55	..	..
3 years	54	54	48	49	44	47	34	39	23	32	34	40	33	40	34	41	..	..
5 years	49	50	43	45	37	41	26	34	16	30	27	36	27	36	27	37	..	..
8 years	48	49	39	42	31	37	20	30	11	33	21	35	21	35	..	..	..	..
10 years	48	49	39	43	29	37	17	30	11	42	20	38	20	37	..	..	..	..

RELATIVE SURVIVAL (%) BY AGE AND PERIOD

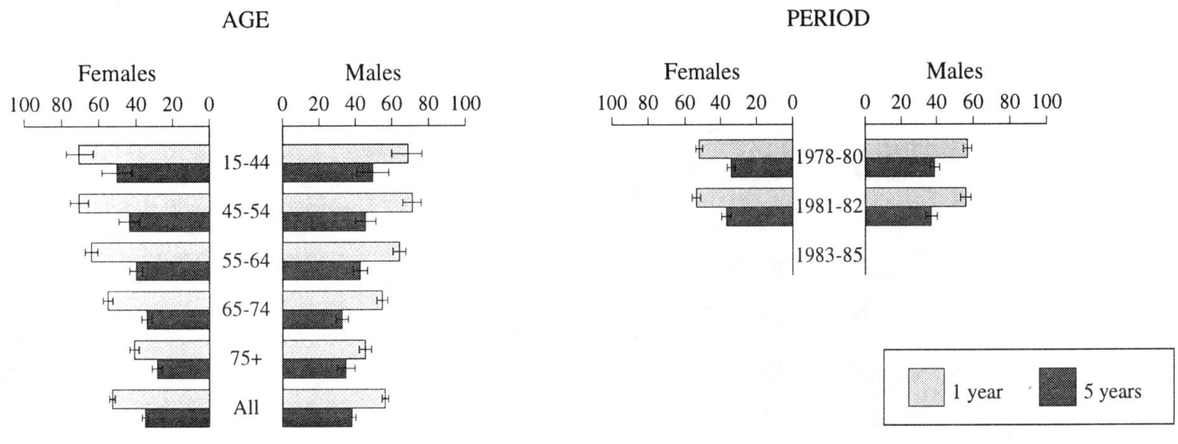

COLON

SPANISH REGISTRIES

REGISTRY	NUMBER OF CASES			PERIOD OF DIAGNOSIS
	Males	Females	All	
Mallorca	120	126	246	1982-1984
Tarragona	40	59	99	1985-1985
Mean age (years)	66.8	67.8	67.3	

RELATIVE SURVIVAL (%)

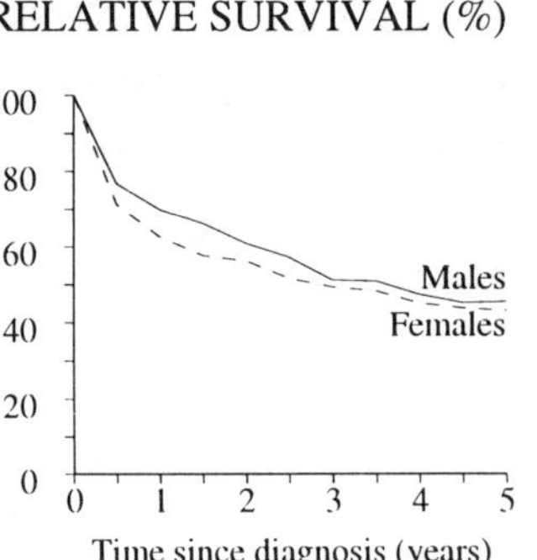

OBSERVED AND RELATIVE SURVIVAL (%) BY AGE AND PERIOD
(Number of cases in parentheses)

	AGE CLASS												PERIOD					
	15-44		45-54		55-64		65-74		75+		All		1978-80		1981-82		1983-85	
	obs	rel	obs	rel	obs	rel	obs	rel	obs	rel	obs	rel	obs	rel	obs	rel	obs	rel
Males	(7)		(20)		(33)		(52)		(48)		(160)		(0)		(35)		(125)	
1 year	100	100	65	65	67	68	65	68	65	71	67	70	..	..	71	75	66	69
3 years	86	86	45	46	45	47	38	43	45	61	45	51	..	..	51	59	43	49
5 years	71	72	45	47	41	46	28	35	32	53	36	46	..	..	45	58	33	42
8 years	71	73	27	29	16	19	25	39	19	48	22	33	..	..	27	42	24	34
10 years	..	..	..	..	..	..	..	..	..	..	..	..	..	..	..	..	..	..
Females	(11)		(17)		(33)		(62)		(62)		(185)		(0)		(41)		(144)	
1 year	55	55	76	77	78	78	59	60	49	53	60	63	..	..	58	60	61	63
3 years	45	46	53	53	62	63	44	47	33	42	44	49	..	..	45	49	44	49
5 years	27	27	47	48	52	54	37	42	25	39	36	43	..	..	37	44	36	43
8 years	27	28	34	35	52	55	32	41	14	30	29	39	..	..	34	46	24	32
10 years	..	..	..	..	..	..	..	..	..	..	..	..	..	..	..	..	..	..
Overall	(18)		(37)		(66)		(114)		(110)		(345)		(0)		(76)		(269)	
1 year	72	72	70	71	72	73	62	64	56	61	63	66	..	..	64	67	63	66
3 years	61	61	49	49	53	55	41	45	38	50	44	50	..	..	48	54	44	49
5 years	44	45	46	47	47	50	33	39	28	45	36	44	..	..	41	50	35	43
8 years	44	45	28	30	27	31	29	39	16	38	26	36	..	..	31	44	22	31
10 years	..	..	..	..	..	..	..	..	..	..	..	..	..	..	..	..	..	..

RELATIVE SURVIVAL (%) BY AGE AND PERIOD

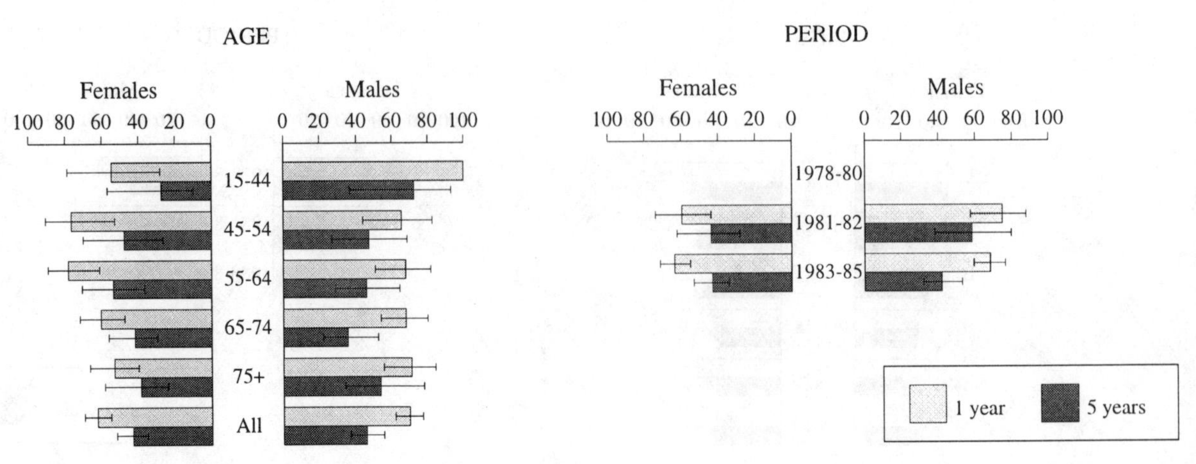

COLON

SWISS REGISTRIES

REGISTRY	NUMBER OF CASES			PERIOD OF DIAGNOSIS
	Males	Females	All	
Basel	231	231	462	1981-1984
Geneva	319	368	687	1978-1984
Mean age (years)	67.9	72.0	70.0	

RELATIVE SURVIVAL (%)

100
80
60
40
20
0
Females
Males
0 1 2 3 4 5
Time since diagnosis (years)

OBSERVED AND RELATIVE SURVIVAL (%) BY AGE AND PERIOD
(Number of cases in parentheses)

	AGE CLASS												PERIOD					
	15-44		45-54		55-64		65-74		75+		All		1978-80		1981-82		1983-85	
	obs	rel	obs	rel	obs	rel	obs	rel	obs	rel	obs	rel	obs	rel	obs	rel	obs	rel
Males	(29)		(52)		(113)		(161)		(195)		(550)		(142)		(200)		(208)	
1 year	67	67	86	87	70	71	73	75	60	66	69	72	70	73	69	72	68	71
3 years	52	53	71	72	52	54	51	58	34	46	47	55	47	54	51	59	44	51
5 years	45	45	58	60	48	53	42	52	25	45	39	51	39	50	40	53	38	50
8 years	45	46	44	46	41	48	30	45	18	49	29	47	..	..	29	47	..	..
10 years	..	..	..	..	..	..	..	..	..	..	..	..	..	..	..	..	..	..
Females	(16)		(34)		(102)		(148)		(299)		(599)		(157)		(203)		(239)	
1 year	87	87	82	82	72	72	68	69	58	63	65	68	65	69	67	71	62	65
3 years	67	67	69	70	62	63	59	62	42	55	52	60	47	55	57	66	50	57
5 years	67	67	63	64	54	56	50	56	35	55	44	57	40	53	46	59	46	58
8 years	67	68	50	52	51	55	46	57	26	60	37	58	..	..	38	59	..	..
10 years	..	..	..	..	..	..	..	..	..	..	..	..	..	..	..	..	..	..
Overall	(45)		(86)		(215)		(309)		(494)		(1149)		(299)		(403)		(447)	
1 year	74	74	85	85	71	71	70	73	59	64	67	70	67	71	68	72	65	68
3 years	57	58	70	71	56	58	55	60	39	52	49	57	47	55	54	63	47	54
5 years	53	53	60	62	51	54	46	54	31	51	42	54	40	51	43	56	42	54
8 years	53	54	47	49	46	52	37	51	23	56	33	52	..	..	34	53	..	..
10 years	..	..	..	..	..	..	..	..	..	..	..	..	..	..	..	..	..	..

RELATIVE SURVIVAL (%) BY AGE AND PERIOD

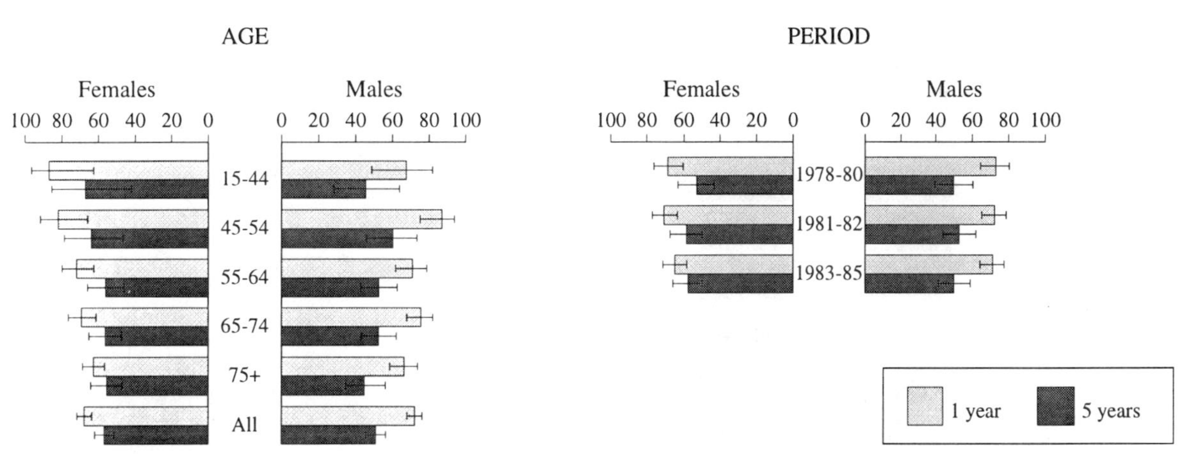

COLON

EUROPEAN REGISTRIES

Weighted analysis

REGISTRY	WEIGHTS (Yearly expected cases in the country) Males	Females	All
DENMARK	754	981	1735
DUTCH REGISTRIES	1891	2392	4283
ENGLISH REGISTRIES	8334	10420	18754
ESTONIA	63	110	173
FINLAND	274	409	683
FRENCH REGISTRIES	8208	8354	16562
GERMAN REGISTRIES	10778	15010	25788
ITALIAN REGISTRIES	6135	6078	12213
POLISH REGISTRIES	1199	1520	2719
SCOTLAND	683	933	1616
SPANISH REGISTRIES	2021	2301	4322
SWISS REGISTRIES	946	992	1938

RELATIVE SURVIVAL (%)
(Age-standardized)

OBSERVED AND RELATIVE SURVIVAL (%) BY AGE AND PERIOD

	AGE CLASS 15-44 obs	15-44 rel	45-54 obs	45-54 rel	55-64 obs	55-64 rel	65-74 obs	65-74 rel	75+ obs	75+ rel	All obs	All rel	PERIOD 1978-80 obs	1978-80 rel	1981-82 obs	1981-82 rel	1983-85 obs	1983-85 rel
Males																		
1 year	76	76	72	73	67	69	59	62	46	52	59	62	55	59	58	62	63	66
3 years	60	60	54	56	47	50	39	46	27	39	40	47	37	44	39	47	43	51
5 years	52	53	49	51	39	43	31	41	19	37	32	43	30	41	32	43	34	45
8 years	49	51	42	46	31	38	24	39	10	33	24	40	23	37	25	41	22	36
10 years	48	50	40	45	29	38	20	39	8	36	22	41	20	38	21	40	..	..
Females																		
1 year	77	77	72	72	69	69	63	64	45	49	58	61	54	57	59	62	61	63
3 years	58	58	53	54	49	51	44	48	28	38	40	46	37	42	41	47	42	48
5 years	51	52	47	48	43	45	36	42	21	34	33	41	30	38	33	42	35	44
8 years	50	50	42	43	39	42	30	39	15	37	27	40	24	37	27	40	27	39
10 years	50	51	40	42	36	41	27	39	12	41	24	41	22	37	22	37	..	..
Overall																		
1 year	77	77	72	73	68	69	61	63	45	50	58	61	55	58	59	62	62	65
3 years	59	59	54	55	48	50	42	47	28	38	40	46	37	43	40	47	43	50
5 years	52	52	48	49	41	44	34	42	20	36	32	42	30	39	33	43	35	45
8 years	50	50	42	44	35	40	27	39	13	35	26	40	24	37	26	40	25	38
10 years	49	51	40	44	33	40	23	39	10	39	23	41	21	38	22	38	..	..

RELATIVE SURVIVAL (%) BY AGE AND PERIOD

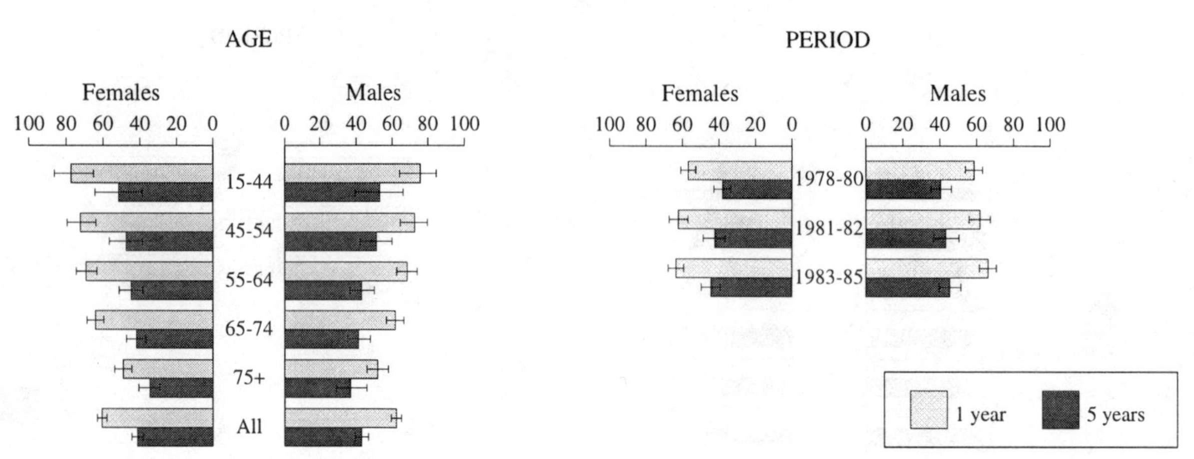

RECTUM

DENMARK

REGISTRY	NUMBER OF CASES			PERIOD OF DIAGNOSIS
	Males	Females	All	
Denmark	5242	4198	9440	1978-1984
Mean age (years)	69.2	69.4	69.3	

RELATIVE SURVIVAL (%)

OBSERVED AND RELATIVE SURVIVAL (%) BY AGE AND PERIOD
(Number of cases in parentheses)

AGE CLASS	15-44		45-54		55-64		65-74		75+	
	obs	rel	obs	rel	obs	rel	obs	rel	obs	rel
Males	(112)		(388)		(1077)		(1934)		(1731)	
1 year	78	78	69	70	75	76	66	69	50	56
3 years	49	49	47	48	48	51	41	47	22	33
5 years	37	38	38	39	36	41	30	39	14	27
8 years	34	34	28	30	28	34	22	35	8	26
10 years	34	35	26	29	25	32	19	36	6	27
Females	(128)		(360)		(807)		(1362)		(1541)	
1 year	77	77	87	87	77	78	68	70	53	58
3 years	59	59	61	62	54	56	47	51	30	39
5 years	53	54	49	50	42	45	36	41	20	32
8 years	49	50	39	41	35	39	26	33	11	27
10 years	49	50	37	40	32	37	21	30	7	23
Overall	(240)		(748)		(1884)		(3296)		(3272)	
1 year	77	77	78	78	76	77	67	69	51	57
3 years	54	54	54	55	50	53	44	49	26	36
5 years	46	46	43	45	39	43	33	40	17	30
8 years	42	42	33	35	31	36	23	34	10	27
10 years	42	43	32	35	28	35	20	33	6	25

	All	
	obs	rel
Males	(5242)	
1 year	63	67
3 years	37	44
5 years	27	37
8 years	19	33
10 years	17	33
Females	(4198)	
1 year	66	69
3 years	44	49
5 years	33	41
8 years	24	35
10 years	21	34
Overall	(9440)	
1 year	64	68
3 years	40	47
5 years	29	39
8 years	21	34
10 years	18	34

PERIOD	1978-80		1981-82		1983-85	
	obs	rel	obs	rel	obs	rel
Males	(2196)		(1533)		(1513)	
1 year	62	65	63	67	64	68
3 years	36	43	38	46	37	44
5 years	26	36	27	37	27	38
8 years	19	33	19	32	..	..
10 years	17	33	..	..	..	..
Females	(1734)		(1209)		(1255)	
1 year	67	70	66	68	66	69
3 years	45	50	42	47	44	50
5 years	34	42	32	39	33	41
8 years	26	37	22	32	..	..
10 years	22	36	..	..	..	..
Overall	(3930)		(2742)		(2768)	
1 year	64	67	64	68	65	69
3 years	40	47	40	46	40	47
5 years	30	39	29	38	30	39
8 years	22	35	20	32	..	..
10 years	19	34	..	..	..	..

RELATIVE SURVIVAL (%) BY AGE AND PERIOD

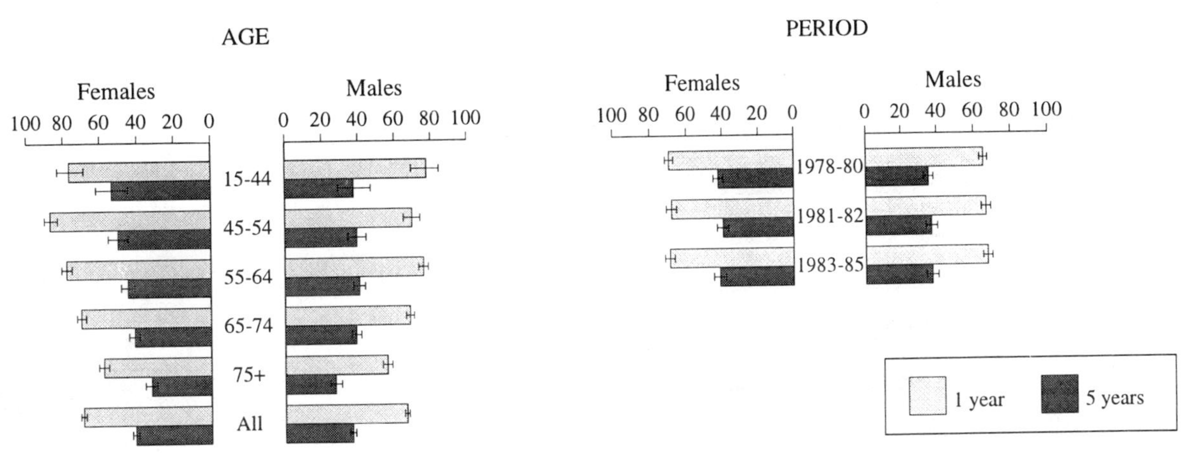

RECTUM

DUTCH REGISTRIES

REGISTRY	NUMBER OF CASES			PERIOD OF DIAGNOSIS
	Males	Females	All	
Eindhoven	544	396	940	1978-1985
Mean age (years)	66.0	67.4	66.6	

RELATIVE SURVIVAL (%)

Females
Males
Time since diagnosis (years)

OBSERVED AND RELATIVE SURVIVAL (%) BY AGE AND PERIOD
(Number of cases in parentheses)

	AGE CLASS												PERIOD					
	15-44		45-54		55-64		65-74		75+		All		1978-80		1981-82		1983-85	
	obs	rel	obs	rel	obs	rel	obs	rel	obs	rel	obs	rel	obs	rel	obs	rel	obs	rel
Males	(30)		(56)		(126)		(212)		(120)		(544)		(188)		(120)		(236)	
1 year	80	80	71	72	79	81	67	70	60	67	69	73	65	68	68	71	74	78
3 years	50	50	55	56	54	57	46	53	33	48	46	53	37	44	52	60	49	57
5 years	43	43	35	36	38	42	33	43	18	34	31	41	24	32	37	47	35	46
8 years	43	43	29	31	18	22	23	39	9	29	20	32	16	26	..	..	..	..
10 years	..	..	29	32	18	24	19	38	..	..	18	33	15	27	..	..	..	..
Females	(10)		(44)		(104)		(125)		(113)		(396)		(138)		(90)		(168)	
1 year	60	60	80	80	79	79	73	74	65	71	73	75	74	76	73	76	71	74
3 years	60	60	54	55	58	59	51	54	33	43	48	53	54	60	48	52	43	48
5 years	48	48	52	53	46	48	43	50	24	38	40	47	45	53	39	46	38	46
8 years	0	0	52	54	45	48	36	47	18	43	35	47	39	52	..	..	..	..
10 years	0	0	26	27	45	50	26	38	..	..	25	37	28	41	..	..	..	..
Overall	(40)		(100)		(230)		(337)		(233)		(940)		(326)		(210)		(404)	
1 year	75	75	75	75	79	80	69	72	63	69	71	74	69	72	70	73	73	76
3 years	52	53	54	55	56	58	47	54	33	45	47	53	44	51	50	57	47	53
5 years	43	44	43	45	42	45	37	46	21	37	35	44	33	41	38	46	36	46
8 years	29	29	41	43	31	36	28	42	14	38	27	40	26	38	..	..	..	..
10 years	..	..	25	26	31	39	20	36	..	..	20	34	20	33	..	..	..	..

RELATIVE SURVIVAL (%) BY AGE AND PERIOD

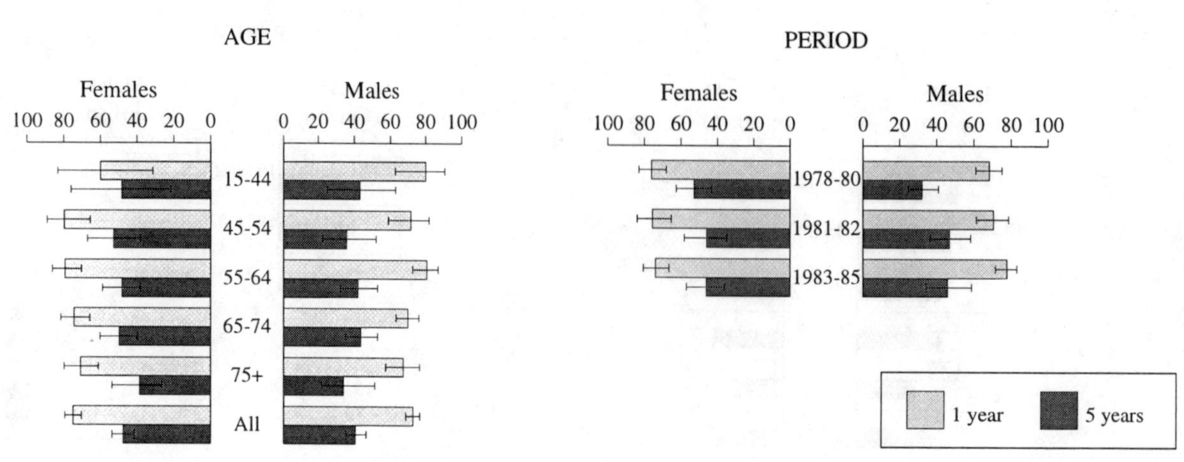

RECTUM

ENGLISH REGISTRIES

REGISTRY	NUMBER OF CASES			PERIOD OF DIAGNOSIS
	Males	Females	All	
East Anglia	1341	1040	2381	1979-1984
Mersey	1731	1529	3260	1978-1984
South Thames	4039	3936	7975	1978-1984
Wessex	520	474	994	1983-1984
West Midlands	3477	2411	5888	1979-1984
Yorkshire	2869	2381	5250	1978-1984
Mean age (years)	68.1	70.8	69.4	

RELATIVE SURVIVAL (%)

OBSERVED AND RELATIVE SURVIVAL (%) BY AGE AND PERIOD
(Number of cases in parentheses)

	AGE CLASS												PERIOD					
	15-44		45-54		55-64		65-74		75+		All		1978-80		1981-82		1983-85	
	obs	rel	obs	rel	obs	rel	obs	rel	obs	rel	obs	rel	obs	rel	obs	rel	obs	rel
Males	(362)		(1192)		(3185)		(5116)		(4122)		(13977)		(5205)		(4048)		(4724)	
1 year	73	73	72	72	71	73	61	64	46	52	60	64	58	61	60	64	63	66
3 years	47	47	45	46	46	49	37	44	25	36	36	44	34	41	37	44	39	46
5 years	36	36	34	36	35	39	27	36	16	33	27	36	24	33	26	36	29	39
8 years	31	32	28	31	27	34	19	32	10	32	19	32	18	30	19	32	21	34
10 years	29	30	26	29	25	33	16	32	7	33	17	32	15	30	16	31	..	..
Females	(284)		(845)		(2132)		(3554)		(4956)		(11771)		(4613)		(3401)		(3757)	
1 year	70	71	77	77	70	71	64	66	42	47	57	60	55	58	56	59	61	64
3 years	48	48	51	52	47	48	41	44	24	32	36	42	33	39	34	40	39	46
5 years	38	39	41	42	38	41	32	38	17	29	28	36	25	34	27	35	31	40
8 years	35	36	36	38	33	37	25	34	11	30	22	34	20	32	21	33	25	38
10 years	34	35	32	34	31	36	23	34	9	33	20	35	18	32	19	33	..	..
Overall	(646)		(2037)		(5317)		(8670)		(9078)		(25748)		(9818)		(7449)		(8481)	
1 year	72	72	74	74	71	72	62	65	44	49	59	62	56	60	58	62	62	65
3 years	47	48	47	48	46	49	39	44	24	34	36	43	34	40	36	42	39	46
5 years	37	37	37	38	36	40	29	37	17	31	27	36	25	34	26	35	30	40
8 years	33	33	32	34	30	35	22	33	11	31	21	33	19	31	20	33	23	36
10 years	31	32	28	31	27	34	19	33	8	33	18	33	17	31	18	32	..	..

RELATIVE SURVIVAL (%) BY AGE AND PERIOD

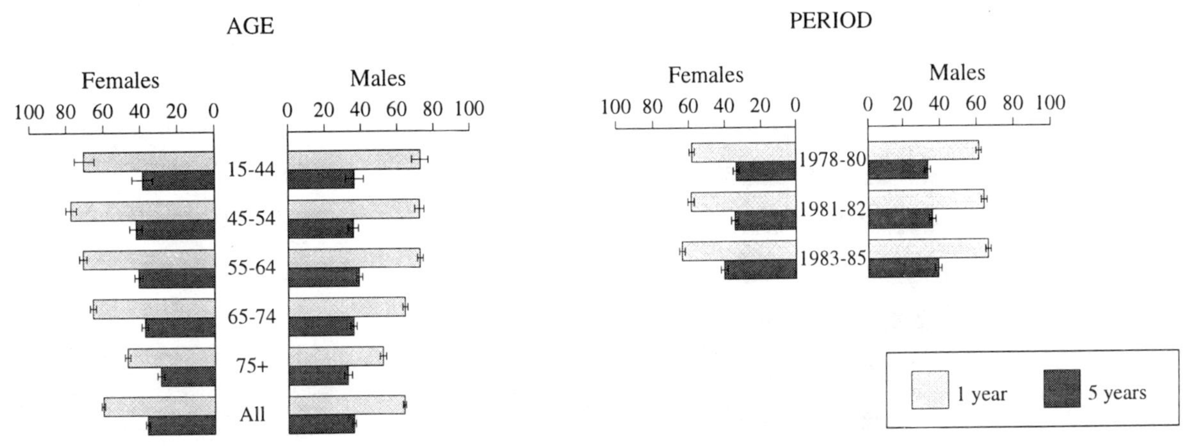

RECTUM

ESTONIA

REGISTRY	NUMBER OF CASES			PERIOD OF DIAGNOSIS
	Males	Females	All	
Estonia	452	719	1171	1978-1984
Mean age (years)	64.6	66.0	65.5	

RELATIVE SURVIVAL (%)

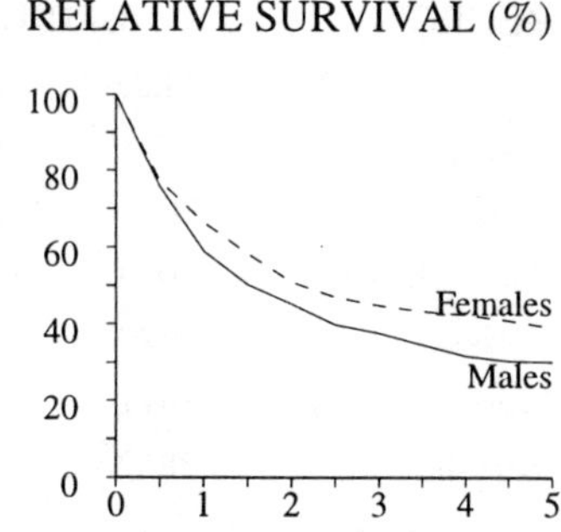

OBSERVED AND RELATIVE SURVIVAL (%) BY AGE AND PERIOD
(Number of cases in parentheses)

	AGE CLASS												PERIOD					
	15-44		45-54		55-64		65-74		75+		All		1978-80		1981-82		1983-85	
	obs	rel	obs	rel	obs	rel	obs	rel	obs	rel	obs	rel	obs	rel	obs	rel	obs	rel
Males	(27)		(65)		(108)		(152)		(100)		(452)		(174)		(133)		(145)	
1 year	63	63	66	67	61	63	54	57	44	50	56	59	60	63	50	53	56	59
3 years	55	56	43	45	35	38	29	35	18	27	32	38	31	37	29	34	36	42
5 years	35	37	31	33	31	36	18	25	12	24	22	30	22	29	20	28	26	34
8 years	35	38	27	31	29	39	14	25	4	14	19	31	17	29	18	31	..	..
10 years	35	39	27	33	27	40	14	31	..	..	18	35	17	32	..	..	..	..
Females	(34)		(95)		(162)		(237)		(191)		(719)		(282)		(220)		(217)	
1 year	82	83	75	75	70	71	65	67	49	54	64	66	69	72	64	66	57	59
3 years	56	56	54	55	55	57	39	44	17	23	40	45	40	45	42	47	38	43
5 years	44	45	47	49	46	48	29	36	12	22	32	39	29	35	37	47	30	37
8 years	40	41	45	47	40	45	22	32	10	27	27	39	23	33	33	48	..	..
10 years	40	41	40	43	37	44	19	33	7	30	24	39	21	33	..	..	..	..
Overall	(61)		(160)		(270)		(389)		(291)		(1171)		(456)		(353)		(362)	
1 year	74	74	71	72	67	68	61	63	47	52	61	63	66	69	59	61	57	59
3 years	55	56	49	51	47	50	35	40	17	24	37	42	36	42	37	42	37	42
5 years	40	41	41	43	40	44	25	32	12	22	28	36	26	33	31	40	28	36
8 years	38	39	38	41	36	43	19	30	8	25	24	36	21	32	27	42	..	..
10 years	38	40	35	39	33	43	17	33	6	28	22	38	19	33	..	..	..	..

RELATIVE SURVIVAL (%) BY AGE AND PERIOD

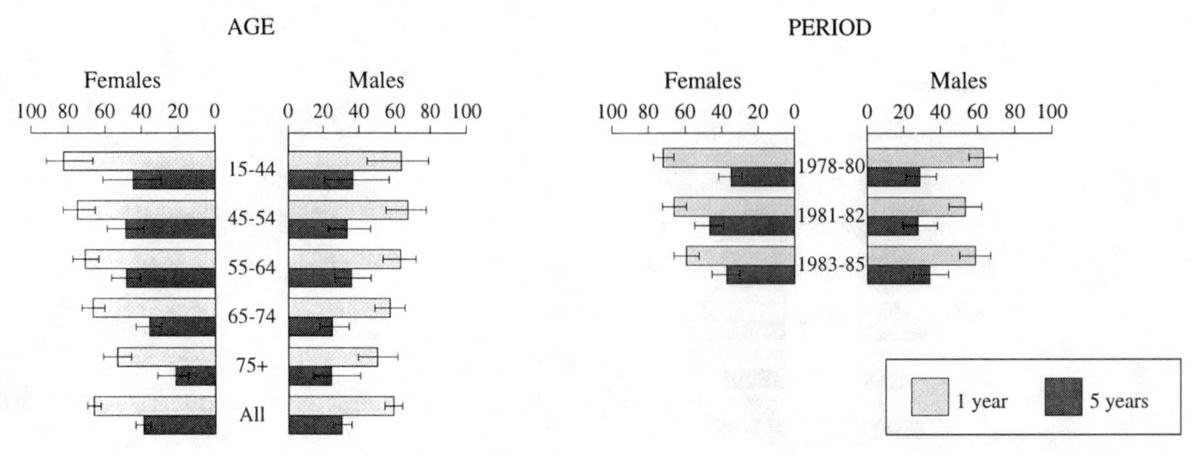

RECTUM

FINLAND

REGISTRY	NUMBER OF CASES			PERIOD OF DIAGNOSIS
	Males	Females	All	
Finland	1908	1952	3860	1978-1984
Mean age (years)	67.3	69.4	68.4	

RELATIVE SURVIVAL (%)

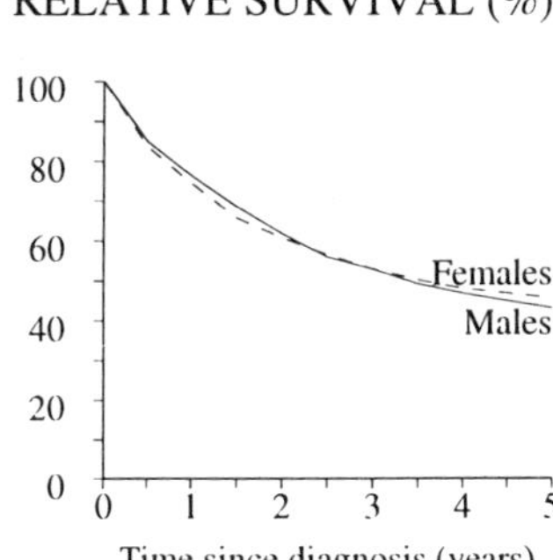

OBSERVED AND RELATIVE SURVIVAL (%) BY AGE AND PERIOD
(Number of cases in parentheses)

	AGE CLASS												PERIOD					
	15-44		45-54		55-64		65-74		75+		All		1978-80		1981-82		1983-85	
	obs	rel	obs	rel	obs	rel	obs	rel	obs	rel	obs	rel	obs	rel	obs	rel	obs	rel
Males	(73)		(166)		(420)		(754)		(495)		(1908)		(808)		(537)		(563)	
1 year	86	87	77	78	81	83	73	76	61	69	72	77	72	77	72	77	72	77
3 years	67	68	53	55	55	59	45	53	28	41	44	53	46	54	42	51	45	53
5 years	56	57	42	44	42	48	32	43	16	32	32	43	33	45	29	40	33	44
8 years	47	49	35	39	34	43	22	37	9	30	23	39	24	39	23	38	23	37
10 years	43	45	33	38	30	40	19	38	6	29	20	38	20	38	21	40	..	..
Females	(76)		(148)		(363)		(626)		(739)		(1952)		(838)		(540)		(574)	
1 year	88	88	81	81	83	84	74	76	60	66	72	75	72	75	72	75	70	73
3 years	72	73	51	52	62	64	49	53	33	44	46	53	49	55	46	53	43	50
5 years	61	61	45	45	53	56	39	46	21	35	36	46	37	46	36	46	34	44
8 years	56	57	39	40	47	52	31	42	12	31	29	43	29	43	29	43	27	41
10 years	56	57	39	41	47	53	27	41	7	23	25	42	26	43	25	42	..	..
Overall	(149)		(314)		(783)		(1380)		(1234)		(3860)		(1646)		(1077)		(1137)	
1 year	87	87	79	79	82	83	73	76	60	67	72	76	72	76	72	76	71	75
3 years	70	70	52	53	58	61	47	53	31	43	45	53	47	55	44	52	44	52
5 years	58	59	43	45	47	52	35	45	19	34	34	44	35	46	33	43	33	44
8 years	52	53	37	39	40	47	26	40	11	31	26	41	27	41	26	41	25	39
10 years	50	51	36	39	38	47	22	39	7	25	23	40	23	41	23	41	..	..

RELATIVE SURVIVAL (%) BY AGE AND PERIOD

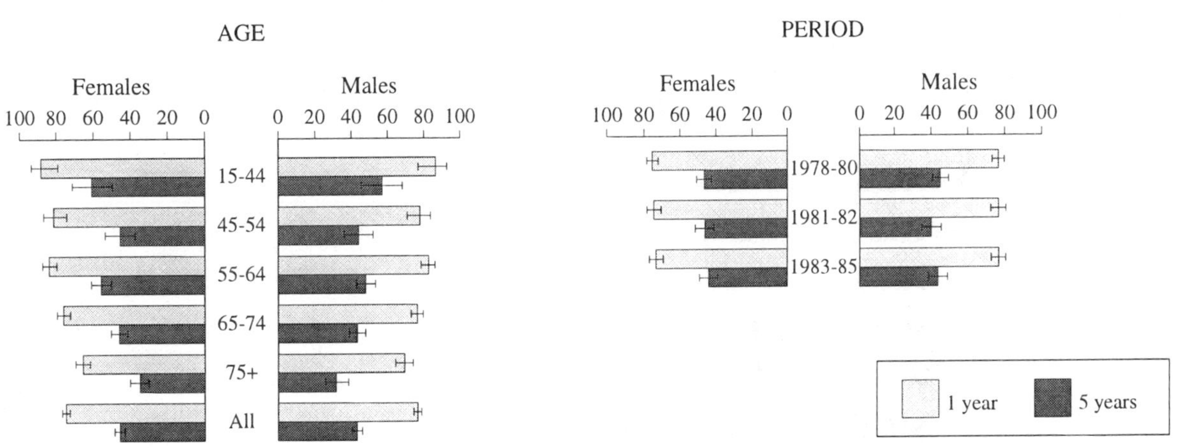

RECTUM

FRENCH REGISTRIES

REGISTRY	NUMBER OF CASES			PERIOD OF DIAGNOSIS
	Males	Females	All	
Amiens	114	96	210	1983-1984
Calvados	391	309	700	1978-1985
Côte-d'Or	432	332	764	1978-1985
Doubs	378	293	671	1978-1985
Mean age (years)	68.1	69.6	68.7	

RELATIVE SURVIVAL (%)

100
80
60
40
20
0
0 1 2 3 4 5
Females
Males
Time since diagnosis (years)

OBSERVED AND RELATIVE SURVIVAL (%) BY AGE AND PERIOD
(Number of cases in parentheses)

	AGE CLASS												PERIOD					
	15-44		45-54		55-64		65-74		75+		All		1978-80		1981-82		1983-85	
	obs	rel	obs	rel	obs	rel	obs	rel	obs	rel	obs	rel	obs	rel	obs	rel	obs	rel
Males	(45)		(106)		(289)		(471)		(404)		(1315)		(454)		(325)		(536)	
1 year	80	80	76	77	71	73	70	73	52	59	66	70	61	65	70	74	67	71
3 years	50	51	53	54	51	53	44	51	24	35	41	48	39	46	41	48	42	49
5 years	48	48	43	45	36	40	32	41	16	30	30	39	28	37	31	41	30	40
8 years	45	46	35	38	28	33	22	35	8	24	21	34	20	33	22	35	..	..
10 years	45	47	29	32	28	35	20	36	6	26	19	35	18	33	22	39	..	..
Females	(42)		(85)		(195)		(287)		(421)		(1030)		(362)		(220)		(448)	
1 year	76	76	83	84	77	77	75	76	60	66	70	73	68	72	73	76	69	72
3 years	52	53	63	64	58	59	51	54	37	49	48	54	45	51	49	56	49	56
5 years	50	50	51	52	47	49	37	42	26	43	36	45	33	41	41	51	36	45
8 years	42	43	43	44	36	38	32	40	16	40	28	40	25	36	32	47	30	44
10 years	42	43	41	43	36	39	27	36	12	42	24	39	22	36	..	..	..	..
Overall	(87)		(191)		(484)		(758)		(825)		(2345)		(816)		(545)		(984)	
1 year	78	78	79	80	74	74	72	74	56	62	68	71	65	68	71	75	68	71
3 years	51	52	57	59	54	56	47	52	31	43	44	51	41	48	44	51	45	53
5 years	49	49	46	48	41	44	34	41	21	37	32	42	30	39	35	45	33	42
8 years	43	44	38	41	31	35	26	37	12	33	24	37	22	34	26	40	24	37
10 years	43	44	34	37	31	37	22	36	9	35	21	37	20	35	19	33	..	..

RELATIVE SURVIVAL (%) BY AGE AND PERIOD

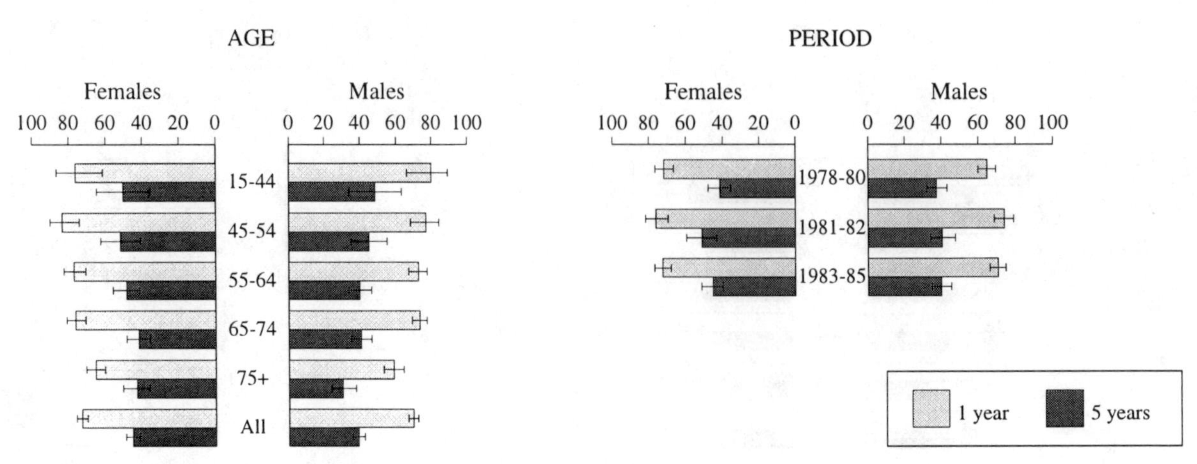

RECTUM

GERMAN REGISTRIES

REGISTRY	NUMBER OF CASES			PERIOD OF DIAGNOSIS
	Males	Females	All	
Saarland	917	883	1800	1978-1984
Mean age (years)	66.5	67.7	67.1	

RELATIVE SURVIVAL (%)

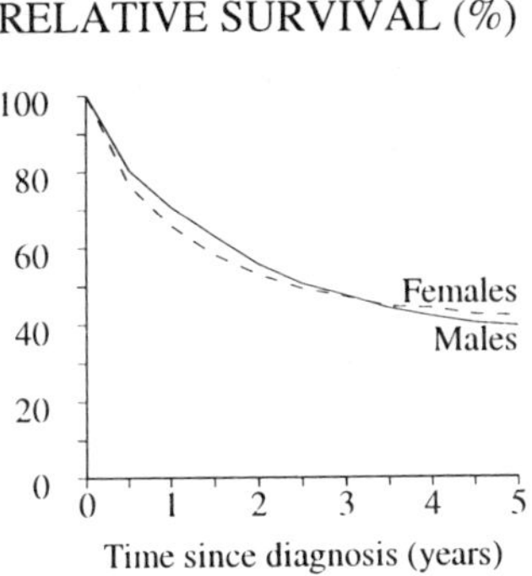

OBSERVED AND RELATIVE SURVIVAL (%) BY AGE AND PERIOD
(Number of cases in parentheses)

	AGE CLASS												PERIOD					
	15-44		45-54		55-64		65-74		75+		All		1978-80		1981-82		1983-85	
	obs	rel	obs	rel	obs	rel	obs	rel	obs	rel	obs	rel	obs	rel	obs	rel	obs	rel
Males	(43)		(114)		(179)		(316)		(265)		(917)		(426)		(289)		(202)	
1 year	77	77	75	75	75	76	69	73	54	61	67	71	67	71	65	69	69	73
3 years	60	61	54	56	44	46	41	49	26	39	40	48	37	45	41	50	43	51
5 years	51	52	41	43	35	39	30	41	16	31	29	40	27	37	30	41	33	43
8 years	45	46	36	40	32	40	21	38	12	38	24	39	23	38	23	38	..	..
10 years	45	47	36	41	30	40	14	31	10	45	20	38	19	36	..	..	..	..
Females	(37)		(94)		(172)		(301)		(279)		(883)		(377)		(272)		(234)	
1 year	86	87	80	80	76	77	64	66	46	50	63	66	62	64	67	69	62	65
3 years	62	62	53	54	51	52	45	49	27	35	42	47	39	44	42	47	46	52
5 years	57	57	49	50	44	46	37	44	18	28	34	42	34	42	33	40	36	45
8 years	53	54	39	41	41	46	28	38	13	29	28	39	27	39	28	38	..	..
10 years	53	54	39	41	36	41	24	37	9	28	24	38	24	38	..	..	..	..
Overall	(80)		(208)		(351)		(617)		(544)		(1800)		(803)		(561)		(436)	
1 year	81	81	77	77	75	77	66	69	50	56	65	68	64	68	66	69	66	69
3 years	61	62	54	55	47	49	43	49	26	37	41	47	38	44	42	48	45	51
5 years	54	54	45	46	39	42	33	43	17	29	32	41	30	39	31	40	35	44
8 years	49	50	38	40	37	43	24	38	13	33	26	39	25	39	25	38	..	..
10 years	49	50	38	41	33	40	19	34	10	34	22	38	21	37	..	..	..	..

RELATIVE SURVIVAL (%) BY AGE AND PERIOD

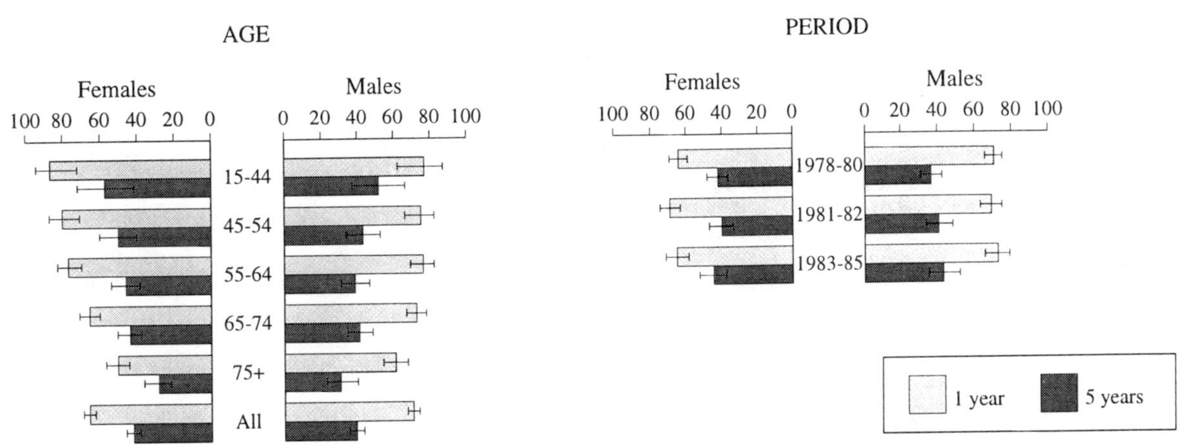

RECTUM

ITALIAN REGISTRIES

REGISTRY	NUMBER OF CASES Males	Females	All	PERIOD OF DIAGNOSIS
Latina	40	37	77	1983-1984
Modena	33	26	59	1984-1984
Ragusa	62	49	111	1981-1984
Varese	488	391	879	1978-1984
Mean age (years)	66.5	67.1	66.8	

RELATIVE SURVIVAL (%)

100 80 60 40 20 0

Females

Males

0 1 2 3 4 5

Time since diagnosis (years)

OBSERVED AND RELATIVE SURVIVAL (%) BY AGE AND PERIOD
(Number of cases in parentheses)

AGE CLASS

	15-44 obs	15-44 rel	45-54 obs	45-54 rel	55-64 obs	55-64 rel	65-74 obs	65-74 rel	75+ obs	75+ rel	All obs	All rel
Males	(29)		(66)		(145)		(221)		(162)		(623)	
1 year	83	83	83	84	72	73	61	64	44	49	62	66
3 years	62	62	56	58	43	46	33	39	21	30	36	43
5 years	52	52	39	41	37	41	22	29	13	25	26	35
8 years	41	42	33	36	33	40	15	26	7	21	21	33
10 years	41	43	33	37	31	40	15	29	7	31	20	35
Females	(28)		(64)		(86)		(175)		(150)		(503)	
1 year	79	79	83	83	74	75	65	66	59	64	68	70
3 years	43	43	53	54	47	48	42	46	25	33	39	44
5 years	39	40	45	46	37	39	33	37	15	25	30	36
8 years	39	40	44	45	31	34	27	34	11	27	26	35
10 years	39	40	41	43	21	24	25	35	10	32	23	33
Overall	(57)		(130)		(231)		(396)		(312)		(1126)	
1 year	81	81	83	84	73	74	63	65	51	56	65	68
3 years	53	53	55	56	45	47	37	42	23	31	38	43
5 years	46	46	42	44	37	40	27	33	14	25	28	35
8 years	40	41	38	41	32	38	20	30	9	25	23	34
10 years	40	41	37	40	26	33	19	32	8	32	21	34

PERIOD

	1978-80 obs	1978-80 rel	1981-82 obs	1981-82 rel	1983-85 obs	1983-85 rel
Males	(209)		(185)		(229)	
1 year	58	61	59	62	69	73
3 years	30	36	33	39	45	52
5 years	22	30	23	31	32	42
8 years	17	28	18	30	26	40
10 years	17	30	18	32	..	..
Females	(169)		(130)		(204)	
1 year	62	64	66	68	73	76
3 years	37	41	32	36	46	51
5 years	30	35	25	29	34	42
8 years	26	35	21	28	29	41
10 years	23	34	18	26	..	..
Overall	(378)		(315)		(433)	
1 year	60	63	62	65	71	74
3 years	33	38	33	37	45	52
5 years	26	32	24	30	33	42
8 years	21	31	19	29	28	40
10 years	20	32	18	29	..	..

RELATIVE SURVIVAL (%) BY AGE AND PERIOD

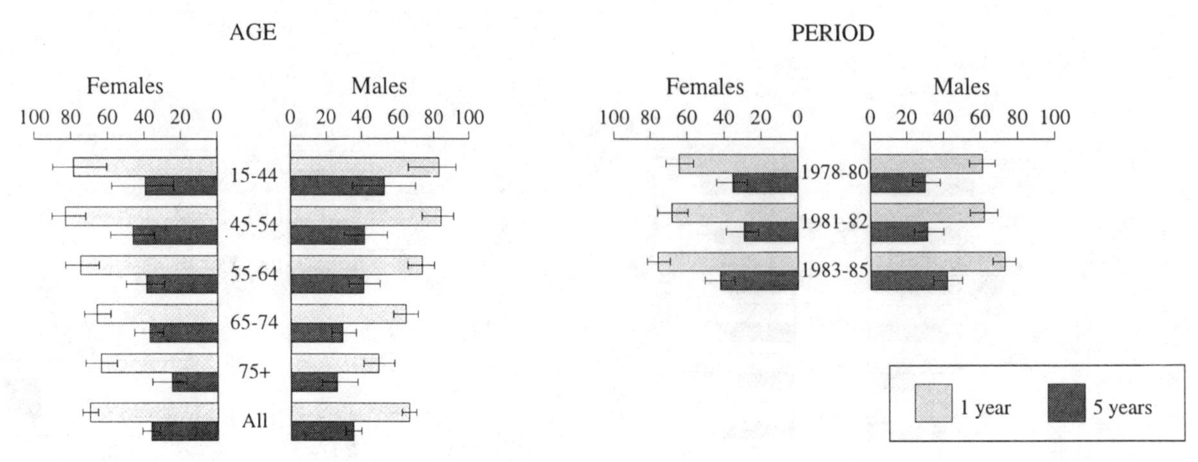

RECTUM

POLISH REGISTRIES

REGISTRY	NUMBER OF CASES			PERIOD OF DIAGNOSIS
	Males	Females	All	
Cracow	215	217	432	1978-1984
Mean age (years)	64.3	65.7	65.0	

RELATIVE SURVIVAL (%)

Females
Males
Time since diagnosis (years)

OBSERVED AND RELATIVE SURVIVAL (%) BY AGE AND PERIOD
(Number of cases in parentheses)

	AGE CLASS												PERIOD					
	15-44		45-54		55-64		65-74		75+		All		1978-80		1981-82		1983-85	
	obs	rel	obs	rel	obs	rel	obs	rel	obs	rel	obs	rel	obs	rel	obs	rel	obs	rel
Males	(15)		(26)		(49)		(83)		(42)		(215)		(102)		(56)		(57)	
1 year	53	54	51	51	48	49	35	37	25	28	39	41	47	49	28	30	36	38
3 years	27	27	34	35	17	18	16	19	7	11	17	20	20	24	9	11	19	23
5 years	20	20	25	27	15	17	8	11	2	5	11	15	11	14	9	13	13	18
8 years	13	14	25	29	9	12	3	6	..	..	8	13	7	11	9	15	10	15
10 years	13	14	20	24	9	13	3	7	..	..	7	13	6	11	9	17	..	..
Females	(12)		(29)		(50)		(65)		(61)		(217)		(87)		(64)		(66)	
1 year	74	74	72	73	55	55	46	47	26	28	47	49	52	54	43	45	44	46
3 years	55	56	38	39	27	28	30	33	15	19	27	31	33	36	21	23	27	31
5 years	46	47	31	32	25	27	19	23	13	21	22	26	26	30	16	19	22	28
8 years	46	47	26	28	22	25	11	16	9	21	17	24	21	28	11	15	..	..
10 years	46	47	9	9	22	26	11	18	6	19	14	21	17	26	9	13	..	..
Overall	(27)		(55)		(99)		(148)		(103)		(432)		(189)		(120)		(123)	
1 year	62	62	63	63	52	52	40	42	26	28	43	45	50	51	36	38	41	43
3 years	39	39	36	37	22	23	22	25	12	16	22	26	26	29	16	18	23	27
5 years	31	31	28	30	20	22	13	17	9	15	17	21	18	22	13	16	18	23
8 years	27	28	26	28	16	19	7	11	6	16	12	18	13	19	10	15	15	22
10 years	27	28	16	18	16	20	7	13	4	15	10	17	11	18	9	14	..	..

RELATIVE SURVIVAL (%) BY AGE AND PERIOD

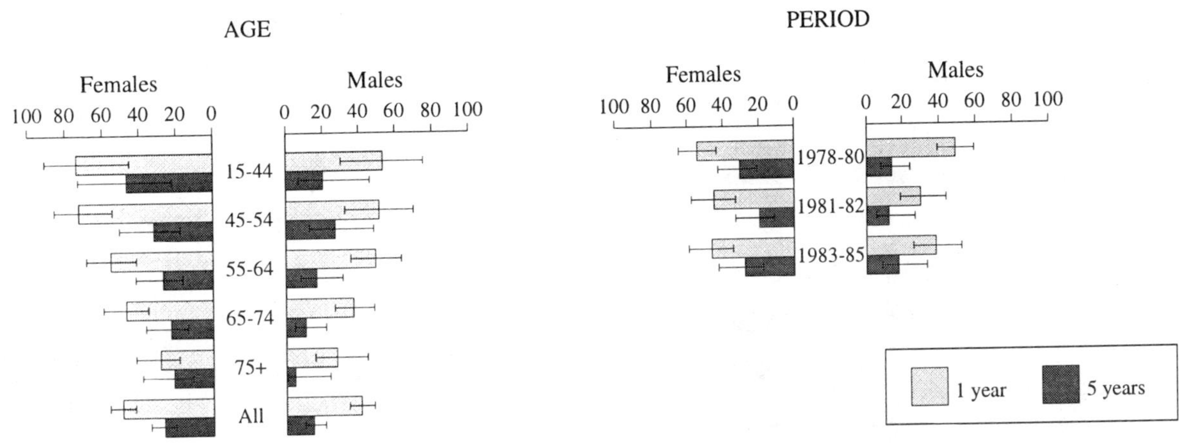

RECTUM

SCOTLAND

REGISTRY	NUMBER OF CASES			PERIOD OF DIAGNOSIS
	Males	Females	All	
Scotland	2223	2036	4259	1978-1982
Mean age (years)	67.7	69.5	68.6	

RELATIVE SURVIVAL (%)

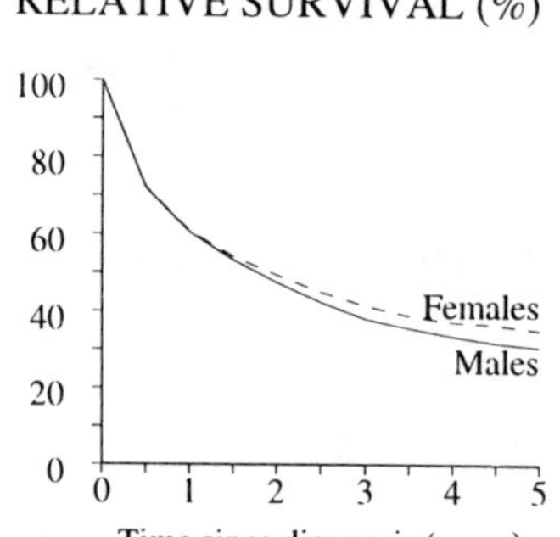

OBSERVED AND RELATIVE SURVIVAL (%) BY AGE AND PERIOD
(Number of cases in parentheses)

	AGE CLASS												PERIOD					
	15-44		45-54		55-64		65-74		75+		All		1978-80		1981-82		1983-85	
	obs	rel	obs	rel	obs	rel	obs	rel	obs	rel	obs	rel	obs	rel	obs	rel	obs	rel
Males	(45)		(205)		(538)		(826)		(609)		(2223)		(1338)		(885)		(0)	
1 year	58	58	73	73	67	69	58	61	41	47	57	60	56	59	58	62	..	..
3 years	47	47	38	39	42	45	31	37	19	30	31	38	30	37	33	40	..	..
5 years	36	36	29	31	32	36	20	28	12	26	22	31	22	30	23	31	..	..
8 years	30	31	25	28	25	32	13	24	6	23	16	27	16	27	..	..	..	..
10 years	30	32	25	29	23	32	7	15	5	28	13	26	13	26	..	..	..	..
Females	(61)		(157)		(426)		(624)		(768)		(2036)		(1256)		(780)		(0)	
1 year	70	71	75	75	72	73	63	64	42	46	58	61	57	60	59	62	..	..
3 years	49	49	53	54	50	52	38	42	21	29	36	41	35	41	36	42	..	..
5 years	38	38	43	44	39	42	30	36	14	24	27	35	28	36	26	33	..	..
8 years	36	36	35	37	34	39	23	31	9	23	21	33	22	34	..	..	..	..
10 years	36	37	33	36	31	37	19	29	6	21	18	32	19	33	..	..	..	..
Overall	(106)		(362)		(964)		(1450)		(1377)		(4259)		(2594)		(1665)		(0)	
1 year	65	65	73	74	69	71	60	62	41	47	57	61	56	60	59	62	..	..
3 years	48	48	44	46	45	48	34	39	20	29	33	40	33	39	35	41	..	..
5 years	37	37	35	37	35	39	25	32	13	25	25	33	25	33	24	32	..	..
8 years	33	34	30	32	29	35	18	28	8	23	19	30	19	31	..	..	..	..
10 years	33	35	29	32	26	34	13	23	6	23	16	29	16	30	..	..	..	..

RELATIVE SURVIVAL (%) BY AGE AND PERIOD

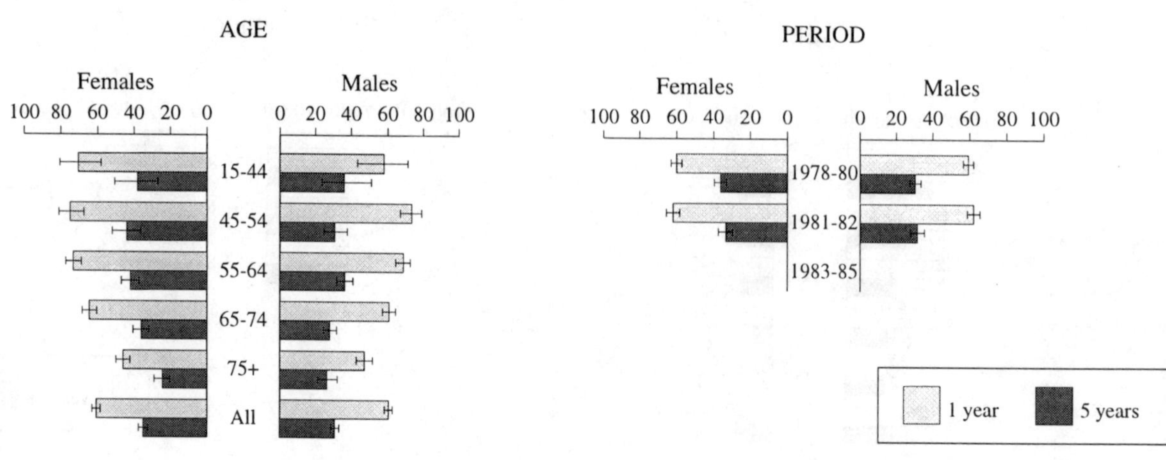

RECTUM

SPANISH REGISTRIES

REGISTRY	NUMBER OF CASES			PERIOD OF DIAGNOSIS
	Males	Females	All	
Mallorca	121	82	203	1982-1984
Tarragona	49	35	84	1985-1985
Mean age (years)	67.8	68.4	68.0	

RELATIVE SURVIVAL (%)

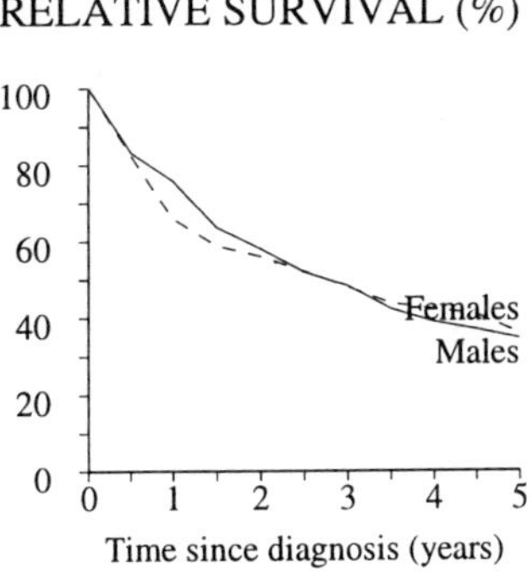

OBSERVED AND RELATIVE SURVIVAL (%) BY AGE AND PERIOD
(Number of cases in parentheses)

	AGE CLASS												PERIOD					
	15-44		45-54		55-64		65-74		75+		All		1978-80		1981-82		1983-85	
	obs	rel	obs	rel	obs	rel	obs	rel	obs	rel	obs	rel	obs	rel	obs	rel	obs	rel
Males	(7)		(16)		(36)		(57)		(54)		(170)		(0)		(36)		(134)	
1 year	86	86	81	81	86	87	70	73	61	68	72	76	..	..	80	85	70	73
3 years	38	38	34	34	46	48	47	54	34	48	41	48	..	..	49	57	39	46
5 years	19	19	34	35	40	43	30	37	13	24	27	35	..	..	33	44	25	32
8 years	..	..	34	36	..	..	14	21	10	28	17	26	..	..	12	19	23	35
10 years	..	..	..	..	..	..	0	0	..	..	0	0	..	..	0	0	..	..
Females	(1)		(9)		(33)		(39)		(35)		(117)		(0)		(27)		(90)	
1 year	100	100	67	67	70	70	56	58	65	70	64	66	..	..	56	57	66	69
3 years	100	100	56	56	57	59	38	40	31	40	44	48	..	..	28	31	48	53
5 years	0	0	56	56	38	40	26	29	21	33	30	36	..	..	15	17	35	41
8 years	0	0	56	57	25	27	18	23	..	..	22	29	..	..	15	19	22	30
10 years	0	0	..	..	..	..	..	..	..	..	..	..	..	..	..	..	..	..
Overall	(8)		(25)		(69)		(96)		(89)		(287)		(0)		(63)		(224)	
1 year	88	88	75	76	78	79	65	67	62	69	69	72	..	..	70	73	68	71
3 years	47	47	42	43	52	53	44	48	33	45	42	48	..	..	40	45	43	49
5 years	16	16	42	43	39	42	28	34	16	27	28	35	..	..	25	32	29	36
8 years	..	..	42	44	27	30	15	21	11	27	19	27	..	..	13	18	22	32
10 years	..	..	..	..	..	..	0	0	..	..	..	..	..	..	..	..	..	..

RELATIVE SURVIVAL (%) BY AGE AND PERIOD

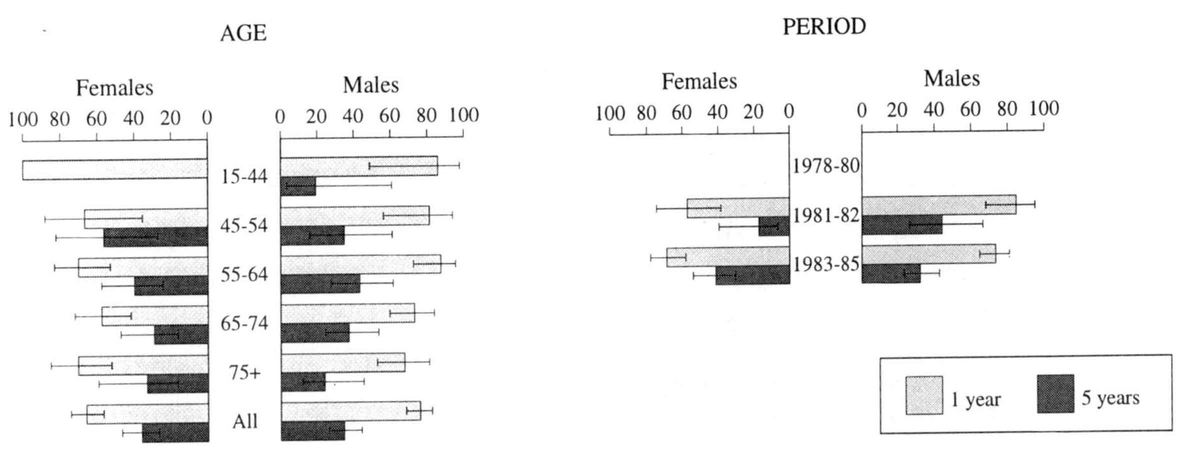

RECTUM

SWISS REGISTRIES

REGISTRY	NUMBER OF CASES			PERIOD OF DIAGNOSIS
	Males	Females	All	
Basel	182	129	311	1981-1984
Geneva	216	226	442	1978-1984
Mean age (years)	68.1	69.0	68.5	

RELATIVE SURVIVAL (%)

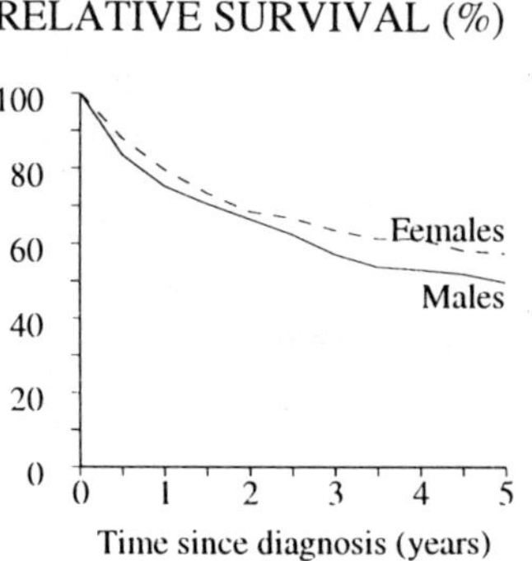

OBSERVED AND RELATIVE SURVIVAL (%) BY AGE AND PERIOD
(Number of cases in parentheses)

	AGE CLASS												PERIOD					
	15-44		45-54		55-64		65-74		75+		All		1978-80		1981-82		1983-85	
	obs	rel	obs	rel	obs	rel	obs	rel	obs	rel	obs	rel	obs	rel	obs	rel	obs	rel
Males	(15)		(40)		(80)		(134)		(129)		(398)		(98)		(145)		(155)	
1 year	93	93	88	88	85	86	75	78	52	58	72	75	69	73	75	78	70	74
3 years	60	60	70	71	64	67	51	58	30	42	49	57	47	54	52	60	48	56
5 years	60	61	51	53	52	57	37	47	24	43	38	50	38	49	39	50	37	50
8 years	60	61	51	55	50	59	22	33	16	48	29	46	..	..	31	48	..	..
10 years	..	..	..	..	..	..	..	..	..	..	..	..	..	..	..	..	..	..
Females	(15)		(41)		(61)		(97)		(141)		(355)		(89)		(131)		(135)	
1 year	87	87	90	91	90	91	80	82	63	69	77	80	70	73	82	86	76	79
3 years	80	80	71	71	72	74	61	64	40	53	56	64	52	59	63	71	53	60
5 years	80	80	59	60	60	63	55	61	28	45	47	57	46	57	52	64	42	51
8 years	55	55	59	60	60	65	49	60	22	51	41	59	..	..	46	65	..	..
10 years	..	..	..	..	..	..	..	..	..	..	..	..	..	..	..	..	..	..
Overall	(30)		(81)		(141)		(231)		(270)		(753)		(187)		(276)		(290)	
1 year	90	90	89	89	87	88	77	80	58	63	74	77	70	73	79	82	72	76
3 years	69	70	70	71	68	70	55	61	35	48	53	60	49	56	57	65	50	58
5 years	69	70	55	57	56	59	45	53	26	44	42	53	42	53	45	57	39	51
8 years	55	56	55	58	55	61	33	45	19	50	34	52	..	..	39	57	..	..
10 years	..	..	..	..	..	..	..	..	..	..	..	..	..	..	..	..	..	..

RELATIVE SURVIVAL (%) BY AGE AND PERIOD

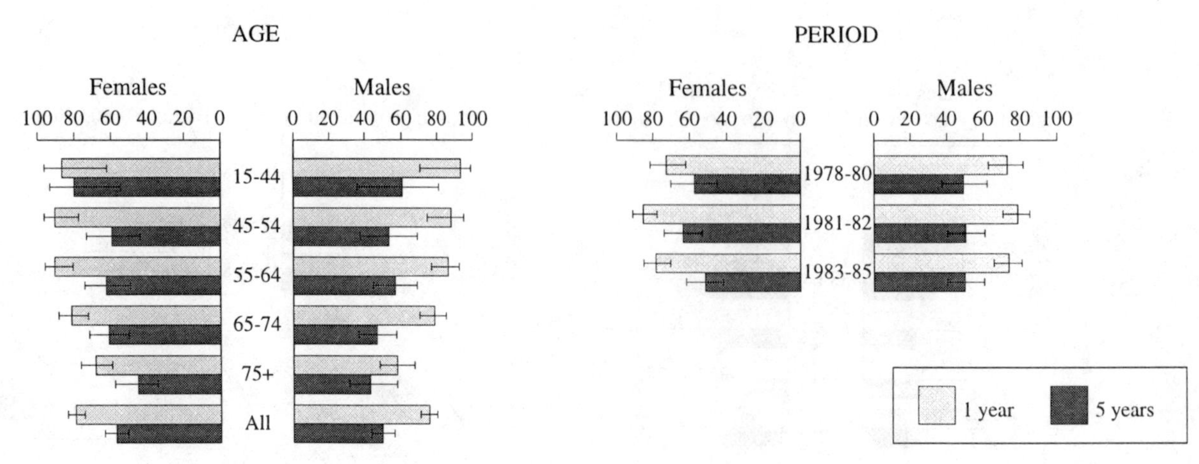

RECTUM

EUROPEAN REGISTRIES

Weighted analysis

REGISTRY	WEIGHTS (Yearly expected cases in the country) Males	Females	All
DENMARK	748	599	1347
DUTCH REGISTRIES	944	743	1687
ENGLISH REGISTRIES	5124	4065	9189
ESTONIA	64	102	166
FINLAND	273	279	552
FRENCH REGISTRIES	3850	2862	6712
GERMAN REGISTRIES	5412	5275	10687
ITALIAN REGISTRIES	3729	3034	6763
POLISH REGISTRIES	1652	1361	3013
SCOTLAND	444	407	851
SPANISH REGISTRIES	1722	1540	3262
SWISS REGISTRIES	660	583	1243

RELATIVE SURVIVAL (%)
(Age-standardized)

Females 100 80 60 40 20 0 — Males 0 20 40 60 80 100

DK, NL, ENG, EST, FIN, F, D, I, PL, SCO, E, CH, EUR

OBSERVED AND RELATIVE SURVIVAL (%) BY AGE AND PERIOD

	AGE CLASS 15-44		45-54		55-64		65-74		75+		All		PERIOD 1978-80		1981-82		1983-85	
	obs	rel	obs	rel	obs	rel	obs	rel	obs	rel	obs	rel	obs	rel	obs	rel	obs	rel
Males																		
1 year	77	77	74	75	72	74	64	67	49	55	63	67	61	64	63	66	65	69
3 years	52	52	49	51	45	47	39	45	24	35	38	45	35	41	38	45	41	48
5 years	42	43	38	40	35	39	27	36	15	28	27	36	25	33	27	37	30	39
8 years	39	40	33	36	28	35	18	30	9	30	20	33	19	31	20	32	21	33
10 years	37	39	30	34	26	34	14	28	7	34	16	31	16	31	16	29	..	..
Females																		
1 year	79	80	79	79	73	74	65	66	51	55	63	66	62	64	64	66	65	67
3 years	58	58	54	55	50	52	44	47	27	36	41	46	39	44	38	43	44	50
5 years	45	45	47	48	41	43	34	39	19	31	32	40	31	39	30	37	34	42
8 years	39	40	41	43	35	39	27	35	13	31	26	37	25	36	24	34	27	39
10 years	39	40	35	37	32	36	23	34	9	31	22	35	22	35	17	28	..	..
Overall																		
1 year	78	78	77	77	73	74	64	67	50	55	63	66	61	64	63	66	65	68
3 years	54	55	52	53	47	49	41	46	26	36	39	45	37	43	38	44	42	49
5 years	43	44	42	43	38	41	30	37	17	29	29	38	28	36	28	37	32	41
8 years	39	40	37	39	32	37	22	33	11	30	23	35	21	33	22	33	24	36
10 years	38	39	32	35	29	35	18	31	8	33	19	33	19	33	16	28	..	..

RELATIVE SURVIVAL (%) BY AGE AND PERIOD

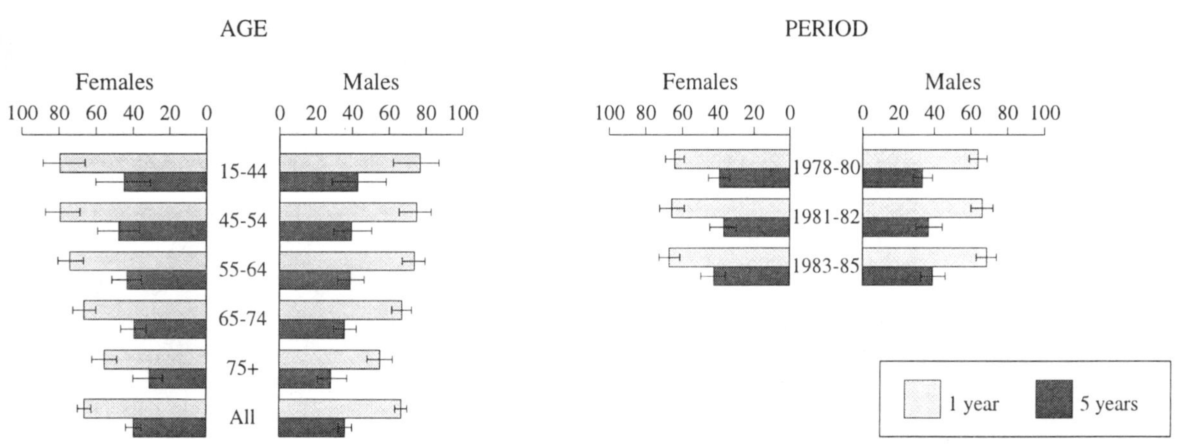

PANCREAS

DENMARK

REGISTRY	NUMBER OF CASES			PERIOD OF DIAGNOSIS
	Males	Females	All	
Denmark	2329	2398	4727	1978-1984
Mean age (years)	68.8	70.9	69.9	

RELATIVE SURVIVAL (%)

OBSERVED AND RELATIVE SURVIVAL (%) BY AGE AND PERIOD
(Number of cases in parentheses)

	AGE CLASS												PERIOD					
	15-44		45-54		55-64		65-74		75+		All		1978-80		1981-82		1983-85	
	obs	rel	obs	rel	obs	rel	obs	rel	obs	rel	obs	rel	obs	rel	obs	rel	obs	rel
Males	(55)		(168)		(490)		(891)		(725)		(2329)		(957)		(674)		(698)	
1 year	15	15	15	15	9	9	10	10	7	8	9	10	9	10	9	9	9	10
3 years	7	7	5	5	2	3	2	3	2	3	3	3	3	3	2	3	3	3
5 years	5	6	5	5	1	2	1	2	2	3	2	2	2	3	2	2	2	2
8 years	5	6	5	5	1	2	1	2	1	2	1	2	2	3	1	2	..	..
10 years	..	..	5	5	1	2	1	1	..	..	1	2	1	3	..	..	..	..
Females	(41)		(141)		(442)		(814)		(960)		(2398)		(980)		(693)		(725)	
1 year	17	17	14	14	14	14	10	10	7	8	10	10	9	9	11	11	10	10
3 years	5	5	4	4	2	2	2	2	2	2	2	2	2	2	2	2	2	2
5 years	5	5	3	3	1	1	1	1	1	1	1	1	1	1	1	1	1	1
8 years	5	5	3	3	..	..	..	..	0	1	1	1	1	1	1	2	..	..
10 years	5	5	2	2	..	..	..	..	..	..	1	1	0	1	..	..	..	..
Overall	(96)		(309)		(932)		(1705)		(1685)		(4727)		(1937)		(1367)		(1423)	
1 year	16	16	15	15	11	11	10	10	7	8	9	10	9	10	10	10	10	10
3 years	6	6	4	4	2	2	2	2	2	2	2	3	2	3	2	3	2	3
5 years	5	5	4	4	1	1	1	1	1	2	1	2	1	2	1	2	1	2
8 years	5	5	4	4	1	1	1	1	1	1	1	2	1	2	1	2	..	..
10 years	5	5	3	3	1	1	0	1	..	..	1	2	1	2	..	..	..	..

RELATIVE SURVIVAL (%) BY AGE AND PERIOD

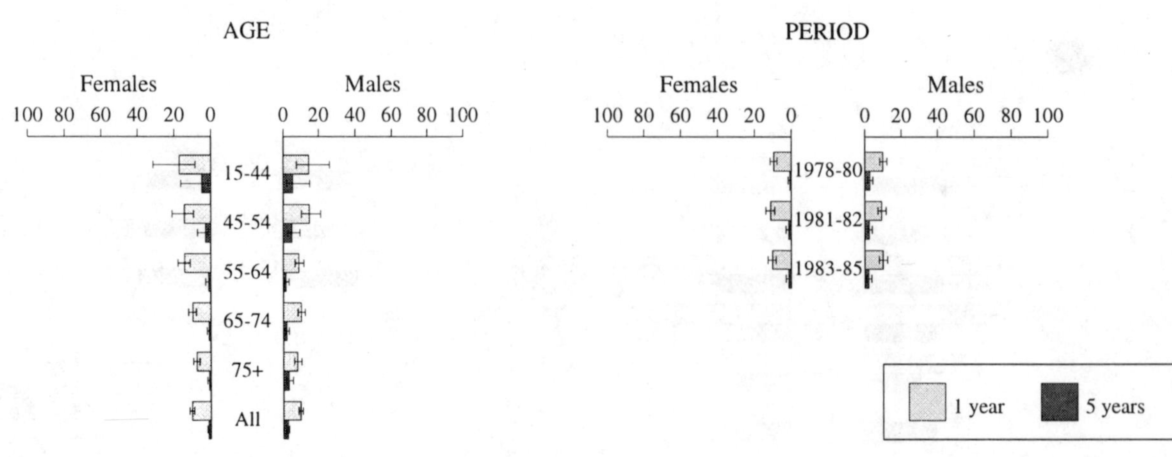

PANCREAS

DUTCH REGISTRIES

REGISTRY	NUMBER OF CASES			PERIOD OF DIAGNOSIS
	Males	Females	All	
Eindhoven	228	197	425	1978-1985
Mean age (years)	65.6	68.8	67.1	

RELATIVE SURVIVAL (%)

— Males
- - Females

Time since diagnosis (years)

OBSERVED AND RELATIVE SURVIVAL (%) BY AGE AND PERIOD

(Number of cases in parentheses)

	AGE CLASS												PERIOD					
	15-44		45-54		55-64		65-74		75+		All		1978-80		1981-82		1983-85	
	obs	rel	obs	rel	obs	rel	obs	rel	obs	rel	obs	rel	obs	rel	obs	rel	obs	rel
Males	(9)		(28)		(62)		(78)		(51)		(228)		(84)		(62)		(82)	
1 year	22	22	25	25	32	33	10	11	12	13	19	20	14	15	23	24	21	22
3 years	0	0	7	7	6	7	1	1	2	3	4	4	2	3	5	6	4	4
5 years	0	0	7	7	6	7	1	2	2	4	4	5	2	3	5	6	4	5
8 years	0	0	..	..	..	..	..	..	0	0	..	..	..	..	..	..	..	..
10 years	0	0	..	..	..	..	..	..	0	0	..	..	..	..	..	..	..	..
Females	(6)		(17)		(37)		(64)		(73)		(197)		(65)		(47)		(85)	
1 year	33	33	6	6	11	11	14	14	10	10	12	12	15	16	13	13	8	9
3 years	33	33	6	6	3	3	2	2	5	7	5	5	8	8	6	7	1	1
5 years	33	34	6	6	3	3	2	2	5	8	5	6	8	9	6	8	1	1
8 years	33	34	..	..	3	3	0	0	5	12	4	6	6	8	..	..	..	..
10 years	..	..	..	..	..	..	0	0	0	0	0	0	0	0	..	..	..	..
Overall	(15)		(45)		(99)		(142)		(124)		(425)		(149)		(109)		(167)	
1 year	27	27	18	18	24	25	12	12	10	11	16	16	15	15	18	19	14	15
3 years	13	13	7	7	5	5	1	2	4	5	4	5	5	5	6	6	2	3
5 years	13	13	7	7	5	5	1	2	4	7	4	5	5	6	6	7	2	3
8 years	13	14	..	..	5	6	..	..	3	7	3	5	3	5	..	..	..	..
10 years	..	..	..	..	..	..	..	..	0	0	0	0	0	0	..	..	..	..

RELATIVE SURVIVAL (%) BY AGE AND PERIOD

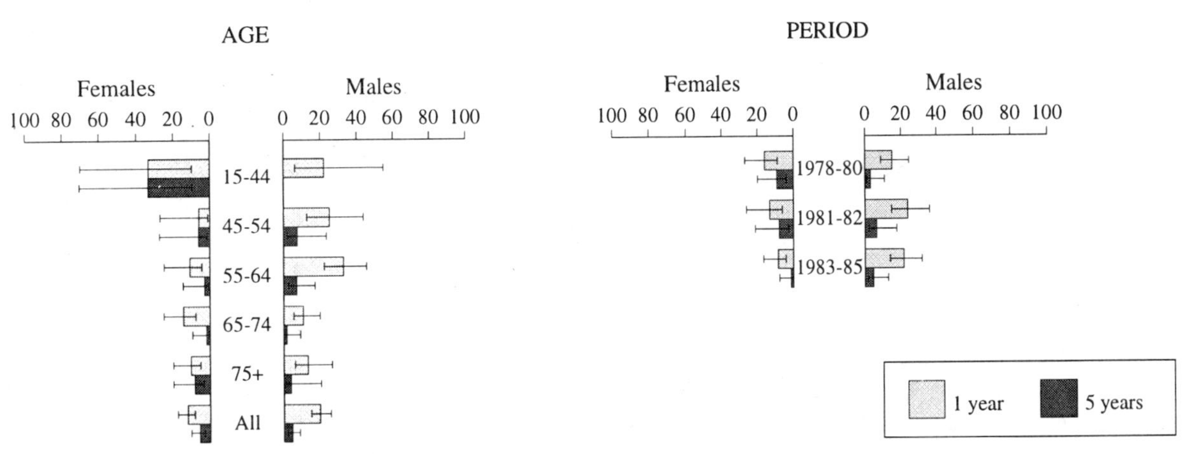

PANCREAS

ENGLISH REGISTRIES

REGISTRY	NUMBER OF CASES			PERIOD OF DIAGNOSIS
	Males	Females	All	
East Anglia	695	678	1373	1979-1984
Mersey	869	839	1708	1978-1984
South Thames	2785	2706	5491	1978-1984
Wessex	273	344	617	1983-1984
West Midlands	1451	1242	2693	1979-1984
Yorkshire	1444	1359	2803	1978-1984
Mean age (years)	68.3	72.4	70.3	

RELATIVE SURVIVAL (%)

100, 80, 60, 40, 20, 0 — Males, - - Females

0 1 2 3 4 5

Time since diagnosis (years)

OBSERVED AND RELATIVE SURVIVAL (%) BY AGE AND PERIOD
(Number of cases in parentheses)

	AGE CLASS												PERIOD					
	15-44		45-54		55-64		65-74		75+		All		1978-80		1981-82		1983-85	
	obs	rel	obs	rel	obs	rel	obs	rel	obs	rel	obs	rel	obs	rel	obs	rel	obs	rel
Males	(181)		(593)		(1753)		(2820)		(2170)		(7517)		(3160)		(2128)		(2229)	
1 year	16	16	15	15	13	14	10	10	7	8	10	11	9	10	10	10	12	13
3 years	6	6	4	4	3	4	2	3	2	2	3	3	2	3	2	3	3	3
5 years	4	4	3	4	3	3	1	2	1	2	2	2	1	2	2	2	2	3
8 years	4	4	3	3	2	2	1	2	1	2	1	2	1	2	1	2	2	3
10 years	4	4	3	3	2	2	1	2	0	2	1	2	1	2	1	3	..	..
Females	(90)		(341)		(1124)		(2295)		(3318)		(7168)		(2947)		(2001)		(2220)	
1 year	21	21	17	17	16	16	12	12	8	9	11	12	10	11	11	12	12	13
3 years	11	11	6	6	4	4	2	3	2	3	3	3	2	3	3	3	3	4
5 years	9	9	4	5	2	2	1	2	1	2	2	2	1	2	2	2	2	3
8 years	6	7	4	4	2	2	1	2	1	3	1	2	1	2	1	2	1	2
10 years	6	7	4	4	2	2	1	1	1	3	1	2	1	2	1	2	..	..
Overall	(271)		(934)		(2877)		(5115)		(5488)		(14685)		(6107)		(4129)		(4449)	
1 year	18	18	16	16	14	15	11	11	8	8	11	11	10	11	10	11	12	13
3 years	7	7	5	5	3	4	2	3	2	3	3	3	2	3	2	3	3	4
5 years	5	6	4	4	2	3	1	2	1	2	2	2	1	2	2	2	2	3
8 years	5	5	3	3	2	2	1	2	1	2	1	2	1	2	1	2	2	3
10 years	5	5	3	3	2	2	1	2	1	3	1	2	1	2	1	2	..	..

RELATIVE SURVIVAL (%) BY AGE AND PERIOD

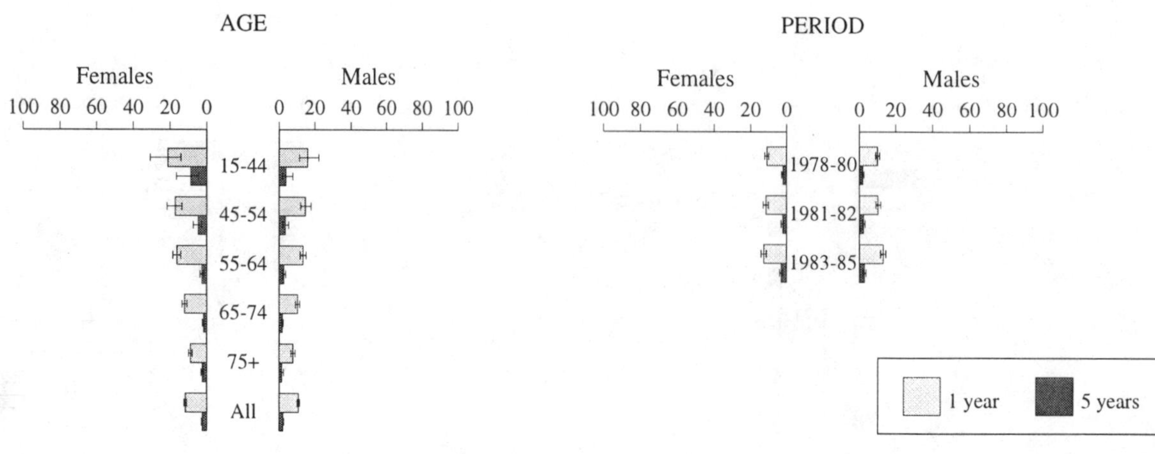

PANCREAS

ESTONIA

REGISTRY	NUMBER OF CASES			PERIOD OF DIAGNOSIS
	Males	Females	All	
Estonia	382	430	812	1978-1984
Mean age (years)	62.6	69.2	66.1	

RELATIVE SURVIVAL (%)

OBSERVED AND RELATIVE SURVIVAL (%) BY AGE AND PERIOD
(Number of cases in parentheses)

	AGE CLASS												PERIOD					
	15-44		45-54		55-64		65-74		75+		All		1978-80		1981-82		1983-85	
	obs	rel	obs	rel	obs	rel	obs	rel	obs	rel	obs	rel	obs	rel	obs	rel	obs	rel
Males	(21)		(67)		(124)		(112)		(58)		(382)		(132)		(117)		(133)	
1 year	0	0	10	11	2	2	11	11	5	6	6	7	6	6	6	6	7	7
3 years	0	0	0	0	1	1	1	1	2	3	1	1	2	2	0	0	1	1
5 years	0	0	0	0	0	0	1	1	2	4	1	1	2	2	0	0	0	0
8 years	0	0	0	0	0	0	0	0	0	0	0	0	0	0	0	0	0	0
10 years	0	0	0	0	0	0	0	0	0	0	0	0	0	0	0	0	0	0
Females	(8)		(37)		(90)		(141)		(154)		(430)		(192)		(111)		(127)	
1 year	17	17	19	19	14	15	10	11	8	9	11	12	10	10	9	9	16	17
3 years	0	0	8	8	3	3	1	1	2	3	3	3	2	2	2	2	4	5
5 years	0	0	5	6	1	1	0	0	1	2	1	2	1	1	0	0	3	3
8 years	0	0	..	..	0	0	0	0	..	..	..	..	0	0	0	0	..	..
10 years	0	0	..	..	0	0	0	0	..	..	..	..	0	0	0	0	..	..
Overall	(29)		(104)		(214)		(253)		(212)		(812)		(324)		(228)		(260)	
1 year	4	4	13	14	7	7	11	11	7	8	9	9	8	9	7	8	11	12
3 years	0	0	3	3	2	2	1	1	2	3	2	2	2	2	1	1	2	3
5 years	0	0	2	2	0	1	1	1	1	2	1	1	1	1	0	0	1	2
8 years	0	0	..	..	0	0	0	0	..	..	0	0	0	0	0	0	..	..
10 years	0	0	..	..	0	0	0	0	..	..	0	0	0	0	0	0	..	..

RELATIVE SURVIVAL (%) BY AGE AND PERIOD

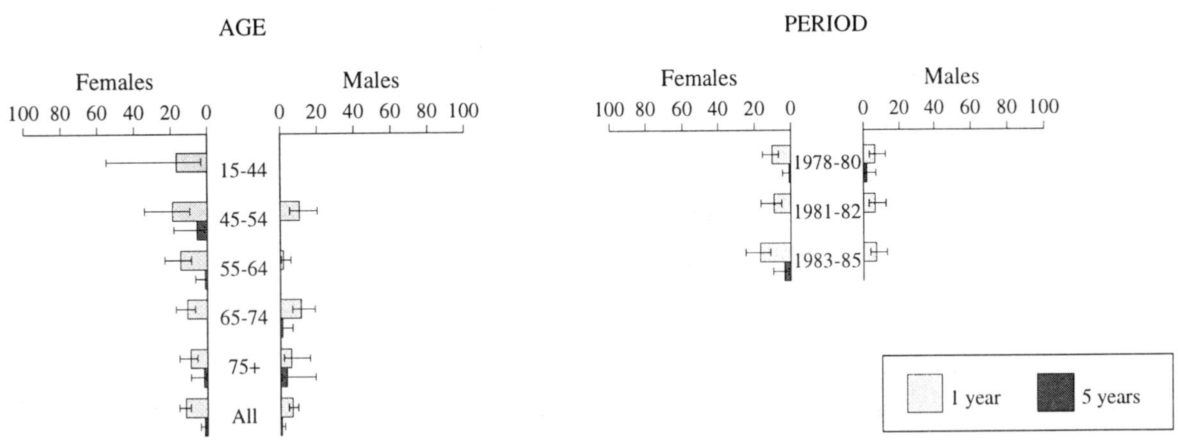

PANCREAS

FINLAND

REGISTRY	NUMBER OF CASES			PERIOD OF DIAGNOSIS
	Males	Females	All	
Finland	1697	1841	3538	1978-1984
Mean age (years)	66.4	70.7	68.7	

RELATIVE SURVIVAL (%)

OBSERVED AND RELATIVE SURVIVAL (%) BY AGE AND PERIOD
(Number of cases in parentheses)

	AGE CLASS											
	15-44		45-54		55-64		65-74		75+		All	
	obs	rel	obs	rel	obs	rel	obs	rel	obs	rel	obs	rel
Males	(57)		(185)		(454)		(610)		(391)		(1697)	
1 year	25	25	15	15	15	16	14	14	14	15	15	15
3 years	14	14	4	4	4	4	2	3	3	5	3	4
5 years	11	11	2	2	2	3	1	2	1	2	2	2
8 years	11	11	2	2	2	2	1	1	1	2	1	2
10 years	11	11	0	0	2	2	0	0	1	2	1	2
Females	(31)		(95)		(345)		(636)		(734)		(1841)	
1 year	23	23	20	20	17	17	14	15	9	10	13	14
3 years	13	13	6	6	3	3	3	3	1	1	3	3
5 years	13	13	3	3	1	2	2	2	0	0	1	2
8 years	13	13	2	2	1	2	1	2	0	0	1	2
10 years	..	..	2	2	1	2	0	1	0	0	1	1
Overall	(88)		(280)		(799)		(1246)		(1125)		(3538)	
1 year	24	24	17	17	16	16	14	14	10	12	14	14
3 years	14	14	5	5	3	4	3	3	2	2	3	4
5 years	11	12	3	3	2	2	1	2	0	1	2	2
8 years	11	12	2	2	2	2	1	2	0	1	1	2
10 years	11	12	1	1	2	2	0	0	0	1	1	1

	PERIOD					
	1978-80		1981-82		1983-85	
	obs	rel	obs	rel	obs	rel
Males	(674)		(468)		(555)	
1 year	13	13	13	14	18	19
3 years	3	3	3	3	5	6
5 years	1	2	1	1	3	4
8 years	1	2	1	1	2	3
10 years	1	1	1	2	..	..
Females	(720)		(554)		(567)	
1 year	13	14	13	14	13	13
3 years	2	3	3	3	3	3
5 years	1	1	1	1	2	3
8 years	1	1	1	1	2	3
10 years	0	1	..	..	..	..
Overall	(1394)		(1022)		(1122)	
1 year	13	14	13	14	15	16
3 years	3	3	3	3	4	5
5 years	1	1	1	1	3	3
8 years	1	2	1	1	2	3
10 years	1	1	1	1	..	..

RELATIVE SURVIVAL (%) BY AGE AND PERIOD

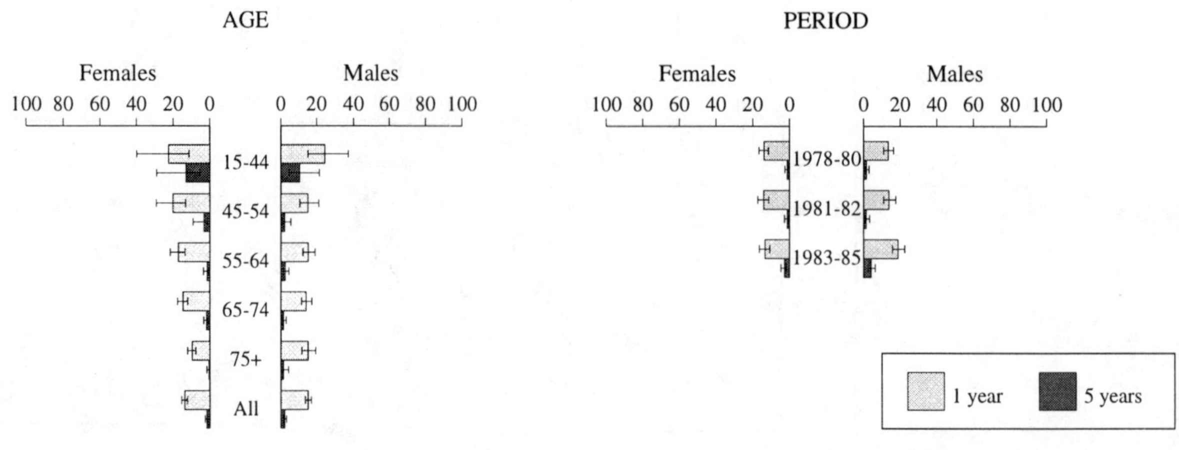

PANCREAS

FRENCH REGISTRIES

REGISTRY	NUMBER OF CASES			PERIOD OF DIAGNOSIS
	Males	Females	All	
Amiens	52	24	76	1983-1984
Calvados	159	118	277	1978-1985
Côte-d'Or	208	151	359	1978-1985
Doubs	102	71	173	1978-1985
Mean age (years)	66.5	71.0	68.3	

RELATIVE SURVIVAL (%)

— Males
- - Females

Time since diagnosis (years)

OBSERVED AND RELATIVE SURVIVAL (%) BY AGE AND PERIOD
(Number of cases in parentheses)

	AGE CLASS												PERIOD					
	15-44		45-54		55-64		65-74		75+		All		1978-80		1981-82		1983-85	
	obs	rel	obs	rel	obs	rel	obs	rel	obs	rel	obs	rel	obs	rel	obs	rel	obs	rel
Males	(21)		(67)		(119)		(162)		(152)		(521)		(199)		(103)		(219)	
1 year	16	16	14	14	14	15	12	12	11	12	12	13	12	12	11	11	14	15
3 years	11	11	0	0	2	2	4	4	2	3	3	3	2	2	2	2	4	4
5 years	11	11	0	0	1	1	4	5	1	3	2	3	1	1	1	1	4	5
8 years	..	..	0	0	1	1	3	4	1	4	2	3	1	2	..	..	3	5
10 years	..	..	0	0	..	..	..	..	0	0	0	0	0	0	..	..	..	..
Females	(10)		(30)		(56)		(113)		(155)		(364)		(135)		(80)		(149)	
1 year	40	40	17	17	25	25	17	17	14	15	18	19	13	13	15	16	23	24
3 years	30	30	10	10	9	9	5	5	4	5	6	7	4	4	4	4	10	11
5 years	30	30	10	10	4	5	3	3	2	4	4	6	3	4	1	2	7	9
8 years	30	30	5	5	4	5	..	..	..	..	3	5	2	2	1	2	7	11
10 years	..	..	..	..	4	5	..	..	..	..	3	6	2	3	..	..	..	..
Overall	(31)		(97)		(175)		(275)		(307)		(885)		(334)		(183)		(368)	
1 year	24	24	15	15	18	18	14	14	12	14	15	15	12	13	13	13	18	19
3 years	17	17	3	3	4	4	4	5	3	4	4	5	2	3	3	3	6	7
5 years	17	17	3	3	2	2	4	4	2	3	3	4	2	2	1	1	5	7
8 years	17	18	2	2	2	2	3	4	1	4	2	4	1	2	1	2	5	7
10 years	..	..	..	..	2	2	..	..	0	0	1	2	1	1	..	..	..	..

RELATIVE SURVIVAL (%) BY AGE AND PERIOD

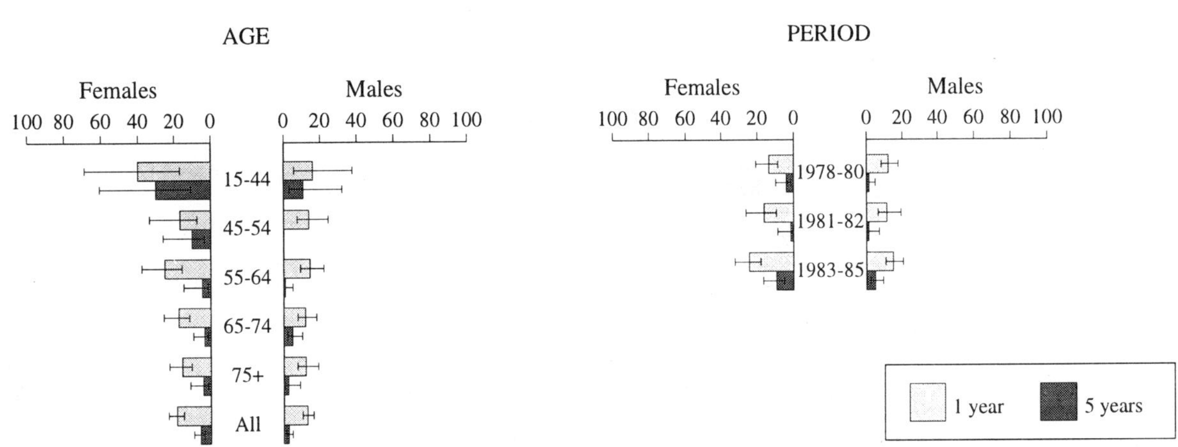

PANCREAS

GERMAN REGISTRIES

REGISTRY	NUMBER OF CASES			PERIOD OF DIAGNOSIS
	Males	Females	All	
Saarland	253	224	477	1978-1984
Mean age (years)	66.1	70.4	68.1	

RELATIVE SURVIVAL (%)

— Males
- - Females

Time since diagnosis (years)

OBSERVED AND RELATIVE SURVIVAL (%) BY AGE AND PERIOD
(Number of cases in parentheses)

	AGE CLASS												PERIOD					
	15-44		45-54		55-64		65-74		75+		All		1978-80		1981-82		1983-85	
	obs	rel	obs	rel	obs	rel	obs	rel	obs	rel	obs	rel	obs	rel	obs	rel	obs	rel
Males	(8)		(34)		(59)		(92)		(60)		(253)		(102)		(81)		(70)	
1 year	50	50	21	21	15	16	9	9	10	11	13	14	14	14	12	13	14	15
3 years	38	38	9	9	5	5	1	1	7	10	6	7	7	8	5	6	4	5
5 years	38	38	6	6	3	4	1	1	5	10	4	6	6	8	2	3	4	6
8 years	38	39	6	6	..	..	1	2	5	17	4	7	6	9	2	4	..	..
10 years	38	39	..	..	..	..	1	2	5	24	4	8	6	11	..	..	..	..
Females	(5)		(11)		(47)		(72)		(89)		(224)		(91)		(66)		(67)	
1 year	40	40	9	9	17	17	7	7	11	12	12	12	10	10	17	17	9	9
3 years	20	20	0	0	4	4	1	2	3	5	3	4	3	4	6	7	0	0
5 years	20	20	0	0	4	4	1	2	3	6	3	4	3	4	6	8	0	0
8 years	20	20	0	0	4	5	..	..	3	8	3	5	3	5	6	9	0	0
10 years	..	..	0	0	0	0	..	..	3	11	2	4	2	4	..	..	0	0
Overall	(13)		(45)		(106)		(164)		(149)		(477)		(193)		(147)		(137)	
1 year	46	46	18	18	16	16	8	8	11	12	13	13	12	13	14	15	12	12
3 years	31	31	7	7	5	5	1	1	5	7	4	5	5	6	5	6	2	3
5 years	31	31	4	5	4	4	1	2	4	7	4	5	5	6	4	5	2	3
8 years	31	32	4	5	4	4	1	2	4	11	4	6	5	7	4	6	..	..
10 years	31	32	..	..	0	0	1	2	4	15	3	6	4	7	..	..	..	..

RELATIVE SURVIVAL (%) BY AGE AND PERIOD

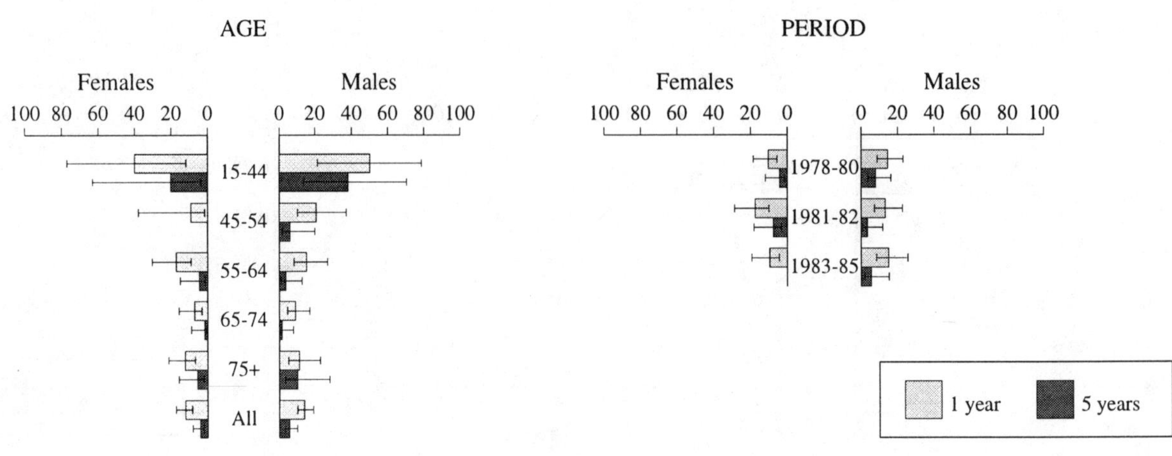

PANCREAS

ITALIAN REGISTRIES

REGISTRY	NUMBER OF CASES			PERIOD OF DIAGNOSIS
	Males	Females	All	
Latina	24	15	39	1983-1984
Ragusa	41	38	79	1981-1984
Varese	245	213	458	1978-1984
Mean age (years)	66.1	69.8	67.8	

RELATIVE SURVIVAL (%)

Males
Females

Time since diagnosis (years)

OBSERVED AND RELATIVE SURVIVAL (%) BY AGE AND PERIOD
(Number of cases in parentheses)

	AGE CLASS												PERIOD					
	15-44		45-54		55-64		65-74		75+		All		1978-80		1981-82		1983-85	
	obs	rel	obs	rel	obs	rel	obs	rel	obs	rel	obs	rel	obs	rel	obs	rel	obs	rel
Males	(12)		(42)		(72)		(115)		(69)		(310)		(108)		(86)		(116)	
1 year	25	25	14	14	13	13	21	22	12	13	16	17	14	15	13	13	21	22
3 years	0	0	0	0	4	4	4	5	4	6	4	4	4	4	2	3	4	5
5 years	0	0	0	0	0	0	1	1	3	6	1	1	1	1	1	1	1	1
8 years	0	0	0	0	0	0	0	0	3	9	1	1	0	0	1	2	1	1
10 years	0	0	0	0	0	0	0	0	..	..	..	..	0	0	..	..	..	..
Females	(8)		(20)		(47)		(99)		(92)		(266)		(93)		(63)		(110)	
1 year	25	25	25	25	26	26	17	18	11	12	17	18	16	17	19	20	17	18
3 years	25	25	20	20	13	13	4	4	4	6	8	9	3	4	6	7	12	14
5 years	25	25	15	15	11	11	4	5	2	4	6	8	3	4	6	8	8	10
8 years	25	25	15	15	11	12	4	5	0	0	5	8	2	3	6	10	7	9
10 years	..	..	15	16	11	12	4	6	0	0	5	8	2	3	6	11	..	..
Overall	(20)		(62)		(119)		(214)		(161)		(576)		(201)		(149)		(226)	
1 year	25	25	18	18	18	18	19	20	11	12	17	17	15	16	15	16	19	20
3 years	10	10	6	7	8	8	4	5	4	6	5	6	3	4	4	5	8	9
5 years	10	10	5	5	4	5	2	3	2	5	3	4	2	3	3	4	4	6
8 years	10	10	5	5	4	5	2	3	1	4	3	4	1	2	3	5	4	5
10 years	..	..	5	5	4	5	2	3	..	..	3	5	1	2	3	6	..	..

RELATIVE SURVIVAL (%) BY AGE AND PERIOD

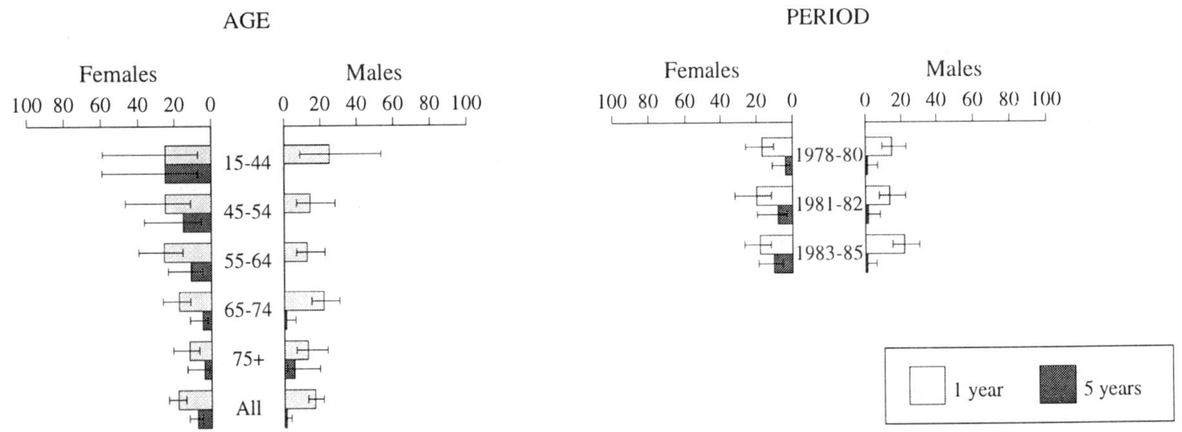

PANCREAS

POLISH REGISTRIES

REGISTRY	NUMBER OF CASES			PERIOD OF DIAGNOSIS
	Males	Females	All	
Cracow	170	184	354	1978-1984
Mean age (years)	62.8	68.3	65.7	

RELATIVE SURVIVAL (%)

— Males
- - Females

Time since diagnosis (years)

OBSERVED AND RELATIVE SURVIVAL (%) BY AGE AND PERIOD
(Number of cases in parentheses)

	AGE CLASS												PERIOD					
	15-44		45-54		55-64		65-74		75+		All		1978-80		1981-82		1983-85	
	obs	rel	obs	rel	obs	rel	obs	rel	obs	rel	obs	rel	obs	rel	obs	rel	obs	rel
Males	(14)		(25)		(45)		(57)		(29)		(170)		(92)		(37)		(41)	
1 year	33	33	36	36	7	7	11	12	7	8	15	15	16	16	19	20	8	8
3 years	24	25	4	4	4	5	7	9	0	0	6	7	7	8	8	9	3	3
5 years	24	25	4	4	4	5	6	8	0	0	5	7	7	9	5	7	3	3
8 years	24	26	4	4	2	3	4	6	0	0	4	6	6	9	5	8	0	0
10 years	24	26	4	5	0	0	4	8	0	0	4	6	4	8	..	..	0	0
Females	(6)		(13)		(39)		(70)		(56)		(184)		(89)		(36)		(59)	
1 year	42	42	23	23	14	14	8	8	8	9	11	12	7	8	11	12	18	19
3 years	42	43	15	16	5	6	2	2	4	5	5	6	7	8	0	0	6	7
5 years	42	43	15	16	3	3	2	2	4	7	5	6	6	8	0	0	6	7
8 years	..	..	15	16	..	..	2	2	4	11	4	6	5	7	0	0	..	..
10 years	..	..	15	16	..	..	2	3	4	15	4	7	5	8	0	0	..	..
Overall	(20)		(38)		(84)		(127)		(85)		(354)		(181)		(73)		(100)	
1 year	36	36	32	32	10	10	9	10	7	8	13	13	12	12	15	16	14	14
3 years	30	30	8	8	5	5	4	5	2	3	6	7	7	8	4	5	5	5
5 years	30	30	8	8	4	4	3	4	2	4	5	6	6	8	3	3	5	6
8 years	24	25	8	9	2	2	3	4	2	7	4	6	5	8	3	4	..	..
10 years	24	25	8	9	0	0	3	5	2	10	4	6	5	8	..	..	..	..

RELATIVE SURVIVAL (%) BY AGE AND PERIOD

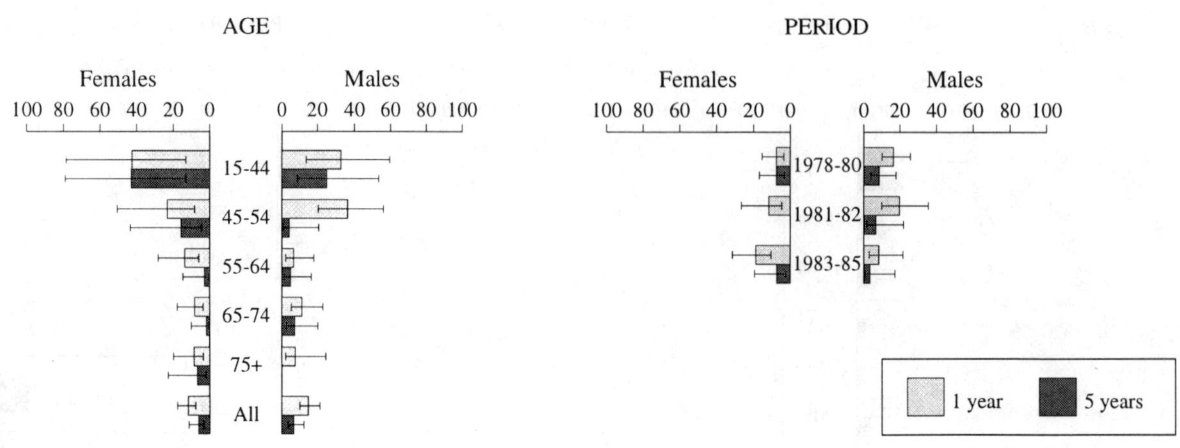

PANCREAS

SCOTLAND

REGISTRY	NUMBER OF CASES			PERIOD OF DIAGNOSIS
	Males	Females	All	
Scotland	1360	1493	2853	1978-1982
Mean age (years)	67.9	71.1	69.6	

RELATIVE SURVIVAL (%)

100
80
60
40
20
0
— Males
- - Females
0 1 2 3 4 5
Time since diagnosis (years)

OBSERVED AND RELATIVE SURVIVAL (%) BY AGE AND PERIOD
(Number of cases in parentheses)

	AGE CLASS												PERIOD					
	15-44		45-54		55-64		65-74		75+		All		1978-80		1981-82		1983-85	
	obs	rel	obs	rel	obs	rel	obs	rel	obs	rel	obs	rel	obs	rel	obs	rel	obs	rel
Males	(34)		(106)		(291)		(553)		(376)		(1360)		(836)		(524)		(0)	
1 year	24	24	11	11	12	12	10	11	13	14	11	12	11	12	11	12	..	..
3 years	15	15	6	6	4	4	2	3	3	4	3	4	4	5	2	3	..	..
5 years	15	15	6	6	4	4	2	2	3	6	3	4	4	5	2	3	..	..
8 years	15	15	5	5	3	4	1	1	2	6	2	3	2	4	..	..	..	..
10 years	..	..	5	5	3	4	..	..	0	0	2	4	2	4	..	..	..	..
Females	(30)		(85)		(248)		(504)		(626)		(1493)		(903)		(590)		(0)	
1 year	23	23	16	17	15	15	11	11	10	11	12	13	11	12	13	14	..	..
3 years	10	10	7	7	5	5	2	3	4	6	4	5	4	5	4	4	..	..
5 years	10	10	4	4	4	4	2	2	4	6	3	4	3	4	3	4	..	..
8 years	10	10	2	2	4	5	2	2	2	6	3	4	3	4	..	..	..	..
10 years	10	10	..	..	4	5	..	..	2	8	3	5	3	5	..	..	..	..
Overall	(64)		(191)		(539)		(1057)		(1002)		(2853)		(1739)		(1114)		(0)	
1 year	23	23	14	14	13	13	10	11	11	13	12	12	11	12	12	13	..	..
3 years	13	13	6	6	4	5	2	3	4	5	4	4	4	5	3	4	..	..
5 years	13	13	5	5	4	4	2	2	3	6	3	4	3	5	3	4	..	..
8 years	13	13	4	4	4	4	1	2	2	6	2	4	2	4	..	..	..	..
10 years	13	13	4	4	4	4	..	..	2	7	2	4	2	4	..	..	..	..

RELATIVE SURVIVAL (%) BY AGE AND PERIOD

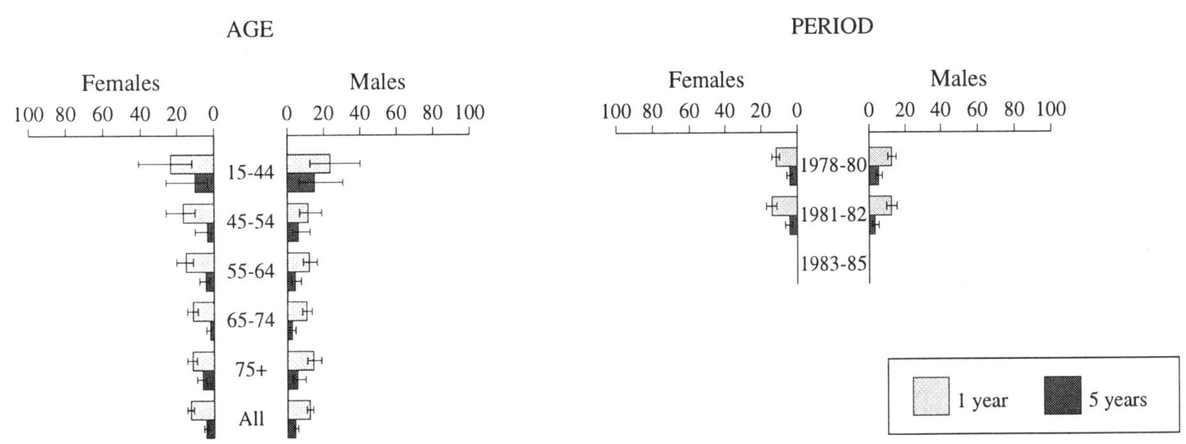

PANCREAS

SPANISH REGISTRIES

REGISTRY	NUMBER OF CASES			PERIOD OF DIAGNOSIS
	Males	Females	All	
Tarragona	17	12	29	1985-1985
Mean age (years)	68.7	71.7	69.9	

Not enough cases for reliable estimation

PANCREAS

SWISS REGISTRIES

REGISTRY	NUMBER OF CASES			PERIOD OF DIAGNOSIS
	Males	Females	All	
Basel	70	62	132	1981-1984
Geneva	113	127	240	1978-1984
Mean age (years)	66.5	72.8	69.7	

RELATIVE SURVIVAL (%)

OBSERVED AND RELATIVE SURVIVAL (%) BY AGE AND PERIOD
(Number of cases in parentheses)

	AGE CLASS												PERIOD					
	15-44		45-54		55-64		65-74		75+		All		1978-80		1981-82		1983-85	
	obs	rel	obs	rel	obs	rel	obs	rel	obs	rel	obs	rel	obs	rel	obs	rel	obs	rel
Males	(9)		(19)		(44)		(63)		(48)		(183)		(45)		(63)		(75)	
1 year	56	56	11	11	7	7	16	16	10	12	14	14	7	7	14	15	17	18
3 years	11	11	0	0	5	5	6	7	0	0	4	4	0	0	6	7	4	4
5 years	11	11	0	0	2	2	5	6	0	0	3	3	0	0	3	4	4	5
8 years	..	..	0	0	..	..	..	..	0	0	..	..	0	0	..	..	..	..
10 years	..	..	0	0	..	..	..	..	0	0	..	..	0	0	..	..	..	..
Females	(4)		(5)		(30)		(59)		(91)		(189)		(43)		(78)		(68)	
1 year	50	50	40	40	27	27	13	13	10	11	15	16	23	24	11	12	15	15
3 years	50	50	20	20	10	10	0	0	1	1	4	4	9	11	3	3	1	2
5 years	50	50	0	0	3	3	0	0	0	0	2	2	5	6	1	2	0	0
8 years	..	..	0	0	3	4	0	0	0	0	2	3	..	..	1	2	0	0
10 years	..	..	0	0	..	..	0	0	0	0	..	..	..	..	..	..	0	0
Overall	(13)		(24)		(74)		(122)		(139)		(372)		(88)		(141)		(143)	
1 year	54	54	17	17	15	15	15	15	10	11	14	15	15	16	13	13	16	17
3 years	23	23	4	4	7	7	3	4	1	1	4	4	5	5	4	5	3	3
5 years	23	23	0	0	3	3	3	3	0	0	2	3	2	3	2	3	2	3
8 years	..	..	0	0	3	3	..	..	0	0	2	3	..	..	2	3	..	..
10 years	..	..	0	0	..	..	..	..	0	0	..	..	..	..	..	..	..	..

RELATIVE SURVIVAL (%) BY AGE AND PERIOD

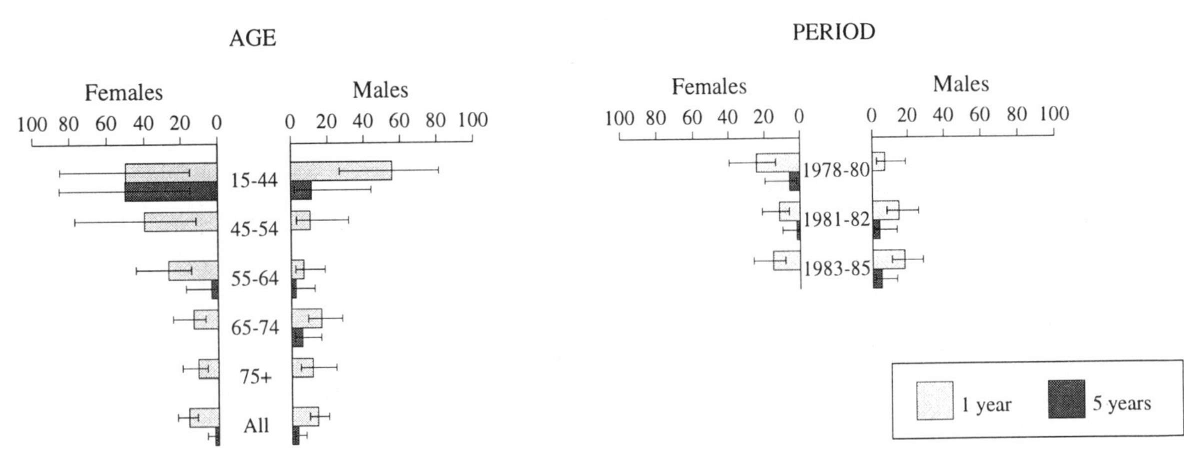

PANCREAS

EUROPEAN REGISTRIES

Weighted analysis

REGISTRY	WEIGHTS (Yearly expected cases in the country)		
	Males	Females	All
DENMARK	332	342	674
DUTCH REGISTRIES	841	696	1537
ENGLISH REGISTRIES	3198	3078	6276
ESTONIA	54	61	115
FINLAND	242	263	505
FRENCH REGISTRIES	2796	2195	4991
GERMAN REGISTRIES	3620	4072	7692
ITALIAN REGISTRIES	2660	2105	4765
POLISH REGISTRIES	1493	1278	2771
SCOTLAND	272	299	571
SWISS REGISTRIES	346	340	686

RELATIVE SURVIVAL (%)
(Age-standardized)

Females 100 80 60 40 20 0 — Males 0 20 40 60 80 100

DK, NL, ENG, EST, FIN, F, D, I, PL, SCO, CH, EUR

OBSERVED AND RELATIVE SURVIVAL (%) BY AGE AND PERIOD

	AGE CLASS												PERIOD					
	15-44		45-54		55-64		65-74		75+		All		1978-80		1981-82		1983-85	
	obs	rel	obs	rel	obs	rel	obs	rel	obs	rel	obs	rel	obs	rel	obs	rel	obs	rel
Males																		
1 year	27	27	17	17	13	13	12	13	10	11	13	14	12	13	13	13	15	15
3 years	14	14	4	4	4	4	3	3	3	4	4	4	4	5	4	4	3	4
5 years	13	14	3	3	2	2	2	3	2	4	3	3	3	4	2	3	3	3
8 years	14	15	2	3	1	1	1	2	2	6	2	4	2	4	2	3	1	2
10 years	14	15	1	2	1	1	1	2	1	7	2	4	2	4	1	2	..	..
Females																		
1 year	33	33	16	16	23	23	12	12	11	12	14	15	12	12	15	15	15	15
3 years	23	23	8	8	11	11	3	4	3	4	5	6	4	4	4	5	5	6
5 years	22	23	6	6	9	10	2	2	2	4	4	5	3	4	4	5	4	5
8 years	19	19	5	5	5	5	2	2	2	5	3	5	3	4	3	5	3	4
10 years	7	7	5	6	3	4	2	2	2	6	3	4	2	3	3	5	..	..
Overall																		
1 year	30	30	16	17	18	18	12	13	10	12	14	14	12	13	14	14	15	15
3 years	18	18	6	6	7	7	3	4	3	4	4	5	4	4	4	5	4	5
5 years	18	18	4	5	6	6	2	2	2	4	3	4	3	4	3	4	3	4
8 years	17	17	4	4	3	3	2	2	2	6	3	4	3	4	3	4	2	3
10 years	11	11	3	3	2	2	1	2	2	6	2	4	2	4	2	3	..	..

RELATIVE SURVIVAL (%) BY AGE AND PERIOD

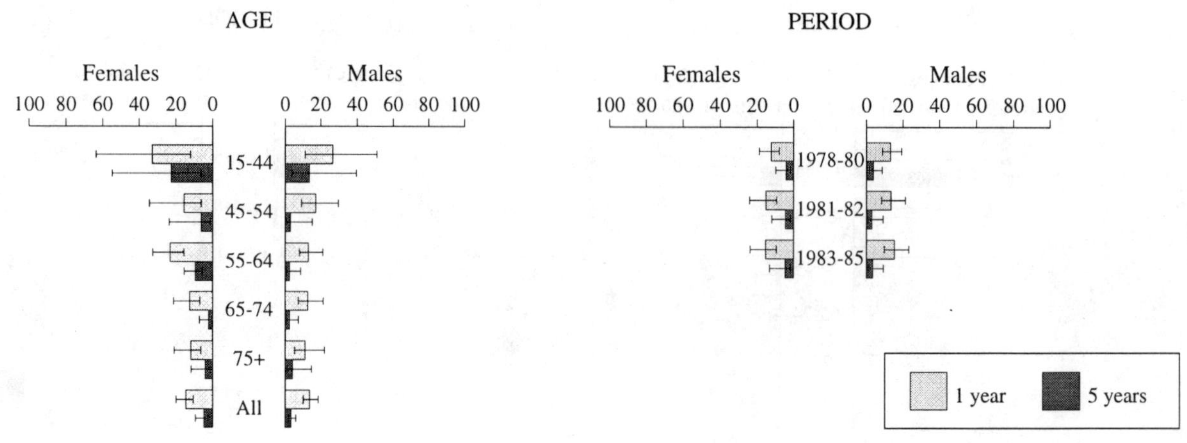

LARYNX

DENMARK

REGISTRY	NUMBER OF CASES			PERIOD OF DIAGNOSIS
	Males	Females	All	
Denmark	1346	258	1604	1978-1984
Mean age (years)	64.1	62.4	63.8	

RELATIVE SURVIVAL (%)

100, 80, 60, 40, 20, 0
Females
Males
0 1 2 3 4 5
Time since diagnosis (years)

OBSERVED AND RELATIVE SURVIVAL (%) BY AGE AND PERIOD
(Number of cases in parentheses)

	AGE CLASS												PERIOD					
	15-44		45-54		55-64		65-74		75+		All		1978-80		1981-82		1983-85	
	obs	rel	obs	rel	obs	rel	obs	rel	obs	rel	obs	rel	obs	rel	obs	rel	obs	rel
Males	(45)		(192)		(453)		(434)		(222)		(1346)		(574)		(383)		(389)	
1 year	93	94	84	85	85	86	80	84	69	77	81	84	80	84	85	88	78	81
3 years	71	72	62	63	65	69	56	64	42	60	58	65	57	65	58	65	60	67
5 years	60	61	58	61	56	63	43	55	27	50	48	59	46	57	46	57	52	64
8 years	60	61	49	53	41	49	35	55	15	45	36	52	35	51	36	51	..	..
10 years	60	62	47	52	32	42	23	42	10	44	29	46	28	45	..	..	..	..
Females	(11)		(51)		(83)		(76)		(37)		(258)		(89)		(78)		(91)	
1 year	91	91	96	97	88	89	82	83	78	83	86	88	91	93	85	86	84	85
3 years	73	73	86	88	71	73	67	72	49	59	70	74	70	74	69	74	70	74
5 years	73	73	74	76	60	63	63	72	38	55	61	68	64	72	60	68	58	64
8 years	73	74	61	64	34	38	45	58	20	40	41	50	42	51	49	61	..	..
10 years	73	74	45	49	34	39	37	53	12	31	34	45	35	45	..	..	..	..
Overall	(56)		(243)		(536)		(510)		(259)		(1604)		(663)		(461)		(480)	
1 year	93	93	87	87	85	87	80	84	70	78	82	85	82	85	85	88	79	82
3 years	71	72	67	69	66	69	58	66	43	60	60	67	59	66	60	66	62	69
5 years	62	63	62	64	57	63	46	58	28	51	50	60	48	59	49	59	53	64
8 years	62	64	52	56	40	48	37	55	16	44	37	52	36	51	38	53	..	..
10 years	62	64	47	52	33	42	25	44	11	42	30	46	29	45	..	..	..	..

RELATIVE SURVIVAL (%) BY AGE AND PERIOD

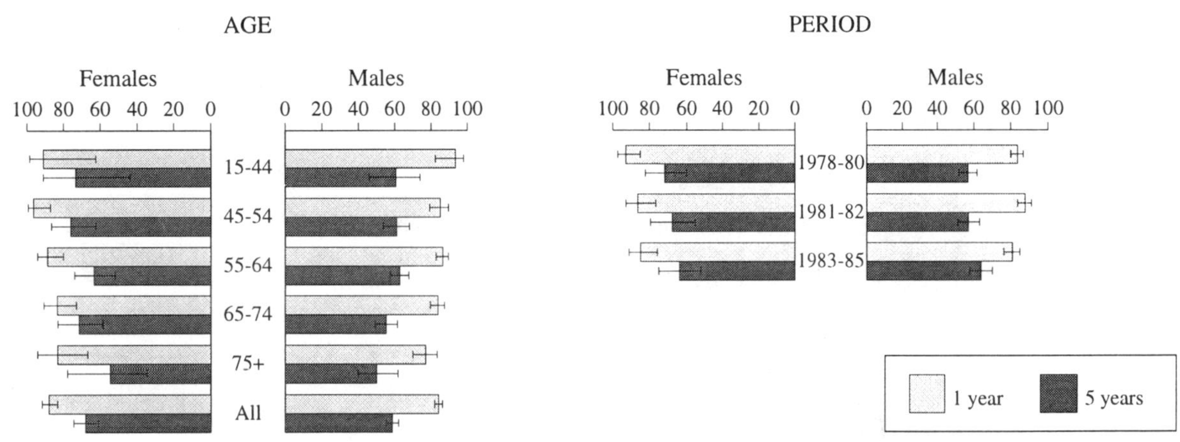

LARYNX

DUTCH REGISTRIES

REGISTRY	NUMBER OF CASES			PERIOD OF DIAGNOSIS
	Males	Females	All	
Eindhoven	219	22	241	1978-1985
Mean age (years)	63.7	60.4	63.4	

RELATIVE SURVIVAL (%)

100, 80, 60, 40, 20, 0 — Males, Females — 0 1 2 3 4 5 — Time since diagnosis (years)

OBSERVED AND RELATIVE SURVIVAL (%) BY AGE AND PERIOD
(Number of cases in parentheses)

	AGE CLASS												PERIOD					
	15-44		45-54		55-64		65-74		75+		All		1978-80		1981-82		1983-85	
	obs	rel	obs	rel	obs	rel	obs	rel	obs	rel	obs	rel	obs	rel	obs	rel	obs	rel
Males	(5)		(34)		(84)		(64)		(32)		(219)		(87)		(64)		(68)	
1 year	80	80	94	95	94	96	87	92	63	70	87	90	90	93	89	92	82	86
3 years	60	60	88	90	76	80	78	90	47	67	74	83	74	84	72	78	74	85
5 years	60	61	81	84	64	71	67	88	16	31	61	74	58	72	66	76	57	74
8 years	60	61	71	76	52	64	44	72	4	13	45	65	42	62	..	..	..	..
10 years	..	..	71	77	52	69	44	88	..	..	45	74	42	70	..	..	..	..
Females	(0)		(7)		(8)		(5)		(2)		(22)		(7)		(4)		(11)	
1 year	..	..	100	100	100	100	80	82	50	53	91	92	71	73	100	100	100	100
3 years	..	..	86	87	52	53	80	86	50	61	72	75	57	62	100	100	67	69
5 years	..	..	69	70	52	54	60	68	0	0	54	58	43	50	75	80	51	52
8 years	..	..	69	71	..	..	60	77	0	0	54	64	43	57	..	..	..	..
10 years	..	..	..	..	..	..	..	..	0	0	..	..	..	..	..	..	..	..
Overall	(5)		(41)		(92)		(69)		(34)		(241)		(94)		(68)		(79)	
1 year	80	80	95	96	95	96	87	91	62	69	88	91	88	92	90	92	85	88
3 years	60	60	88	89	74	78	78	90	47	67	73	82	73	83	74	80	74	83
5 years	60	61	79	82	63	70	67	86	15	28	60	73	57	70	66	77	57	71
8 years	60	61	70	75	52	63	46	74	4	11	46	65	42	61	..	..	..	..
10 years	..	..	70	76	52	67	46	89	..	..	46	73	42	70	..	..	..	..

RELATIVE SURVIVAL (%) BY AGE AND PERIOD

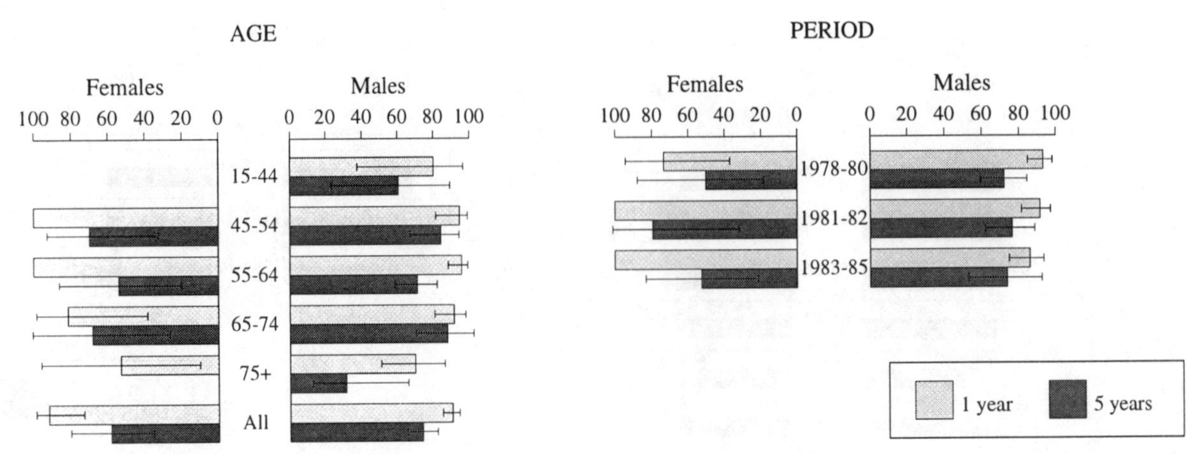

LARYNX

ENGLISH REGISTRIES

REGISTRY	NUMBER OF CASES			PERIOD OF DIAGNOSIS
	Males	Females	All	
East Anglia	338	60	398	1979-1984
Mersey	532	143	675	1978-1984
South Thames	1168	256	1424	1978-1984
Wessex	149	36	185	1983-1984
West Midlands	763	118	881	1979-1984
Yorkshire	816	160	976	1978-1984
Mean age (years)	64.9	65.3	65.0	

RELATIVE SURVIVAL (%)

100
80
60
40
20
0
Males
Females
0 1 2 3 4 5
Time since diagnosis (years)

OBSERVED AND RELATIVE SURVIVAL (%) BY AGE AND PERIOD
(Number of cases in parentheses)

	AGE CLASS												PERIOD					
	15-44		45-54		55-64		65-74		75+		All		1978-80		1981-82		1983-85	
	obs	rel	obs	rel	obs	rel	obs	rel	obs	rel	obs	rel	obs	rel	obs	rel	obs	rel
Males	(121)		(447)		(1201)		(1329)		(668)		(3766)		(1413)		(1097)		(1256)	
1 year	88	89	87	88	86	88	78	82	63	70	79	83	79	82	81	84	79	83
3 years	77	77	68	70	68	72	56	66	43	62	60	68	59	69	62	70	59	67
5 years	74	75	64	67	61	68	45	59	33	62	51	65	51	65	54	67	50	63
8 years	70	71	60	65	50	62	35	57	20	62	41	61	41	62	43	62	41	60
10 years	66	69	55	61	45	60	27	53	12	53	35	58	35	60	36	57	..	..
Females	(32)		(85)		(266)		(220)		(170)		(773)		(305)		(219)		(249)	
1 year	88	88	86	86	77	78	72	74	57	63	73	75	72	74	68	70	78	81
3 years	78	78	72	73	61	63	50	55	37	50	55	60	52	57	53	57	59	66
5 years	78	79	69	71	56	60	43	50	31	52	49	58	48	56	46	53	53	64
8 years	71	72	65	68	46	51	31	41	22	55	40	52	37	49	39	49	47	63
10 years	63	64	62	66	40	46	25	37	16	53	34	48	33	47	31	42	..	..
Overall	(153)		(532)		(1467)		(1549)		(838)		(4539)		(1718)		(1316)		(1505)	
1 year	88	88	87	87	84	86	77	81	62	69	78	82	77	81	79	82	79	82
3 years	77	78	69	70	67	71	55	64	42	59	59	67	58	67	60	68	59	67
5 years	75	76	65	67	60	66	45	58	33	60	51	63	50	63	53	64	50	63
8 years	70	71	61	65	50	60	34	54	21	60	41	59	41	59	42	60	42	60
10 years	66	68	56	62	44	57	27	50	13	54	35	56	35	57	35	55	..	..

RELATIVE SURVIVAL (%) BY AGE AND PERIOD

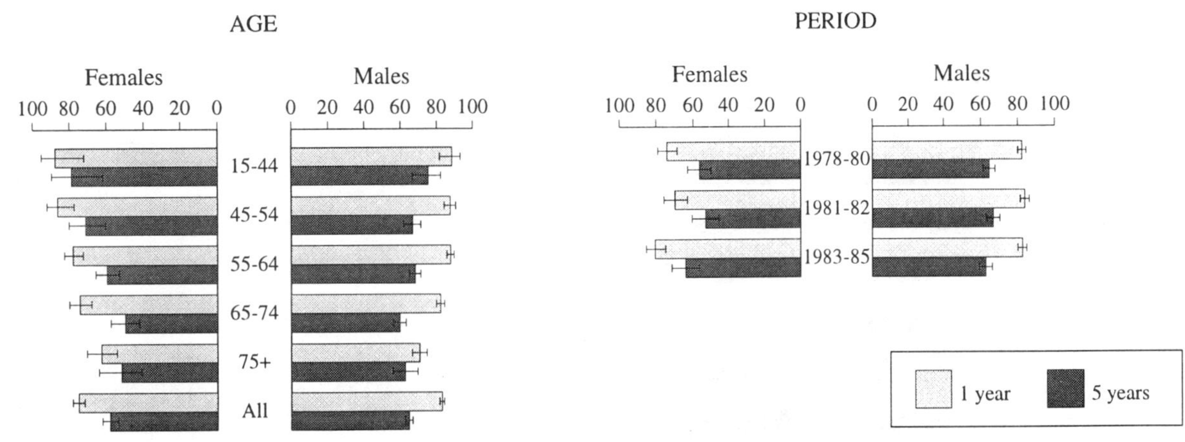

LARYNX

ESTONIA

REGISTRY	NUMBER OF CASES Males	Females	All	PERIOD OF DIAGNOSIS
Estonia	373	33	406	1978-1984
Mean age (years)	57.9	59.4	58.0	

RELATIVE SURVIVAL (%)

100 80 60 40 20 0

Males

Females

0 1 2 3 4 5

Time since diagnosis (years)

OBSERVED AND RELATIVE SURVIVAL (%) BY AGE AND PERIOD
(Number of cases in parentheses)

	AGE CLASS 15-44		45-54		55-64		65-74		75+		All		PERIOD 1978-80		1981-82		1983-85	
	obs	rel	obs	rel	obs	rel	obs	rel	obs	rel	obs	rel	obs	rel	obs	rel	obs	rel
Males	(32)		(133)		(108)		(74)		(26)		(373)		(157)		(106)		(110)	
1 year	88	88	86	88	80	82	70	74	42	48	78	81	79	82	77	80	78	81
3 years	69	70	60	63	56	61	36	44	27	40	53	59	50	56	54	60	55	61
5 years	63	65	51	55	43	50	22	30	23	47	42	50	38	46	39	47	50	60
8 years	58	62	43	50	33	44	17	31	4	14	33	46	30	40	32	45	..	..
10 years	52	57	43	53	23	34	15	34	4	22	30	45	26	39	..	..	..	..
Females	(3)		(7)		(11)		(9)		(3)		(33)		(11)		(9)		(13)	
1 year	67	67	86	86	73	73	67	68	33	37	70	71	64	65	89	90	62	63
3 years	67	67	86	87	45	47	33	36	33	45	52	55	64	69	56	58	38	41
5 years	67	67	57	59	36	39	33	39	33	58	42	48	55	63	56	61	23	26
8 years	67	67	38	40	27	31	22	31	33	95	32	40	55	69	33	40	..	..
10 years	67	68	38	41	27	32	..	..	33	100	32	43	55	74	..	..	..	..
Overall	(35)		(140)		(119)		(83)		(29)		(406)		(168)		(115)		(123)	
1 year	86	86	86	88	79	81	70	74	41	47	78	80	78	81	78	81	76	79
3 years	69	70	61	64	55	60	36	43	28	41	53	58	51	57	54	60	54	59
5 years	63	65	51	55	42	49	23	31	24	48	42	50	39	47	40	48	47	56
8 years	59	63	43	50	33	43	17	31	7	24	33	45	31	42	32	44	..	..
10 years	54	59	43	52	25	35	15	34	7	38	30	45	28	42	..	..	..	..

RELATIVE SURVIVAL (%) BY AGE AND PERIOD

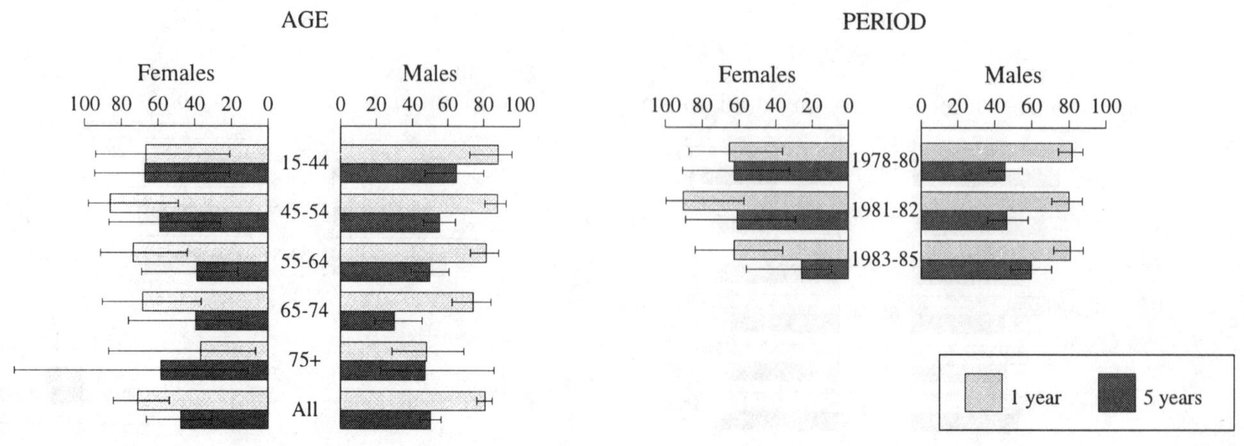

LARYNX

FINLAND

REGISTRY	NUMBER OF CASES			PERIOD OF DIAGNOSIS
	Males	Females	All	
Finland	848	79	927	1978-1984
Mean age (years)	63.2	63.3	63.2	

RELATIVE SURVIVAL (%)

Females
Males
Time since diagnosis (years)

OBSERVED AND RELATIVE SURVIVAL (%) BY AGE AND PERIOD
(Number of cases in parentheses)

	AGE CLASS												PERIOD					
	15-44		45-54		55-64		65-74		75+		All		1978-80		1981-82		1983-85	
	obs	rel	obs	rel	obs	rel	obs	rel	obs	rel	obs	rel	obs	rel	obs	rel	obs	rel
Males	(32)		(114)		(317)		(284)		(101)		(848)		(370)		(248)		(230)	
1 year	94	94	88	89	87	89	87	91	70	79	85	89	86	90	85	88	86	89
3 years	69	70	72	74	64	69	64	75	42	59	63	71	61	69	64	72	64	72
5 years	66	67	64	68	54	61	47	63	28	52	50	62	50	62	50	62	51	62
8 years	66	68	49	55	43	54	30	50	13	37	37	53	37	53	35	51	39	53
10 years	59	62	37	43	37	49	22	43	7	29	29	46	28	46	27	42	..	..
Females	(4)		(11)		(33)		(17)		(14)		(79)		(34)		(27)		(18)	
1 year	100	100	100	100	91	92	76	78	57	63	84	86	85	87	93	95	67	69
3 years	75	75	100	100	73	75	65	70	29	39	67	72	71	76	81	88	39	42
5 years	75	76	100	100	70	73	41	47	14	25	58	66	62	70	67	76	39	45
8 years	75	76	91	94	60	66	25	32	14	39	50	63	50	62	59	75	39	49
10 years	75	77	91	95	60	68	0	0	14	58	48	64	50	65	53	70	..	..
Overall	(36)		(125)		(350)		(301)		(115)		(927)		(404)		(275)		(248)	
1 year	94	95	89	90	88	90	86	91	69	77	85	89	86	89	85	89	84	87
3 years	69	70	74	77	65	70	64	74	40	57	63	71	62	70	65	74	62	69
5 years	67	68	67	71	55	62	47	62	26	48	51	62	51	63	52	64	50	61
8 years	67	69	53	59	45	55	30	49	13	37	38	53	38	54	38	53	39	53
10 years	62	64	43	49	39	52	21	41	8	33	31	48	30	48	30	46	..	..

RELATIVE SURVIVAL (%) BY AGE AND PERIOD

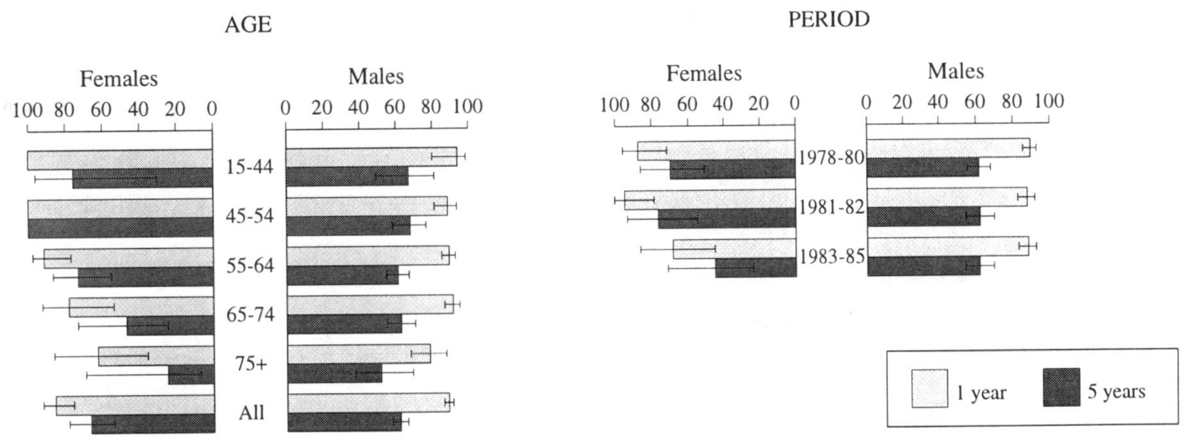

LARYNX

FRENCH REGISTRIES

REGISTRY	NUMBER OF CASES Males	Females	All	PERIOD OF DIAGNOSIS
Amiens	103	4	107	1983-1984
Doubs	271	8	279	1978-1985
Mean age (years)	60.8	62.2	60.9	

RELATIVE SURVIVAL (%)

100, 80, 60, 40, 20, 0

Females

Males

0 1 2 3 4 5

Time since diagnosis (years)

OBSERVED AND RELATIVE SURVIVAL (%) BY AGE AND PERIOD
(Number of cases in parentheses)

	AGE CLASS												PERIOD					
	15-44		45-54		55-64		65-74		75+		All		1978-80		1981-82		1983-85	
	obs	rel	obs	rel	obs	rel	obs	rel	obs	rel	obs	rel	obs	rel	obs	rel	obs	rel
Males	(23)		(106)		(110)		(90)		(45)		(374)		(98)		(68)		(208)	
1 year	77	78	80	80	86	88	71	73	63	74	77	80	75	77	81	85	77	80
3 years	43	43	58	60	51	53	45	51	28	42	48	53	41	45	54	60	50	55
5 years	36	37	48	51	45	49	37	46	19	36	40	47	34	39	47	57	41	48
8 years	27	28	33	36	40	48	28	43	13	39	31	41	24	31	41	55	..	..
10 years	14	14	28	31	40	50	21	38	13	58	27	38	20	28	..	..	..	..
Females	(0)		(5)		(3)		(2)		(2)		(12)		(3)		(4)		(5)	
1 year	..	..	80	80	67	67	50	51	0	0	58	61	33	33	75	76	60	66
3 years	..	..	80	81	67	68	50	54	0	0	58	65	33	34	75	77	60	77
5 years	..	..	60	61	67	70	0	0	0	0	42	49	33	34	50	53	40	58
8 years	..	..	..	..	..	..	0	0	0	0	..	..	0	0	..	..	..	..
10 years	..	..	..	..	..	..	0	0	0	0	..	..	0	0	..	..	..	..
Overall	(23)		(111)		(113)		(92)		(47)		(386)		(101)		(72)		(213)	
1 year	77	78	80	80	86	87	70	73	60	71	77	80	74	76	80	84	77	80
3 years	43	43	59	61	51	54	45	51	27	41	49	53	41	44	55	61	50	55
5 years	36	37	49	51	45	50	36	45	18	35	40	47	34	39	48	57	41	48
8 years	27	28	32	35	41	48	28	42	12	39	31	41	23	30	42	55	..	..
10 years	14	14	28	31	41	51	21	36	12	56	27	38	20	27	..	..	..	..

RELATIVE SURVIVAL (%) BY AGE AND PERIOD

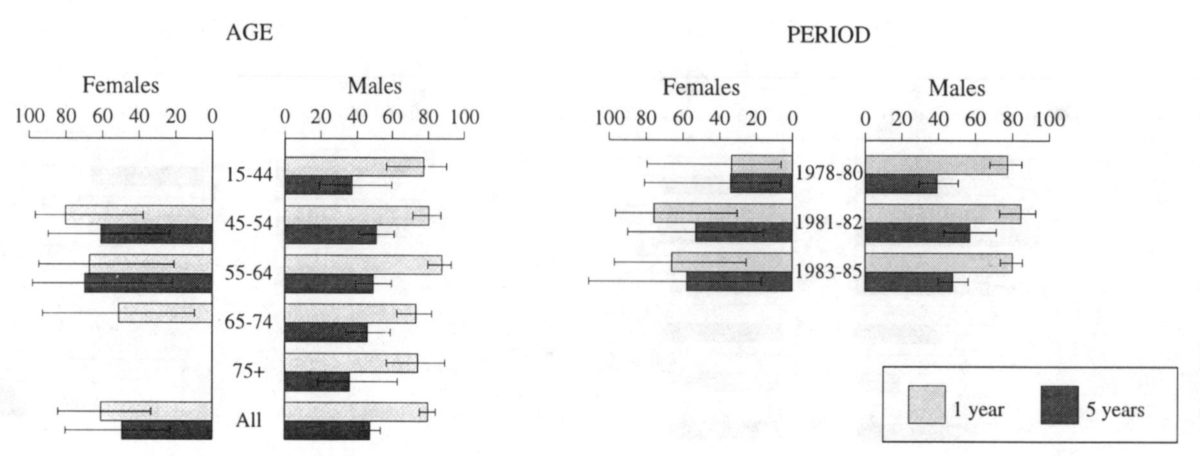

LARYNX

GERMAN REGISTRIES

REGISTRY	NUMBER OF CASES			PERIOD OF DIAGNOSIS
	Males	Females	All	
Saarland	315	28	343	1978-1984
Mean age (years)	60.9	56.9	60.6	

RELATIVE SURVIVAL (%)

Females
Males
Time since diagnosis (years)

OBSERVED AND RELATIVE SURVIVAL (%) BY AGE AND PERIOD
(Number of cases in parentheses)

	AGE CLASS												PERIOD					
	15-44		45-54		55-64		65-74		75+		All		1978-80		1981-82		1983-85	
	obs	rel	obs	rel	obs	rel	obs	rel	obs	rel	obs	rel	obs	rel	obs	rel	obs	rel
Males	(22)		(73)		(95)		(84)		(41)		(315)		(150)		(73)		(92)	
1 year	86	87	79	80	86	88	80	84	66	74	80	83	79	82	81	84	82	84
3 years	59	60	62	63	65	69	58	69	39	56	59	66	57	63	60	68	61	68
5 years	55	56	58	60	54	60	48	65	32	60	50	61	46	56	53	66	54	65
8 years	50	52	52	57	46	57	31	53	23	70	40	56	39	53	39	55	..	..
10 years	50	52	49	54	39	51	26	54	23	98	35	54	34	51	..	..	..	..
Females	(3)		(9)		(10)		(6)		(0)		(28)		(13)		(5)		(10)	
1 year	100	100	89	89	80	81	83	86	..	..	86	87	69	70	100	100	100	100
3 years	100	100	56	56	80	82	33	37	..	..	64	67	46	48	100	100	70	72
5 years	100	100	56	57	80	84	33	40	..	..	64	68	46	50	100	100	70	74
8 years	100	100	56	58	69	76	17	23	..	..	52	59	31	35	100	100	..	..
10 years	100	100	56	58	69	79	..	..	..	..	52	61	31	36	..	..	..	..
Overall	(25)		(82)		(105)		(90)		(41)		(343)		(163)		(78)		(102)	
1 year	88	88	80	81	86	87	80	84	66	74	81	84	79	81	82	85	83	86
3 years	64	65	61	62	67	71	57	67	39	56	59	66	56	62	63	71	62	68
5 years	60	61	57	60	56	62	47	63	32	60	51	62	46	55	56	69	56	66
8 years	56	58	52	57	48	58	30	50	23	70	41	56	38	52	43	59	..	..
10 years	56	59	49	55	41	53	25	51	23	98	37	54	34	50	..	..	..	..

RELATIVE SURVIVAL (%) BY AGE AND PERIOD

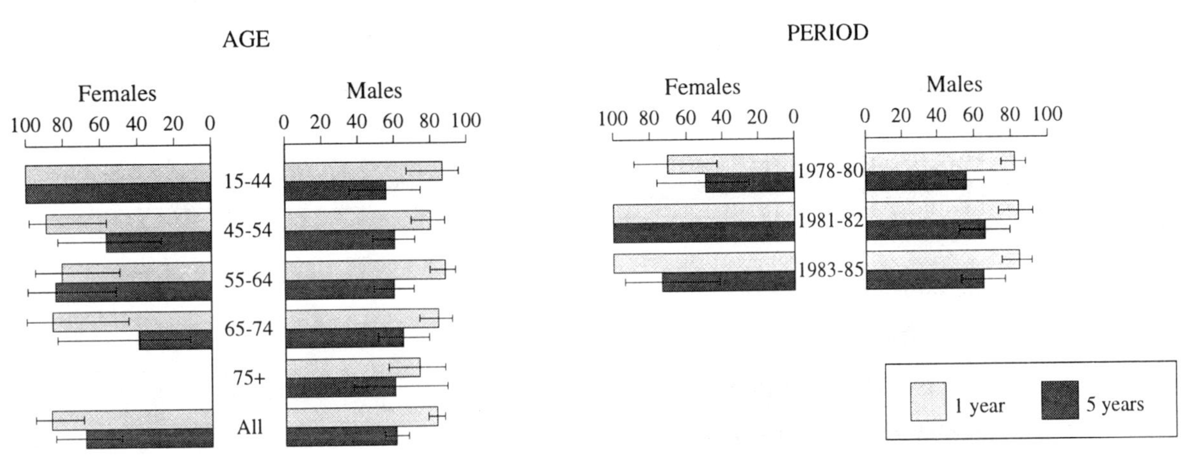

LARYNX

ITALIAN REGISTRIES

REGISTRY	NUMBER OF CASES			PERIOD OF DIAGNOSIS
	Males	Females	All	
Latina	38	2	40	1983-1984
Ragusa	64	6	70	1981-1984
Varese	566	30	596	1978-1985
Mean age (years)	60.8	63.4	60.9	

RELATIVE SURVIVAL (%)

Females
Males
Time since diagnosis (years)

OBSERVED AND RELATIVE SURVIVAL (%) BY AGE AND PERIOD
(Number of cases in parentheses)

	AGE CLASS												PERIOD					
	15-44		45-54		55-64		65-74		75+		All		1978-80		1981-82		1983-85	
	obs	rel	obs	rel	obs	rel	obs	rel	obs	rel	obs	rel	obs	rel	obs	rel	obs	rel
Males	(34)		(160)		(232)		(178)		(64)		(668)		(208)		(181)		(279)	
1 year	94	94	94	95	89	91	82	86	66	73	86	89	83	85	88	90	88	91
3 years	88	89	77	79	70	74	58	67	36	50	66	73	62	68	67	73	68	76
5 years	82	84	73	76	60	67	40	52	20	37	55	65	54	63	54	64	57	68
8 years	75	77	64	70	45	55	30	48	7	20	44	58	43	56	44	57	43	57
10 years	69	72	62	70	37	48	25	46	0	0	38	55	38	55	32	45	..	..
Females	(1)		(11)		(9)		(8)		(9)		(38)		(11)		(9)		(18)	
1 year	100	100	100	100	89	90	100	100	78	87	92	95	100	100	78	81	94	98
3 years	100	100	91	92	67	68	88	93	56	77	76	84	91	96	44	51	83	92
5 years	100	100	91	92	67	70	38	42	33	61	61	71	82	90	44	56	56	65
8 years	100	100	72	74	53	58	38	47	33	89	52	66	82	96	44	65	31	39
10 years	100	100	59	61	36	40	38	53	33	100	42	57	73	89	..	..	..	..
Overall	(35)		(171)		(241)		(186)		(73)		(706)		(219)		(190)		(297)	
1 year	94	95	95	95	89	91	83	86	67	75	87	89	84	86	87	90	89	91
3 years	89	89	78	80	70	74	59	68	38	54	67	73	63	69	66	72	69	77
5 years	83	84	74	77	60	67	40	51	22	40	55	65	55	64	54	63	57	67
8 years	76	78	65	70	45	55	31	48	11	30	44	58	45	59	44	57	42	56
10 years	70	73	62	69	36	47	25	46	5	20	39	55	40	57	32	44	..	..

RELATIVE SURVIVAL (%) BY AGE AND PERIOD

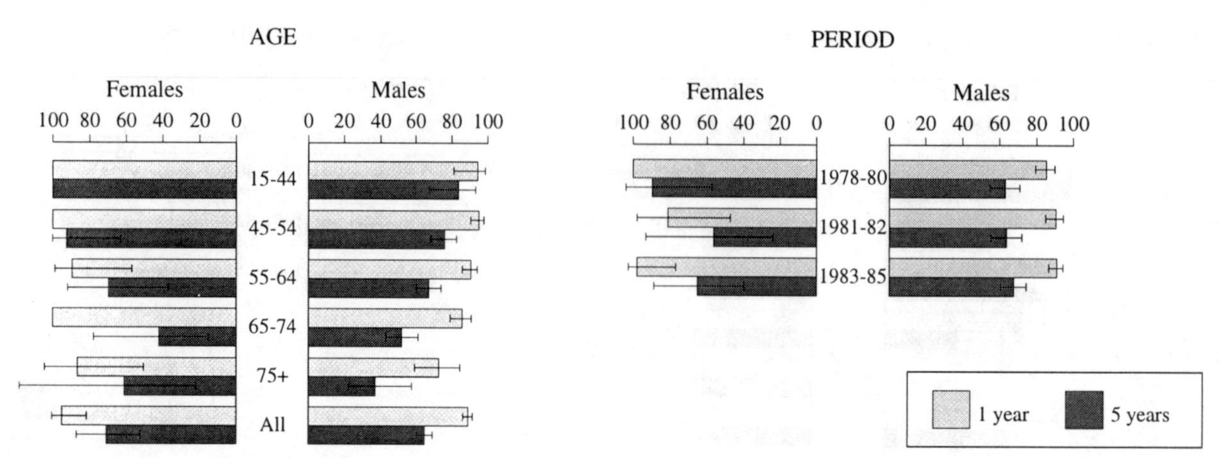

LARYNX

POLISH REGISTRIES

REGISTRY	NUMBER OF CASES			PERIOD OF DIAGNOSIS
	Males	Females	All	
Cracow	255	28	283	1978-1984
Mean age (years)	58.1	58.2	58.1	

RELATIVE SURVIVAL (%)

100
80
60
40
20
0
Females
Males
0 1 2 3 4 5
Time since diagnosis (years)

OBSERVED AND RELATIVE SURVIVAL (%) BY AGE AND PERIOD
(Number of cases in parentheses)

	AGE CLASS										All		PERIOD					
	15-44		45-54		55-64		65-74		75+		All		1978-80		1981-82		1983-85	
	obs	rel	obs	rel	obs	rel	obs	rel	obs	rel	obs	rel	obs	rel	obs	rel	obs	rel
Males	(21)		(79)		(90)		(47)		(18)		(255)		(97)		(76)		(82)	
1 year	70	70	80	81	82	84	60	64	77	85	76	78	74	77	76	78	79	81
3 years	55	56	71	74	63	68	43	51	53	74	61	66	58	64	61	66	63	69
5 years	55	56	63	67	52	59	31	44	30	53	50	59	50	60	51	58	50	59
8 years	55	58	61	68	39	49	26	49	..	..	43	57	43	59	44	56	43	56
10 years	55	59	52	61	23	33	16	37	..	..	34	49	34	51	32	44	..	..
Females	(4)		(7)		(7)		(5)		(5)		(28)		(10)		(8)		(10)	
1 year	100	100	86	86	85	85	40	41	60	63	74	75	68	70	75	76	78	80
3 years	100	100	86	87	85	87	40	44	40	48	70	75	68	74	75	79	67	71
5 years	100	100	71	73	68	72	40	48	40	56	62	70	68	79	50	55	67	75
8 years	100	100	57	60	68	75	20	28	0	0	47	58	57	74	38	44	45	55
10 years	100	100	57	62	68	78	0	0	0	0	38	51	46	65	38	47	..	..
Overall	(25)		(86)		(97)		(52)		(23)		(283)		(107)		(84)		(92)	
1 year	74	74	81	82	82	84	58	62	73	80	76	78	74	76	76	78	79	81
3 years	61	62	72	75	65	70	42	51	50	68	61	67	59	65	63	68	63	69
5 years	61	62	64	68	53	60	32	45	32	54	51	60	52	62	51	58	52	61
8 years	61	64	60	67	40	51	26	46	..	..	44	57	45	61	44	55	43	56
10 years	61	65	53	61	27	37	14	30	..	..	34	49	35	52	33	44	..	..

RELATIVE SURVIVAL (%) BY AGE AND PERIOD

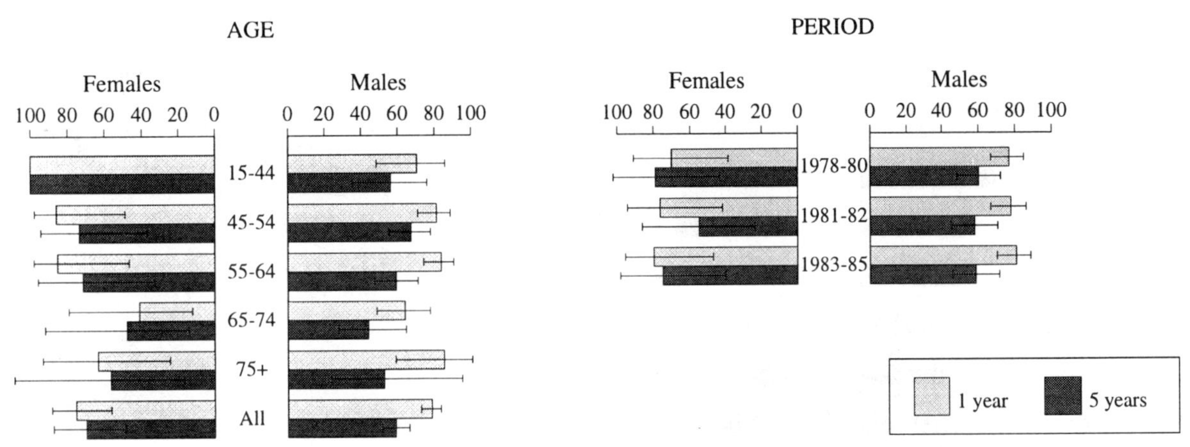

LARYNX

SCOTLAND

REGISTRY	NUMBER OF CASES			PERIOD OF DIAGNOSIS
	Males	Females	All	
Scotland	739	211	950	1978-1982
Mean age (years)	64.1	64.8	64.3	

RELATIVE SURVIVAL (%)

100
80
60
40
20
0
Males
Females
0 1 2 3 4 5
Time since diagnosis (years)

OBSERVED AND RELATIVE SURVIVAL (%) BY AGE AND PERIOD
(Number of cases in parentheses)

	AGE CLASS												PERIOD					
	15-44		45-54		55-64		65-74		75+		All		1978-80		1981-82		1983-85	
	obs	rel	obs	rel	obs	rel	obs	rel	obs	rel	obs	rel	obs	rel	obs	rel	obs	rel
Males	(24)		(115)		(234)		(256)		(110)		(739)		(418)		(321)		(0)	
1 year	88	88	82	82	88	90	77	82	65	74	80	84	78	82	82	86	..	..
3 years	71	72	65	67	71	76	53	63	45	71	60	69	58	68	63	72	..	..
5 years	71	72	59	62	65	74	42	58	31	66	51	66	50	65	53	66	..	..
8 years	61	63	56	62	49	62	31	54	23	82	40	61	40	61	..	..	..	..
10 years	61	64	49	56	46	63	27	58	..	..	37	64	36	64	..	..	..	..
Females	(9)		(30)		(68)		(62)		(42)		(211)		(128)		(83)		(0)	
1 year	89	89	87	87	85	86	71	73	50	56	74	77	77	79	71	74	..	..
3 years	89	89	80	81	69	72	44	48	36	50	57	64	59	65	55	62	..	..
5 years	78	79	67	69	57	62	39	46	26	47	48	57	51	60	43	52	..	..
8 years	78	79	60	64	50	57	21	28	10	26	37	49	40	53	..	..	..	..
10 years	78	80	60	65	43	51	21	31	..	..	35	51	38	55	..	..	..	..
Overall	(33)		(145)		(302)		(318)		(152)		(950)		(546)		(404)		(0)	
1 year	88	88	83	83	87	89	76	80	61	69	79	82	77	81	80	83	..	..
3 years	76	76	68	70	71	75	51	60	43	65	59	68	58	67	61	70	..	..
5 years	73	74	61	64	63	71	42	55	30	60	51	64	50	64	51	63	..	..
8 years	66	68	57	62	49	61	29	48	19	65	39	58	40	59	..	..	..	..
10 years	66	69	52	59	45	60	26	51	..	..	36	60	37	62	..	..	..	..

RELATIVE SURVIVAL (%) BY AGE AND PERIOD

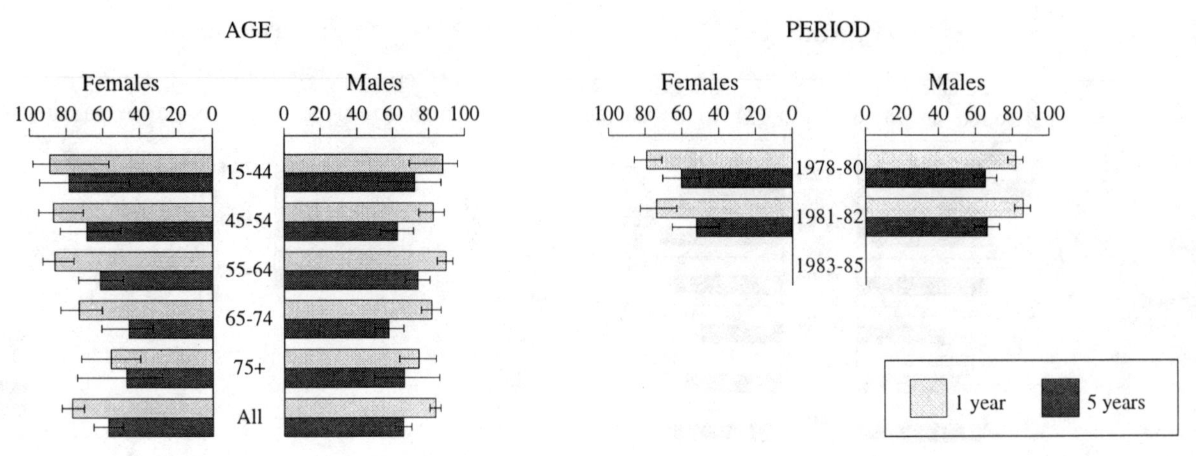

LARYNX

SPANISH REGISTRIES

REGISTRY	NUMBER OF CASES			PERIOD OF DIAGNOSIS
	Males	Females	All	
Tarragona	30	2	32	1985-1985
Mean age (years)	62.8	64.5	62.9	

RELATIVE SURVIVAL (%)

100 80 60 40 20 0
Males
Females
0 1 2 3 4 5
Time since diagnosis (years)

OBSERVED AND RELATIVE SURVIVAL (%) BY AGE AND PERIOD
(Number of cases in parentheses)

	AGE CLASS												PERIOD					
	15-44		45-54		55-64		65-74		75+		All		1978-80		1981-82		1983-85	
	obs	rel	obs	rel	obs	rel	obs	rel	obs	rel	obs	rel	obs	rel	obs	rel	obs	rel
Males	(0)		(4)		(13)		(11)		(2)		(30)		(0)		(0)		(30)	
1 year	..	..	100	100	92	93	91	94	100	100	93	95	..	..	..	..	93	95
3 years	..	..	100	100	62	64	64	71	50	66	67	72	..	..	..	..	67	72
5 years	..	..	100	100	46	49	45	55	50	81	53	60	..	..	..	..	53	60
8 years	..	..	..	..	..	..	..	..	..	..	..	..	..	..	..	..	..	..
10 years	..	..	..	..	..	..	..	..	..	..	..	..	..	..	..	..	..	..
Females	(0)		(0)		(1)		(1)		(0)		(2)		(0)		(0)		(2)	
1 year	..	..	..	..	0	0	100	100	..	..	50	51	..	..	..	..	50	51
3 years	..	..	..	..	0	0	100	100	..	..	50	53	..	..	..	..	50	53
5 years	..	..	..	..	0	0	100	100	..	..	50	55	..	..	..	..	50	55
8 years	..	..	..	..	0	0	..	..	..	..	..	..	..	..	..	..	..	..
10 years	..	..	..	..	0	0	..	..	..	..	..	..	..	..	..	..	..	..
Overall	(0)		(4)		(14)		(12)		(2)		(32)		(0)		(0)		(32)	
1 year	..	..	100	100	86	87	92	95	100	100	91	93	..	..	..	..	91	93
3 years	..	..	100	100	57	59	67	74	50	66	66	70	..	..	..	..	66	70
5 years	..	..	100	100	43	45	50	60	50	81	53	60	..	..	..	..	53	60
8 years	..	..	..	..	..	..	..	..	..	..	..	..	..	..	..	..	..	..
10 years	..	..	..	..	..	..	..	..	..	..	..	..	..	..	..	..	..	..

RELATIVE SURVIVAL (%) BY AGE AND PERIOD

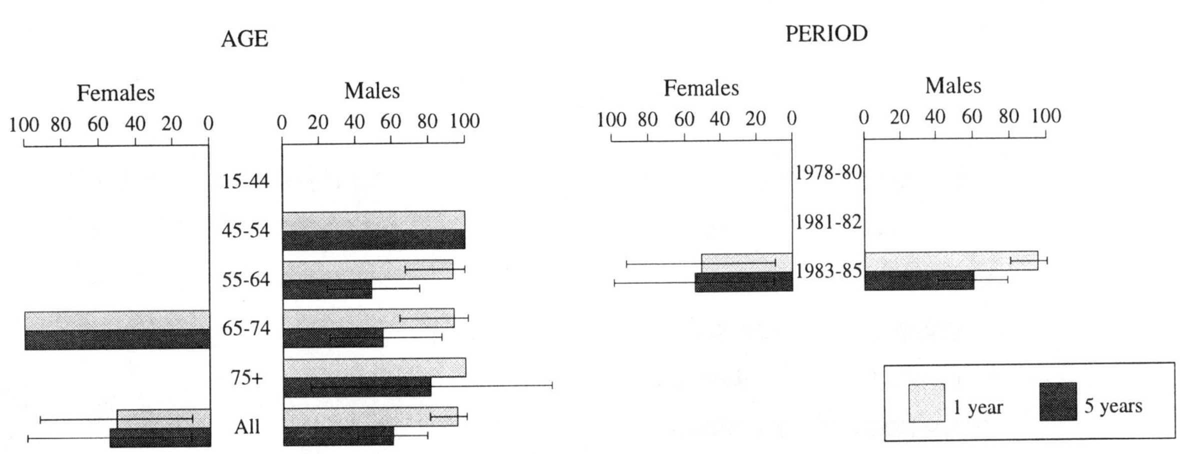

LARYNX

SWISS REGISTRIES

REGISTRY	NUMBER OF CASES			PERIOD OF DIAGNOSIS
	Males	Females	All	
Basel	48	6	54	1981-1984
Geneva	118	23	141	1978-1984
Mean age (years)	60.7	59.9	60.6	

RELATIVE SURVIVAL (%)

Females

Males

Time since diagnosis (years)

OBSERVED AND RELATIVE SURVIVAL (%) BY AGE AND PERIOD
(Number of cases in parentheses)

	AGE CLASS												PERIOD					
	15-44		45-54		55-64		65-74		75+		All		1978-80		1981-82		1983-85	
	obs	rel	obs	rel	obs	rel	obs	rel	obs	rel	obs	rel	obs	rel	obs	rel	obs	rel
Males	(9)		(39)		(61)		(36)		(21)		(166)		(51)		(54)		(61)	
1 year	100	100	95	95	85	86	78	81	57	63	83	85	88	90	81	84	80	82
3 years	78	78	74	75	70	74	50	56	47	63	64	69	67	72	63	68	63	69
5 years	78	79	61	63	58	63	42	52	37	61	53	61	51	58	55	63	55	63
8 years	39	40	57	60	56	64	35	52	19	48	43	55	..	..	47	61	..	..
10 years	..	..	..	..	..	..	..	..	..	..	..	..	..	..	..	..	..	..
Females	(5)		(3)		(11)		(6)		(4)		(29)		(9)		(10)		(10)	
1 year	80	80	100	100	91	91	100	100	75	81	90	91	89	90	90	92	90	92
3 years	60	60	33	34	82	83	50	53	50	65	62	66	67	70	60	63	60	64
5 years	60	60	33	34	82	85	50	56	50	81	62	68	67	73	60	66	60	67
8 years	60	61	..	..	..	..	..	..	..	..	62	74	..	..	60	70	..	..
10 years	..	..	..	..	..	..	..	..	..	..	..	..	..	..	..	..	..	..
Overall	(14)		(42)		(72)		(42)		(25)		(195)		(60)		(64)		(71)	
1 year	93	93	95	96	86	87	81	84	60	66	84	86	88	90	83	85	81	83
3 years	71	72	71	72	72	75	50	56	47	63	64	69	67	72	62	67	63	68
5 years	71	72	59	60	62	67	43	52	39	65	55	63	53	60	56	64	56	64
8 years	48	48	55	58	60	68	36	52	23	59	45	57	..	..	48	62	..	..
10 years	..	..	..	..	..	..	..	..	..	..	..	..	..	..	..	..	..	..

RELATIVE SURVIVAL (%) BY AGE AND PERIOD

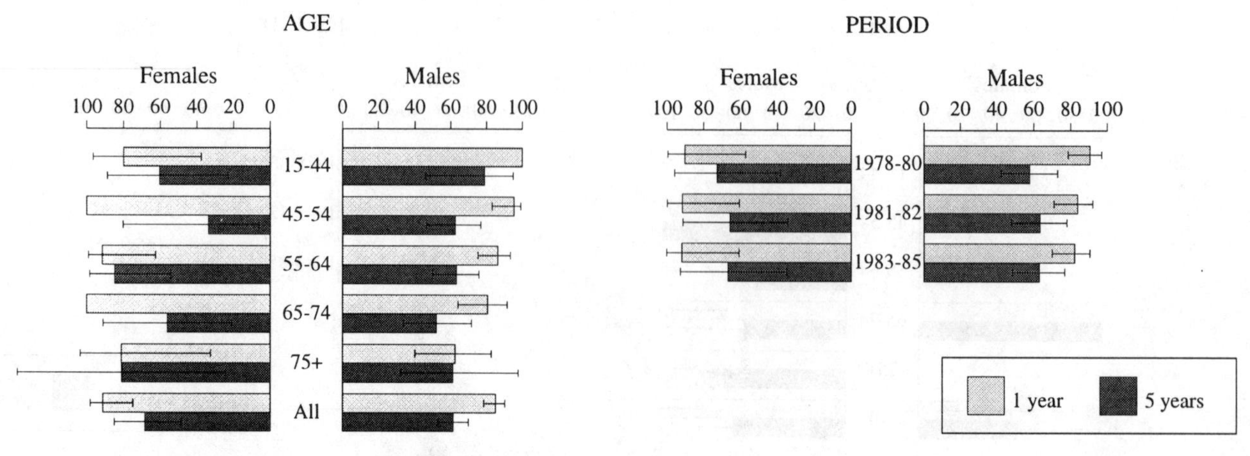

LARYNX

EUROPEAN REGISTRIES

Weighted analysis

REGISTRY	WEIGHTS (Yearly expected cases in the country) Males	Females	All
DENMARK	192	36	228
DUTCH REGISTRIES	293	32	325
ENGLISH REGISTRIES	1203	226	1429
ESTONIA	53	4	57
FINLAND	121	11	132
FRENCH REGISTRIES	8809	231	9040
GERMAN REGISTRIES	2240	148	2388
ITALIAN REGISTRIES	5876	206	6082
POLISH REGISTRIES	2057	186	2243
SCOTLAND	147	42	189
SPANISH REGISTRIES	3866	106	3972
SWISS REGISTRIES	246	29	275

RELATIVE SURVIVAL (%)
(Age-standardized)

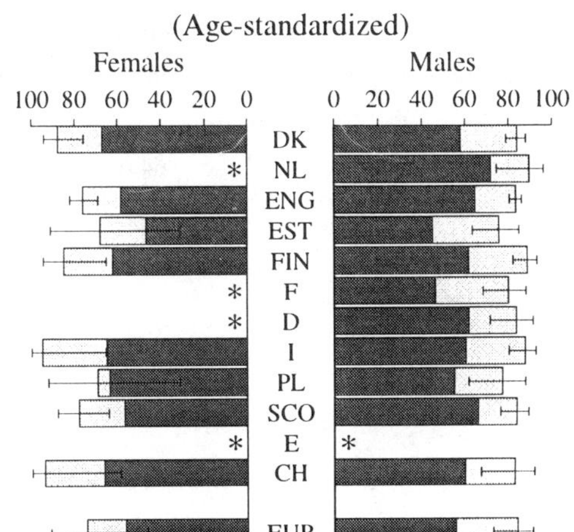

OBSERVED AND RELATIVE SURVIVAL (%) BY AGE AND PERIOD

	AGE CLASS 15-44 obs	rel	45-54 obs	rel	55-64 obs	rel	65-74 obs	rel	75+ obs	rel	All obs	rel	PERIOD 1978-80 obs	rel	1981-82 obs	rel	1983-85 obs	rel
Males																		
1 year	83	84	87	88	87	89	77	81	71	78	82	85	78	81	82	86	83	86
3 years	61	62	71	73	61	64	53	61	38	53	58	64	52	58	60	66	60	66
5 years	57	58	65	68	51	57	40	52	27	48	49	57	44	52	51	61	49	58
8 years	49	51	49	53	43	52	30	47	13	38	38	51	34	46	42	56	43	57
10 years	42	44	45	50	38	49	23	43	10	43	33	47	30	43	33	46	..	..
Females																		
1 year	95	95	89	89	74	74	73	74	49	54	74	76	70	71	79	80	79	81
3 years	91	91	78	78	64	66	58	62	34	45	63	68	59	62	68	71	66	73
5 years	91	91	69	71	60	63	38	43	25	41	54	62	55	62	56	62	55	64
8 years	89	89	63	66	50	55	23	30	14	35	47	58	41	50	52	62	41	53
10 years	88	88	58	62	44	51	17	24	12	37	40	53	36	47	34	45	..	..
Overall																		
1 year	84	84	87	88	87	88	77	80	70	77	82	85	78	80	82	85	83	85
3 years	63	63	72	73	61	64	53	61	38	53	59	64	53	58	60	67	60	66
5 years	58	59	66	68	52	57	40	51	27	48	49	57	45	53	51	61	50	59
8 years	51	53	50	54	43	52	29	47	13	38	38	51	35	46	42	56	43	57
10 years	44	46	45	51	38	49	23	42	10	43	33	48	30	43	33	46	..	..

RELATIVE SURVIVAL (%) BY AGE AND PERIOD

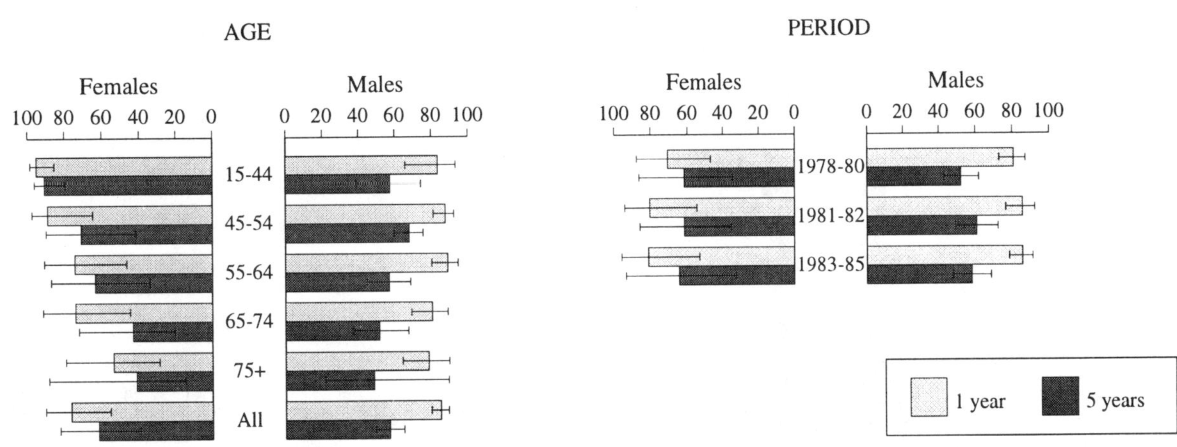

LUNG

DENMARK

REGISTRY	NUMBER OF CASES			PERIOD OF DIAGNOSIS
	Males	Females	All	
Denmark	14084	4820	18904	1978-1984
Mean age (years)	67.1	64.6	66.5	

RELATIVE SURVIVAL (%)

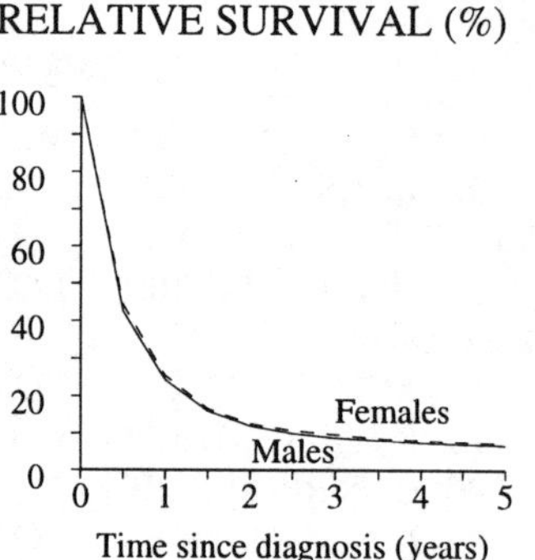

OBSERVED AND RELATIVE SURVIVAL (%) BY AGE AND PERIOD
(Number of cases in parentheses)

	AGE CLASS												PERIOD					
	15-44		45-54		55-64		65-74		75+		All		1978-80		1981-82		1983-85	
	obs	rel	obs	rel	obs	rel	obs	rel	obs	rel	obs	rel	obs	rel	obs	rel	obs	rel
Males	(201)		(1140)		(3921)		(5694)		(3128)		(14084)		(5776)		(4203)		(4105)	
1 year	32	32	32	32	29	29	23	24	14	15	23	24	23	24	23	24	23	24
3 years	18	19	14	14	10	11	7	8	2	3	8	9	8	9	8	9	7	8
5 years	15	15	10	10	8	9	4	6	1	2	5	7	6	8	5	6	4	6
8 years	15	15	8	9	5	6	3	5	0	1	4	5	4	6	3	5	..	..
10 years	15	15	7	8	4	6	2	4	0	2	3	5	4	6	..	..	..	..
Females	(191)		(743)		(1417)		(1509)		(960)		(4820)		(1738)		(1438)		(1644)	
1 year	36	36	35	35	29	29	22	23	13	14	25	25	25	25	27	28	23	24
3 years	15	15	13	13	11	11	8	8	4	5	9	10	10	11	9	10	8	8
5 years	13	13	9	10	8	8	5	6	2	3	6	7	7	8	7	8	5	6
8 years	11	12	8	8	5	6	4	5	0	1	5	6	5	6	5	7	..	..
10 years	9	9	7	7	4	5	4	6	0	1	4	5	4	6	..	..	..	..
Overall	(392)		(1883)		(5338)		(7203)		(4088)		(18904)		(7514)		(5641)		(5749)	
1 year	34	34	33	33	29	29	23	23	14	15	24	25	24	25	24	25	23	24
3 years	17	17	13	14	11	11	7	8	3	4	8	9	9	10	8	9	7	8
5 years	14	14	10	10	8	8	5	6	1	2	5	7	6	8	5	7	5	6
8 years	13	13	8	8	5	6	3	5	0	1	4	6	4	6	4	5	..	..
10 years	12	12	7	8	4	5	3	4	0	1	3	5	4	6	..	..	..	..

RELATIVE SURVIVAL (%) BY AGE AND PERIOD

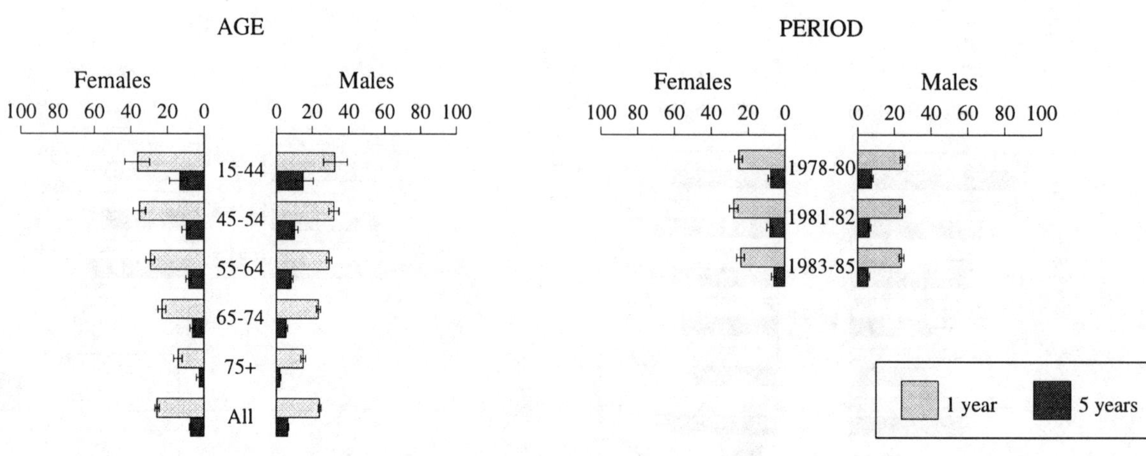

LUNG

DUTCH REGISTRIES

REGISTRY	NUMBER OF CASES			PERIOD OF DIAGNOSIS
	Males	Females	All	
Eindhoven	3138	243	3381	1978-1985
Mean age (years)	66.1	60.6	65.7	

RELATIVE SURVIVAL (%)

OBSERVED AND RELATIVE SURVIVAL (%) BY AGE AND PERIOD
(Number of cases in parentheses)

	AGE CLASS												PERIOD					
	15-44		45-54		55-64		65-74		75+		All		1978-80		1981-82		1983-85	
	obs	rel	obs	rel	obs	rel	obs	rel	obs	rel	obs	rel	obs	rel	obs	rel	obs	rel
Males	(63)		(333)		(864)		(1252)		(626)		(3138)		(1153)		(811)		(1174)	
1 year	31	31	44	44	43	44	38	39	28	31	38	39	36	37	37	39	40	42
3 years	14	15	22	22	18	19	12	14	5	8	14	16	12	14	14	16	14	17
5 years	13	13	19	19	13	15	8	10	2	3	9	12	8	10	10	13	10	13
8 years	..	..	17	18	9	11	4	6	1	3	6	10	5	8	..	..	..	..
10 years	..	..	16	17	8	11	3	6	1	3	6	10	4	8	..	..	..	..
Females	(24)		(57)		(68)		(59)		(35)		(243)		(71)		(66)		(106)	
1 year	67	67	44	44	49	49	37	38	17	18	42	43	41	42	39	40	44	45
3 years	37	37	22	23	16	16	23	25	3	4	19	20	17	18	26	27	17	18
5 years	37	37	18	19	12	13	18	20	..	..	16	18	14	16	20	22	17	19
8 years	37	37	18	19	10	10	13	16	..	..	14	16	11	14	..	..	..	..
10 years	37	37	..	..	..	..	4	6	..	..	8	10	6	8	..	..	..	..
Overall	(87)		(390)		(932)		(1311)		(661)		(3381)		(1224)		(877)		(1280)	
1 year	41	41	44	44	44	44	38	39	27	30	38	40	36	37	38	39	40	42
3 years	21	21	22	23	18	19	13	15	5	7	14	16	13	14	15	17	15	17
5 years	19	20	19	19	13	14	8	10	2	3	10	12	8	10	11	14	11	14
8 years	19	20	17	18	9	11	4	7	1	3	7	10	5	8	..	..	..	..
10 years	19	20	16	17	8	11	2	4	1	3	5	9	4	7	..	..	..	..

RELATIVE SURVIVAL (%) BY AGE AND PERIOD

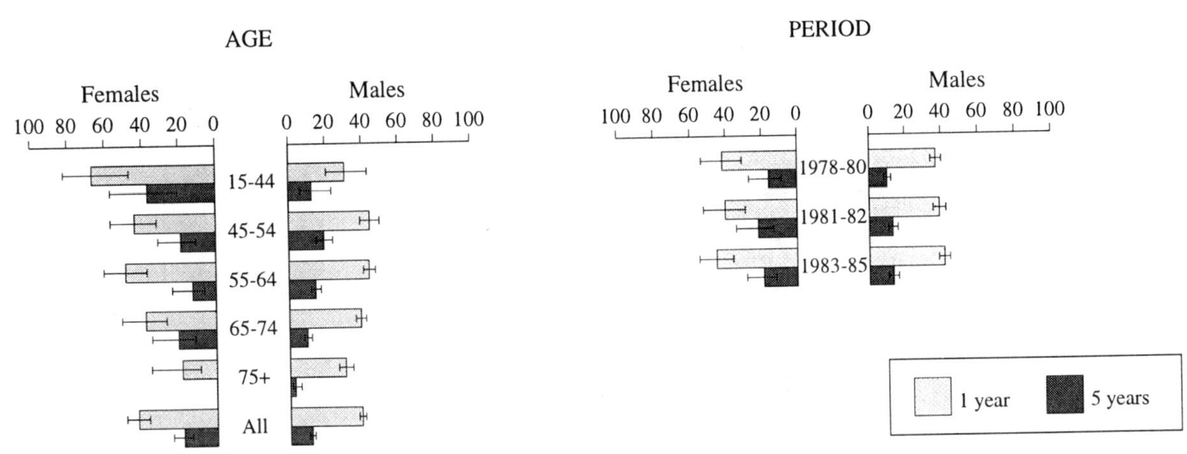

LUNG

ENGLISH REGISTRIES

REGISTRY	NUMBER OF CASES			PERIOD OF DIAGNOSIS
	Males	Females	All	
East Anglia	6279	2002	8281	1979-1984
Mersey	9565	3409	12974	1978-1984
South Thames	23674	8755	32429	1978-1984
Wessex	2453	930	3383	1983-1984
West Midlands	14659	3858	18517	1979-1984
Yorkshire	13621	4434	18055	1978-1984
Mean age (years)	67.9	67.8	67.9	

RELATIVE SURVIVAL (%)

100
80
60
40
20
0
Males
Females
0 1 2 3 4 5
Time since diagnosis (years)

OBSERVED AND RELATIVE SURVIVAL (%) BY AGE AND PERIOD
(Number of cases in parentheses)

	AGE CLASS												PERIOD					
	15-44		45-54		55-64		65-74		75+		All		1978-80		1981-82		1983-85	
	obs	rel	obs	rel	obs	rel	obs	rel	obs	rel	obs	rel	obs	rel	obs	rel	obs	rel
Males	(957)		(5038)		(18083)		(28472)		(17701)		(70251)		(28373)		(20429)		(21449)	
1 year	32	32	29	29	25	26	19	20	12	14	20	21	19	20	20	21	20	21
3 years	14	15	12	12	9	10	6	7	2	4	6	8	6	7	6	8	7	8
5 years	12	12	10	10	7	8	4	5	1	2	5	6	4	6	5	6	5	6
8 years	10	11	8	9	5	7	3	4	1	2	3	5	3	5	3	5	4	6
10 years	10	11	7	8	4	6	2	4	1	3	3	5	3	5	3	5	..	..
Females	(439)		(1906)		(6182)		(8588)		(6273)		(23388)		(8843)		(6900)		(7645)	
1 year	31	31	25	26	24	24	19	19	11	11	19	19	17	18	19	19	20	20
3 years	16	16	11	11	9	9	6	6	3	4	6	7	6	7	6	7	7	8
5 years	13	13	9	9	7	7	4	5	1	2	5	6	4	5	4	5	5	6
8 years	12	13	7	8	5	6	3	4	1	2	4	5	3	5	4	5	4	5
10 years	11	12	6	7	5	5	3	4	1	3	3	5	3	5	3	5	..	..
Overall	(1396)		(6944)		(24265)		(37060)		(23974)		(93639)		(37216)		(27329)		(29094)	
1 year	31	32	28	28	25	25	19	20	12	13	20	20	19	20	20	21	20	21
3 years	15	15	12	12	9	10	6	7	3	4	6	7	6	7	6	7	7	8
5 years	12	13	9	10	7	8	4	5	1	2	5	6	4	6	5	6	5	6
8 years	11	11	8	8	5	6	3	4	1	2	3	5	3	5	3	5	4	6
10 years	11	11	7	8	5	6	2	4	1	3	3	5	3	5	3	5	..	..

RELATIVE SURVIVAL (%) BY AGE AND PERIOD

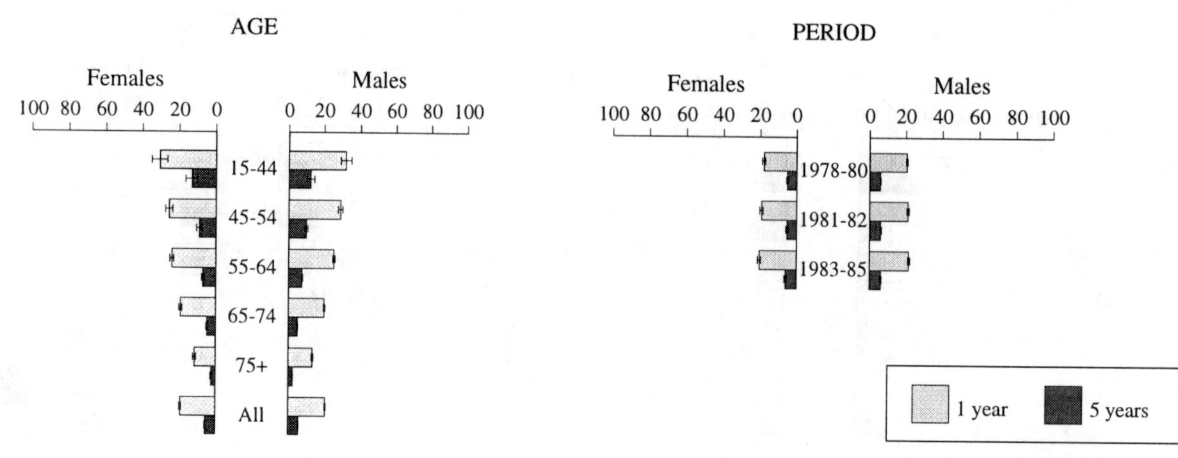

LUNG

ESTONIA

REGISTRY	NUMBER OF CASES			PERIOD OF DIAGNOSIS
	Males	Females	All	
Estonia	2731	500	3231	1978-1984
Mean age (years)	61.9	65.0	62.4	

RELATIVE SURVIVAL (%)

OBSERVED AND RELATIVE SURVIVAL (%) BY AGE AND PERIOD
(Number of cases in parentheses)

	AGE CLASS												PERIOD					
	15-44		45-54		55-64		65-74		75+		All		1978-80		1981-82		1983-85	
	obs	rel	obs	rel	obs	rel	obs	rel	obs	rel	obs	rel	obs	rel	obs	rel	obs	rel
Males	(123)		(570)		(871)		(849)		(318)		(2731)		(1090)		(830)		(811)	
1 year	33	33	35	35	32	33	23	24	27	31	29	30	30	32	29	30	28	29
3 years	18	18	15	15	11	12	4	5	5	8	9	11	10	11	11	12	8	9
5 years	14	15	9	10	8	9	2	3	2	3	6	8	6	8	7	9	5	6
8 years	13	14	7	8	6	8	1	3	1	2	4	7	5	7	5	8	..	..
10 years	9	10	7	8	4	6	1	2	..	..	4	6	4	6	..	..	..	..
Females	(12)		(89)		(129)		(167)		(103)		(500)		(208)		(140)		(152)	
1 year	33	33	26	26	25	25	27	28	36	39	28	29	30	31	29	30	25	26
3 years	33	34	19	19	11	11	10	11	14	19	13	15	14	15	14	16	11	13
5 years	33	34	17	17	7	7	5	6	4	7	8	10	7	9	11	13	7	8
8 years	33	34	10	10	7	8	3	4	3	7	6	8	4	6	8	11	..	..
10 years	..	..	10	10	7	8	3	5	..	..	5	8	4	6	..	..	..	..
Overall	(135)		(659)		(1000)		(1016)		(421)		(3231)		(1298)		(970)		(963)	
1 year	33	33	34	34	31	32	24	25	29	33	29	30	30	32	29	30	27	28
3 years	19	19	15	16	11	12	5	6	7	11	10	11	10	12	11	13	8	9
5 years	16	16	10	11	8	9	3	4	2	4	6	8	6	8	8	9	5	6
8 years	15	16	7	8	6	8	2	3	1	4	5	7	5	7	6	8	..	..
10 years	11	12	7	8	5	6	1	3	..	..	4	6	4	6	..	..	..	..

RELATIVE SURVIVAL (%) BY AGE AND PERIOD

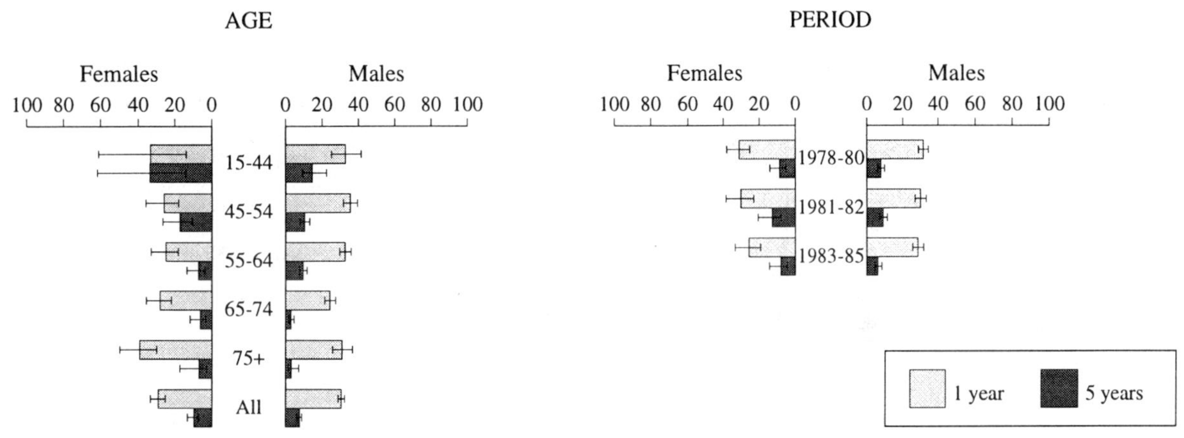

LUNG

FINLAND

REGISTRY	NUMBER OF CASES			PERIOD OF DIAGNOSIS
	Males	Females	All	
Finland	12509	1710	14219	1978-1984
Mean age (years)	65.8	66.6	65.9	

RELATIVE SURVIVAL (%)

100
80
60
40
20
0
Females
Males
0 1 2 3 4 5
Time since diagnosis (years)

OBSERVED AND RELATIVE SURVIVAL (%) BY AGE AND PERIOD
(Number of cases in parentheses)

	AGE CLASS											
	15-44		45-54		55-64		65-74		75+		All	
	obs	rel	obs	rel	obs	rel	obs	rel	obs	rel	obs	rel
Males	(197)		(1246)		(3927)		(4867)		(2272)		(12509)	
1 year	39	39	45	45	44	45	38	40	30	33	39	41
3 years	18	18	17	18	18	19	10	12	5	8	13	15
5 years	14	14	13	14	12	14	6	8	2	3	8	10
8 years	11	11	9	10	8	10	3	6	0	1	5	8
10 years	9	9	8	9	6	9	2	5	0	1	4	7
Females	(64)		(179)		(440)		(599)		(428)		(1710)	
1 year	47	47	51	52	49	49	40	41	25	27	40	41
3 years	25	25	24	24	21	21	14	15	5	7	15	17
5 years	19	19	21	21	14	14	8	9	1	2	10	11
8 years	16	16	15	15	10	11	5	7	0	0	7	9
10 years	8	8	14	15	7	8	4	6	0	0	5	8
Overall	(261)		(1425)		(4367)		(5466)		(2700)		(14219)	
1 year	41	41	46	46	45	46	38	40	29	32	39	41
3 years	20	20	18	19	18	20	11	13	5	8	13	15
5 years	15	15	14	15	12	14	6	8	2	3	8	10
8 years	12	12	10	11	8	10	4	6	0	1	5	8
10 years	9	9	9	10	6	9	3	5	0	1	4	7

	PERIOD					
	1978-80		1981-82		1983-85	
	obs	rel	obs	rel	obs	rel
Males	(5473)		(3539)		(3497)	
1 year	39	41	39	41	39	41
3 years	13	15	13	15	13	15
5 years	8	10	8	10	8	11
8 years	5	7	5	8	6	9
10 years	4	6	5	8	..	..
Females	(696)		(473)		(541)	
1 year	40	42	39	40	40	41
3 years	16	17	15	16	15	17
5 years	10	12	9	10	9	11
8 years	6	9	7	9	8	10
10 years	5	7	5	7	..	..
Overall	(6169)		(4012)		(4038)	
1 year	39	41	39	41	39	41
3 years	13	15	13	15	13	15
5 years	8	10	8	10	9	11
8 years	5	7	5	8	6	9
10 years	4	6	5	8	..	..

RELATIVE SURVIVAL (%) BY AGE AND PERIOD

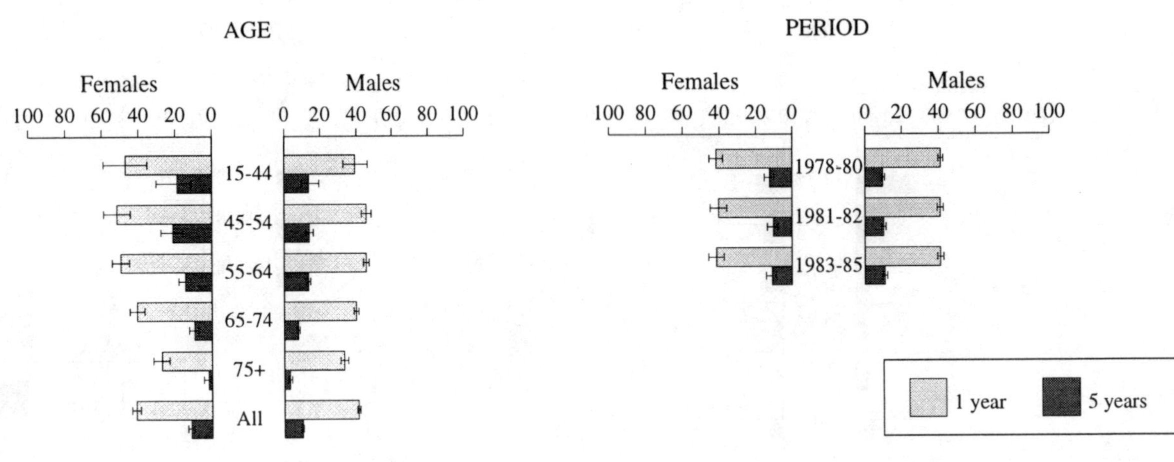

LUNG

FRENCH REGISTRIES

REGISTRY	NUMBER OF CASES			PERIOD OF DIAGNOSIS
	Males	Females	All	
Amiens	426	33	459	1983-1984
Doubs	1100	81	1181	1978-1985
Mean age (years)	63.3	62.9	63.3	

RELATIVE SURVIVAL (%)

Females
Males
Time since diagnosis (years)

OBSERVED AND RELATIVE SURVIVAL (%) BY AGE AND PERIOD
(Number of cases in parentheses)

	AGE CLASS												PERIOD					
	15-44		45-54		55-64		65-74		75+		All		1978-80		1981-82		1983-85	
	obs	rel	obs	rel	obs	rel	obs	rel	obs	rel	obs	rel	obs	rel	obs	rel	obs	rel
Males	(75)		(258)		(478)		(476)		(239)		(1526)		(424)		(276)		(826)	
1 year	51	52	48	48	40	41	36	38	29	32	39	41	40	41	42	43	38	39
3 years	20	21	22	22	14	15	10	11	5	7	13	15	13	14	15	17	12	14
5 years	16	16	18	19	11	12	6	7	2	3	9	11	9	10	13	15	9	10
8 years	15	15	14	15	6	8	5	7	..	..	7	9	6	8	11	16	5	7
10 years	15	15	14	15	6	8	5	8	..	..	7	10	6	8	..	..	..	..
Females	(10)		(15)		(36)		(31)		(22)		(114)		(28)		(22)		(64)	
1 year	50	50	67	67	36	36	23	23	36	39	38	38	39	40	36	37	38	38
3 years	40	40	40	40	13	13	13	14	9	11	18	19	25	26	5	5	20	22
5 years	40	40	40	41	10	10	10	11	5	7	15	17	25	27	0	0	17	19
8 years	..	..	40	41	10	10	5	6	5	10	14	17	25	29	0	0	..	..
10 years	..	..	40	42	0	0	5	6	5	14	11	15	20	24	0	0	..	..
Overall	(85)		(273)		(514)		(507)		(261)		(1640)		(452)		(298)		(890)	
1 year	51	51	49	50	40	40	36	37	29	33	39	40	40	41	41	43	38	39
3 years	23	23	23	23	14	15	10	11	6	8	13	15	14	15	14	16	13	14
5 years	19	19	19	20	11	12	6	8	2	3	10	12	10	12	12	14	9	11
8 years	17	18	15	16	7	8	5	7	2	5	7	10	7	9	10	14	6	8
10 years	17	18	15	17	5	6	5	8	2	7	7	10	7	9	..	..	..	..

RELATIVE SURVIVAL (%) BY AGE AND PERIOD

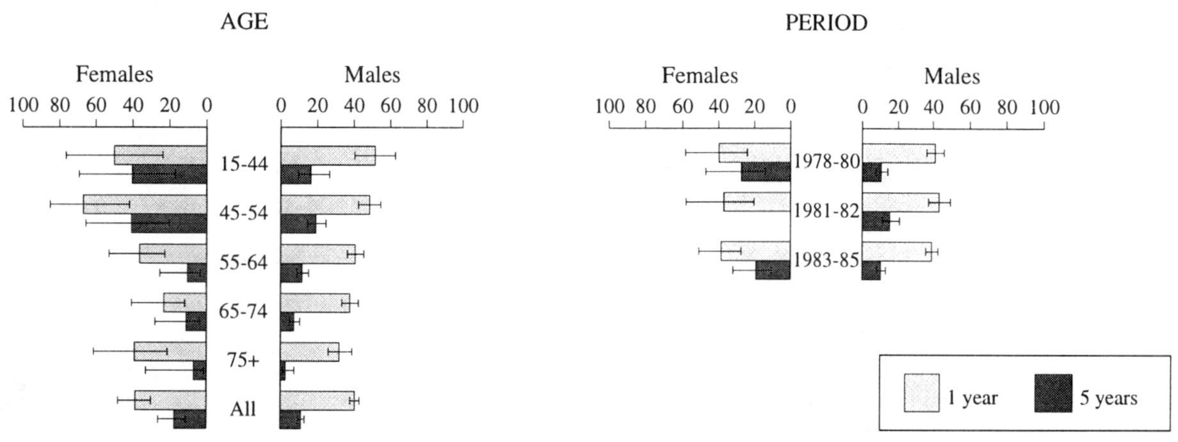

LUNG

GERMAN REGISTRIES

REGISTRY	NUMBER OF CASES			PERIOD OF DIAGNOSIS
	Males	Females	All	
Saarland	2871	391	3262	1978-1984
Mean age (years)	65.1	64.5	65.0	

RELATIVE SURVIVAL (%)

OBSERVED AND RELATIVE SURVIVAL (%) BY AGE AND PERIOD
(Number of cases in parentheses)

	AGE CLASS												PERIOD					
	15-44		45-54		55-64		65-74		75+		All		1978-80		1981-82		1983-85	
	obs	rel	obs	rel	obs	rel	obs	rel	obs	rel	obs	rel	obs	rel	obs	rel	obs	rel
Males	(89)		(396)		(771)		(1082)		(533)		(2871)		(1255)		(807)		(809)	
1 year	38	38	40	40	29	29	25	26	19	21	27	29	26	28	29	30	28	29
3 years	19	19	17	18	12	13	6	8	4	6	10	11	9	11	11	13	9	10
5 years	17	17	14	15	10	11	4	6	3	5	7	9	7	9	8	10	7	9
8 years	13	14	12	13	7	9	4	6	2	6	6	9	5	9	6	10	..	..
10 years	13	14	9	10	6	8	3	7	2	9	5	9	5	9	..	..	..	..
Females	(21)		(44)		(117)		(139)		(70)		(391)		(165)		(109)		(117)	
1 year	48	48	41	41	35	35	27	28	17	19	30	31	35	36	33	34	22	23
3 years	19	19	18	18	13	13	11	12	7	9	12	13	13	15	13	14	9	10
5 years	19	19	18	19	9	10	8	9	4	7	9	11	10	12	11	13	8	9
8 years	19	19	18	19	9	10	6	8	2	5	8	11	8	10	10	13	..	..
10 years	19	19	18	19	9	11	6	9	2	6	8	12	8	11	..	..	..	..
Overall	(110)		(440)		(888)		(1221)		(603)		(3262)		(1420)		(916)		(926)	
1 year	40	40	40	41	30	30	25	26	18	21	28	29	27	29	29	30	27	28
3 years	19	19	18	18	13	13	7	8	5	7	10	11	10	11	11	13	9	10
5 years	17	18	14	15	10	11	5	6	3	5	7	10	7	10	8	10	7	9
8 years	14	15	12	13	7	9	4	6	2	6	6	9	6	9	7	10	..	..
10 years	14	15	10	11	6	8	4	7	2	9	5	9	5	9	..	..	..	..

RELATIVE SURVIVAL (%) BY AGE AND PERIOD

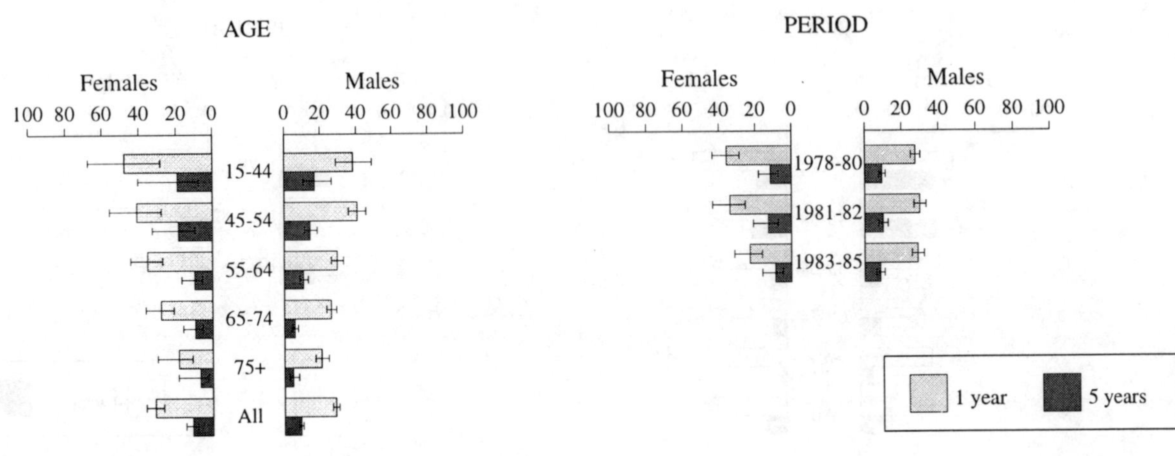

LUNG

ITALIAN REGISTRIES

REGISTRY	NUMBER OF CASES Males	Females	All	PERIOD OF DIAGNOSIS
Florence	580	99	679	1985-1985
Latina	226	32	258	1983-1984
Ragusa	271	36	307	1981-1984
Varese	2534	306	2840	1978-1984
Mean age (years)	63.7	66.9	64.1	

RELATIVE SURVIVAL (%)

OBSERVED AND RELATIVE SURVIVAL (%) BY AGE AND PERIOD
(Number of cases in parentheses)

	AGE CLASS												PERIOD					
	15-44		45-54		55-64		65-74		75+		All		1978-80		1981-82		1983-85	
	obs	rel	obs	rel	obs	rel	obs	rel	obs	rel	obs	rel	obs	rel	obs	rel	obs	rel
Males	(113)		(574)		(1190)		(1206)		(528)		(3611)		(1028)		(872)		(1711)	
1 year	41	41	36	36	33	34	30	31	21	23	31	32	29	30	33	34	31	33
3 years	18	18	11	11	12	13	7	8	4	6	9	10	7	8	10	11	11	12
5 years	14	14	9	9	9	10	4	5	0	1	6	8	4	5	6	7	7	9
8 years	12	13	6	7	6	7	2	4	..	..	4	6	3	4	4	6	5	7
10 years	12	13	5	6	5	6	1	3	..	..	3	5	2	4	3	5	..	..
Females	(16)		(56)		(108)		(159)		(134)		(473)		(117)		(91)		(265)	
1 year	44	44	46	47	37	37	23	24	19	21	29	30	23	24	32	33	30	31
3 years	31	31	20	20	21	22	11	12	7	10	14	16	9	10	13	15	17	18
5 years	25	25	13	13	16	16	6	7	7	11	10	12	3	4	10	12	13	15
8 years	25	25	13	13	13	14	..	..	2	5	8	10	2	2	7	9	12	16
10 years	..	..	..	..	8	9	..	..	..	..	6	8	2	2	..	..	..	..
Overall	(129)		(630)		(1298)		(1365)		(662)		(4084)		(1145)		(963)		(1976)	
1 year	41	41	37	37	34	34	29	31	21	23	31	32	28	29	33	34	31	32
3 years	19	20	12	12	13	13	8	9	5	6	10	11	7	8	10	11	11	13
5 years	16	16	9	9	9	10	4	6	2	3	7	8	4	5	6	8	8	10
8 years	14	14	7	7	7	8	3	4	1	1	5	6	3	4	5	6	6	8
10 years	14	14	6	7	5	6	2	3	..	..	4	6	2	4	3	5	..	..

RELATIVE SURVIVAL (%) BY AGE AND PERIOD

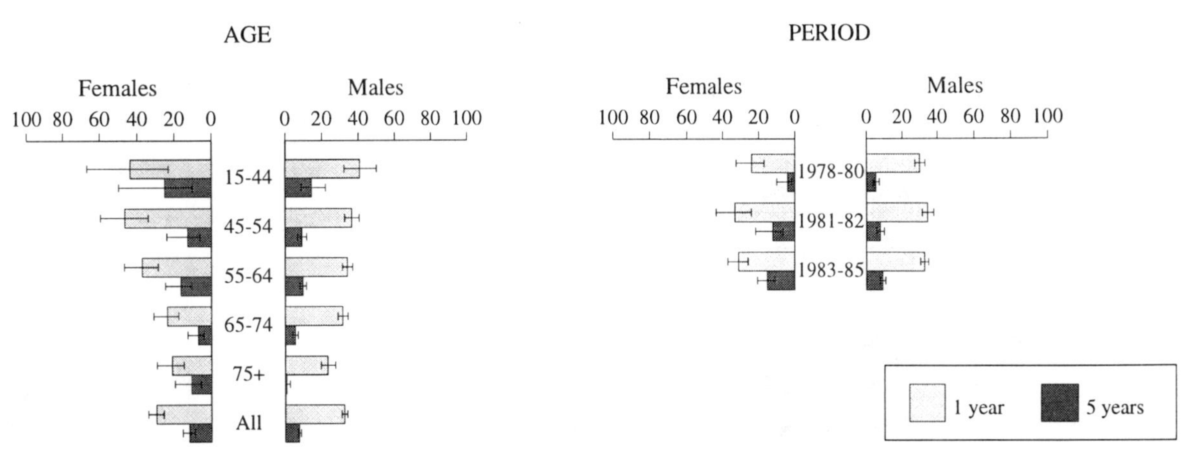

LUNG

POLISH REGISTRIES

REGISTRY	NUMBER OF CASES Males	Females	All	PERIOD OF DIAGNOSIS
Cracow	1625	409	2034	1978-1984
Mean age (years)	62.2	64.3	62.6	

RELATIVE SURVIVAL (%)

100, 80, 60, 40, 20, 0

Females

Males

0 1 2 3 4 5

Time since diagnosis (years)

OBSERVED AND RELATIVE SURVIVAL (%) BY AGE AND PERIOD
(Number of cases in parentheses)

	AGE CLASS												PERIOD					
	15-44		45-54		55-64		65-74		75+		All		1978-80		1981-82		1983-85	
	obs	rel	obs	rel	obs	rel	obs	rel	obs	rel	obs	rel	obs	rel	obs	rel	obs	rel
Males	(75)		(315)		(532)		(503)		(200)		(1625)		(672)		(450)		(503)	
1 year	35	35	27	28	27	27	17	18	13	15	22	23	25	26	20	21	22	23
3 years	19	19	11	12	9	9	3	4	4	6	7	8	8	9	7	7	7	8
5 years	16	16	9	10	6	7	2	2	2	4	5	7	5	7	5	7	5	6
8 years	13	14	7	8	4	5	2	3	2	5	4	6	4	6	5	7	4	5
10 years	13	14	6	7	3	4	2	4	2	7	3	6	3	5	5	8	..	..
Females	(17)		(72)		(106)		(125)		(89)		(409)		(161)		(126)		(122)	
1 year	53	53	30	30	26	27	20	21	17	19	24	25	20	20	30	31	24	25
3 years	35	35	16	16	8	8	10	11	12	15	12	13	10	11	12	13	15	16
5 years	29	30	16	16	6	6	8	9	7	11	9	11	8	9	9	10	12	14
8 years	22	22	14	15	5	5	6	9	6	14	8	10	6	8	9	11	8	11
10 years	..	..	14	15	5	6	6	10	6	19	8	11	6	9	9	12	..	..
Overall	(92)		(387)		(638)		(628)		(289)		(2034)		(833)		(576)		(625)	
1 year	38	38	28	28	27	27	17	18	14	16	23	24	24	25	22	23	22	23
3 years	22	22	12	12	8	9	5	5	6	9	8	9	8	9	8	9	9	10
5 years	19	19	10	11	6	7	3	4	4	7	6	8	6	7	6	8	7	8
8 years	15	15	9	10	4	5	3	4	3	8	5	7	5	7	6	8	5	6
10 years	15	16	8	9	3	4	3	5	3	12	4	7	4	6	6	9	..	..

RELATIVE SURVIVAL (%) BY AGE AND PERIOD

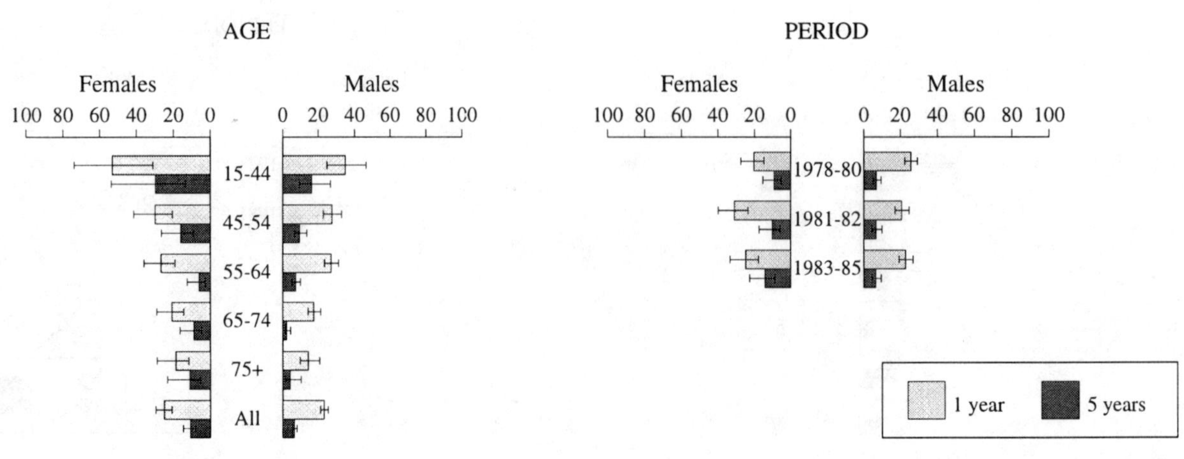

LUNG

SCOTLAND

REGISTRY	NUMBER OF CASES			PERIOD OF DIAGNOSIS
	Males	Females	All	
Scotland	15027	5460	20487	1978-1982
Mean age (years)	66.7	65.6	66.4	

RELATIVE SURVIVAL (%)

100
80
60
40
20
0
Females
Males
0 1 2 3 4 5
Time since diagnosis (years)

OBSERVED AND RELATIVE SURVIVAL (%) BY AGE AND PERIOD
(Number of cases in parentheses)

	AGE CLASS												PERIOD					
	15-44		45-54		55-64		65-74		75+		All		1978-80		1981-82		1983-85	
	obs	rel	obs	rel	obs	rel	obs	rel	obs	rel	obs	rel	obs	rel	obs	rel	obs	rel
Males	(247)		(1389)		(4114)		(6143)		(3134)		(15027)		(9138)		(5889)		(0)	
1 year	30	30	28	29	25	26	19	20	12	14	20	22	20	21	21	22	..	..
3 years	14	14	13	14	10	11	6	7	3	4	7	8	7	8	7	9	..	..
5 years	12	12	10	11	7	8	4	6	1	3	5	7	5	7	5	7	..	..
8 years	11	11	9	9	6	7	2	4	1	3	4	6	4	6	..	..	..	..
10 years	11	12	7	9	4	6	2	4	1	4	3	6	3	6	..	..	..	..
Females	(155)		(645)		(1615)		(1928)		(1117)		(5460)		(3149)		(2311)		(0)	
1 year	39	39	26	27	26	26	19	19	12	13	21	21	20	21	21	22	..	..
3 years	18	18	12	12	10	10	7	7	3	4	8	9	8	9	7	8	..	..
5 years	18	18	9	10	8	8	5	5	2	4	6	7	6	7	6	7	..	..
8 years	17	18	9	9	6	7	4	5	1	3	5	7	5	7	..	..	..	..
10 years	17	18	8	9	6	7	1	2	1	2	4	6	4	6	..	..	..	..
Overall	(402)		(2034)		(5729)		(8071)		(4251)		(20487)		(12287)		(8200)		(0)	
1 year	34	34	28	28	25	26	19	20	12	13	20	22	20	21	21	22	..	..
3 years	16	16	13	13	10	11	6	7	3	4	7	9	7	9	7	9	..	..
5 years	14	15	10	10	7	8	4	6	2	3	5	7	5	7	5	7	..	..
8 years	14	14	9	9	6	7	3	4	1	3	4	6	4	6	..	..	..	..
10 years	14	14	8	9	5	6	2	4	1	3	3	6	3	6	..	..	..	..

RELATIVE SURVIVAL (%) BY AGE AND PERIOD

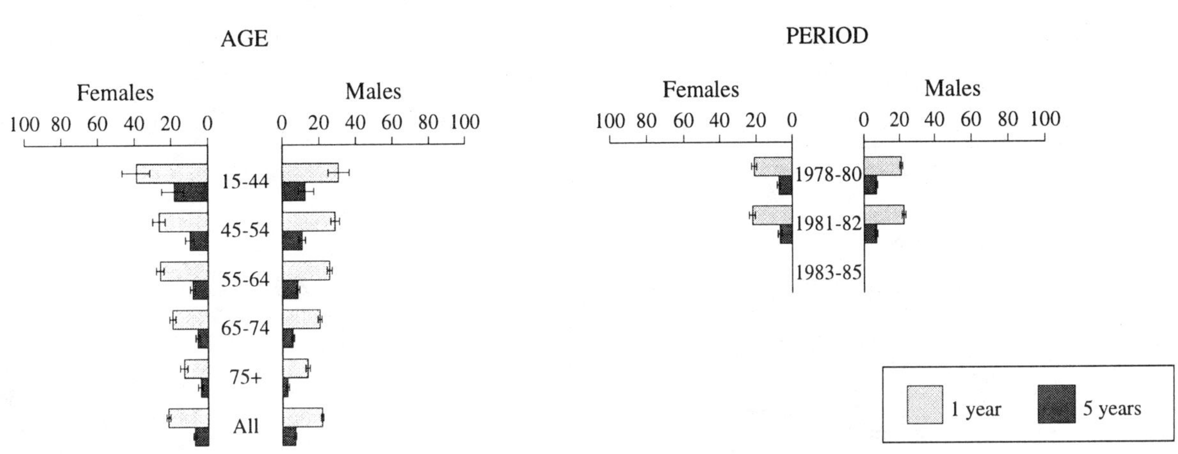

LUNG

SPANISH REGISTRIES

REGISTRY	NUMBER OF CASES			PERIOD OF DIAGNOSIS
	Males	Females	All	
Granada	154	16	170	1985-1985
Tarragona	145	13	158	1985-1985
Mean age (years)	64.3	63.7	64.2	

RELATIVE SURVIVAL (%)

OBSERVED AND RELATIVE SURVIVAL (%) BY AGE AND PERIOD
(Number of cases in parentheses)

	AGE CLASS												PERIOD					
	15-44		45-54		55-64		65-74		75+		All		1978-80		1981-82		1983-85	
	obs	rel	obs	rel	obs	rel	obs	rel	obs	rel	obs	rel	obs	rel	obs	rel	obs	rel
Males	(11)		(39)		(99)		(103)		(47)		(299)		(0)		(0)		(299)	
1 year	18	18	31	31	35	36	19	20	19	21	26	27	..	..	..	..	26	27
3 years	9	9	10	10	9	9	2	2	4	6	6	7	..	..	..	..	6	7
5 years	9	9	8	8	8	8	2	3	2	4	5	6	..	..	..	..	5	6
8 years	..	..	..	..	..	..	..	..	..	..	..	..	..	..	..	..	..	..
10 years	..	..	..	..	..	..	..	..	..	..	..	..	..	..	..	..	..	..
Females	(0)		(6)		(6)		(15)		(2)		(29)		(0)		(0)		(29)	
1 year	..	..	83	84	33	34	20	20	50	53	38	39	..	..	..	..	38	39
3 years	..	..	50	50	17	17	7	7	0	0	17	18	..	..	..	..	17	18
5 years	..	..	50	51	17	17	7	7	0	0	17	19	..	..	..	..	17	19
8 years	..	..	..	..	..	..	..	..	0	0	..	..	..	..	..	..	..	..
10 years	..	..	..	..	..	..	..	..	0	0	..	..	..	..	..	..	..	..
Overall	(11)		(45)		(105)		(118)		(49)		(328)		(0)		(0)		(328)	
1 year	18	18	38	38	35	36	20	20	20	22	27	28	..	..	..	..	27	28
3 years	9	9	16	16	9	10	3	3	4	6	7	8	..	..	..	..	7	8
5 years	9	9	13	14	8	9	3	3	2	3	6	7	..	..	..	..	6	7
8 years	..	..	..	..	..	..	..	..	..	..	..	..	..	..	..	..	..	..
10 years	..	..	..	..	..	..	..	..	..	..	..	..	..	..	..	..	..	..

RELATIVE SURVIVAL (%) BY AGE AND PERIOD

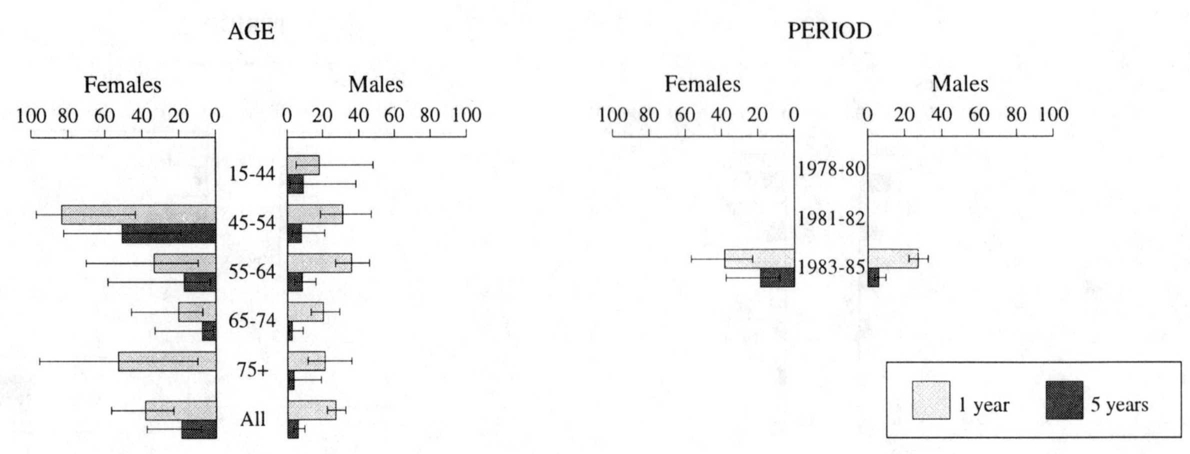

LUNG

SWISS REGISTRIES

REGISTRY	NUMBER OF CASES			PERIOD OF DIAGNOSIS
	Males	Females	All	
Basel	622	115	737	1981-1984
Geneva	937	203	1140	1978-1984
Mean age (years)	65.2	65.3	65.2	

RELATIVE SURVIVAL (%)

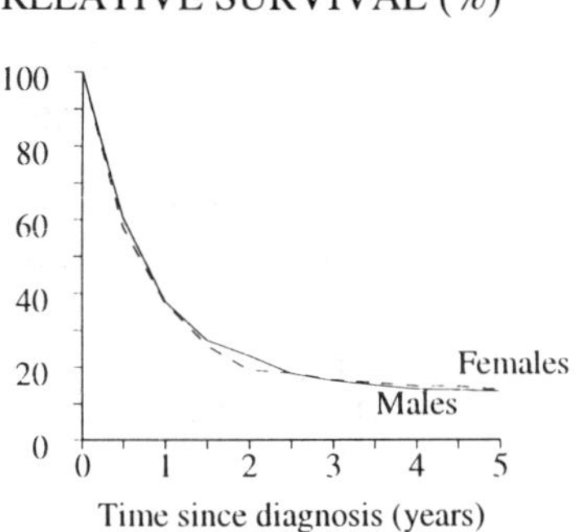

OBSERVED AND RELATIVE SURVIVAL (%) BY AGE AND PERIOD
(Number of cases in parentheses)

	AGE CLASS												PERIOD					
	15-44		45-54		55-64		65-74		75+		All		1978-80		1981-82		1983-85	
	obs	rel	obs	rel	obs	rel	obs	rel	obs	rel	obs	rel	obs	rel	obs	rel	obs	rel
Males	(51)		(184)		(481)		(525)		(318)		(1559)		(399)		(589)		(571)	
1 year	60	60	47	47	41	41	38	39	19	21	36	38	36	38	35	36	38	40
3 years	34	34	20	20	20	21	12	13	4	5	14	16	11	12	14	16	18	20
5 years	30	30	16	16	16	17	9	11	3	4	11	13	8	10	11	13	13	16
8 years	30	31	14	15	13	15	6	10	3	7	9	13	..	..	9	13	..	..
10 years	..	..	..	..	..	..	..	..	..	..	..	..	..	..	..	..	..	..
Females	(21)		(43)		(74)		(102)		(78)		(318)		(88)		(103)		(127)	
1 year	43	43	60	61	42	42	35	36	18	19	36	37	43	44	33	34	35	35
3 years	24	24	23	23	19	19	16	17	5	6	15	17	22	23	16	18	10	11
5 years	24	24	23	23	14	14	13	14	1	2	12	14	17	19	13	15	8	9
8 years	..	..	23	23	8	8	13	16	..	..	9	12	..	..	11	14	..	..
10 years	..	..	..	..	..	..	..	..	..	..	..	..	..	..	..	..	..	..
Overall	(72)		(227)		(555)		(627)		(396)		(1877)		(487)		(692)		(698)	
1 year	55	55	49	49	41	41	37	38	19	20	36	38	38	39	35	36	38	39
3 years	31	31	20	21	20	21	13	14	4	5	15	16	13	14	14	16	16	18
5 years	28	29	17	18	15	17	9	11	2	4	11	14	10	12	11	13	12	15
8 years	28	29	16	17	12	14	7	10	2	6	9	13	..	..	9	13	..	..
10 years	..	..	..	..	..	..	..	..	..	..	..	..	..	..	..	..	..	..

RELATIVE SURVIVAL (%) BY AGE AND PERIOD

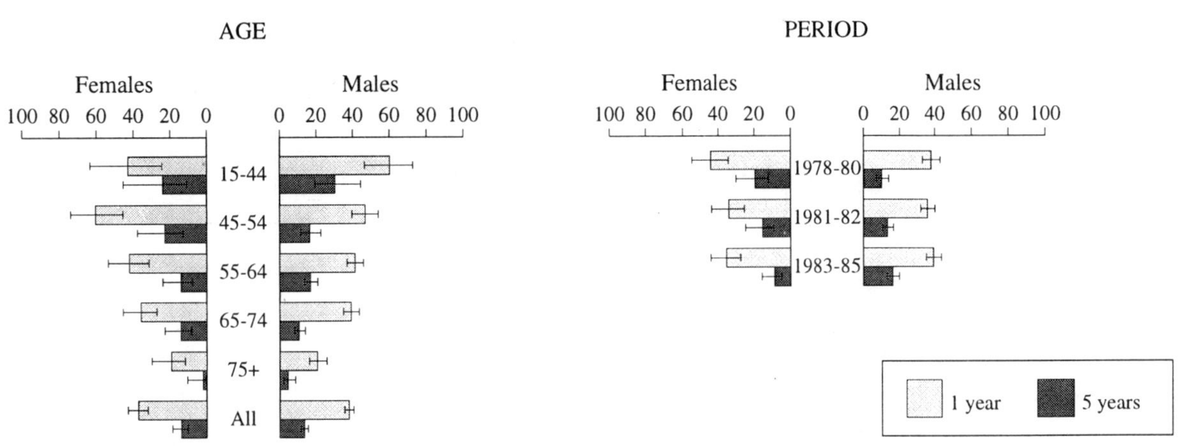

LUNG

EUROPEAN REGISTRIES
Weighted analysis

REGISTRY	WEIGHTS (Yearly expected cases in the country) Males	Females	All
DENMARK	2012	688	2700
DUTCH REGISTRIES	7804	743	8547
ENGLISH REGISTRIES	31149	8559	39708
ESTONIA	390	71	461
FINLAND	1789	245	2034
FRENCH REGISTRIES	18747	1976	20723
GERMAN REGISTRIES	24663	3914	28577
ITALIAN REGISTRIES	25963	3023	28986
POLISH REGISTRIES	11470	2173	13643
SCOTLAND	3006	1092	4098
SPANISH REGISTRIES	9048	1127	10175
SWISS REGISTRIES	2539	453	2992

RELATIVE SURVIVAL (%)
(Age-standardized)

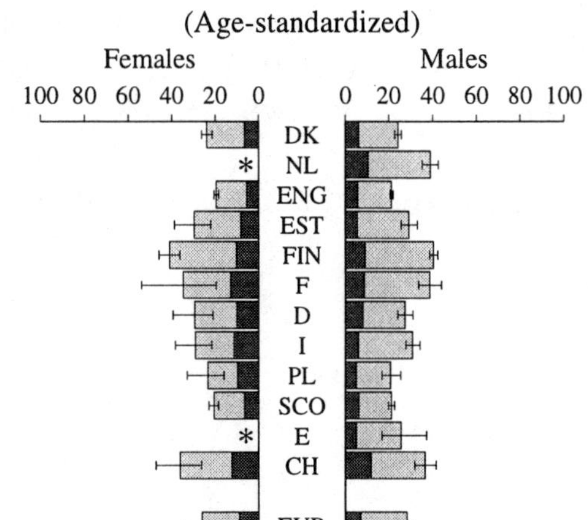

* Not enough cases for reliable estimation

OBSERVED AND RELATIVE SURVIVAL (%) BY AGE AND PERIOD

	AGE CLASS 15-44 obs	15-44 rel	45-54 obs	45-54 rel	55-64 obs	55-64 rel	65-74 obs	65-74 rel	75+ obs	75+ rel	All obs	All rel	PERIOD 1978-80 obs	1978-80 rel	1981-82 obs	1981-82 rel	1983-85 obs	1983-85 rel
Males																		
1 year	37	37	36	37	32	32	26	27	19	21	28	29	28	29	29	30	29	30
3 years	17	17	15	15	12	12	7	8	4	6	9	10	9	10	10	11	9	11
5 years	14	15	12	12	9	10	4	6	2	3	7	8	6	8	7	9	7	8
8 years	13	13	10	11	6	8	3	5	1	4	5	7	4	6	6	8	4	7
10 years	12	13	9	10	5	7	3	5	1	5	4	7	4	6	3	5	..	..
Females																		
1 year	41	41	39	39	31	31	22	23	18	19	26	27	25	26	27	28	26	27
3 years	23	24	19	19	12	13	9	10	5	7	11	12	11	12	10	11	11	13
5 years	21	21	17	17	9	10	7	8	3	5	9	10	8	9	7	8	9	11
8 years	18	18	14	15	8	8	5	6	2	5	7	9	7	8	6	8	6	9
10 years	15	15	13	14	6	6	4	6	2	6	6	8	6	8	4	5	..	..
Overall																		
1 year	38	38	37	37	32	32	26	27	19	21	28	29	27	28	29	30	28	29
3 years	18	18	15	16	12	12	7	8	4	6	9	11	9	10	10	11	10	11
5 years	15	16	13	13	9	10	5	6	2	3	7	8	6	8	7	9	7	9
8 years	14	14	10	11	6	8	3	5	1	4	5	7	5	7	6	8	5	7
10 years	13	13	9	10	5	7	3	5	1	5	4	7	4	6	3	5	..	..

RELATIVE SURVIVAL (%) BY AGE AND PERIOD

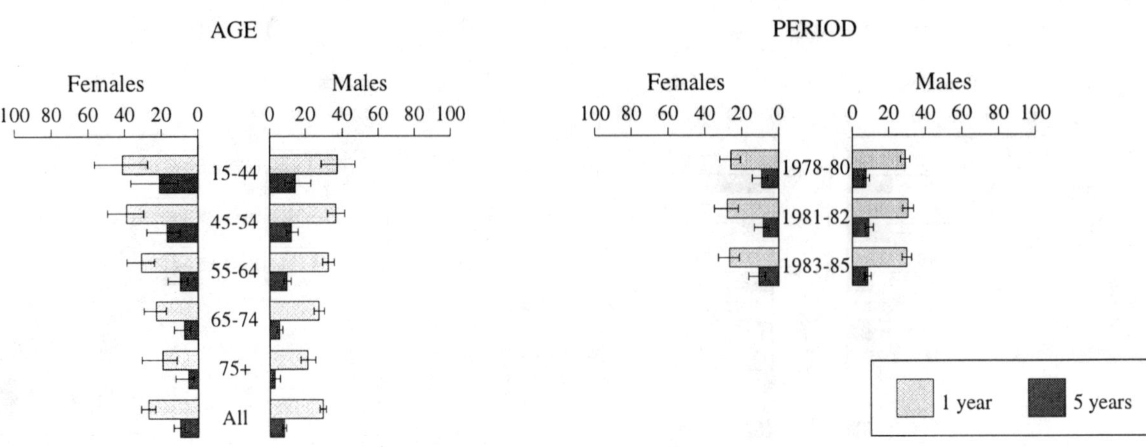

BONE

DENMARK

REGISTRY	NUMBER OF CASES			PERIOD OF DIAGNOSIS
	Males	Females	All	
Denmark	123	71	194	1978-1984
Mean age (years)	49.6	58.8	53.0	

RELATIVE SURVIVAL (%)

100, 80, 60, 40, 20, 0 — Males, Females — 0 1 2 3 4 5 — Time since diagnosis (years)

OBSERVED AND RELATIVE SURVIVAL (%) BY AGE AND PERIOD
(Number of cases in parentheses)

	AGE CLASS												PERIOD					
	20-44		45-54		55-64		65-74		75+		All		1978-80		1981-82		1983-85	
	obs	rel	obs	rel	obs	rel	obs	rel	obs	rel	obs	rel	obs	rel	obs	rel	obs	rel
Males	(54)		(13)		(26)		(16)		(14)		(123)		(45)		(32)		(46)	
1 year	89	89	92	93	69	71	31	33	43	48	72	74	80	82	72	73	65	67
3 years	61	61	77	79	54	57	19	22	29	42	52	56	58	63	44	46	52	56
5 years	53	53	69	72	42	47	13	16	14	28	43	48	49	56	28	31	48	54
8 years	48	49	58	62	34	42	13	21	14	44	38	47	42	53	28	33	..	..
10 years	48	49	..	..	24	32	6	12	..	..	33	43	37	49	..	..	..	..
Females	(14)		(12)		(13)		(15)		(17)		(71)		(35)		(15)		(21)	
1 year	86	86	83	84	62	62	60	61	35	38	63	65	54	56	80	81	67	69
3 years	57	57	58	59	46	47	47	50	24	31	45	49	40	43	53	56	48	53
5 years	50	50	50	51	46	48	39	45	18	28	39	45	34	39	47	51	37	45
8 years	25	25	50	52	37	40	14	18	12	27	27	34	26	32	..	..	..	..
10 years	25	25	..	..	37	42	..	..	..	..	27	37	26	35	..	..	..	..
Overall	(68)		(25)		(39)		(31)		(31)		(194)		(80)		(47)		(67)	
1 year	88	88	88	89	67	68	45	47	39	43	69	71	69	71	74	76	66	68
3 years	60	61	68	69	51	54	32	36	26	35	49	53	50	54	47	49	51	55
5 years	52	52	59	62	44	48	25	31	16	28	41	47	43	49	34	37	45	52
8 years	44	45	53	57	35	41	16	23	13	33	34	42	35	44	29	35	..	..
10 years	44	45	..	..	30	37	9	15	..	..	30	40	32	43	..	..	..	..

RELATIVE SURVIVAL (%) BY AGE AND PERIOD

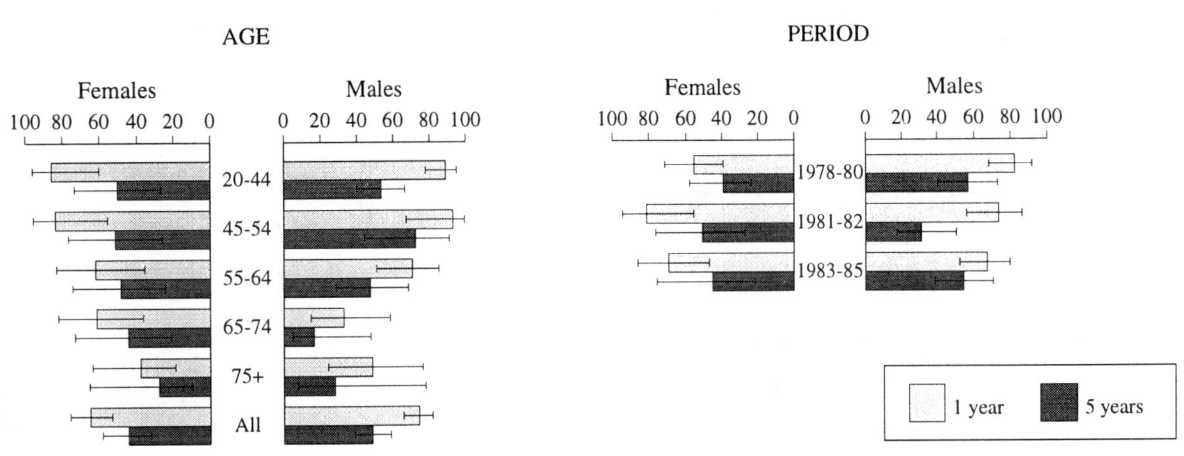

BONE

ENGLISH REGISTRIES

REGISTRY	NUMBER OF CASES			PERIOD OF DIAGNOSIS
	Males	Females	All	
East Anglia	38	27	65	1979-1984
Mersey	30	31	61	1978-1984
South Thames	126	119	245	1978-1984
Wessex	18	15	33	1983-1984
West Midlands	93	70	163	1979-1984
Yorkshire	71	59	130	1978-1984
Mean age (years)	53.9	59.6	56.5	

RELATIVE SURVIVAL (%)

100 80 60 40 20 0
Females
Males
0 1 2 3 4 5
Time since diagnosis (years)

OBSERVED AND RELATIVE SURVIVAL (%) BY AGE AND PERIOD
(Number of cases in parentheses)

	AGE CLASS												PERIOD					
	20-44		45-54		55-64		65-74		75+		All		1978-80		1981-82		1983-85	
	obs	rel	obs	rel	obs	rel	obs	rel	obs	rel	obs	rel	obs	rel	obs	rel	obs	rel
Males	(118)		(53)		(68)		(83)		(54)		(376)		(158)		(99)		(119)	
1 year	81	81	81	82	62	63	36	38	31	36	60	63	55	58	64	65	65	67
3 years	58	58	58	60	44	47	24	28	13	19	41	46	38	43	46	50	42	46
5 years	52	52	55	57	38	42	19	25	9	18	36	43	34	42	39	44	37	43
8 years	47	47	47	50	29	35	16	27	9	30	31	41	30	41	31	38	34	45
10 years	45	46	42	47	26	34	13	26	6	29	29	40	29	43	26	33	..	..
Females	(84)		(17)		(53)		(80)		(87)		(321)		(124)		(94)		(103)	
1 year	86	86	71	71	64	65	48	49	29	32	56	58	53	55	49	51	67	69
3 years	69	69	47	48	47	49	35	38	18	25	42	47	42	47	38	43	46	50
5 years	64	65	35	36	43	46	29	34	16	28	37	45	39	47	33	40	40	47
8 years	59	60	35	37	24	27	19	25	15	40	30	41	35	47	25	34	15	20
10 years	57	57	26	28	21	24	16	24	12	45	27	39	30	44	25	36	..	..
Overall	(202)		(70)		(121)		(163)		(141)		(697)		(282)		(193)		(222)	
1 year	83	83	79	79	63	64	42	43	30	33	59	61	54	57	56	58	66	68
3 years	62	63	56	57	45	48	29	33	16	23	42	46	40	45	42	46	44	48
5 years	57	57	50	52	40	44	24	30	13	25	37	44	36	44	36	42	38	45
8 years	52	52	44	47	27	32	17	26	13	37	31	41	32	44	28	36	27	35
10 years	50	51	38	42	24	29	15	25	9	39	28	40	29	43	25	34	..	..

RELATIVE SURVIVAL (%) BY AGE AND PERIOD

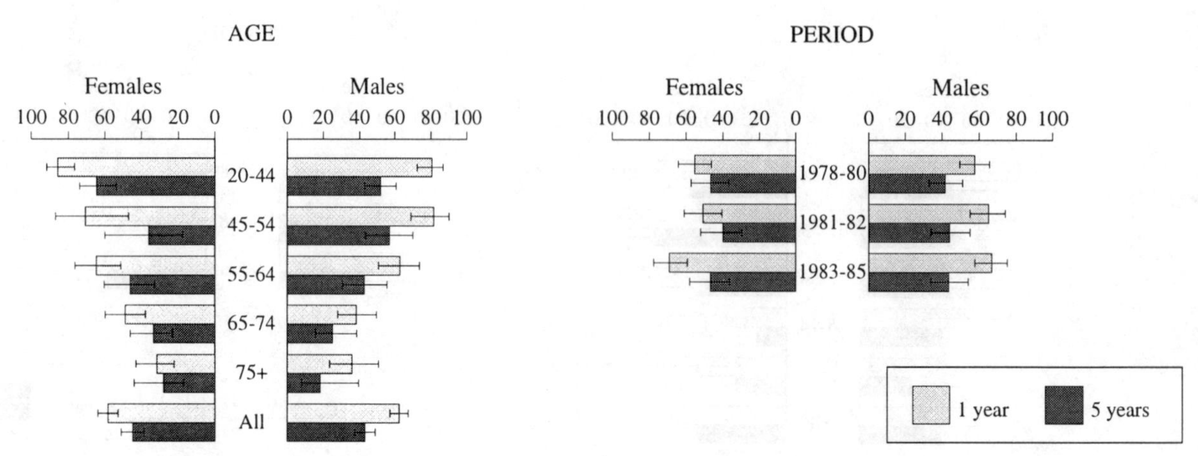

BONE

FINLAND

REGISTRY	NUMBER OF CASES			PERIOD OF DIAGNOSIS
	Males	Females	All	
Finland	137	90	227	1978-1984
Mean age (years)	48.6	56.1	51.6	

RELATIVE SURVIVAL (%)

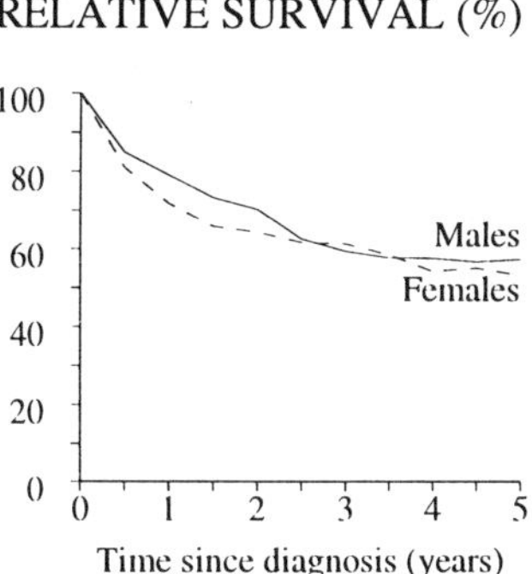

OBSERVED AND RELATIVE SURVIVAL (%) BY AGE AND PERIOD
(Number of cases in parentheses)

	AGE CLASS												PERIOD					
	20-44		45-54		55-64		65-74		75+		All		1978-80		1981-82		1983-85	
	obs	rel	obs	rel	obs	rel	obs	rel	obs	rel	obs	rel	obs	rel	obs	rel	obs	rel
Males	(61)		(23)		(21)		(21)		(11)		(137)		(57)		(36)		(44)	
1 year	89	89	91	92	71	73	52	55	45	51	77	79	77	79	75	77	80	81
3 years	69	69	78	80	52	56	24	28	0	0	55	59	47	51	58	62	64	67
5 years	67	68	74	78	48	54	10	13	0	0	51	57	44	50	58	65	55	60
8 years	54	55	61	66	33	42	5	8	0	0	40	48	33	42	50	60	42	48
10 years	54	56	61	69	28	37	..	..	0	0	39	49	32	42	50	62	..	..
Females	(29)		(10)		(12)		(20)		(19)		(90)		(37)		(28)		(25)	
1 year	93	93	90	90	75	76	55	56	37	40	70	72	65	67	71	73	76	78
3 years	86	86	70	71	58	60	35	38	26	35	57	61	49	53	64	69	60	64
5 years	79	80	60	61	33	35	25	29	21	35	47	53	43	51	46	53	52	58
8 years	72	73	45	46	25	27	20	26	21	53	41	50	38	49	39	49	31	37
10 years	72	73	45	47	0	0	10	15	13	44	33	44	35	48	..	..	..	..
Overall	(90)		(33)		(33)		(41)		(30)		(227)		(94)		(64)		(69)	
1 year	90	90	91	92	73	74	54	56	40	44	74	76	72	74	73	75	78	80
3 years	74	75	76	77	55	58	29	33	17	23	56	60	48	52	61	65	62	66
5 years	71	72	70	72	42	47	17	21	13	24	49	56	44	50	53	60	54	59
8 years	60	61	56	60	29	35	12	18	13	37	40	49	35	44	45	55	36	42
10 years	60	61	56	62	21	27	6	10	8	31	36	47	33	44	40	50	..	..

RELATIVE SURVIVAL (%) BY AGE AND PERIOD

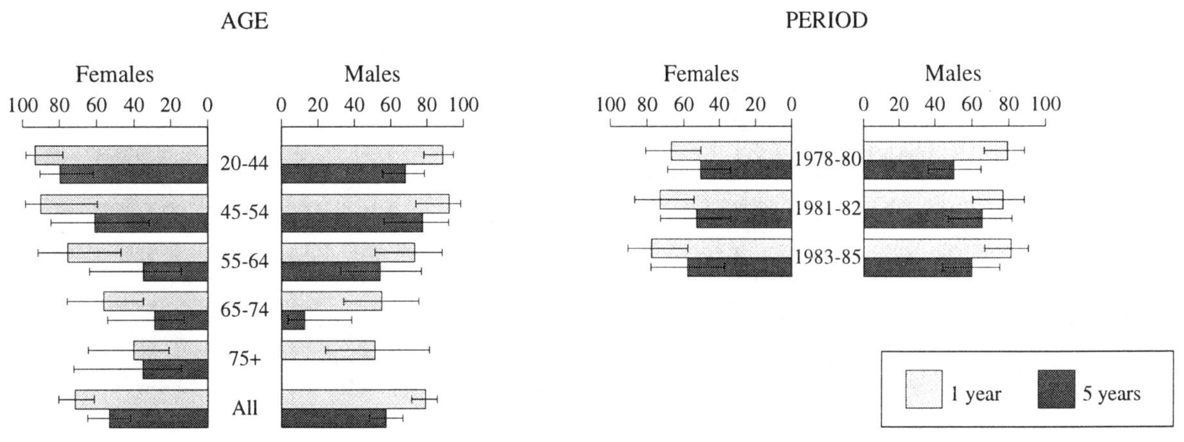

BONE

DUTCH REGISTRIES

REGISTRY	NUMBER OF CASES			PERIOD OF DIAGNOSIS
	Males	Females	All	
Eindhoven	22	7	29	1979-1985
Mean age (years)	48.0	44.9	47.2	

RELATIVE SURVIVAL (%)
(Both sexes)

Time since diagnosis (years)

OBSERVED AND RELATIVE SURVIVAL (%) BY PERIOD AND SEX
(Number of cases in parentheses)

	PERIOD						SEX					
	1978-80		1981-82		1983-85		Males		Females		All	
	obs	rel	obs	rel	obs	rel	obs	rel	obs	rel	obs	rel
N. Cases	(7)		(13)		(9)		(22)		(7)		(29)	
1 year	71	73	69	70	67	67	68	69	71	72	69	70
3 years	57	60	62	65	56	56	59	61	57	59	59	61
5 years	43	46	54	59	56	57	48	52	57	61	50	54
8 years	43	49	..	..	..	..	48	56	..	..	50	58
10 years	..	..	..	..	..	..	..	..	..	..	..	..

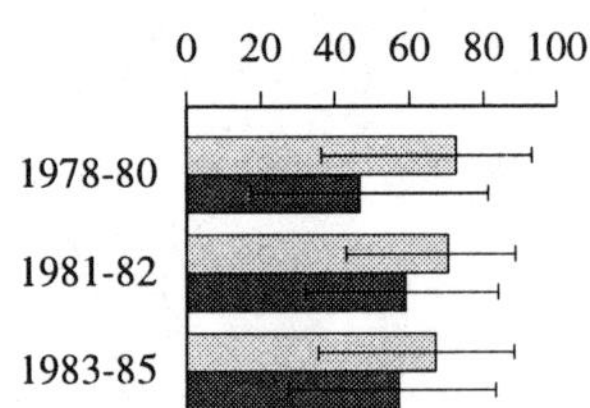

ESTONIA

REGISTRY	NUMBER OF CASES			PERIOD OF DIAGNOSIS
	Males	Females	All	
Estonia	38	36	74	1978-1984
Mean age (years)	58.3	60.2	59.2	

RELATIVE SURVIVAL (%)
(Both sexes)

Time since diagnosis (years)

OBSERVED AND RELATIVE SURVIVAL (%) BY PERIOD AND SEX
(Number of cases in parentheses)

	PERIOD						SEX					
	1978-80		1981-82		1983-85		Males		Females		All	
	obs	rel	obs	rel	obs	rel	obs	rel	obs	rel	obs	rel
N. Cases	(31)		(17)		(26)		(38)		(36)		(74)	
1 year	58	60	41	43	46	49	39	41	61	64	50	52
3 years	32	35	18	20	23	27	18	21	33	38	26	29
5 years	23	26	18	23	19	25	18	23	22	27	20	25
8 years	16	21	12	19	..	..	16	23	13	18	14	19
10 years	12	17	..	..	..	..	16	25	8	12	10	16

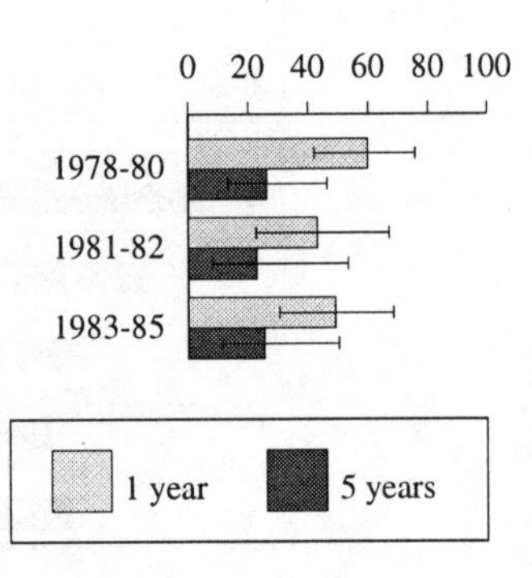

BONE

FRENCH REGISTRIES

REGISTRY	NUMBER OF CASES			PERIOD OF DIAGNOSIS
	Males	Females	All	
Amiens	7	5	12	1983-1984
Doubs	17	9	26	1978-1985
Mean age (years)	52.8	65.6	57.5	

RELATIVE SURVIVAL (%)
(Both sexes)

Time since diagnosis (years)

OBSERVED AND RELATIVE SURVIVAL (%) BY PERIOD AND SEX
(Number of cases in parentheses)

	PERIOD						SEX					
	1978-80		1981-82		1983-85		Males		Females		All	
	obs	rel	obs	rel	obs	rel	obs	rel	obs	rel	obs	rel
N. Cases	(13)		(6)		(19)		(24)		(14)		(38)	
1 year	46	50	17	17	67	68	57	58	43	46	52	54
3 years	15	18	0	0	50	53	44	47	7	8	30	32
5 years	15	19	0	0	44	49	39	45	7	9	27	31
8 years	15	21	0	0	..	..	39	50	..	..	27	34
10 years	..	..	0	0	..	..	..	..	..	..	..	..

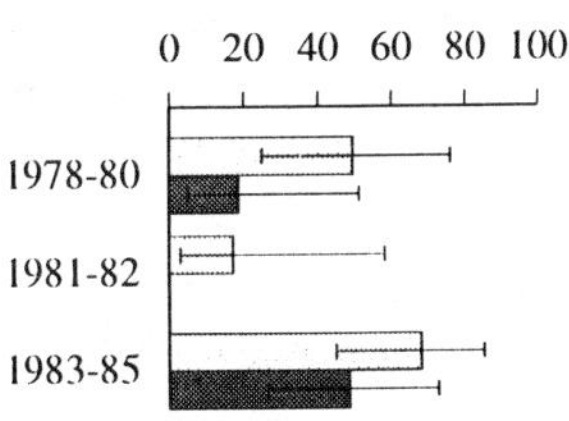

GERMAN REGISTRIES

REGISTRY	NUMBER OF CASES			PERIOD OF DIAGNOSIS
	Males	Females	All	
Saarland	32	19	51	1978-1984
Mean age (years)	54.5	53.9	54.3	

RELATIVE SURVIVAL (%)
(Both sexes)

Time since diagnosis (years)

OBSERVED AND RELATIVE SURVIVAL (%) BY PERIOD AND SEX
(Number of cases in parentheses)

	PERIOD						SEX					
	1978-80		1981-82		1983-85		Males		Females		All	
	obs	rel	obs	rel	obs	rel	obs	rel	obs	rel	obs	rel
N. Cases	(26)		(8)		(17)		(32)		(19)		(51)	
1 year	62	64	75	77	65	67	66	68	63	65	65	67
3 years	42	47	50	55	53	58	41	45	58	63	47	52
5 years	35	41	38	44	41	48	28	34	53	60	37	44
8 years	23	31	25	33	..	..	15	20	44	56	25	33
10 years	23	33	..	..	..	..	15	21	44	61	25	35

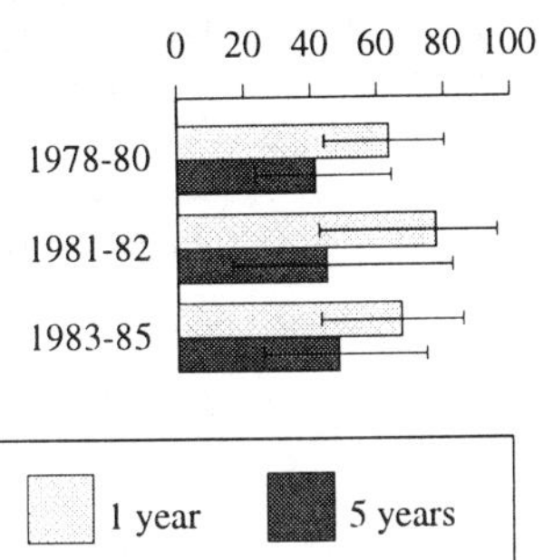

BONE

ITALIAN REGISTRIES

REGISTRY	NUMBER OF CASES			PERIOD OF DIAGNOSIS
	Males	Females	All	
Latina	2	3	5	1983-1984
Ragusa	7	2	9	1981-1984
Varese	19	17	36	1978-1984
Mean age (years)	58.4	52.5	55.8	

RELATIVE SURVIVAL (%)

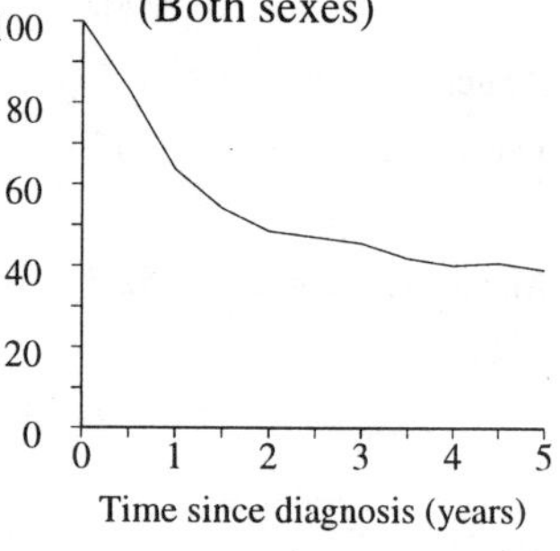

OBSERVED AND RELATIVE SURVIVAL (%) BY PERIOD AND SEX
(Number of cases in parentheses)

	PERIOD						SEX					
	1978-80		1981-82		1983-85		Males		Females		All	
	obs	rel	obs	rel	obs	rel	obs	rel	obs	rel	obs	rel
N. Cases	(14)		(12)		(24)		(28)		(22)		(50)	
1 year	50	52	67	68	67	68	61	63	64	65	62	64
3 years	43	47	25	27	50	54	32	36	55	58	42	46
5 years	36	42	17	19	42	47	25	30	45	50	34	39
8 years	29	37	8	11	42	50	25	33	35	41	29	37
10 years	29	40	..	..	..	..	25	36	35	43	29	40

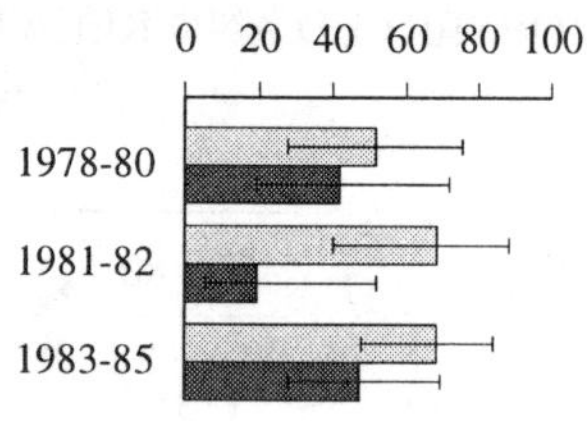

POLISH REGISTRIES

REGISTRY	NUMBER OF CASES			PERIOD OF DIAGNOSIS
	Males	Females	All	
Cracow	15	17	32	1978-1984
Mean age (years)	45.1	53.5	49.6	

RELATIVE SURVIVAL (%)

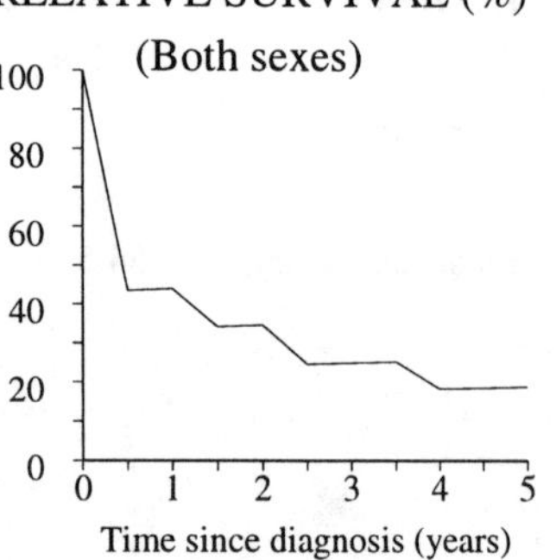

OBSERVED AND RELATIVE SURVIVAL (%) BY PERIOD AND SEX
(Number of cases in parentheses)

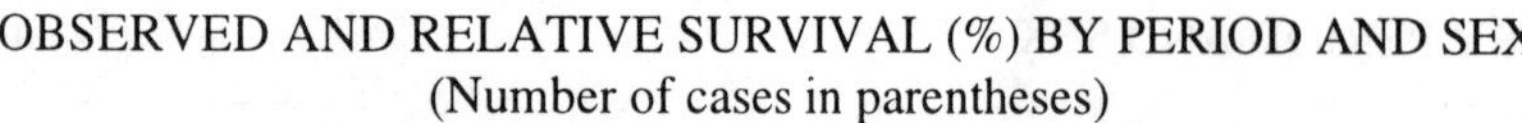

	PERIOD						SEX					
	1978-80		1981-82		1983-85		Males		Females		All	
	obs	rel	obs	rel	obs	rel	obs	rel	obs	rel	obs	rel
N. Cases	(13)		(8)		(11)		(15)		(17)		(32)	
1 year	54	54	25	26	43	44	38	39	47	48	43	44
3 years	23	24	13	15	32	35	23	24	24	26	23	25
5 years	23	24	13	17	11	12	15	17	18	20	16	19
8 years	23	25	13	20	..	..	15	18	18	23	16	21
10 years	23	26	..	..	..	..	..	..	18	24	16	22

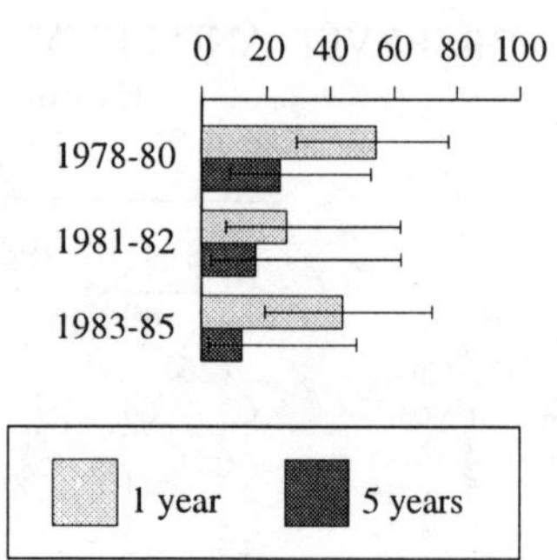

BONE

SCOTLAND

REGISTRY	NUMBER OF CASES			PERIOD OF DIAGNOSIS
	Males	Females	All	
Scotland	78	67	145	1978-1982
Mean age (years)	55.6	55.0	55.3	

RELATIVE SURVIVAL (%)
(Both sexes)

Time since diagnosis (years)

OBSERVED AND RELATIVE SURVIVAL (%) BY PERIOD AND SEX
(Number of cases in parentheses)

	PERIOD						SEX					
	1978-80		1981-82		1983-85		Males		Females		All	
	obs	rel	obs	rel	obs	rel	obs	rel	obs	rel	obs	rel
N. Cases	(97)		(48)		(0)		(78)		(67)		(145)	
1 year	60	62	58	60	..	..	62	64	57	58	59	61
3 years	37	42	35	39	..	..	33	38	40	44	37	41
5 years	29	35	31	36	..	..	24	30	36	42	30	35
8 years	26	35	..	..	..	..	19	26	36	46	27	36
10 years	24	36	..	..	..	..	19	29	32	46	25	37

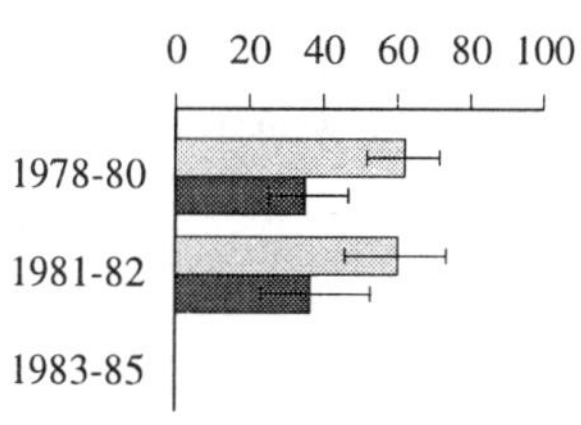

SWISS REGISTRIES

REGISTRY	NUMBER OF CASES			PERIOD OF DIAGNOSIS
	Males	Females	All	
Basel	4	9	13	1981-1984
Geneva	5	5	10	1978-1983
Mean age (years)	56.0	56.3	56.2	

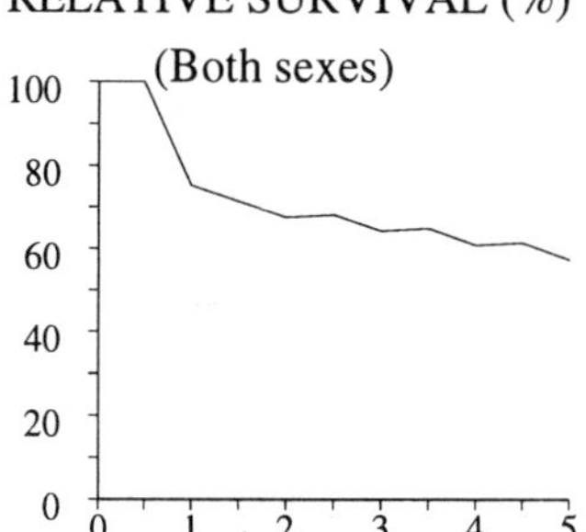

OBSERVED AND RELATIVE SURVIVAL (%) BY PERIOD AND SEX
(Number of cases in parentheses)

	PERIOD						SEX					
	1978-80		1981-82		1983-85		Males		Females		All	
	obs	rel	obs	rel	obs	rel	obs	rel	obs	rel	obs	rel
N. Cases	(4)		(11)		(8)		(9)		(14)		(23)	
1 year	75	76	55	56	100	100	78	79	71	73	74	75
3 years	50	52	45	49	88	90	56	59	64	68	61	64
5 years	50	54	36	42	75	78	44	50	57	62	52	57
8 years	..	..	36	47	..	..	44	55	57	68	52	63
10 years	..	..	..	..	..	..	..	..	..	..	..	..

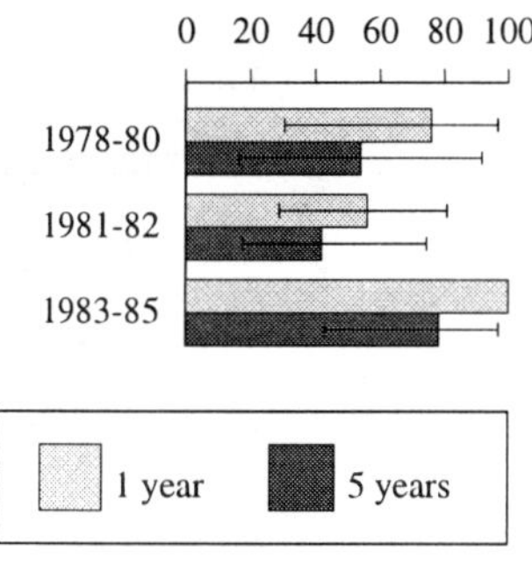

BONE

EUROPEAN REGISTRIES

Unweighted analysis

REGISTRY	CASES Males	CASES Females	CASES All
DENMARK	123	71	194
DUTCH REGISTRIES	22	7	29
ENGLISH REGISTRIES	376	321	697
ESTONIA	38	36	74
FINLAND	137	90	227
FRENCH REGISTRIES	24	14	38
GERMAN REGISTRIES	32	19	51
ITALIAN REGISTRIES	28	22	50
POLISH REGISTRIES	15	17	32
SCOTLAND	78	67	145
SWISS REGISTRIES	9	14	23
Mean age (years)	52.7	58.0	55.0

RELATIVE SURVIVAL (%)
(Age-standardized)

Females — 100 80 60 40 20 0 — Males — 0 20 40 60 80 100

DK
ENG
FIN
EUR

OBSERVED AND RELATIVE SURVIVAL (%) BY AGE AND PERIOD
(Number of cases in parentheses)

	20-44 obs	20-44 rel	45-54 obs	45-54 rel	55-64 obs	55-64 rel	65-74 obs	65-74 rel	75+ obs	75+ rel	All obs	All rel	1978-80 obs	1978-80 rel	1981-82 obs	1981-82 rel	1983-85 obs	1983-85 rel
Males	(304)		(127)		(166)		(172)		(113)		(882)		(369)		(238)		(275)	
1 year	83	83	81	82	61	62	40	42	35	39	64	66	62	64	65	67	66	68
3 years	60	60	60	61	42	44	22	26	16	24	43	48	40	45	43	46	48	52
5 years	55	55	54	56	33	37	16	21	10	19	37	43	35	41	37	42	41	48
8 years	47	48	45	49	25	31	13	22	9	27	31	40	29	38	31	39	35	45
10 years	47	48	43	49	21	28	10	21	7	34	29	40	27	39	29	37	..	..
Females	(192)		(58)		(101)		(160)		(167)		(678)		(292)		(189)		(197)	
1 year	85	85	86	87	64	65	48	49	30	33	60	61	58	60	54	56	67	69
3 years	68	68	64	65	47	49	33	35	19	25	44	48	42	46	43	48	48	52
5 years	62	62	57	58	40	43	26	30	14	25	38	45	37	44	36	42	41	48
8 years	56	57	49	51	27	30	17	23	13	34	31	41	32	42	27	36	22	27
10 years	55	55	44	47	23	26	11	17	10	34	28	39	29	41	23	33	..	..
Overall	(496)		(185)		(267)		(332)		(280)		(1560)		(661)		(427)		(472)	
1 year	84	84	83	83	62	63	44	45	32	35	62	64	60	62	60	62	67	69
3 years	63	63	61	62	44	46	27	31	18	25	44	48	41	45	43	47	48	52
5 years	58	58	55	57	36	39	21	26	13	23	38	44	36	42	36	42	41	48
8 years	51	52	47	50	26	31	15	22	11	31	31	40	30	40	29	37	30	38
10 years	50	51	44	48	22	28	11	18	9	34	28	39	28	40	26	35	..	..

RELATIVE SURVIVAL (%) BY AGE AND PERIOD

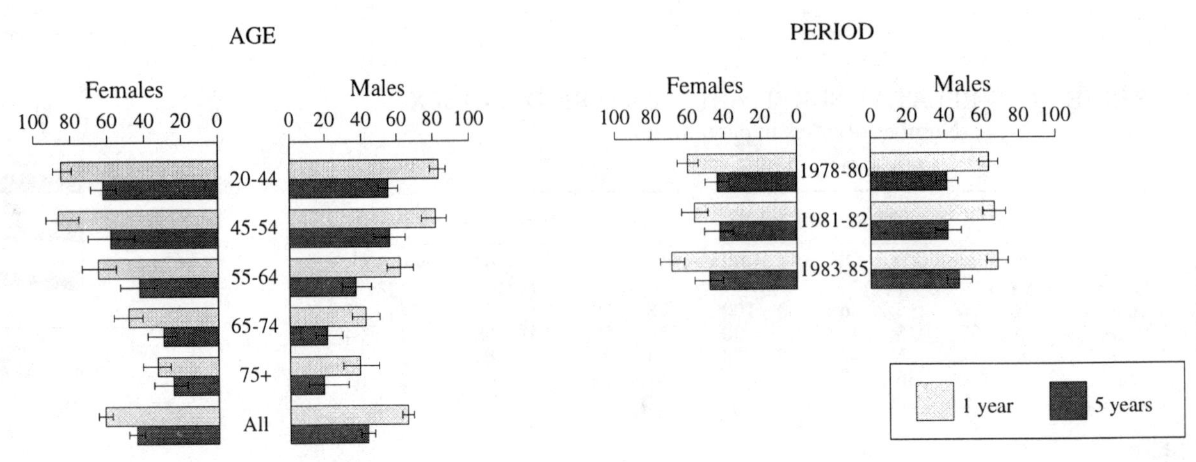

BREAST

DENMARK

REGISTRY	NUMBER OF CASES	PERIOD OF DIAGNOSIS
Denmark	17498	1978-1984
Mean age (years)	61.9	

RELATIVE SURVIVAL (%)

100 80 60 40 20 0

0 1 2 3 4 5

Time since diagnosis (years)

OBSERVED AND RELATIVE SURVIVAL (%) BY AGE AND PERIOD
(Number of cases in parentheses)

	AGE CLASS												PERIOD					
	15-44		45-54		55-64		65-74		75+		All		1978-80		1981-82		1983-85	
	obs	rel	obs	rel	obs	rel	obs	rel	obs	rel	obs	rel	obs	rel	obs	rel	obs	rel
Females	(2321)		(3372)		(3952)		(4033)		(3820)		(17498)		(7166)		(5060)		(5272)	
1 year	97	97	95	96	92	93	88	90	76	82	89	91	89	91	89	91	89	92
3 years	84	85	83	84	77	80	71	77	52	68	72	79	72	79	72	78	73	79
5 years	75	76	72	74	66	70	58	67	35	56	60	69	60	69	60	69	60	69
8 years	65	66	63	66	54	60	43	56	20	47	47	60	47	60	46	59	..	..
10 years	61	62	56	60	48	55	36	52	13	42	41	56	41	56	..	..	..	..

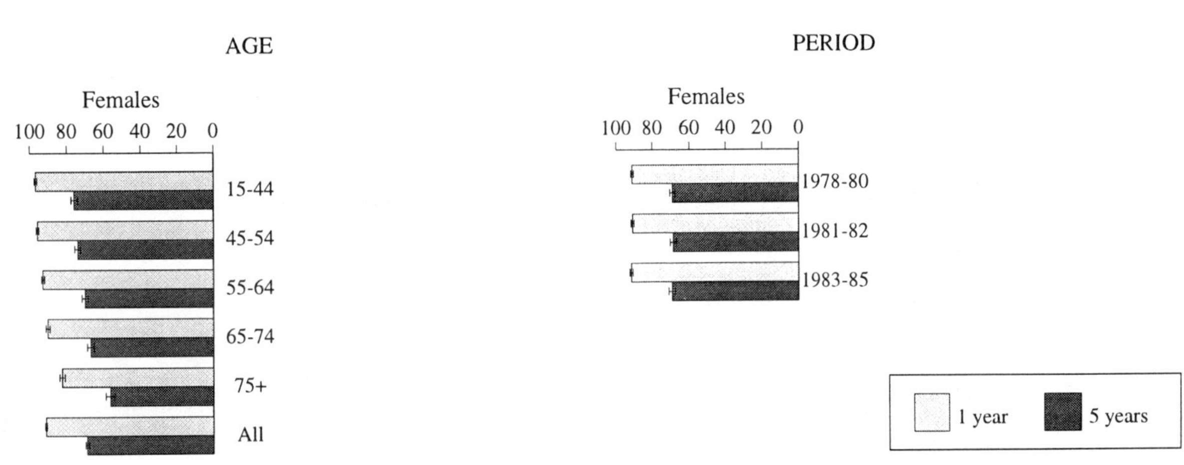

BREAST

DUTCH REGISTRIES

REGISTRY	NUMBER OF CASES	PERIOD OF DIAGNOSIS
Eindhoven	2653	1978-1985
Mean age (years)	58.6	

RELATIVE SURVIVAL (%)

OBSERVED AND RELATIVE SURVIVAL (%) BY AGE AND PERIOD
(Number of cases in parentheses)

	AGE CLASS												PERIOD					
	15-44		45-54		55-64		65-74		75+		All		1978-80		1981-82		1983-85	
	obs	rel	obs	rel	obs	rel	obs	rel	obs	rel	obs	rel	obs	rel	obs	rel	obs	rel
Females	(463)		(622)		(610)		(561)		(397)		(2653)		(940)		(692)		(1021)	
1 year	97	97	97	97	94	95	91	93	82	88	93	94	92	93	93	95	93	95
3 years	86	86	85	86	79	81	74	79	56	72	77	81	75	79	80	84	77	82
5 years	77	77	78	80	65	68	59	67	40	62	65	72	62	68	69	76	64	72
8 years	66	66	69	72	53	57	43	54	24	53	53	63	50	59	..	..	..	..
10 years	57	58	63	66	47	53	39	55	10	29	46	58	43	54	..	..	..	..

RELATIVE SURVIVAL (%) BY AGE AND PERIOD

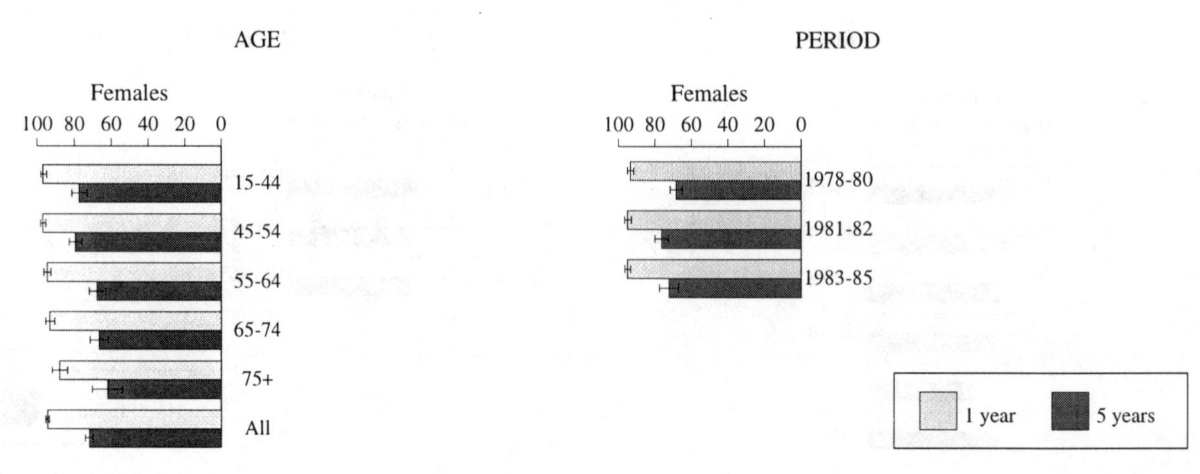

BREAST

ENGLISH REGISTRIES

REGISTRY	NUMBER OF CASES	PERIOD OF DIAGNOSIS
East Anglia	5699	1979-1984
Mersey	7220	1978-1984
South Thames	20535	1978-1984
Wessex	2684	1983-1984
West Midlands	13261	1979-1984
Yorkshire	10991	1978-1984
Mean age (years)	62.5	

RELATIVE SURVIVAL (%)

100 80 60 40 20 0

0 1 2 3 4 5

Time since diagnosis (years)

OBSERVED AND RELATIVE SURVIVAL (%) BY AGE AND PERIOD
(Number of cases in parentheses)

	AGE CLASS												PERIOD					
	15-44		45-54		55-64		65-74		75+		All		1978-80		1981-82		1983-85	
	obs	rel	obs	rel	obs	rel	obs	rel	obs	rel	obs	rel	obs	rel	obs	rel	obs	rel
Females	(7268)		(10877)		(14024)		(14810)		(13411)		(60390)		(22916)		(17634)		(19840)	
1 year	94	94	92	93	88	89	85	87	68	75	84	87	83	86	84	87	85	88
3 years	78	78	76	77	70	72	67	73	46	62	66	72	65	71	66	72	67	73
5 years	67	67	65	67	58	62	55	64	32	55	54	63	53	62	54	63	55	64
8 years	57	58	55	58	47	53	42	55	20	50	42	55	42	54	42	55	43	56
10 years	53	54	51	54	41	48	35	52	15	50	37	51	37	51	36	50	..	..

RELATIVE SURVIVAL (%) BY AGE AND PERIOD

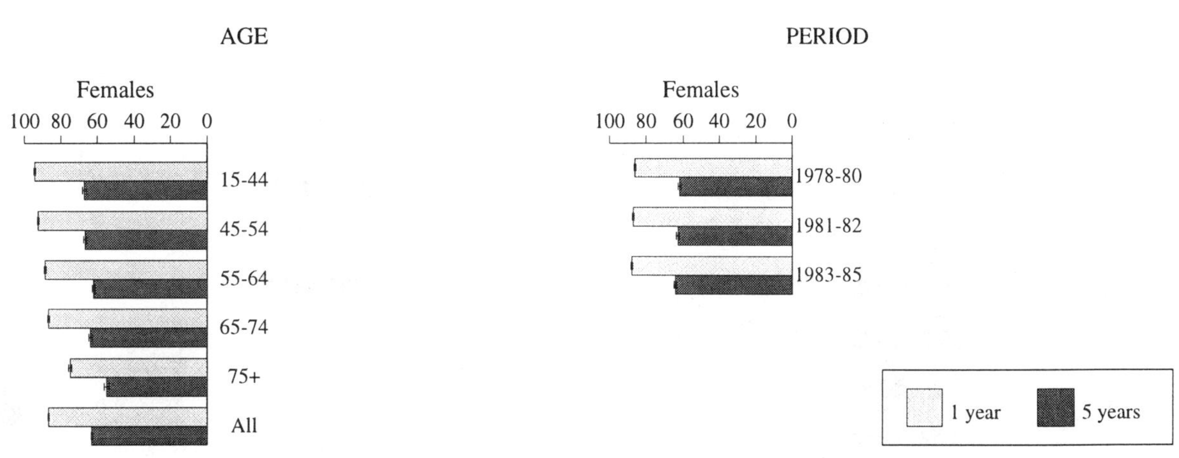

BREAST

ESTONIA

REGISTRY	NUMBER OF CASES	PERIOD OF DIAGNOSIS
Estonia	2387	1978-1984
Mean age (years)	57.3	

RELATIVE SURVIVAL (%)

Time since diagnosis (years)

OBSERVED AND RELATIVE SURVIVAL (%) BY AGE AND PERIOD
(Number of cases in parentheses)

	AGE CLASS												PERIOD					
	15-44		45-54		55-64		65-74		75+		All		1978-80		1981-82		1983-85	
	obs	rel	obs	rel	obs	rel	obs	rel	obs	rel	obs	rel	obs	rel	obs	rel	obs	rel
Females	(441)		(642)		(560)		(457)		(287)		(2387)		(971)		(674)		(742)	
1 year	94	94	91	92	89	89	84	87	71	78	87	89	88	89	85	87	89	91
3 years	74	75	70	71	67	69	63	69	43	59	65	70	65	69	65	69	67	72
5 years	63	63	60	62	56	60	50	60	28	51	54	60	52	58	54	60	56	63
8 years	54	55	51	53	48	54	37	54	13	38	44	53	41	50	45	54	..	..
10 years	52	53	46	49	40	47	28	47	6	24	38	48	35	45	..	..	..	..

RELATIVE SURVIVAL (%) BY AGE AND PERIOD

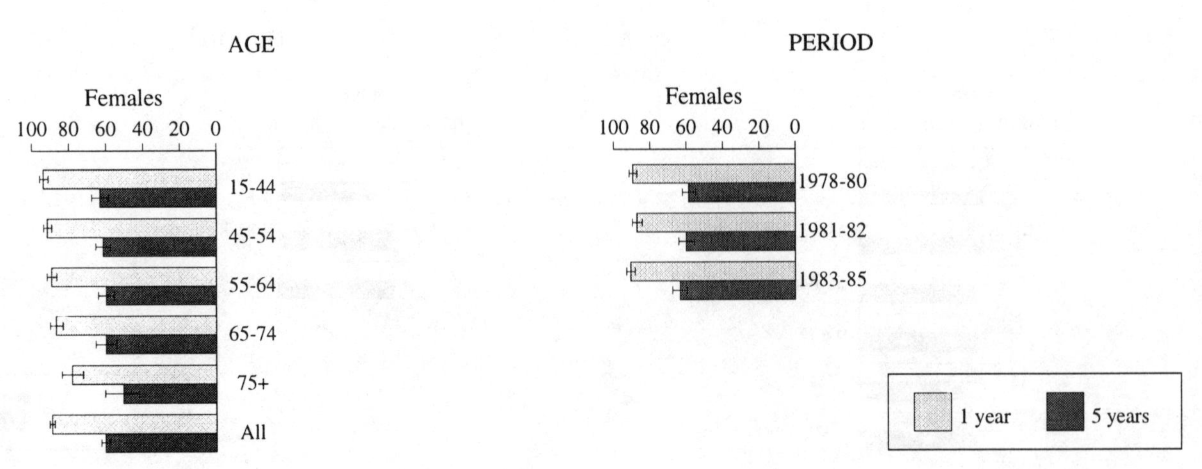

BREAST

FINLAND

REGISTRY	NUMBER OF CASES	PERIOD OF DIAGNOSIS
Finland	11123	1978-1984
Mean age (years)	60.4	

RELATIVE SURVIVAL (%)

Time since diagnosis (years)

OBSERVED AND RELATIVE SURVIVAL (%) BY AGE AND PERIOD
(Number of cases in parentheses)

	AGE CLASS												PERIOD					
	15-44		45-54		55-64		65-74		75+		All		1978-80		1981-82		1983-85	
	obs	rel	obs	rel	obs	rel	obs	rel	obs	rel	obs	rel	obs	rel	obs	rel	obs	rel
Females	(1617)		(2388)		(2484)		(2628)		(2006)		(11123)		(4419)		(3210)		(3494)	
1 year	96	96	96	97	94	95	91	93	82	89	92	94	92	94	92	95	92	94
3 years	86	86	86	87	81	83	76	82	59	78	78	83	77	83	79	85	78	84
5 years	77	78	77	79	71	74	64	74	40	65	66	75	65	73	67	77	66	75
8 years	67	68	69	71	59	65	48	62	21	52	53	65	52	63	54	67	54	66
10 years	63	64	65	68	52	59	37	55	13	44	46	60	46	59	47	61	..	..

RELATIVE SURVIVAL (%) BY AGE AND PERIOD

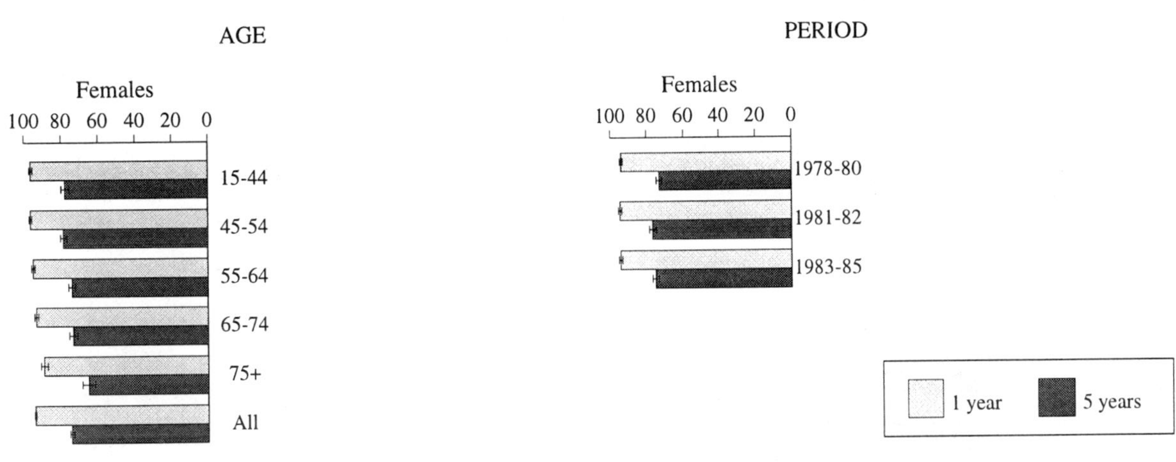

BREAST

FRENCH REGISTRIES

REGISTRY	NUMBER OF CASES	PERIOD OF DIAGNOSIS
Amiens	397	1983-1984
Côte-d'Or	762	1982-1985
Doubs	1339	1978-1985
Mean age (years)	60.4	

RELATIVE SURVIVAL (%)

Time since diagnosis (years)

OBSERVED AND RELATIVE SURVIVAL (%) BY AGE AND PERIOD
(Number of cases in parentheses)

	AGE CLASS												PERIOD					
	15-44		45-54		55-64		65-74		75+		All		1978-80		1981-82		1983-85	
	obs	rel	obs	rel	obs	rel	obs	rel	obs	rel	obs	rel	obs	rel	obs	rel	obs	rel
Females	(336)		(610)		(572)		(481)		(499)		(2498)		(488)		(500)		(1510)	
1 year	97	97	97	97	94	95	92	94	80	88	92	94	89	92	93	95	93	95
3 years	84	85	84	85	79	80	75	79	57	76	76	81	74	79	76	82	77	82
5 years	76	76	74	75	70	72	62	69	41	67	64	72	63	71	63	72	65	73
8 years	66	67	66	68	55	59	41	51	28	65	52	62	49	59	52	64	54	64
10 years	60	61	63	66	50	55	39	52	24	76	48	61	45	58	..	..	..	..

RELATIVE SURVIVAL (%) BY AGE AND PERIOD

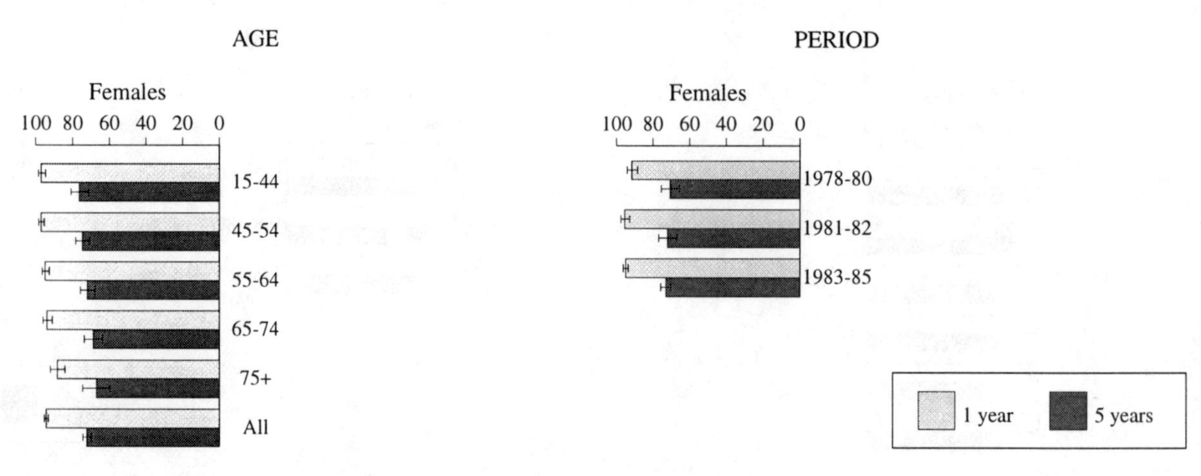

BREAST

GERMAN REGISTRIES

REGISTRY	NUMBER OF CASES	PERIOD OF DIAGNOSIS
Saarland	3359	1978-1984
Mean age (years)	60.6	

RELATIVE SURVIVAL (%)

100
80
60
40
20
0
0 1 2 3 4 5
Time since diagnosis (years)

OBSERVED AND RELATIVE SURVIVAL (%) BY AGE AND PERIOD
(Number of cases in parentheses)

	AGE CLASS												PERIOD					
	15-44		45-54		55-64		65-74		75+		All		1978-80		1981-82		1983-85	
	obs	rel	obs	rel	obs	rel	obs	rel	obs	rel	obs	rel	obs	rel	obs	rel	obs	rel
Females	(465)		(666)		(816)		(874)		(538)		(3359)		(1363)		(973)		(1023)	
1 year	96	96	92	92	91	92	87	90	77	84	89	91	89	91	88	91	89	91
3 years	82	82	76	77	74	76	70	77	56	75	72	77	71	77	72	78	72	77
5 years	70	71	66	67	63	67	60	70	41	68	60	68	60	69	60	69	60	68
8 years	61	62	56	59	55	61	46	62	31	72	50	62	50	63	49	62	..	..
10 years	59	60	53	56	50	57	39	58	24	73	45	58	45	59	..	..	..	..

RELATIVE SURVIVAL (%) BY AGE AND PERIOD

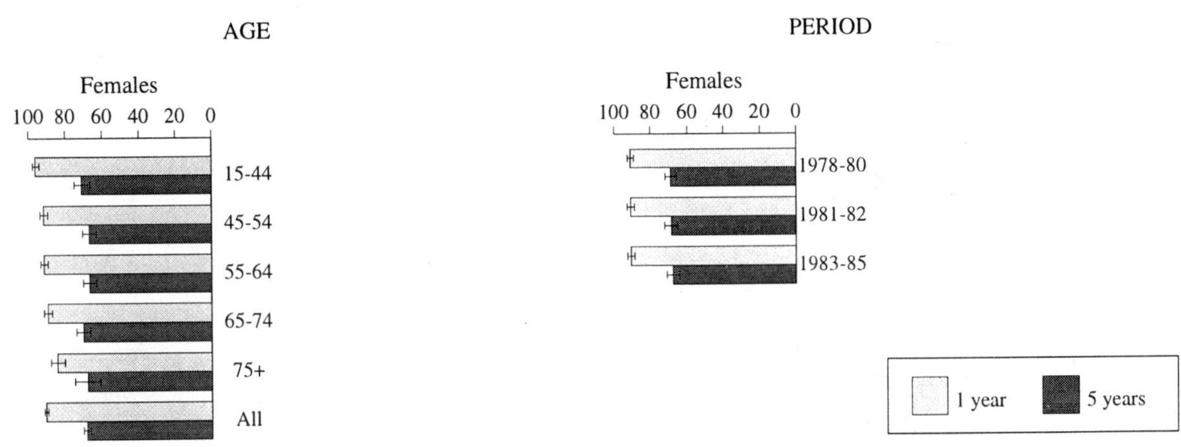

BREAST

ITALIAN REGISTRIES

REGISTRY	NUMBER OF CASES	PERIOD OF DIAGNOSIS
Florence	595	1985-1985
Latina	200	1983-1984
Ragusa	353	1981-1984
Varese	2447	1978-1984
Mean age (years)	59.4	

RELATIVE SURVIVAL (%)

100
80
60
40
20
0
0 1 2 3 4 5
Time since diagnosis (years)

OBSERVED AND RELATIVE SURVIVAL (%) BY AGE AND PERIOD
(Number of cases in parentheses)

	AGE CLASS												PERIOD					
	15-44		45-54		55-64		65-74		75+		All		1978-80		1981-82		1983-85	
	obs	rel	obs	rel	obs	rel	obs	rel	obs	rel	obs	rel	obs	rel	obs	rel	obs	rel
Females	(582)		(833)		(789)		(804)		(587)		(3595)		(963)		(902)		(1730)	
1 year	98	98	97	98	95	96	90	92	80	87	92	94	92	94	92	94	93	95
3 years	87	87	86	87	77	79	73	79	55	71	76	81	76	81	75	80	77	82
5 years	78	79	76	77	67	70	59	67	41	65	65	72	63	71	65	72	66	73
8 years	68	69	65	66	56	61	46	59	27	61	53	63	52	63	52	62	57	67
10 years	64	65	61	64	51	56	39	55	19	57	48	60	47	60	47	59	..	..

RELATIVE SURVIVAL (%) BY AGE AND PERIOD

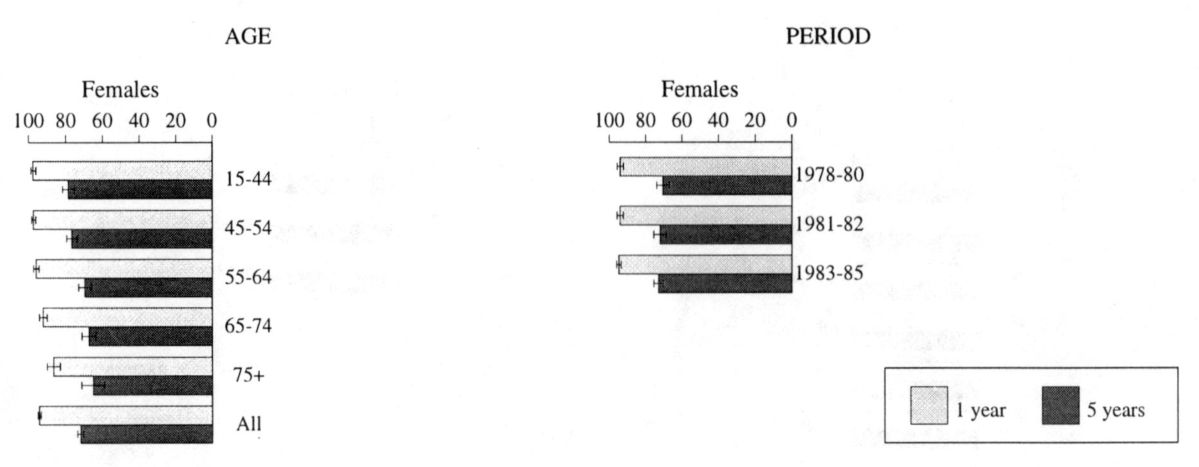

BREAST

POLISH REGISTRIES

REGISTRY	NUMBER OF CASES	PERIOD OF DIAGNOSIS
Cracow	1089	1978-1984
Mean age (years)	58.5	

RELATIVE SURVIVAL (%)

Time since diagnosis (years)

OBSERVED AND RELATIVE SURVIVAL (%) BY AGE AND PERIOD
(Number of cases in parentheses)

	AGE CLASS												PERIOD					
	15-44		45-54		55-64		65-74		75+		All		1978-80		1981-82		1983-85	
	obs	rel	obs	rel	obs	rel	obs	rel	obs	rel	obs	rel	obs	rel	obs	rel	obs	rel
Females	(168)		(259)		(281)		(243)		(138)		(1089)		(407)		(320)		(362)	
1 year	85	85	84	84	80	81	75	77	58	63	78	79	73	74	78	80	83	85
3 years	63	63	58	59	58	60	51	56	32	42	54	58	44	47	57	60	64	68
5 years	52	52	44	45	46	49	37	44	19	32	41	46	29	32	47	53	51	57
8 years	46	46	37	39	37	42	24	33	8	21	32	39	21	25	38	46	41	50
10 years	39	40	33	35	31	36	18	29	..	..	27	35	17	22	34	43	..	..

RELATIVE SURVIVAL (%) BY AGE AND PERIOD

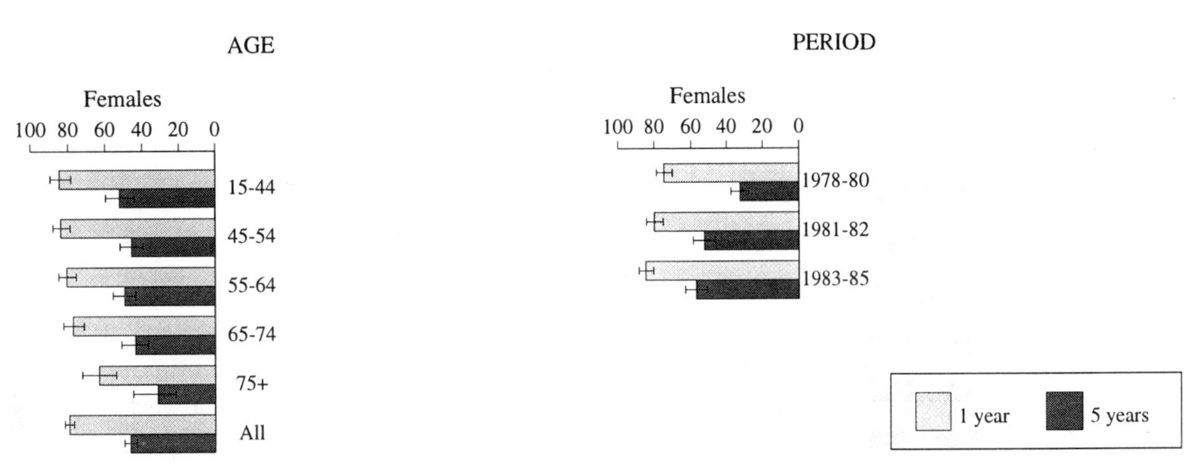

BREAST

SCOTLAND

REGISTRY	NUMBER OF CASES	PERIOD OF DIAGNOSIS	RELATIVE SURVIVAL (%)
Scotland	11261	1978-1982	
Mean age (years)	61.2		

OBSERVED AND RELATIVE SURVIVAL (%) BY AGE AND PERIOD
(Number of cases in parentheses)

	AGE CLASS												PERIOD					
	15-44		45-54		55-64		65-74		75+		All		1978-80		1981-82		1983-85	
	obs	rel	obs	rel	obs	rel	obs	rel	obs	rel	obs	rel	obs	rel	obs	rel	obs	rel
Females	(1482)		(2289)		(2611)		(2710)		(2169)		(11261)		(6692)		(4569)		(0)	
1 year	94	94	91	92	88	89	84	86	69	76	85	87	85	88	84	87	..	..
3 years	78	79	73	74	69	72	66	72	48	65	66	72	66	73	66	72	..	..
5 years	66	67	62	64	58	62	52	62	33	56	54	62	54	62	54	62	..	..
8 years	57	58	52	55	46	52	37	51	18	45	41	53	41	53	..	..	..	..
10 years	50	51	48	52	39	46	32	49	13	46	36	49	36	50	..	..	..	..

RELATIVE SURVIVAL (%) BY AGE AND PERIOD

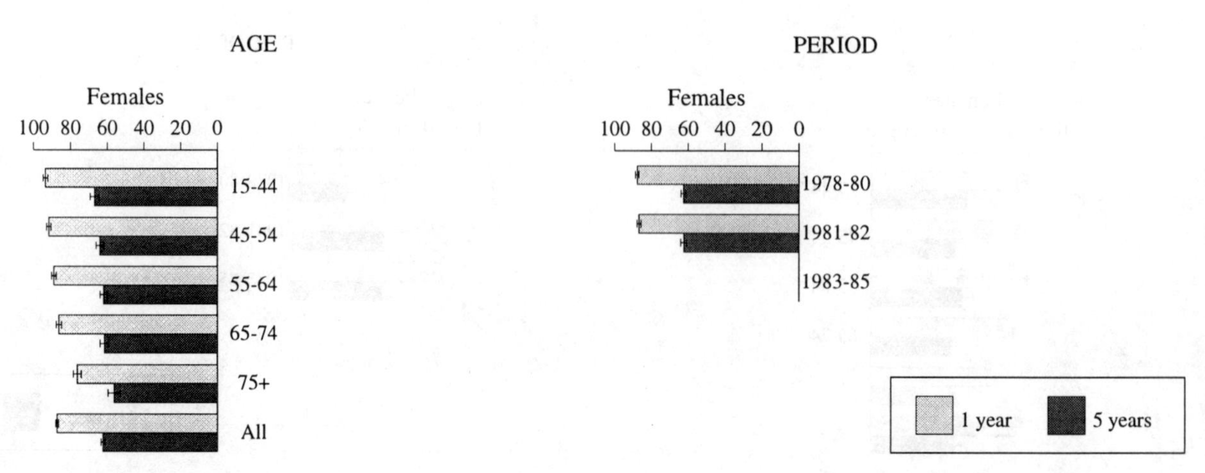

BREAST

SPANISH REGISTRIES

REGISTRY	NUMBER OF CASES	PERIOD OF DIAGNOSIS
Girona	734	1980-1985
Granada	154	1985-1985
Tarragona	155	1985-1985
Mean age (years)	59.4	

RELATIVE SURVIVAL (%)

Time since diagnosis (years)

OBSERVED AND RELATIVE SURVIVAL (%) BY AGE AND PERIOD
(Number of cases in parentheses)

	AGE CLASS												PERIOD					
	15-44		45-54		55-64		65-74		75+		All		1978-80		1981-82		1983-85	
	obs	rel	obs	rel	obs	rel	obs	rel	obs	rel	obs	rel	obs	rel	obs	rel	obs	rel
Females	(156)		(237)		(253)		(251)		(146)		(1043)		(113)		(239)		(691)	
1 year	97	97	96	96	93	94	88	89	74	80	90	92	92	93	91	93	90	92
3 years	82	82	78	78	76	77	70	74	55	70	73	77	69	72	77	80	72	76
5 years	64	64	66	67	65	67	52	59	37	56	58	64	61	65	60	66	57	63
8 years	47	48	50	51	43	46	38	47	27	55	42	48	43	47	43	49	47	55
10 years	47	48	45	46	34	37	35	47	24	63	38	46	38	44	39	47	..	..

RELATIVE SURVIVAL (%) BY AGE AND PERIOD

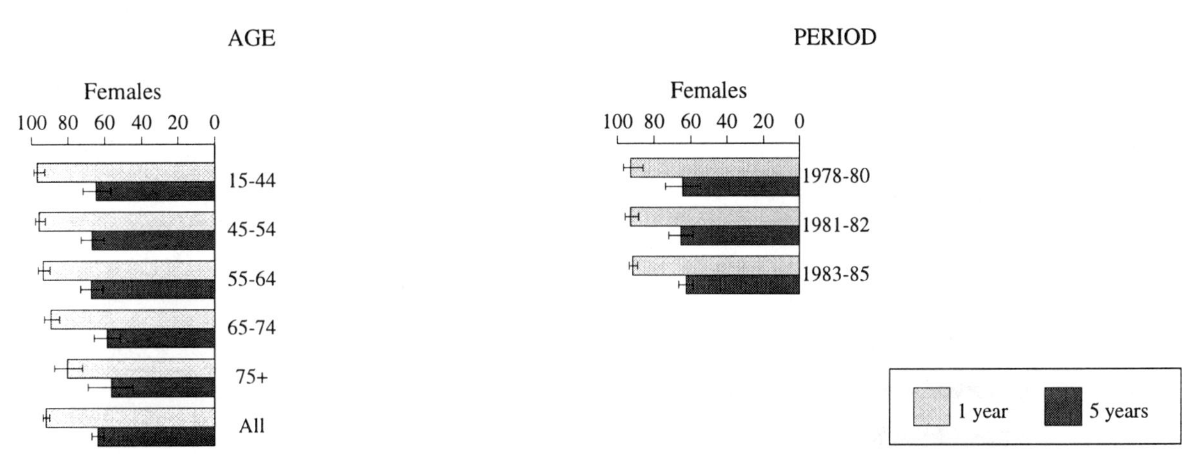

BREAST

SWISS REGISTRIES

REGISTRY	NUMBER OF CASES	PERIOD OF DIAGNOSIS
Basel	845	1981-1984
Geneva	1398	1978-1984
Mean age (years)	61.9	

RELATIVE SURVIVAL (%)

100 80 60 40 20 0

0 1 2 3 4 5

Time since diagnosis (years)

OBSERVED AND RELATIVE SURVIVAL (%) BY AGE AND PERIOD
(Number of cases in parentheses)

	AGE CLASS												PERIOD					
	15-44		45-54		55-64		65-74		75+		All		1978-80		1981-82		1983-85	
	obs	rel	obs	rel	obs	rel	obs	rel	obs	rel	obs	rel	obs	rel	obs	rel	obs	rel
Females	(304)		(461)		(445)		(524)		(509)		(2243)		(589)		(786)		(868)	
1 year	99	99	97	97	96	97	93	95	83	90	93	95	94	97	93	95	93	95
3 years	89	89	86	86	85	87	79	84	60	77	78	84	79	86	77	83	79	85
5 years	78	79	75	76	74	77	68	76	45	72	67	76	68	78	65	73	68	77
8 years	72	73	70	72	68	73	63	77	26	58	58	73	..	..	58	71	..	..
10 years	..	..	..	..	..	..	..	..	..	..	..	..	..	..	..	..	..	..

RELATIVE SURVIVAL (%) BY AGE AND PERIOD

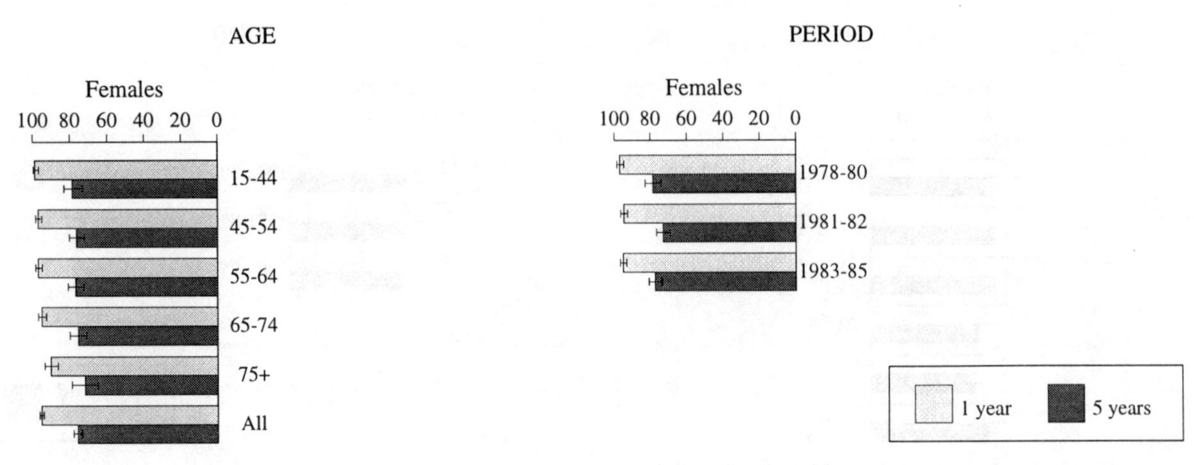

BREAST

EUROPEAN REGISTRIES

Weighted analysis

REGISTRY	WEIGHTS (Yearly expected cases in the country)
DENMARK	2499
DUTCH REGISTRIES	6602
ENGLISH REGISTRIES	30501
ESTONIA	341
FINLAND	1591
FRENCH REGISTRIES	20311
GERMAN REGISTRIES	29382
ITALIAN REGISTRIES	21784
POLISH REGISTRIES	6266
SCOTLAND	2252
SPANISH REGISTRIES	9329
SWISS REGISTRIES	3339

RELATIVE SURVIVAL (%)
(Age-standardized)

OBSERVED AND RELATIVE SURVIVAL (%) BY AGE AND PERIOD

	AGE CLASS												PERIOD					
	15-44		45-54		55-64		65-74		75+		All		1978-80		1981-82		1983-85	
	obs	rel	obs	rel	obs	rel	obs	rel	obs	rel	obs	rel	obs	rel	obs	rel	obs	rel
Females																		
1 year	96	96	94	94	91	92	88	90	75	82	89	91	88	90	89	91	89	91
3 years	82	82	79	80	74	76	70	76	52	69	71	77	70	75	72	77	72	78
5 years	71	71	68	70	63	67	57	66	38	61	60	67	58	66	60	68	61	68
8 years	61	62	59	61	52	57	43	56	25	58	48	59	46	57	48	59	49	60
10 years	57	58	54	57	46	51	37	52	19	60	42	55	41	54	40	52	..	..

RELATIVE SURVIVAL (%) BY AGE AND PERIOD

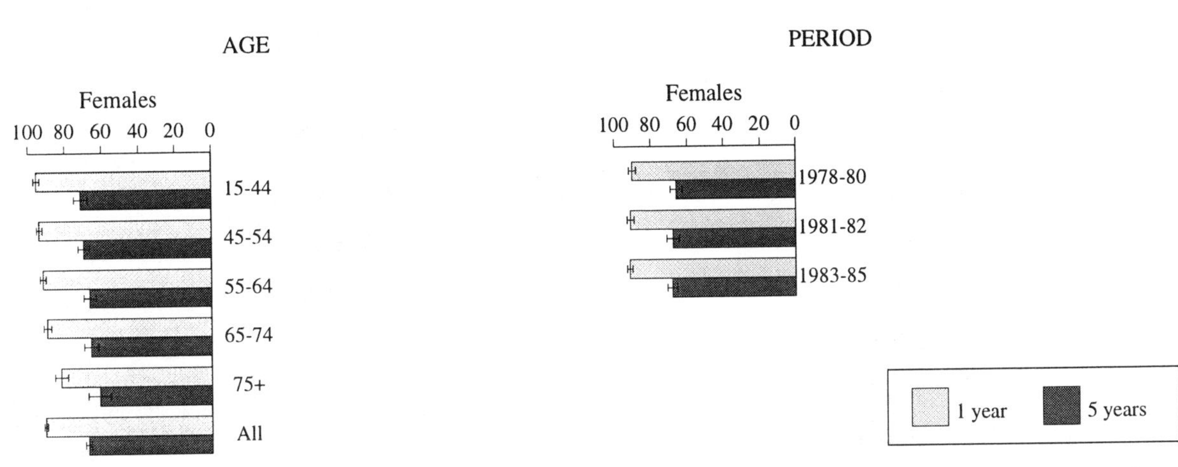

CERVIX UTERI

DENMARK

REGISTRY	NUMBER OF CASES	PERIOD OF DIAGNOSIS
Denmark	4199	1978-1984
Mean age (years)	54.1	

RELATIVE SURVIVAL (%)

Time since diagnosis (years)

OBSERVED AND RELATIVE SURVIVAL (%) BY AGE AND PERIOD
(Number of cases in parentheses)

	AGE CLASS												PERIOD					
	15-44		45-54		55-64		65-74		75+		All		1978-80		1981-82		1983-85	
	obs	rel	obs	rel	obs	rel	obs	rel	obs	rel	obs	rel	obs	rel	obs	rel	obs	rel
Females	(1281)		(792)		(924)		(788)		(414)		(4199)		(1851)		(1261)		(1087)	
1 year	92	92	85	85	82	83	77	79	55	59	82	83	83	84	83	84	81	82
3 years	81	81	68	69	62	64	56	60	30	38	65	68	64	67	66	69	64	68
5 years	79	79	63	64	53	56	46	52	22	34	58	63	57	62	59	64	59	64
8 years	78	79	59	62	45	50	35	45	15	33	53	61	52	60	54	63	..	..
10 years	77	79	57	61	41	47	30	42	9	27	50	60	49	59	..	..	..	..

RELATIVE SURVIVAL (%) BY AGE AND PERIOD

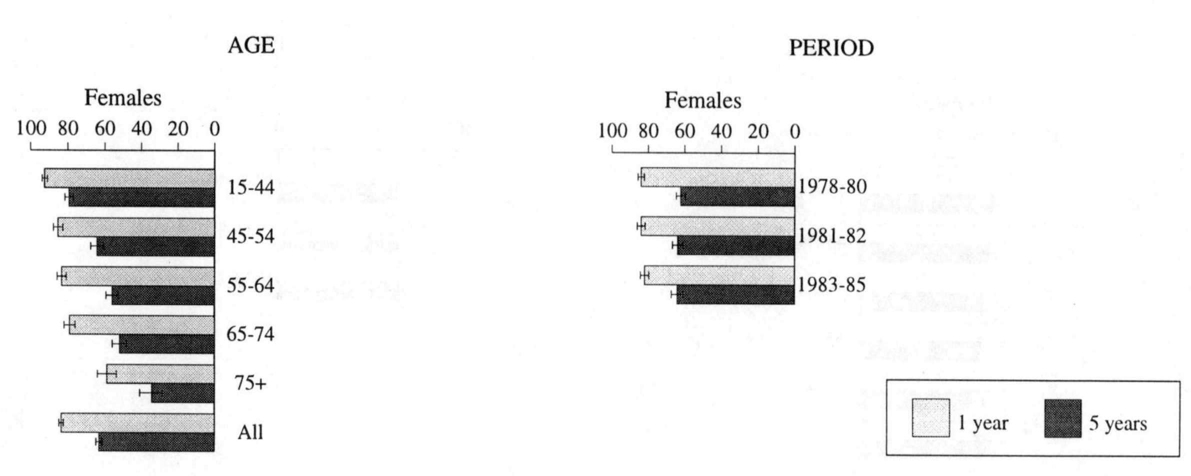

CERVIX UTERI

DUTCH REGISTRIES

REGISTRY	NUMBER OF CASES	PERIOD OF DIAGNOSIS
Eindhoven	249	1978-1985
Mean age (years)	53.6	

RELATIVE SURVIVAL (%)

100
80
60
40
20
0
0 1 2 3 4 5
Time since diagnosis (years)

OBSERVED AND RELATIVE SURVIVAL (%) BY AGE AND PERIOD
(Number of cases in parentheses)

	AGE CLASS												PERIOD					
	15-44		45-54		55-64		65-74		75+		All		1978-80		1981-82		1983-85	
	obs	rel	obs	rel	obs	rel	obs	rel	obs	rel	obs	rel	obs	rel	obs	rel	obs	rel
Females	(82)		(52)		(46)		(36)		(33)		(249)		(98)		(63)		(88)	
1 year	93	93	83	83	91	92	92	93	70	75	87	88	85	86	87	89	90	91
3 years	74	74	65	66	73	75	66	70	33	43	65	69	65	68	62	65	67	70
5 years	70	70	54	55	70	73	52	58	26	42	58	63	58	63	51	56	67	73
8 years	70	71	54	56	57	62	35	44	19	43	52	60	51	58	..	..	..	..
10 years	70	71	54	57	57	64	35	48	..	..	52	63	51	62	..	..	..	..

RELATIVE SURVIVAL (%) BY AGE AND PERIOD

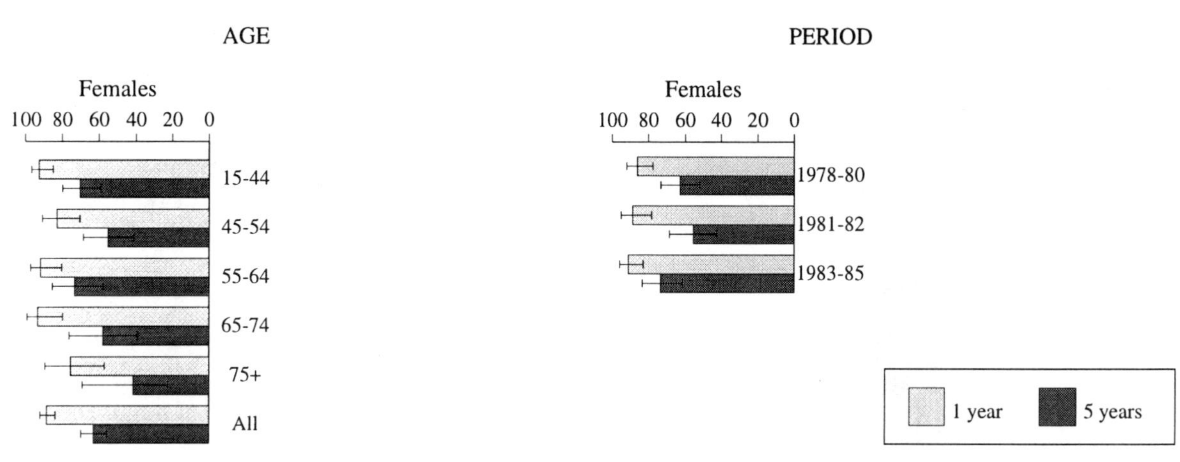

CERVIX UTERI

ENGLISH REGISTRIES

REGISTRY	NUMBER OF CASES	PERIOD OF DIAGNOSIS
East Anglia	914	1979-1984
Mersey	1752	1978-1984
South Thames	2870	1978-1984
Wessex	426	1983-1984
West Midlands	2434	1979-1984
Yorkshire	2382	1978-1984
Mean age (years)	54.2	

RELATIVE SURVIVAL (%)

100 80 60 40 20 0

0 1 2 3 4 5

Time since diagnosis (years)

OBSERVED AND RELATIVE SURVIVAL (%) BY AGE AND PERIOD
(Number of cases in parentheses)

	AGE CLASS												PERIOD					
	15-44		45-54		55-64		65-74		75+		All		1978-80		1981-82		1983-85	
	obs	rel	obs	rel	obs	rel	obs	rel	obs	rel	obs	rel	obs	rel	obs	rel	obs	rel
Females	(3415)		(1723)		(2488)		(2000)		(1152)		(10778)		(4175)		(3093)		(3510)	
1 year	89	89	82	82	80	81	71	73	45	49	78	79	76	77	78	79	80	82
3 years	75	76	60	61	58	60	49	53	25	33	59	62	56	59	59	62	62	65
5 years	72	72	54	56	49	52	39	45	18	30	52	57	49	54	52	56	55	60
8 years	69	70	51	53	41	46	30	39	13	32	46	54	44	52	47	54	49	56
10 years	68	69	47	50	37	42	26	37	10	32	43	53	40	50	45	54	..	..

RELATIVE SURVIVAL (%) BY AGE AND PERIOD

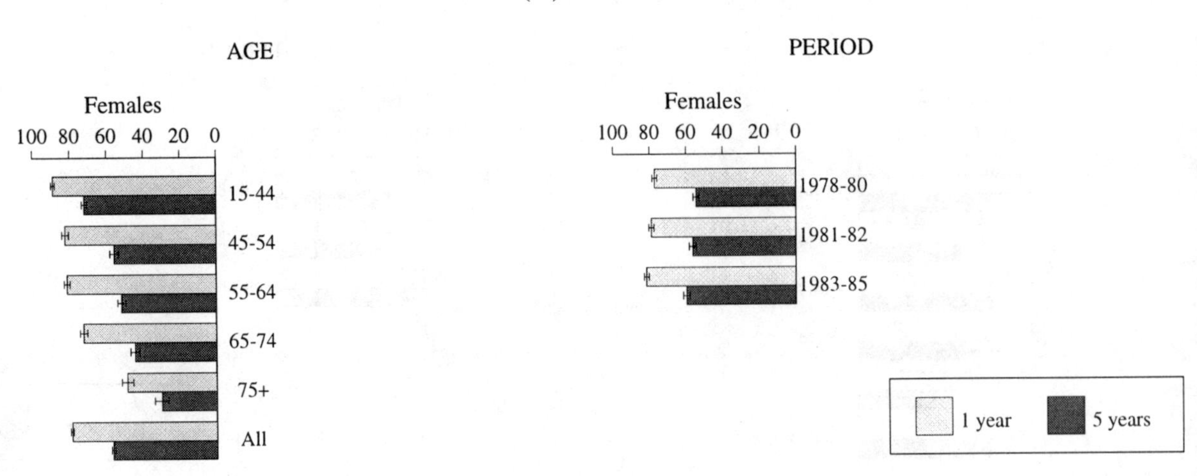

CERVIX UTERI

ESTONIA

REGISTRY	NUMBER OF CASES	PERIOD OF DIAGNOSIS
Estonia	1095	1978-1984
Mean age (years)	58.1	

RELATIVE SURVIVAL (%)

100 80 60 40 20 0

0 1 2 3 4 5

Time since diagnosis (years)

OBSERVED AND RELATIVE SURVIVAL (%) BY AGE AND PERIOD
(Number of cases in parentheses)

	AGE CLASS												PERIOD					
	15-44		45-54		55-64		65-74		75+		All		1978-80		1981-82		1983-85	
	obs	rel	obs	rel	obs	rel	obs	rel	obs	rel	obs	rel	obs	rel	obs	rel	obs	rel
Females	(170)		(233)		(342)		(234)		(116)		(1095)		(465)		(319)		(311)	
1 year	82	82	86	86	84	85	73	75	59	64	79	81	78	79	80	82	80	81
3 years	62	62	68	69	66	68	49	54	23	31	58	61	57	61	62	65	55	59
5 years	58	59	63	64	61	64	40	49	12	21	51	57	50	57	55	61	50	55
8 years	58	59	56	59	51	57	34	49	11	30	45	55	43	54	51	61	..	..
10 years	57	58	54	58	44	52	30	52	9	35	42	55	40	53	..	..	..	..

RELATIVE SURVIVAL (%) BY AGE AND PERIOD

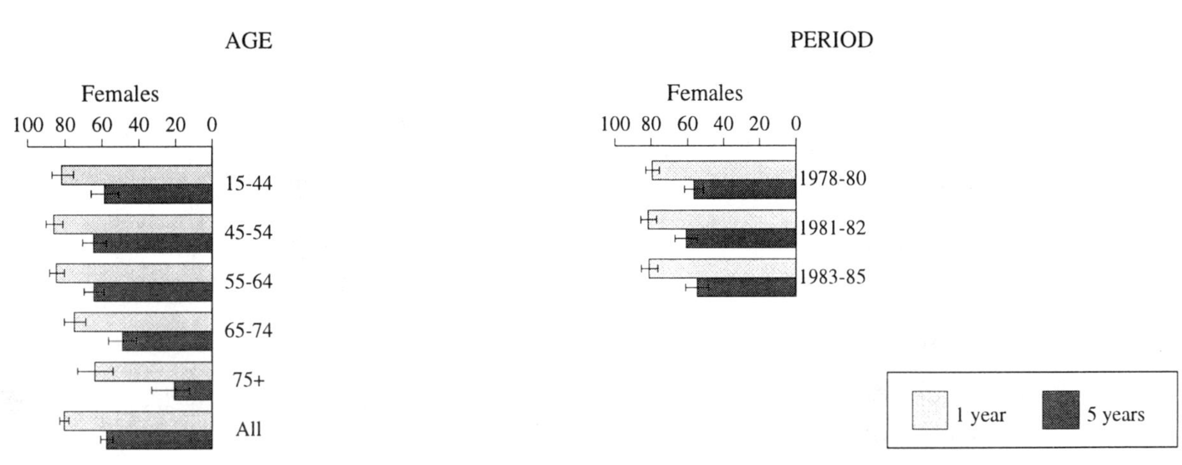

CERVIX UTERI

FINLAND

REGISTRY	NUMBER OF CASES	PERIOD OF DIAGNOSIS
Finland	1290	1978-1984
Mean age (years)	60.4	

RELATIVE SURVIVAL (%)

Time since diagnosis (years)

OBSERVED AND RELATIVE SURVIVAL (%) BY AGE AND PERIOD
(Number of cases in parentheses)

	AGE CLASS												PERIOD					
	15-44		45-54		55-64		65-74		75+		All		1978-80		1981-82		1983-85	
	obs	rel	obs	rel	obs	rel	obs	rel	obs	rel	obs	rel	obs	rel	obs	rel	obs	rel
Females	(230)		(160)		(307)		(387)		(206)		(1290)		(565)		(376)		(349)	
1 year	94	94	91	92	87	88	81	83	66	72	84	86	83	85	85	88	83	85
3 years	83	84	66	66	66	68	54	59	37	49	61	66	62	66	62	67	58	63
5 years	78	79	61	62	59	62	45	52	25	41	53	60	54	60	54	61	50	58
8 years	77	78	56	58	51	56	31	41	12	30	44	55	47	57	43	53	41	51
10 years	75	76	53	56	47	54	25	36	5	17	40	52	42	54	38	50	..	..

RELATIVE SURVIVAL (%) BY AGE AND PERIOD

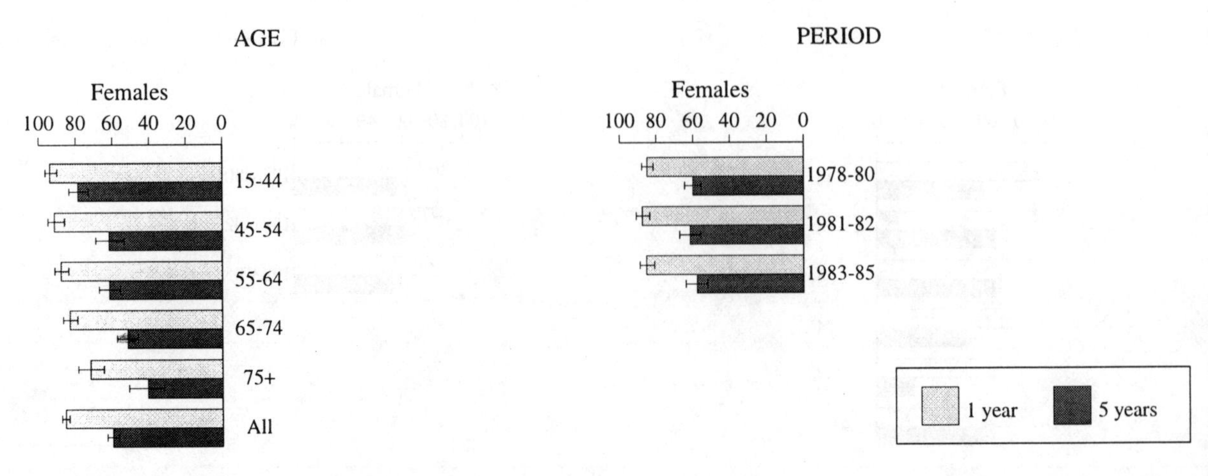

CERVIX UTERI

FRENCH REGISTRIES

REGISTRY	NUMBER OF CASES	PERIOD OF DIAGNOSIS
Amiens	106	1983-1984
Doubs	278	1978-1985
Mean age (years)	58.3	

RELATIVE SURVIVAL (%)

OBSERVED AND RELATIVE SURVIVAL (%) BY AGE AND PERIOD
(Number of cases in parentheses)

	AGE CLASS												PERIOD					
	15-44		45-54		55-64		65-74		75+		All		1978-80		1981-82		1983-85	
	obs	rel	obs	rel	obs	rel	obs	rel	obs	rel	obs	rel	obs	rel	obs	rel	obs	rel
Females	(76)		(82)		(94)		(73)		(59)		(384)		(121)		(64)		(199)	
1 year	99	99	80	80	91	92	86	88	53	61	84	86	82	85	84	86	84	86
3 years	81	81	69	69	74	75	56	60	28	39	64	68	63	69	60	63	66	70
5 years	78	79	61	62	67	69	50	56	19	32	58	64	55	61	55	59	61	67
8 years	72	73	59	61	60	64	36	44	15	34	52	60	50	59	51	58	..	..
10 years	72	74	59	62	57	62	36	48	15	45	51	62	49	61	..	..	..	..

RELATIVE SURVIVAL (%) BY AGE AND PERIOD

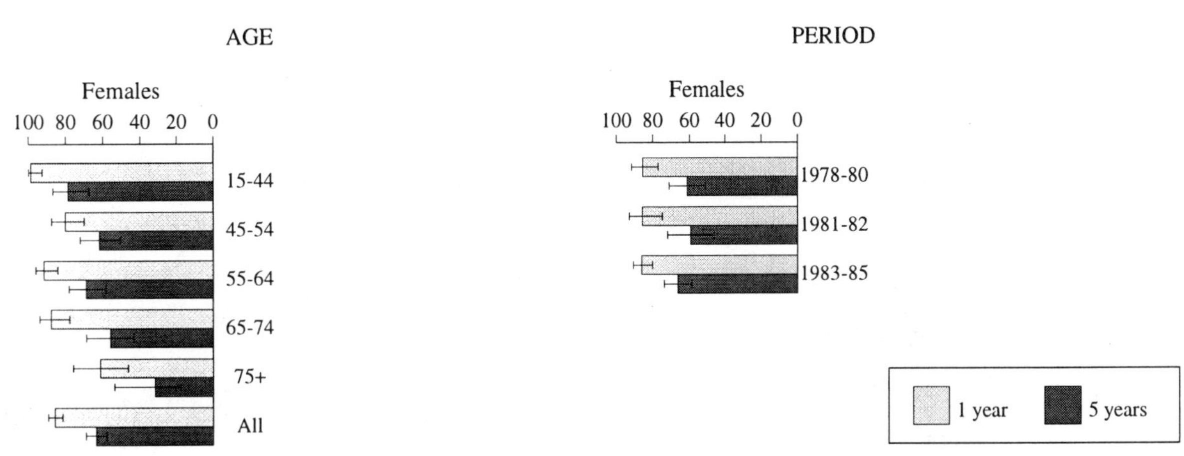

CERVIX UTERI

GERMAN REGISTRIES

REGISTRY	NUMBER OF CASES	PERIOD OF DIAGNOSIS
Saarland	713	1978-1984
Mean age (years)	57.3	

RELATIVE SURVIVAL (%)

100 80 60 40 20 0

0 1 2 3 4 5

Time since diagnosis (years)

OBSERVED AND RELATIVE SURVIVAL (%) BY AGE AND PERIOD
(Number of cases in parentheses)

	AGE CLASS												PERIOD					
	15-44		45-54		55-64		65-74		75+		All		1978-80		1981-82		1983-85	
	obs	rel	obs	rel	obs	rel	obs	rel	obs	rel	obs	rel	obs	rel	obs	rel	obs	rel
Females	(153)		(115)		(194)		(178)		(73)		(713)		(344)		(179)		(190)	
1 year	92	92	91	92	84	85	78	80	66	71	84	85	83	84	85	86	84	86
3 years	76	76	69	70	68	70	51	56	37	47	62	66	64	67	62	65	61	64
5 years	72	72	66	68	62	65	43	50	22	34	56	61	57	63	56	61	54	60
8 years	71	71	59	62	55	61	35	47	18	38	50	59	51	61	50	58	..	..
10 years	71	72	57	59	49	56	33	49	15	41	47	58	48	60	..	..	..	..

RELATIVE SURVIVAL (%) BY AGE AND PERIOD

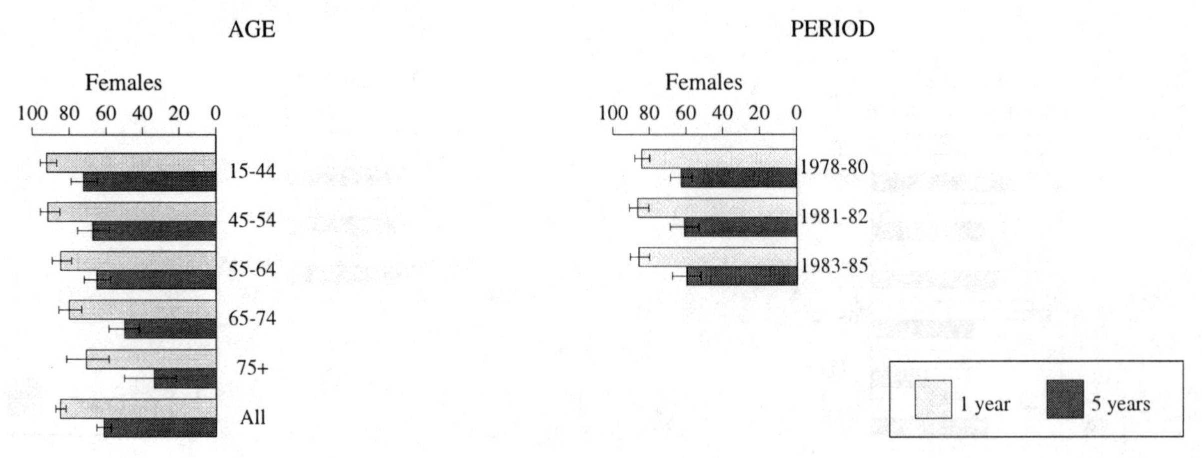

CERVIX UTERI

ITALIAN REGISTRIES

REGISTRY	NUMBER OF CASES	PERIOD OF DIAGNOSIS
Latina	56	1983-1984
Ragusa	74	1981-1984
Varese	349	1978-1984
Mean age (years)	55.0	

RELATIVE SURVIVAL (%)

100
80
60
40
20
0
0 1 2 3 4 5
Time since diagnosis (years)

OBSERVED AND RELATIVE SURVIVAL (%) BY AGE AND PERIOD
(Number of cases in parentheses)

	AGE CLASS											
	15-44		45-54		55-64		65-74		75+		All	
	obs	rel	obs	rel	obs	rel	obs	rel	obs	rel	obs	rel
Females	(135)		(102)		(101)		(95)		(46)		(479)	
1 year	97	97	90	90	91	92	82	84	67	73	89	90
3 years	80	80	71	71	70	72	57	61	39	51	67	71
5 years	76	77	68	69	64	67	48	55	20	31	61	66
8 years	75	75	62	64	56	60	37	48	10	23	54	62
10 years	75	76	59	62	54	60	32	45	0	0	51	61

	PERIOD					
	1978-80		1981-82		1983-85	
	obs	rel	obs	rel	obs	rel
Females	(174)		(125)		(180)	
1 year	83	85	91	93	92	93
3 years	63	67	71	75	69	71
5 years	56	62	65	71	63	66
8 years	49	57	56	64	57	63
10 years	46	56	53	63	..	..

RELATIVE SURVIVAL (%) BY AGE AND PERIOD

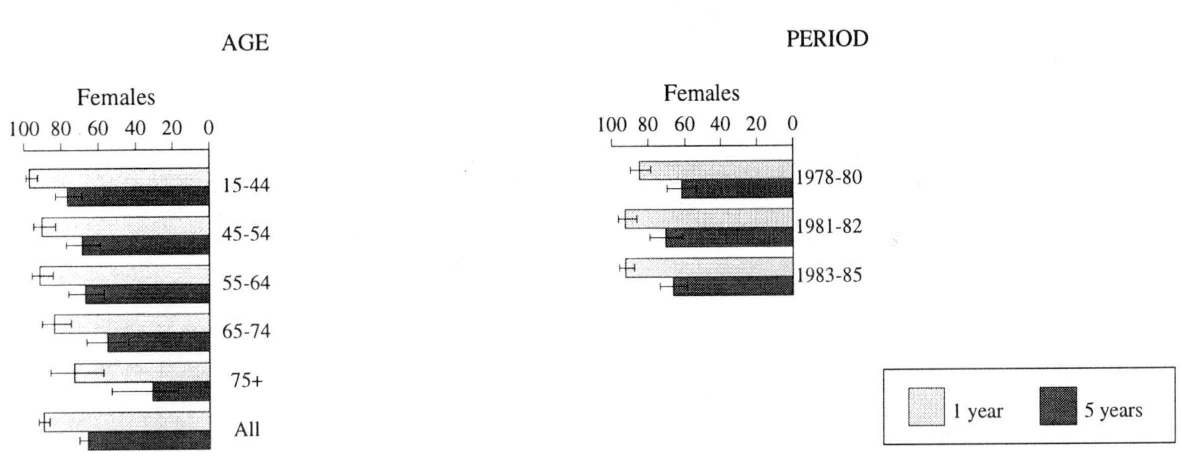

CERVIX UTERI

POLISH REGISTRIES

REGISTRY	NUMBER OF CASES	PERIOD OF DIAGNOSIS
Cracow	618	1978-1984
Mean age (years)	53.4	

RELATIVE SURVIVAL (%)

OBSERVED AND RELATIVE SURVIVAL (%) BY AGE AND PERIOD
(Number of cases in parentheses)

	AGE CLASS												PERIOD					
	15-44		45-54		55-64		65-74		75+		All		1978-80		1981-82		1983-85	
	obs	rel	obs	rel	obs	rel	obs	rel	obs	rel	obs	rel	obs	rel	obs	rel	obs	rel
Females	(164)		(180)		(128)		(103)		(43)		(618)		(253)		(182)		(183)	
1 year	86	86	81	81	73	74	62	63	26	28	74	75	73	74	77	78	71	72
3 years	69	69	59	59	57	59	50	55	16	21	57	59	54	56	61	64	56	59
5 years	66	67	53	54	51	54	36	42	9	15	50	54	47	50	54	58	51	55
8 years	62	63	47	50	45	51	26	35	9	22	45	51	40	46	49	56	48	54
10 years	61	63	43	46	43	51	26	40	9	30	43	51	38	46	46	56	..	..

RELATIVE SURVIVAL (%) BY AGE AND PERIOD

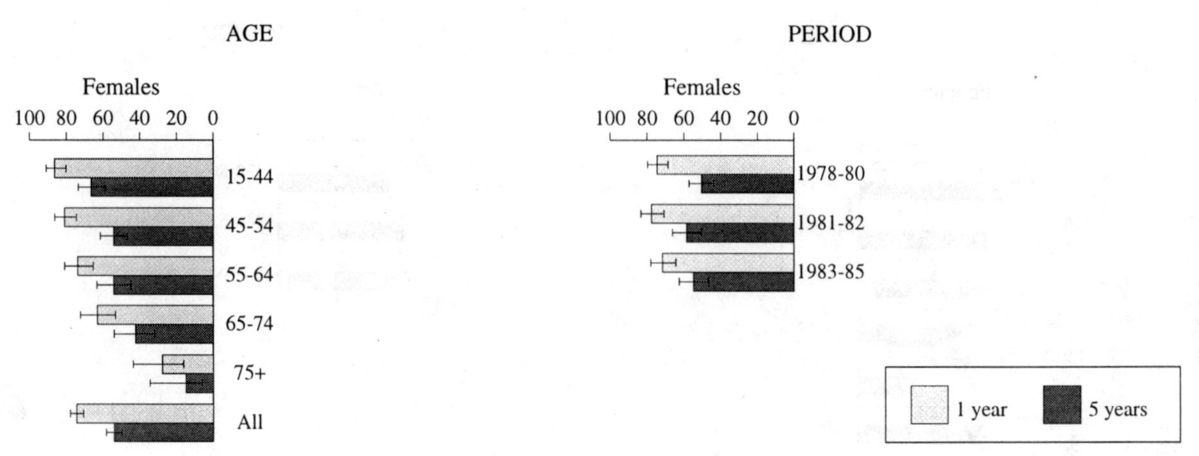

CERVIX UTERI

SCOTLAND

REGISTRY	NUMBER OF CASES	PERIOD OF DIAGNOSIS
Scotland	1955	1978-1982
Mean age (years)	54.1	

RELATIVE SURVIVAL (%)

OBSERVED AND RELATIVE SURVIVAL (%) BY AGE AND PERIOD
(Number of cases in parentheses)

	AGE CLASS												PERIOD					
	15-44		45-54		55-64		65-74		75+		All		1978-80		1981-82		1983-85	
	obs	rel	obs	rel	obs	rel	obs	rel	obs	rel	obs	rel	obs	rel	obs	rel	obs	rel
Females	(583)		(323)		(501)		(357)		(191)		(1955)		(1135)		(820)		(0)	
1 year	88	88	79	79	79	80	69	71	39	43	76	77	75	76	77	79	..	..
3 years	71	72	59	59	56	59	48	53	21	28	56	59	55	58	58	61	..	..
5 years	67	67	54	56	46	49	38	44	15	24	49	54	47	52	51	56	..	..
8 years	63	63	49	52	37	42	29	38	8	20	42	50	41	48	..	..	..	..
10 years	63	64	49	53	33	39	25	37	..	..	40	50	39	48	..	..	..	..

RELATIVE SURVIVAL (%) BY AGE AND PERIOD

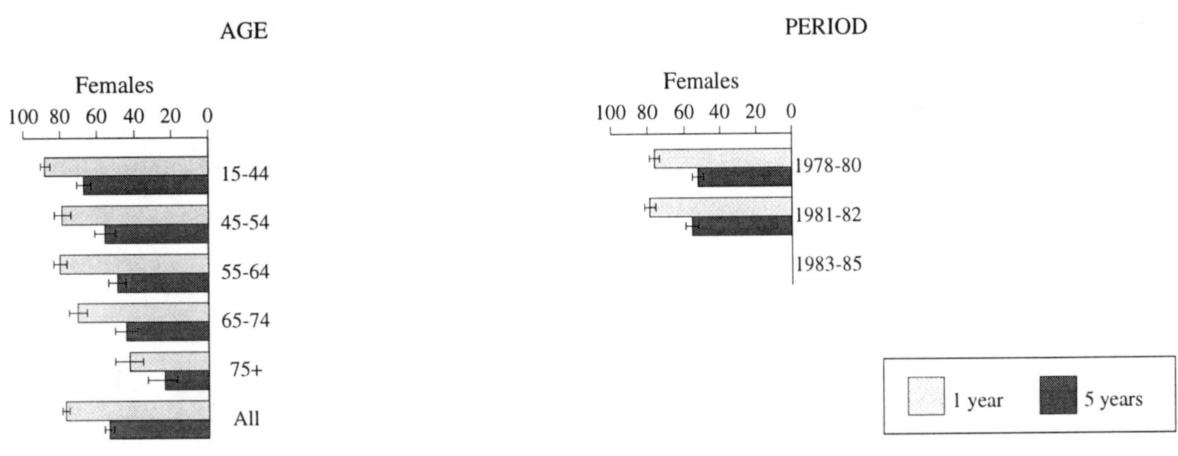

CERVIX UTERI

SPANISH REGISTRIES

REGISTRY	NUMBER OF CASES	PERIOD OF DIAGNOSIS
Girona	97	1980-1985
Tarragona	29	1985-1985
Mean age (years)	58.1	

RELATIVE SURVIVAL (%)

Time since diagnosis (years)

OBSERVED AND RELATIVE SURVIVAL (%) BY AGE AND PERIOD
(Number of cases in parentheses)

	AGE CLASS												PERIOD					
	15-44		45-54		55-64		65-74		75+		All		1978-80		1981-82		1983-85	
	obs	rel	obs	rel	obs	rel	obs	rel	obs	rel	obs	rel	obs	rel	obs	rel	obs	rel
Females	(24)		(24)		(36)		(24)		(18)		(126)		(15)		(34)		(77)	
1 year	78	78	83	84	86	87	60	61	48	52	74	75	87	89	78	79	70	71
3 years	60	60	46	46	64	65	32	34	12	15	47	49	47	51	49	51	46	48
5 years	51	51	33	34	52	54	28	31	6	9	37	41	27	30	39	42	39	42
8 years	51	51	33	34	45	48	28	34	0	0	34	39	27	33	39	43	31	35
10 years	51	52	33	35	34	37	..	..	0	0	30	36	20	26	..	..	..	..

RELATIVE SURVIVAL (%) BY AGE AND PERIOD

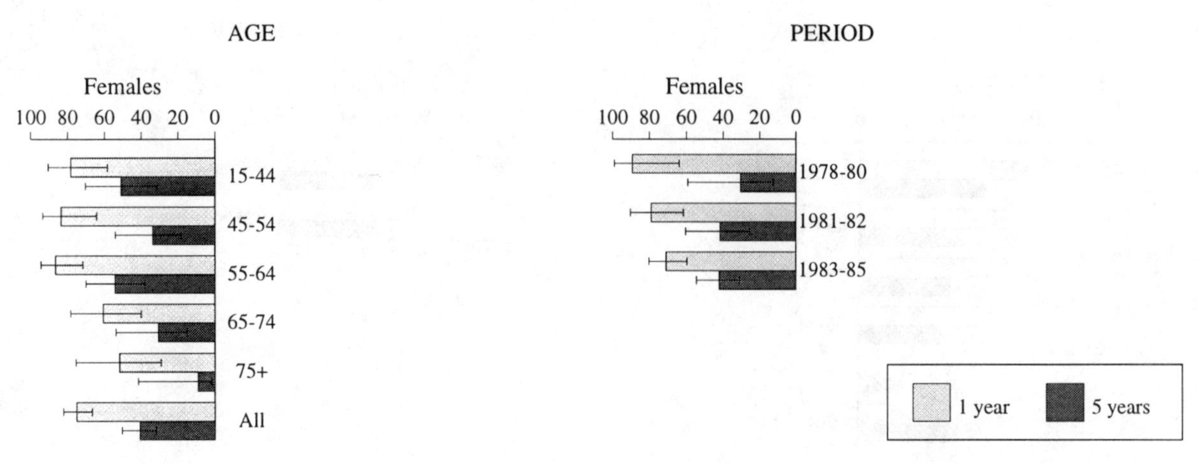

CERVIX UTERI

SWISS REGISTRIES

REGISTRY	NUMBER OF CASES	PERIOD OF DIAGNOSIS
Basel	87	1981-1984
Geneva	146	1978-1984
Mean age (years)	57.5	

RELATIVE SURVIVAL (%)

Time since diagnosis (years)

OBSERVED AND RELATIVE SURVIVAL (%) BY AGE AND PERIOD
(Number of cases in parentheses)

	AGE CLASS												PERIOD					
	15-44		45-54		55-64		65-74		75+		All		1978-80		1981-82		1983-85	
	obs	rel	obs	rel	obs	rel	obs	rel	obs	rel	obs	rel	obs	rel	obs	rel	obs	rel
Females	(63)		(49)		(34)		(43)		(44)		(233)		(76)		(78)		(79)	
1 year	92	92	88	88	85	86	93	95	48	52	82	84	91	93	82	84	73	75
3 years	81	81	69	70	68	69	72	77	23	31	64	68	73	78	68	72	51	55
5 years	79	80	67	68	62	64	56	62	14	23	57	64	64	71	60	66	48	55
8 years	79	80	56	58	62	66	42	51	..	..	52	63	..	..	53	63	..	..
10 years	..	..	..	..	..	..	..	..	..	..	..	..	..	..	..	..	..	..

RELATIVE SURVIVAL (%) BY AGE AND PERIOD

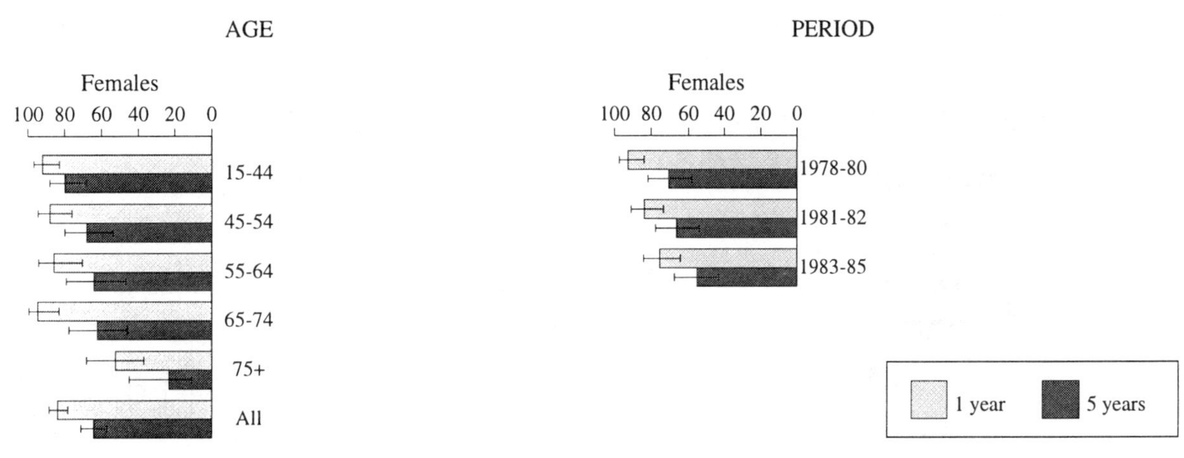

CERVIX UTERI

EUROPEAN REGISTRIES

Weighted analysis

REGISTRY	WEIGHTS (Yearly expected cases in the country)
DENMARK	599
DUTCH REGISTRIES	671
ENGLISH REGISTRIES	4179
ESTONIA	156
FINLAND	184
FRENCH REGISTRIES	3327
GERMAN REGISTRIES	4700
ITALIAN REGISTRIES	3662
POLISH REGISTRIES	3478
SCOTLAND	391
SPANISH REGISTRIES	2080
SWISS REGISTRIES	448

RELATIVE SURVIVAL (%)
(Age-standardized)

Females
100 80 60 40 20 0
DK
NL
ENG
EST
FIN
F
D
I
PL
SCO
E
CH
EUR

OBSERVED AND RELATIVE SURVIVAL (%) BY AGE AND PERIOD

	AGE CLASS												PERIOD					
	15-44		45-54		55-64		65-74		75+		All		1978-80		1981-82		1983-85	
	obs	rel	obs	rel	obs	rel	obs	rel	obs	rel	obs	rel	obs	rel	obs	rel	obs	rel
Females																		
1 year	91	91	85	85	84	85	75	77	52	57	81	82	80	82	82	84	81	83
3 years	75	75	64	64	65	67	51	56	28	37	61	64	59	63	61	64	61	64
5 years	71	71	58	59	58	61	42	48	17	27	54	59	51	56	55	59	55	60
8 years	68	69	54	56	51	55	33	42	12	28	48	56	45	53	50	57	48	54
10 years	68	69	51	54	46	52	30	44	9	27	45	55	42	52	48	57	..	..

RELATIVE SURVIVAL (%) BY AGE AND PERIOD

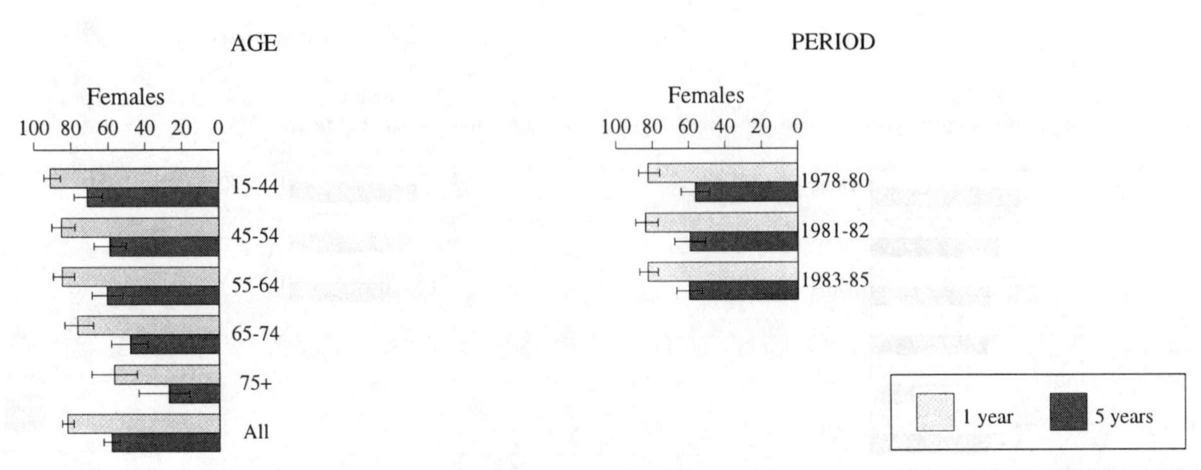

CORPUS UTERI

DENMARK

REGISTRY	NUMBER OF CASES	PERIOD OF DIAGNOSIS
Denmark	4404	1978-1984
Mean age (years)	64.2	

RELATIVE SURVIVAL (%)

Time since diagnosis (years)

OBSERVED AND RELATIVE SURVIVAL (%) BY AGE AND PERIOD

(Number of cases in parentheses)

	AGE CLASS												PERIOD					
	15-44		45-54		55-64		65-74		75+		All		1978-80		1981-82		1983-85	
	obs	rel	obs	rel	obs	rel	obs	rel	obs	rel	obs	rel	obs	rel	obs	rel	obs	rel
Females	(120)		(587)		(1644)		(1276)		(777)		(4404)		(1818)		(1285)		(1301)	
1 year	89	89	94	94	93	94	86	88	66	71	86	88	85	87	88	90	86	88
3 years	83	84	88	89	85	88	72	77	43	54	74	80	73	78	75	80	75	81
5 years	79	80	85	88	81	86	65	74	34	51	68	78	67	76	69	79	69	79
8 years	76	78	83	87	76	85	54	69	23	49	61	77	60	75	63	79	..	..
10 years	74	76	81	87	73	84	49	69	14	41	57	78	56	75	..	..	..	..

RELATIVE SURVIVAL (%) BY AGE AND PERIOD

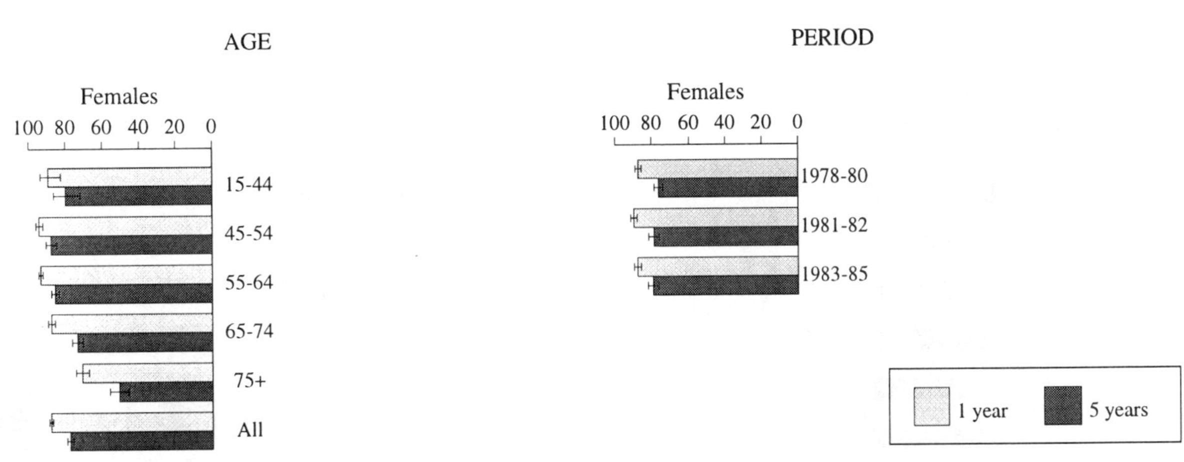

CORPUS UTERI

DUTCH REGISTRIES

REGISTRY	NUMBER OF CASES	PERIOD OF DIAGNOSIS
Eindhoven	410	1978-1985
Mean age (years)	63.2	

RELATIVE SURVIVAL (%)

100 80 60 40 20 0

0 1 2 3 4 5

Time since diagnosis (years)

OBSERVED AND RELATIVE SURVIVAL (%) BY AGE AND PERIOD
(Number of cases in parentheses)

	AGE CLASS												PERIOD					
	15-44		45-54		55-64		65-74		75+		All		1978-80		1981-82		1983-85	
	obs	rel	obs	rel	obs	rel	obs	rel	obs	rel	obs	rel	obs	rel	obs	rel	obs	rel
Females	(17)		(71)		(147)		(106)		(69)		(410)		(134)		(110)		(166)	
1 year	94	94	90	90	95	96	86	88	77	82	89	91	90	91	85	87	90	92
3 years	94	95	80	81	87	89	76	81	53	67	78	83	80	85	68	73	82	88
5 years	94	95	80	82	84	88	66	75	38	57	72	80	72	80	64	71	80	90
8 years	94	95	74	77	80	87	62	79	30	63	67	83	66	81	..	..	..	..
10 years	..	..	74	78	80	90	57	81	20	55	62	85	62	83	..	..	..	..

RELATIVE SURVIVAL (%) BY AGE AND PERIOD

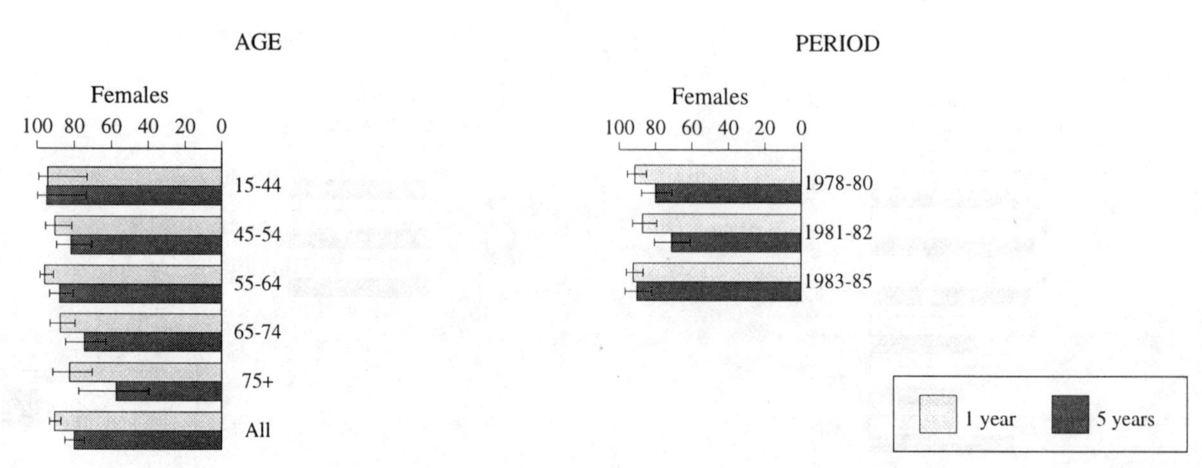

CORPUS UTERI

ENGLISH REGISTRIES

REGISTRY	NUMBER OF CASES	PERIOD OF DIAGNOSIS
East Anglia	1078	1979-1984
Mersey	976	1978-1984
South Thames	3688	1978-1984
Wessex	431	1983-1984
West Midlands	2279	1979-1984
Yorkshire	1655	1978-1984
Mean age (years)	64.8	

RELATIVE SURVIVAL (%)

100
80
60
40
20
0
0 1 2 3 4 5
Time since diagnosis (years)

OBSERVED AND RELATIVE SURVIVAL (%) BY AGE AND PERIOD
(Number of cases in parentheses)

	AGE CLASS												PERIOD					
	15-44		45-54		55-64		65-74		75+		All		1978-80		1981-82		1983-85	
	obs	rel	obs	rel	obs	rel	obs	rel	obs	rel	obs	rel	obs	rel	obs	rel	obs	rel
Females	(335)		(1573)		(3141)		(2853)		(2205)		(10107)		(3840)		(3019)		(3248)	
1 year	90	90	92	93	89	90	78	80	61	66	80	83	79	82	80	82	82	84
3 years	83	83	85	86	78	80	62	68	41	54	67	73	65	71	67	73	68	74
5 years	80	80	82	84	73	77	55	63	32	51	60	71	59	69	61	71	62	72
8 years	77	78	79	83	67	75	47	62	24	57	54	71	53	70	54	71	55	71
10 years	73	75	75	80	63	72	41	60	18	57	49	69	49	69	49	68	..	..

RELATIVE SURVIVAL (%) BY AGE AND PERIOD

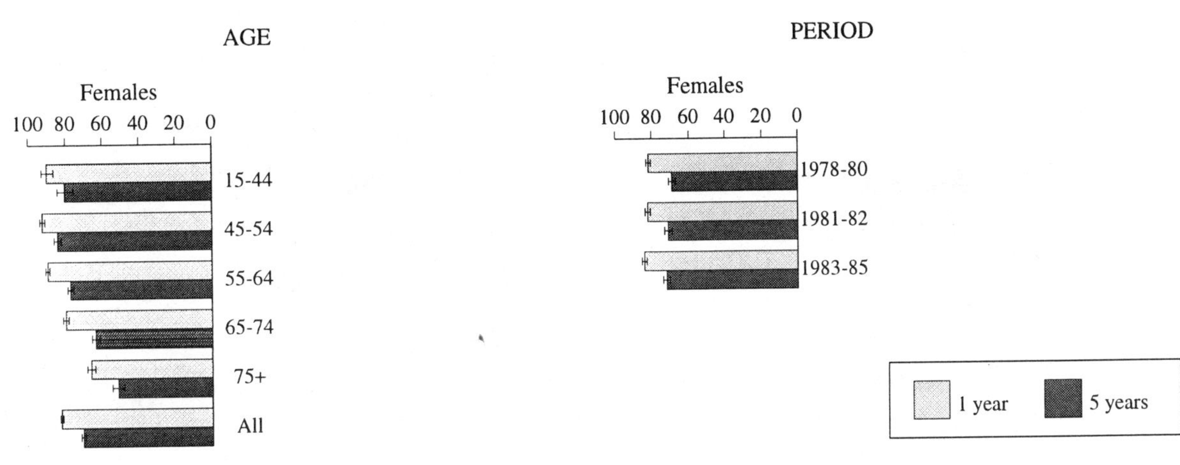

CORPUS UTERI

ESTONIA

REGISTRY	NUMBER OF CASES	PERIOD OF DIAGNOSIS
Estonia	873	1978-1984
Mean age (years)	60.7	

RELATIVE SURVIVAL (%)

100
80
60
40
20
0
0 1 2 3 4 5
Time since diagnosis (years)

OBSERVED AND RELATIVE SURVIVAL (%) BY AGE AND PERIOD
(Number of cases in parentheses)

	AGE CLASS												PERIOD					
	15-44		45-54		55-64		65-74		75+		All		1978-80		1981-82		1983-85	
	obs	rel	obs	rel	obs	rel	obs	rel	obs	rel	obs	rel	obs	rel	obs	rel	obs	rel
Females	(46)		(228)		(284)		(213)		(102)		(873)		(366)		(261)		(246)	
1 year	96	96	90	90	87	88	74	76	60	66	82	84	78	80	86	88	84	86
3 years	84	85	83	85	74	76	52	58	37	50	67	72	63	68	74	79	66	71
5 years	84	85	80	82	68	72	44	53	26	45	61	69	59	66	67	76	59	67
8 years	82	84	77	81	63	70	32	46	15	41	54	68	52	65	60	74	..	..
10 years	78	81	74	80	62	72	29	50	12	47	52	71	50	67	..	..	..	..

RELATIVE SURVIVAL (%) BY AGE AND PERIOD

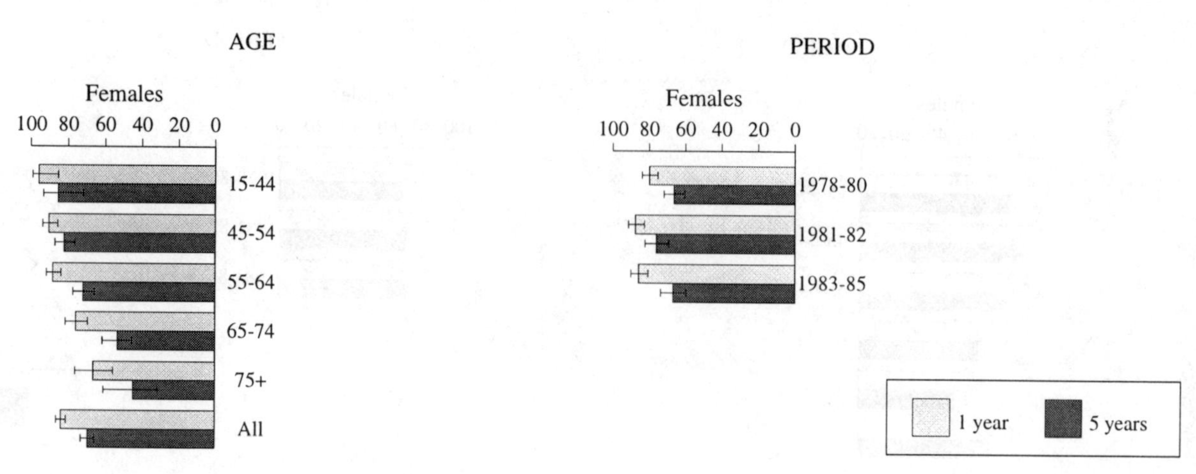

CORPUS UTERI

FINLAND

REGISTRY	NUMBER OF CASES	PERIOD OF DIAGNOSIS
Finland	2867	1978-1984
Mean age (years)	63.1	

RELATIVE SURVIVAL (%)

Time since diagnosis (years)

OBSERVED AND RELATIVE SURVIVAL (%) BY AGE AND PERIOD
(Number of cases in parentheses)

	AGE CLASS												PERIOD					
	15-44		45-54		55-64		65-74		75+		All		1978-80		1981-82		1983-85	
	obs	rel	obs	rel	obs	rel	obs	rel	obs	rel	obs	rel	obs	rel	obs	rel	obs	rel
Females	(112)		(548)		(910)		(830)		(467)		(2867)		(1237)		(806)		(824)	
1 year	100	100	98	98	94	94	85	87	71	77	88	90	87	89	90	91	90	92
3 years	97	98	93	93	84	86	70	75	49	63	76	82	74	80	78	84	77	82
5 years	96	96	89	91	79	83	61	70	39	61	70	79	68	77	72	81	71	80
8 years	94	95	87	90	74	80	53	69	24	55	63	78	62	76	66	81	63	77
10 years	92	94	85	89	71	80	47	67	18	54	59	77	58	76	62	81	..	..

RELATIVE SURVIVAL (%) BY AGE AND PERIOD

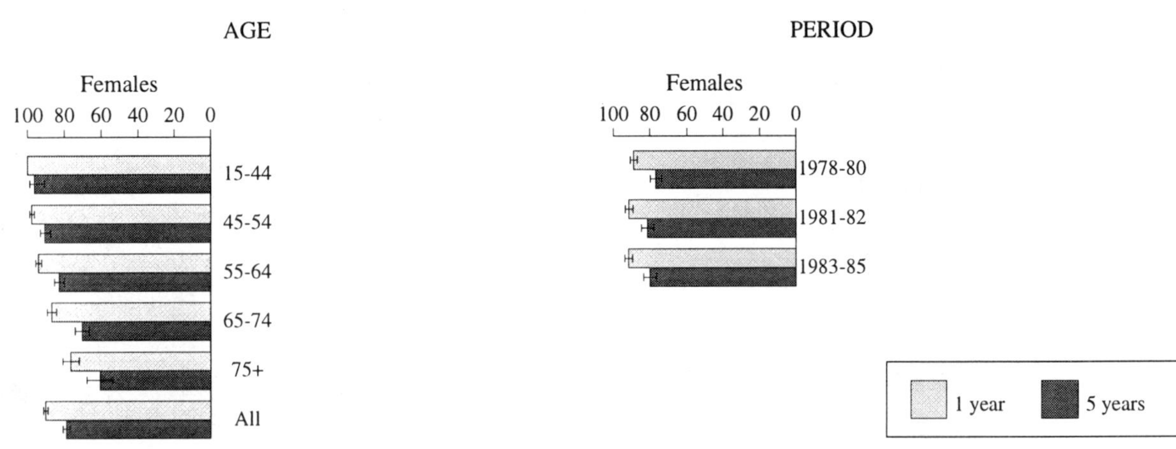

CORPUS UTERI

FRENCH REGISTRIES

REGISTRY	NUMBER OF CASES	PERIOD OF DIAGNOSIS
Amiens	89	1983-1984
Mean age (years)	64.1	

RELATIVE SURVIVAL (%)

100
80
60
40
20
0
0 1 2 3 4 5
Time since diagnosis (years)

OBSERVED AND RELATIVE SURVIVAL (%) BY AGE AND PERIOD
(Number of cases in parentheses)

	AGE CLASS												PERIOD					
	15-44		45-54		55-64		65-74		75+		All		1978-80		1981-82		1983-85	
	obs	rel	obs	rel	obs	rel	obs	rel	obs	rel	obs	rel	obs	rel	obs	rel	obs	rel
Females	(3)		(13)		(32)		(25)		(16)		(89)		(0)		(0)		(89)	
1 year	100	100	92	93	87	88	84	85	69	73	84	86	..	..	..	..	84	86
3 years	67	67	92	94	81	83	67	71	56	69	74	78	..	..	..	..	74	78
5 years	67	67	92	95	65	67	50	56	38	55	60	67	..	..	..	..	60	67
8 years	..	..	..	..	..	..	..	..	..	..	..	..	..	..	..	..	..	..
10 years	..	..	..	..	..	..	..	..	..	..	..	..	..	..	..	..	..	..

RELATIVE SURVIVAL (%) BY AGE AND PERIOD

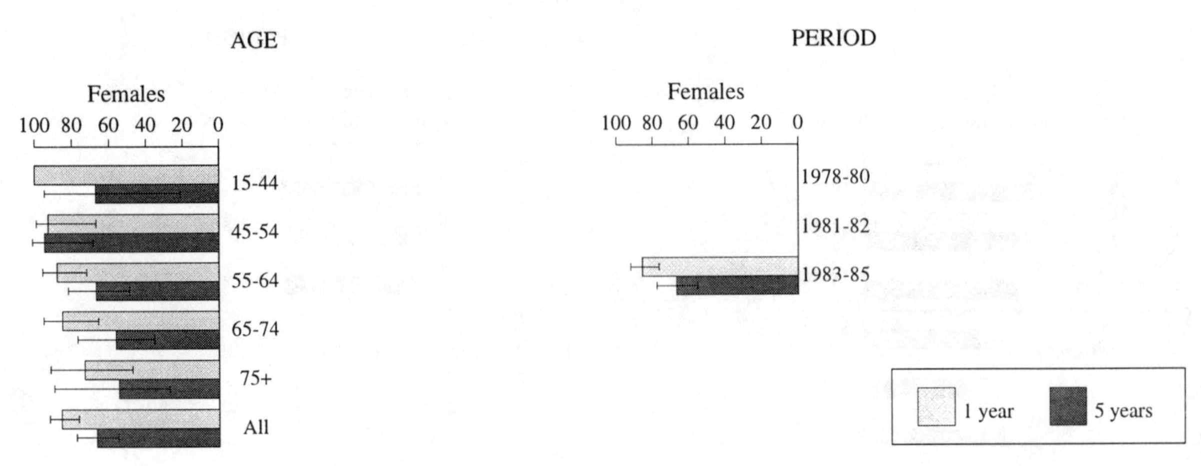

CORPUS UTERI

GERMAN REGISTRIES

REGISTRY	NUMBER OF CASES	PERIOD OF DIAGNOSIS
Saarland	965	1978-1984
Mean age (years)	65.2	

RELATIVE SURVIVAL (%)

Time since diagnosis (years)

OBSERVED AND RELATIVE SURVIVAL (%) BY AGE AND PERIOD
(Number of cases in parentheses)

	AGE CLASS												PERIOD					
	15-44		45-54		55-64		65-74		75+		All		1978-80		1981-82		1983-85	
	obs	rel	obs	rel	obs	rel	obs	rel	obs	rel	obs	rel	obs	rel	obs	rel	obs	rel
Females	(13)		(115)		(327)		(340)		(170)		(965)		(396)		(273)		(296)	
1 year	100	100	91	92	93	93	87	89	76	83	88	90	87	89	85	88	91	94
3 years	100	100	85	86	83	86	69	76	52	67	73	80	73	80	69	75	77	84
5 years	100	100	82	84	76	80	62	73	42	65	66	76	67	77	63	73	68	78
8 years	100	100	76	80	71	78	50	67	33	69	58	74	59	76	54	69	..	..
10 years	100	100	72	77	69	79	44	65	27	74	54	74	55	76	..	..	..	..

RELATIVE SURVIVAL (%) BY AGE AND PERIOD

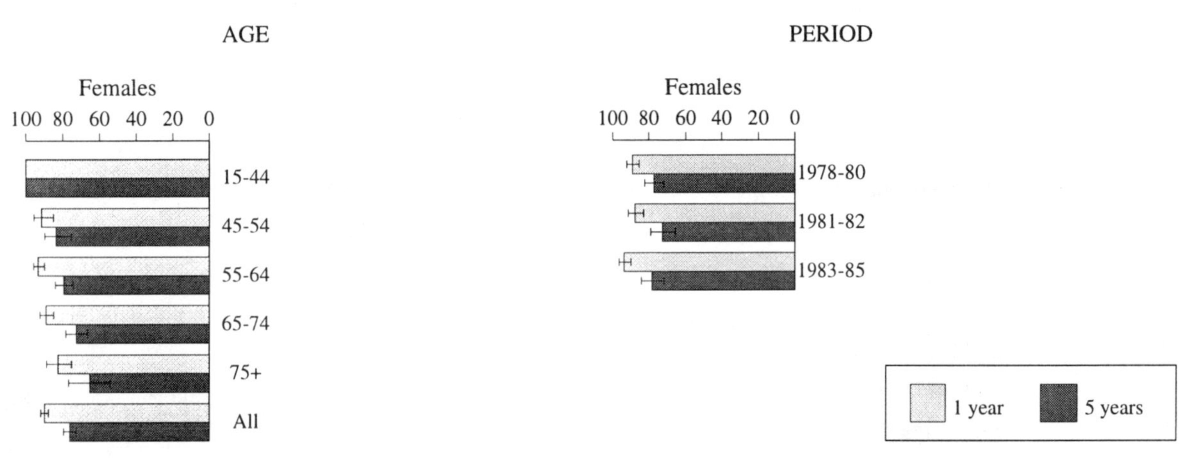

CORPUS UTERI

ITALIAN REGISTRIES

REGISTRY	NUMBER OF CASES	PERIOD OF DIAGNOSIS
Latina	57	1983-1984
Ragusa	98	1981-1984
Varese	518	1978-1984
Mean age (years)	61.9	

RELATIVE SURVIVAL (%)

100
80
60
40
20
0
0 1 2 3 4 5
Time since diagnosis (years)

OBSERVED AND RELATIVE SURVIVAL (%) BY AGE AND PERIOD
(Number of cases in parentheses)

	AGE CLASS												PERIOD					
	15-44		45-54		55-64		65-74		75+		All		1978-80		1981-82		1983-85	
	obs	rel	obs	rel	obs	rel	obs	rel	obs	rel	obs	rel	obs	rel	obs	rel	obs	rel
Females	(30)		(134)		(237)		(191)		(81)		(673)		(218)		(186)		(269)	
1 year	97	97	93	93	90	91	87	89	72	77	88	89	88	89	85	87	90	91
3 years	97	97	86	87	82	84	74	79	46	58	77	81	77	82	73	77	80	84
5 years	93	94	83	84	79	82	62	70	40	60	71	78	69	77	68	75	74	81
8 years	90	91	78	81	75	81	52	65	26	56	64	76	62	76	62	73	64	75
10 years	90	91	76	80	67	75	47	65	24	65	59	74	56	73	62	76	..	..

RELATIVE SURVIVAL (%) BY AGE AND PERIOD

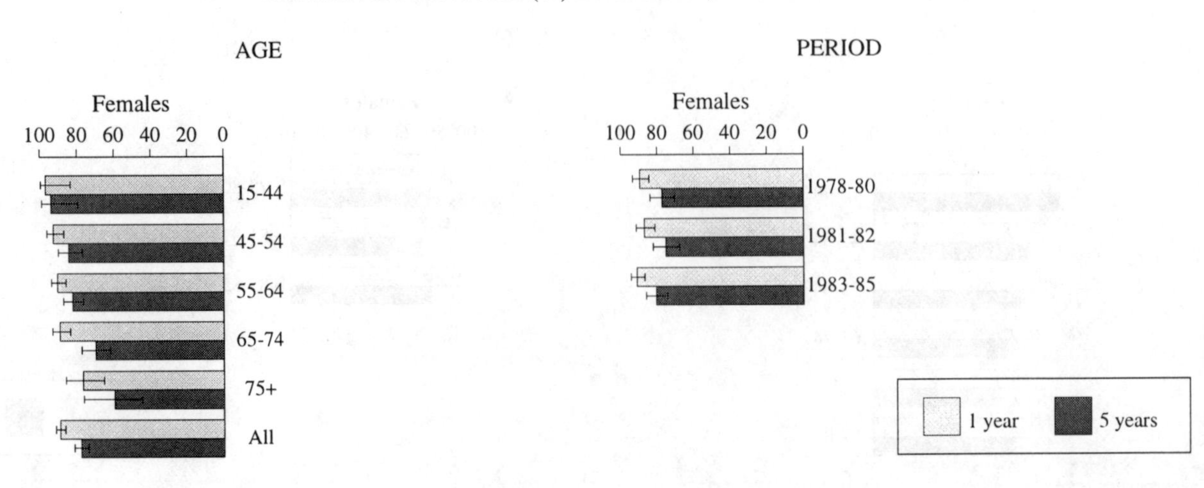

CORPUS UTERI

POLISH REGISTRIES

REGISTRY	NUMBER OF CASES	PERIOD OF DIAGNOSIS
Cracow	317	1978-1984
Mean age (years)	61.2	

RELATIVE SURVIVAL (%)

100, 80, 60, 40, 20, 0

0, 1, 2, 3, 4, 5

Time since diagnosis (years)

OBSERVED AND RELATIVE SURVIVAL (%) BY AGE AND PERIOD
(Number of cases in parentheses)

	AGE CLASS												PERIOD					
	15-44		45-54		55-64		65-74		75+		All		1978-80		1981-82		1983-85	
	obs	rel	obs	rel	obs	rel	obs	rel	obs	rel	obs	rel	obs	rel	obs	rel	obs	rel
Females	(18)		(71)		(106)		(86)		(36)		(317)		(130)		(91)		(96)	
1 year	94	95	85	85	82	82	62	64	45	49	74	75	68	70	77	78	78	80
3 years	89	89	74	76	72	74	40	44	27	36	60	64	56	60	61	65	64	68
5 years	89	90	74	77	70	74	30	36	21	36	56	63	53	60	56	63	60	67
8 years	89	91	73	77	62	69	30	43	14	36	52	65	51	65	50	61	55	67
10 years	89	91	70	75	58	68	30	49	14	51	50	67	49	68	49	63	..	..

RELATIVE SURVIVAL (%) BY AGE AND PERIOD

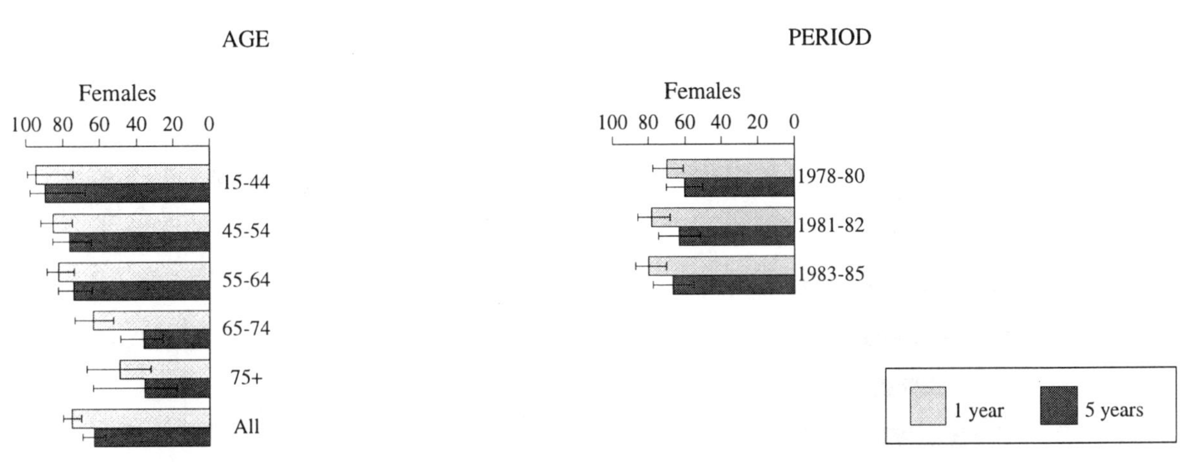

CORPUS UTERI

SCOTLAND

REGISTRY	NUMBER OF CASES	PERIOD OF DIAGNOSIS
Scotland	1368	1978-1982
Mean age (years)	63.8	

RELATIVE SURVIVAL (%)

OBSERVED AND RELATIVE SURVIVAL (%) BY AGE AND PERIOD
(Number of cases in parentheses)

	AGE CLASS												PERIOD					
	15-44		45-54		55-64		65-74		75+		All		1978-80		1981-82		1983-85	
	obs	rel	obs	rel	obs	rel	obs	rel	obs	rel	obs	rel	obs	rel	obs	rel	obs	rel
Females	(49)		(247)		(433)		(367)		(272)		(1368)		(786)		(582)		(0)	
1 year	98	98	96	97	85	86	76	78	61	67	80	83	80	82	81	83	..	..
3 years	96	96	88	90	73	76	57	63	37	49	65	72	65	71	66	73	..	..
5 years	88	88	84	87	69	74	47	56	29	48	59	69	57	67	60	71	..	..
8 years	88	89	78	83	62	71	38	51	21	50	51	67	49	64	..	..	..	..
10 years	..	..	78	84	61	71	35	54	18	54	49	71	47	68	..	..	..	..

RELATIVE SURVIVAL (%) BY AGE AND PERIOD

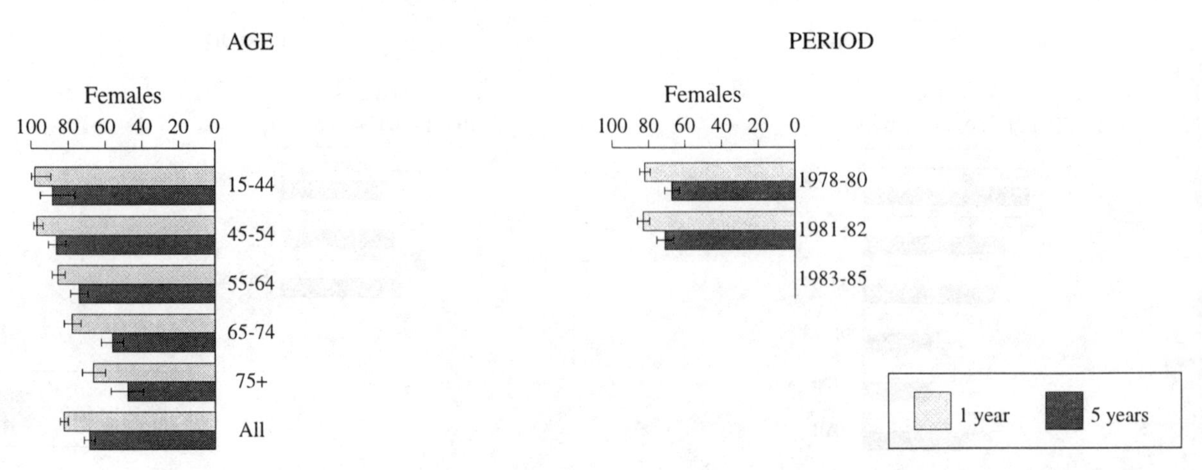

CORPUS UTERI

SPANISH REGISTRIES

REGISTRY	NUMBER OF CASES	PERIOD OF DIAGNOSIS
Girona	173	1980-1985
Tarragona	43	1985-1985
Mean age (years)	61.3	

RELATIVE SURVIVAL (%)

Time since diagnosis (years)

OBSERVED AND RELATIVE SURVIVAL (%) BY AGE AND PERIOD
(Number of cases in parentheses)

	AGE CLASS												PERIOD					
	15-44		45-54		55-64		65-74		75+		All		1978-80		1981-82		1983-85	
	obs	rel	obs	rel	obs	rel	obs	rel	obs	rel	obs	rel	obs	rel	obs	rel	obs	rel
Females	(8)		(44)		(91)		(49)		(24)		(216)		(11)		(66)		(139)	
1 year	100	100	88	88	85	86	78	79	69	74	83	84	78	78	83	83	83	85
3 years	100	100	78	79	68	69	54	57	27	33	63	66	65	66	66	69	62	65
5 years	86	86	72	74	64	66	39	44	15	22	56	60	65	68	59	63	54	59
8 years	86	87	72	74	56	60	39	48	..	..	53	60	65	71	55	61	50	58
10 years	86	87	72	75	51	56	..	..	..	..	51	59	52	59	55	63	..	..

RELATIVE SURVIVAL (%) BY AGE AND PERIOD

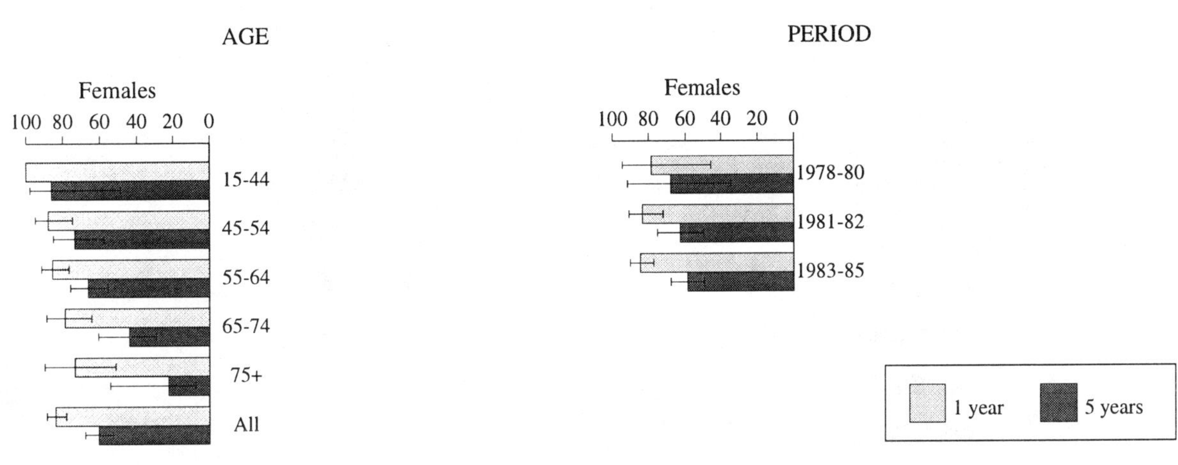

CORPUS UTERI

SWISS REGISTRIES

REGISTRY	NUMBER OF CASES	PERIOD OF DIAGNOSIS
Basel	207	1981-1984
Geneva	272	1978-1984
Mean age (years)	66.0	

RELATIVE SURVIVAL (%)

OBSERVED AND RELATIVE SURVIVAL (%) BY AGE AND PERIOD
(Number of cases in parentheses)

	AGE CLASS												PERIOD					
	15-44		45-54		55-64		65-74		75+		All		1978-80		1981-82		1983-85	
	obs	rel	obs	rel	obs	rel	obs	rel	obs	rel	obs	rel	obs	rel	obs	rel	obs	rel
Females	(16)		(59)		(150)		(130)		(124)		(479)		(121)		(178)		(180)	
1 year	94	94	95	95	95	96	81	82	73	79	86	88	84	86	87	90	85	87
3 years	80	81	93	94	89	91	62	65	50	64	72	78	69	75	75	82	70	76
5 years	80	81	92	93	87	90	57	63	37	58	66	76	64	72	67	78	67	77
8 years	80	81	92	95	86	92	51	62	32	72	62	82	..	..	62	82	..	..
10 years	..	..	..	..	..	..	..	..	..	..	..	..	..	..	..	..	..	..

RELATIVE SURVIVAL (%) BY AGE AND PERIOD

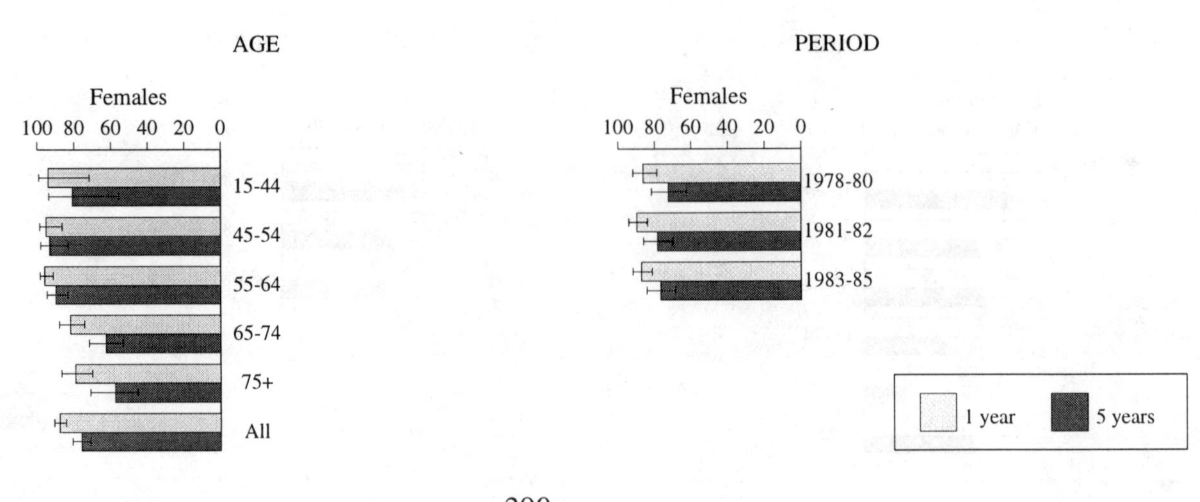

CORPUS UTERI

EUROPEAN REGISTRIES

Weighted analysis

REGISTRY	WEIGHTS (Yearly expected cases in the country)
DENMARK	629
DUTCH REGISTRIES	1022
ENGLISH REGISTRIES	3935
ESTONIA	124
FINLAND	409
FRENCH REGISTRIES	3812
GERMAN REGISTRIES	4782
ITALIAN REGISTRIES	5102
POLISH REGISTRIES	1617
SCOTLAND	273
SPANISH REGISTRIES	2483
SWISS REGISTRIES	840

RELATIVE SURVIVAL (%)
(Age-standardized)

Females
100 80 60 40 20 0
DK
NL
ENG
EST
FIN
F
D
I
PL
SCO
E
CH
EUR

OBSERVED AND RELATIVE SURVIVAL (%) BY AGE AND PERIOD

	AGE CLASS												PERIOD					
	15-44		45-54		55-64		65-74		75+		All		1978-80		1981-82		1983-85	
	obs	rel	obs	rel	obs	rel	obs	rel	obs	rel	obs	rel	obs	rel	obs	rel	obs	rel
Females																		
1 year	97	97	91	92	89	90	82	84	68	74	84	86	83	85	84	85	86	88
3 years	89	90	85	86	80	82	65	70	45	57	71	76	70	75	69	74	73	78
5 years	87	87	83	85	73	77	54	62	34	53	64	72	65	73	63	72	65	74
8 years	89	90	78	81	70	76	48	62	27	59	58	72	59	73	57	70	58	70
10 years	88	89	74	78	65	74	44	64	22	62	54	72	54	71	55	70	..	..

RELATIVE SURVIVAL (%) BY AGE AND PERIOD

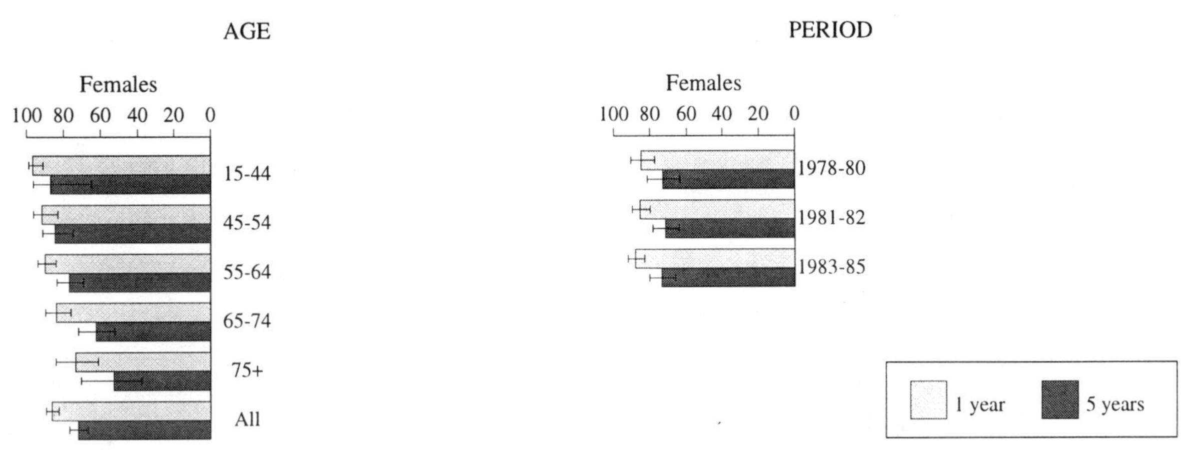

OVARY

DENMARK

REGISTRY	NUMBER OF CASES	PERIOD OF DIAGNOSIS
Denmark	3977	1978-1984
Mean age (years)	62.7	

RELATIVE SURVIVAL (%)

OBSERVED AND RELATIVE SURVIVAL (%) BY AGE AND PERIOD
(Number of cases in parentheses)

	AGE CLASS												PERIOD					
	15-44		45-54		55-64		65-74		75+		All		1978-80		1981-82		1983-85	
	obs	rel	obs	rel	obs	rel	obs	rel	obs	rel	obs	rel	obs	rel	obs	rel	obs	rel
Females	(375)		(631)		(1088)		(1088)		(795)		(3977)		(1697)		(1146)		(1134)	
1 year	84	84	74	75	61	61	48	49	25	27	54	56	52	54	54	56	58	59
3 years	64	64	44	44	31	31	25	27	12	15	30	33	29	31	29	32	34	37
5 years	55	56	34	34	23	24	18	21	7	11	23	27	22	25	21	24	27	31
8 years	51	51	28	29	18	21	12	16	4	10	19	23	18	22	17	22	..	..
10 years	48	49	25	26	15	18	9	13	3	9	16	22	15	20	..	..	..	..

RELATIVE SURVIVAL (%) BY AGE AND PERIOD

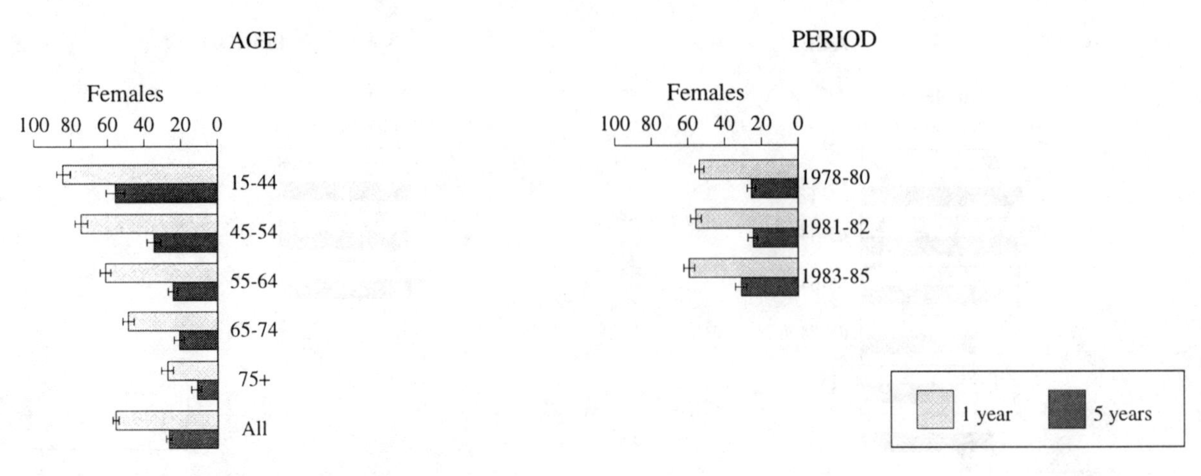

OVARY

DUTCH REGISTRIES

REGISTRY	NUMBER OF CASES	PERIOD OF DIAGNOSIS
Eindhoven	426	1978-1985
Mean age (years)	58.8	

RELATIVE SURVIVAL (%)

100
80
60
40
20
0
0 1 2 3 4 5
Time since diagnosis (years)

OBSERVED AND RELATIVE SURVIVAL (%) BY AGE AND PERIOD
(Number of cases in parentheses)

	AGE CLASS												PERIOD					
	15-44		45-54		55-64		65-74		75+		All		1978-80		1981-82		1983-85	
	obs	rel	obs	rel	obs	rel	obs	rel	obs	rel	obs	rel	obs	rel	obs	rel	obs	rel
Females	(56)		(99)		(102)		(115)		(54)		(426)		(146)		(110)		(170)	
1 year	89	89	76	76	71	71	41	42	37	39	62	63	53	53	66	67	67	68
3 years	78	79	48	49	46	47	21	22	22	27	41	43	33	34	45	47	46	48
5 years	74	74	42	43	34	35	15	16	12	17	33	36	24	26	36	40	41	45
8 years	71	71	40	41	28	31	9	11	12	24	30	36	23	26	..	..	..	..
10 years	71	72	40	42	..	..	..	..	6	15	29	36	21	26	..	..	..	..

RELATIVE SURVIVAL (%) BY AGE AND PERIOD

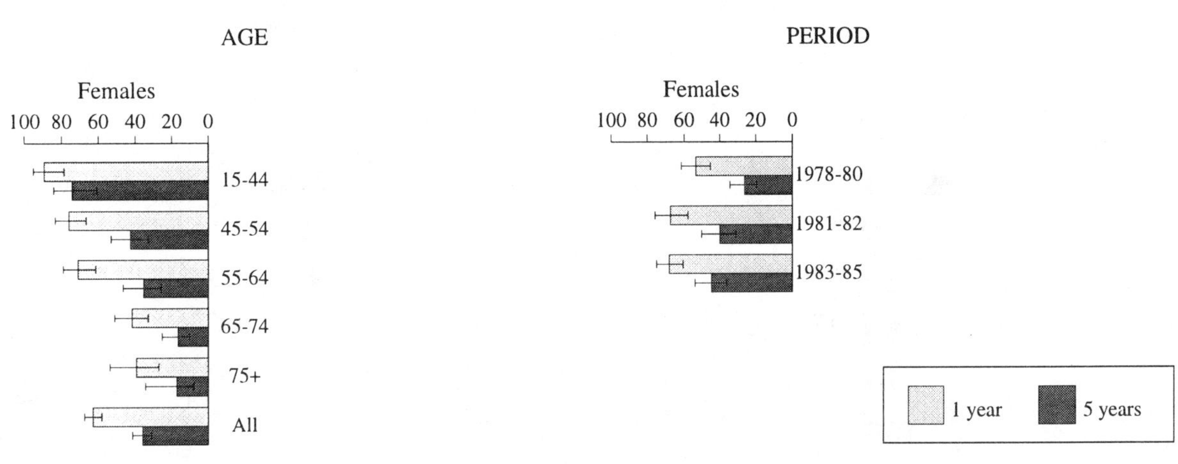

OVARY

ENGLISH REGISTRIES

REGISTRY	NUMBER OF CASES	PERIOD OF DIAGNOSIS
East Anglia	1193	1979-1984
Mersey	1338	1978-1984
South Thames	4410	1978-1984
Wessex	552	1983-1984
West Midlands	2540	1979-1984
Yorkshire	2042	1978-1984
Mean age (years)	62.4	

RELATIVE SURVIVAL (%)

Time since diagnosis (years)

OBSERVED AND RELATIVE SURVIVAL (%) BY AGE AND PERIOD
(Number of cases in parentheses)

	AGE CLASS												PERIOD					
	15-44		45-54		55-64		65-74		75+		All		1978-80		1981-82		1983-85	
	obs	rel	obs	rel	obs	rel	obs	rel	obs	rel	obs	rel	obs	rel	obs	rel	obs	rel
Females	(1150)		(2162)		(3208)		(3131)		(2424)		(12075)		(4562)		(3488)		(4025)	
1 year	79	79	67	67	55	56	40	41	26	29	50	51	48	49	51	52	51	52
3 years	60	60	39	39	29	30	21	23	12	15	28	31	27	29	29	32	30	32
5 years	55	55	32	33	24	25	17	20	8	13	23	27	22	25	24	28	25	29
8 years	52	53	28	29	20	22	13	17	6	15	20	25	18	23	20	26	21	27
10 years	49	50	25	27	18	21	12	17	5	16	18	25	17	23	18	25	..	..

RELATIVE SURVIVAL (%) BY AGE AND PERIOD

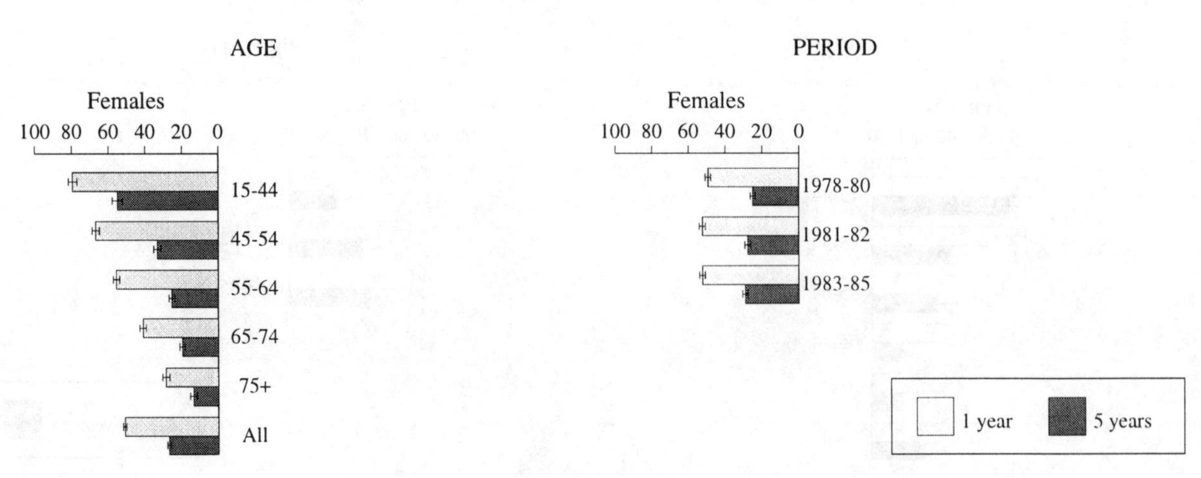

OVARY

ESTONIA

REGISTRY	NUMBER OF CASES	PERIOD OF DIAGNOSIS
Estonia	954	1978-1984
Mean age (years)	61.0	

RELATIVE SURVIVAL (%)

Time since diagnosis (years)

OBSERVED AND RELATIVE SURVIVAL (%) BY AGE AND PERIOD
(Number of cases in parentheses)

	AGE CLASS												PERIOD					
	15-44		45-54		55-64		65-74		75+		All		1978-80		1981-82		1983-85	
	obs	rel	obs	rel	obs	rel	obs	rel	obs	rel	obs	rel	obs	rel	obs	rel	obs	rel
Females	(98)		(201)		(253)		(238)		(164)		(954)		(395)		(262)		(297)	
1 year	74	75	65	65	53	53	33	34	32	35	49	50	50	51	52	54	45	46
3 years	50	50	35	36	25	26	16	17	13	17	25	28	24	27	29	31	23	26
5 years	45	46	27	28	19	20	12	14	9	16	20	23	19	22	23	26	19	22
8 years	39	40	23	24	16	18	9	13	6	16	16	21	15	19	19	24	..	..
10 years	39	40	21	23	14	16	8	13	4	17	15	21	14	19	..	..	..	..

RELATIVE SURVIVAL (%) BY AGE AND PERIOD

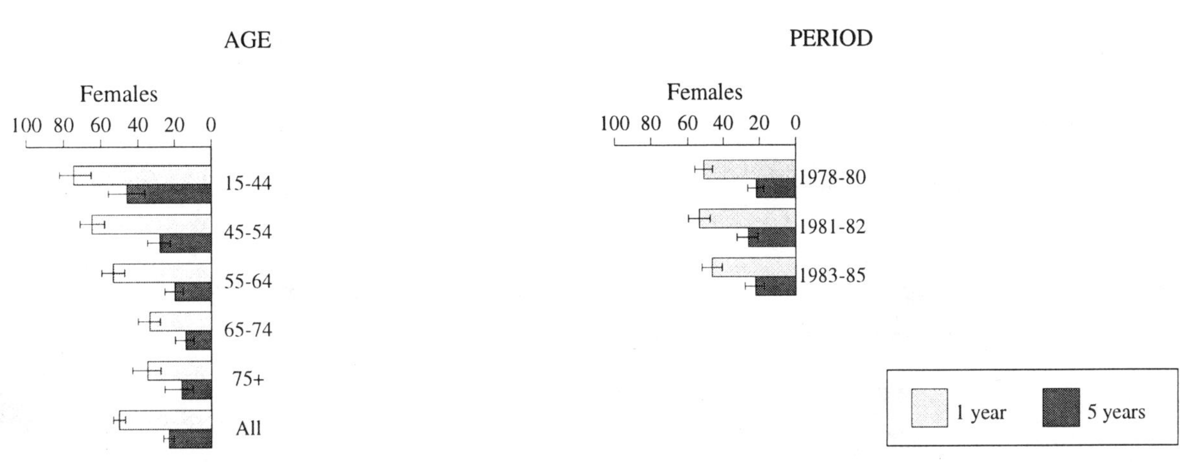

OVARY

FINLAND

REGISTRY	NUMBER OF CASES	PERIOD OF DIAGNOSIS
Finland	2322	1978-1984
Mean age (years)	60.7	

RELATIVE SURVIVAL (%)

100
80
60
40
20
0
0 1 2 3 4 5
Time since diagnosis (years)

OBSERVED AND RELATIVE SURVIVAL (%) BY AGE AND PERIOD
(Number of cases in parentheses)

	AGE CLASS												PERIOD					
	15-44		45-54		55-64		65-74		75+		All		1978-80		1981-82		1983-85	
	obs	rel	obs	rel	obs	rel	obs	rel	obs	rel	obs	rel	obs	rel	obs	rel	obs	rel
Females	(293)		(406)		(625)		(595)		(403)		(2322)		(953)		(669)		(700)	
1 year	86	86	75	75	68	69	59	60	37	40	64	65	61	62	66	67	67	68
3 years	71	72	47	48	41	42	32	34	19	24	40	43	38	41	41	43	41	45
5 years	66	66	37	38	34	36	22	25	14	22	32	36	32	35	32	36	33	37
8 years	63	64	32	33	29	31	15	20	8	18	27	33	26	32	27	32	27	33
10 years	62	63	29	30	25	28	12	18	5	15	24	31	23	30	24	31	..	..

RELATIVE SURVIVAL (%) BY AGE AND PERIOD

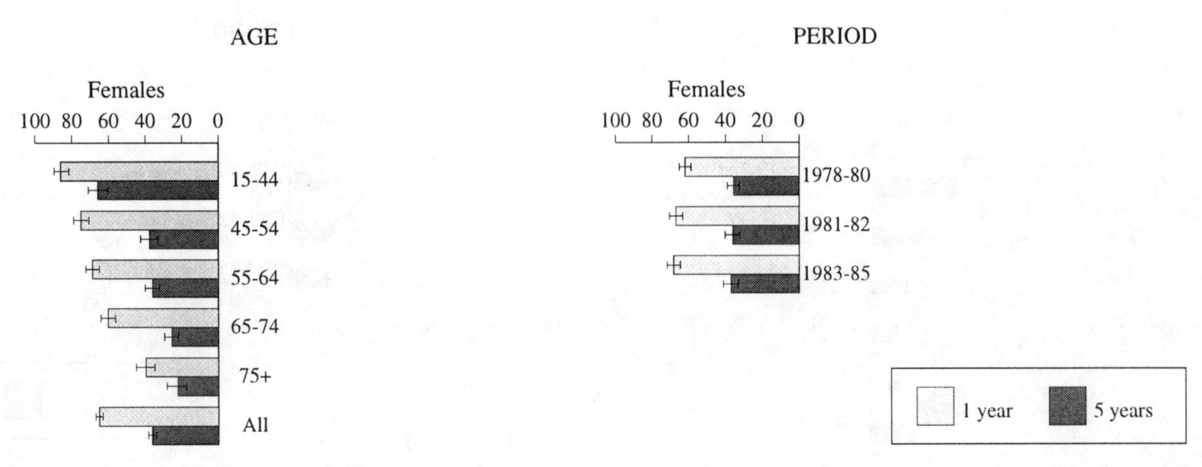

OVARY

FRENCH REGISTRIES

REGISTRY	NUMBER OF CASES	PERIOD OF DIAGNOSIS
Amiens	90	1983-1984
Doubs	213	1978-1985
Mean age (years)	59.3	

RELATIVE SURVIVAL (%)

100
80
60
40
20
0
0 1 2 3 4 5
Time since diagnosis (years)

OBSERVED AND RELATIVE SURVIVAL (%) BY AGE AND PERIOD
(Number of cases in parentheses)

	AGE CLASS												PERIOD					
	15-44		45-54		55-64		65-74		75+		All		1978-80		1981-82		1983-85	
	obs	rel	obs	rel	obs	rel	obs	rel	obs	rel	obs	rel	obs	rel	obs	rel	obs	rel
Females	(41)		(78)		(67)		(68)		(49)		(303)		(88)		(49)		(166)	
1 year	88	88	83	83	71	72	54	55	39	43	67	69	58	60	82	83	68	69
3 years	65	65	61	61	34	34	23	24	20	27	40	43	30	33	48	50	43	46
5 years	57	57	46	47	29	30	18	20	14	22	32	35	27	30	32	34	34	38
8 years	53	54	42	44	23	25	12	15	8	19	27	33	22	27	32	36	..	..
10 years	53	54	42	44	23	26	..	..	..	..	27	35	22	28	..	..	..	..

RELATIVE SURVIVAL (%) BY AGE AND PERIOD

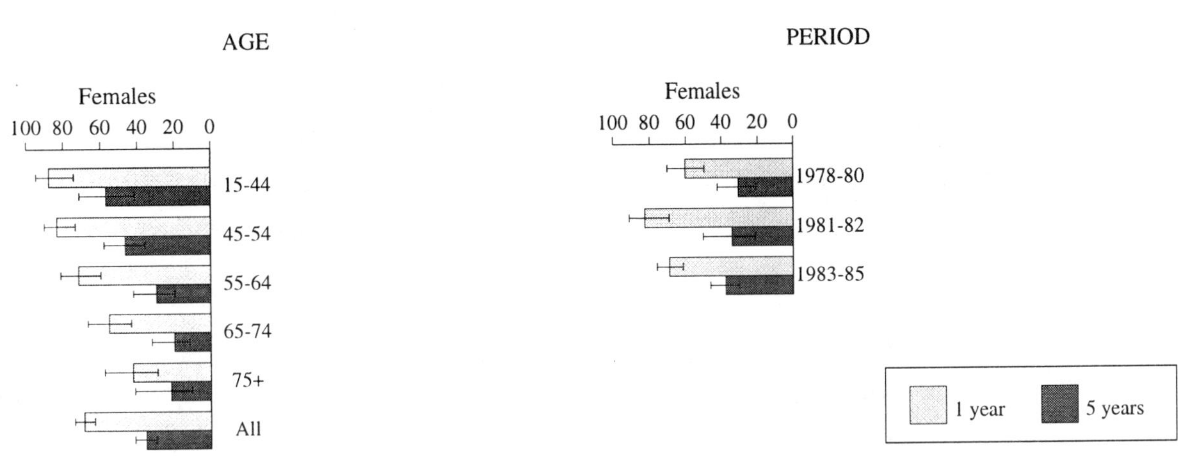

OVARY

GERMAN REGISTRIES

REGISTRY	NUMBER OF CASES	PERIOD OF DIAGNOSIS
Saarland	543	1978-1984
Mean age (years)	61.2	

RELATIVE SURVIVAL (%)

Time since diagnosis (years)

OBSERVED AND RELATIVE SURVIVAL (%) BY AGE AND PERIOD
(Number of cases in parentheses)

	AGE CLASS												PERIOD					
	15-44		45-54		55-64		65-74		75+		All		1978-80		1981-82		1983-85	
	obs	rel	obs	rel	obs	rel	obs	rel	obs	rel	obs	rel	obs	rel	obs	rel	obs	rel
Females	(53)		(94)		(156)		(157)		(83)		(543)		(206)		(163)		(174)	
1 year	83	83	74	75	62	63	49	50	40	43	59	60	55	57	60	61	63	65
3 years	68	68	40	41	39	40	28	31	20	26	36	39	34	37	37	40	37	40
5 years	62	63	31	31	29	31	20	23	18	27	28	32	26	30	29	32	30	34
8 years	58	59	24	25	24	26	16	22	15	31	24	29	22	28	25	30	..	..
10 years	52	53	24	26	22	25	15	22	8	21	21	27	19	26	..	..	..	..

RELATIVE SURVIVAL (%) BY AGE AND PERIOD

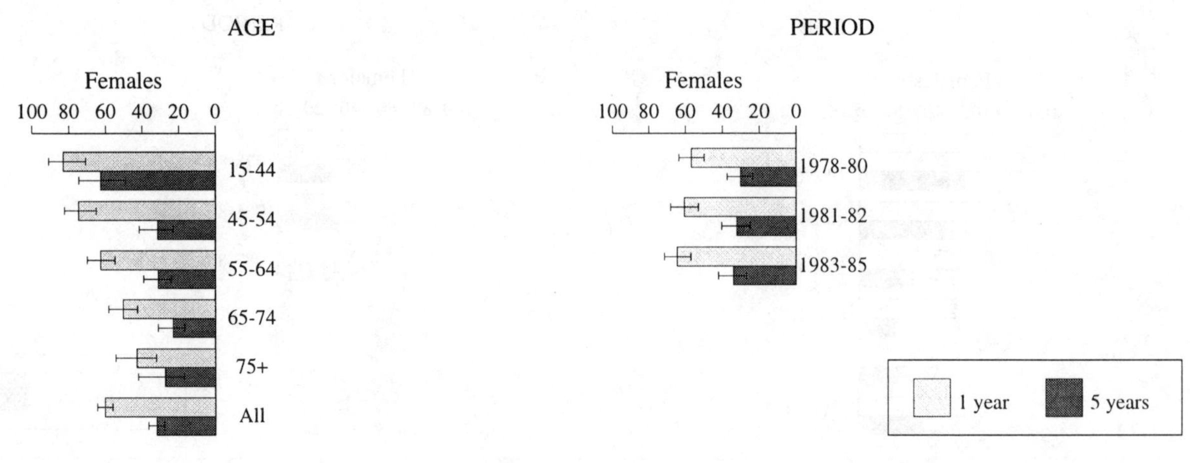

OVARY

ITALIAN REGISTRIES

REGISTRY	NUMBER OF CASES	PERIOD OF DIAGNOSIS
Latina	23	1983-1984
Ragusa	56	1981-1984
Varese	417	1978-1984
Mean age (years)	58.8	

RELATIVE SURVIVAL (%)

100 80 60 40 20 0

0 1 2 3 4 5

Time since diagnosis (years)

OBSERVED AND RELATIVE SURVIVAL (%) BY AGE AND PERIOD
(Number of cases in parentheses)

	AGE CLASS												PERIOD					
	15-44		45-54		55-64		65-74		75+		All		1978-80		1981-82		1983-85	
	obs	rel	obs	rel	obs	rel	obs	rel	obs	rel	obs	rel	obs	rel	obs	rel	obs	rel
Females	(77)		(117)		(123)		(101)		(78)		(496)		(158)		(151)		(187)	
1 year	86	86	79	79	63	63	49	50	26	28	61	63	59	60	58	59	66	68
3 years	66	66	48	48	32	32	26	28	15	20	37	39	35	38	36	39	39	42
5 years	61	61	40	41	24	25	18	20	10	16	30	34	29	32	29	32	32	36
8 years	56	56	35	36	21	23	14	18	6	14	26	31	27	32	26	30	22	27
10 years	56	56	35	37	18	20	14	19	6	18	25	32	27	33	25	31	..	..

RELATIVE SURVIVAL (%) BY AGE AND PERIOD

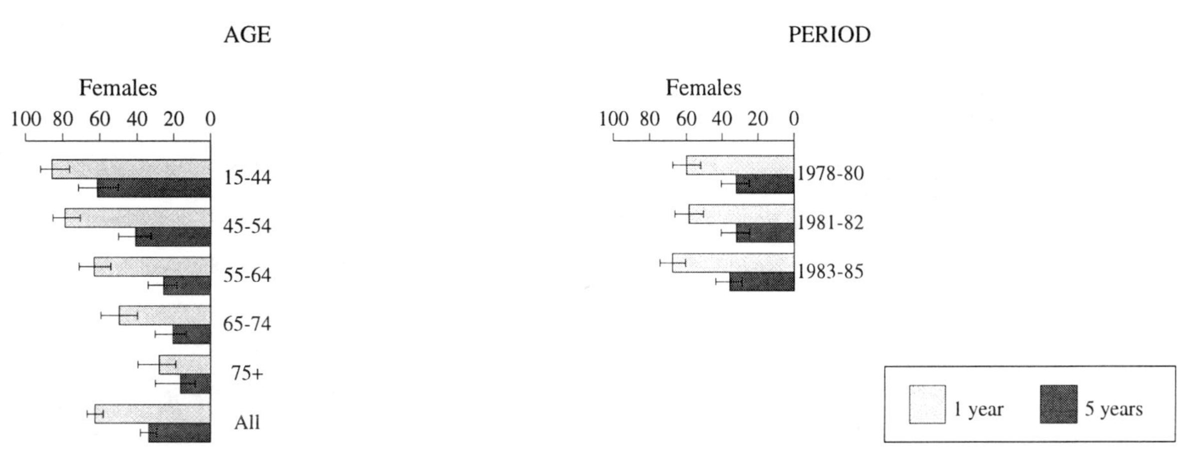

OVARY

POLISH REGISTRIES

REGISTRY	NUMBER OF CASES	PERIOD OF DIAGNOSIS
Cracow	320	1978-1984
Mean age (years)	56.8	

RELATIVE SURVIVAL (%)

Time since diagnosis (years)

OBSERVED AND RELATIVE SURVIVAL (%) BY AGE AND PERIOD
(Number of cases in parentheses)

	AGE CLASS												PERIOD					
	15-44		45-54		55-64		65-74		75+		All		1978-80		1981-82		1983-85	
	obs	rel	obs	rel	obs	rel	obs	rel	obs	rel	obs	rel	obs	rel	obs	rel	obs	rel
Females	(53)		(80)		(88)		(71)		(28)		(320)		(148)		(86)		(86)	
1 year	67	67	56	57	46	47	27	27	24	26	46	47	44	45	46	46	50	51
3 years	55	56	37	37	25	26	19	21	10	12	31	32	27	29	31	33	35	37
5 years	49	50	31	32	23	24	18	21	5	8	27	30	27	30	24	26	30	33
8 years	43	44	29	30	19	21	16	23	5	11	24	28	24	28	19	22	30	36
10 years	37	37	29	31	13	16	14	23	0	0	20	25	19	25	18	22	..	..

RELATIVE SURVIVAL (%) BY AGE AND PERIOD

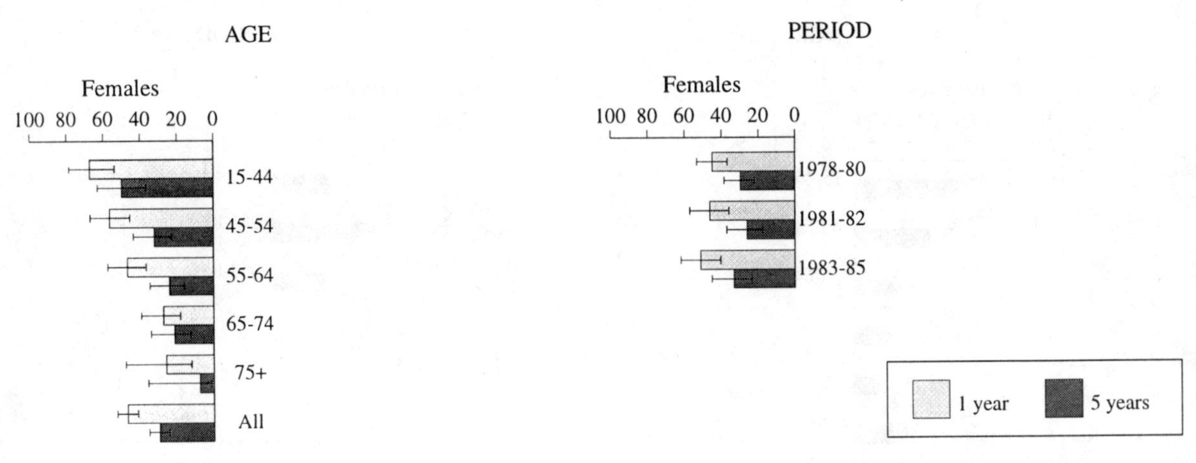

OVARY

SCOTLAND

REGISTRY	NUMBER OF CASES	PERIOD OF DIAGNOSIS
Scotland	2137	1978-1982
Mean age (years)	61.5	

RELATIVE SURVIVAL (%)

100 80 60 40 20 0

0 1 2 3 4 5

Time since diagnosis (years)

OBSERVED AND RELATIVE SURVIVAL (%) BY AGE AND PERIOD
(Number of cases in parentheses)

	AGE CLASS												PERIOD					
	15-44		45-54		55-64		65-74		75+		All		1978-80		1981-82		1983-85	
	obs	rel	obs	rel	obs	rel	obs	rel	obs	rel	obs	rel	obs	rel	obs	rel	obs	rel
Females	(236)		(397)		(551)		(571)		(382)		(2137)		(1242)		(895)		(0)	
1 year	78	78	68	69	54	55	39	41	29	32	51	52	50	51	52	54	..	..
3 years	58	59	45	45	29	31	22	24	14	19	31	33	30	33	32	35	..	..
5 years	52	52	38	39	23	25	18	21	10	16	25	29	25	29	26	30	..	..
8 years	46	47	33	35	19	22	15	21	6	13	21	27	21	26	..	..	..	..
10 years	46	47	33	35	15	18	15	22	..	..	20	28	20	27	..	..	..	..

RELATIVE SURVIVAL (%) BY AGE AND PERIOD

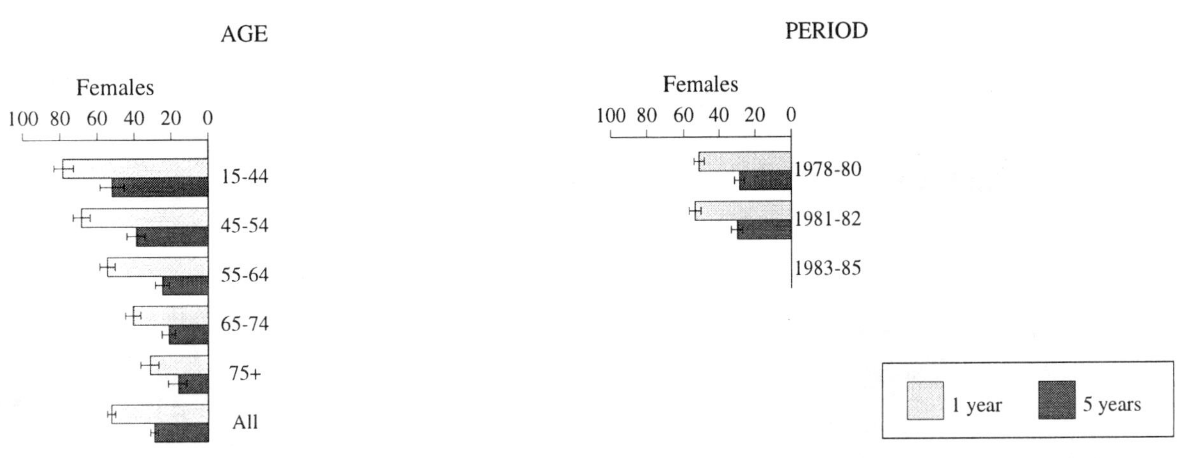

OVARY

SPANISH REGISTRIES

REGISTRY	NUMBER OF CASES	PERIOD OF DIAGNOSIS
Girona	100	1980-1985
Tarragona	24	1985-1985
Mean age (years)	59.3	

RELATIVE SURVIVAL (%)

100
80
60
40
20
0
0 1 2 3 4 5
Time since diagnosis (years)

OBSERVED AND RELATIVE SURVIVAL (%) BY AGE AND PERIOD
(Number of cases in parentheses)

	AGE CLASS												PERIOD					
	15-44		45-54		55-64		65-74		75+		All		1978-80		1981-82		1983-85	
	obs	rel	obs	rel	obs	rel	obs	rel	obs	rel	obs	rel	obs	rel	obs	rel	obs	rel
Females	(10)		(33)		(40)		(26)		(15)		(124)		(9)		(23)		(92)	
1 year	100	100	67	67	70	70	62	63	57	61	68	69	33	34	77	78	69	70
3 years	80	80	45	46	38	38	38	41	41	49	44	45	22	23	55	56	43	45
5 years	80	80	39	40	22	23	19	21	33	46	32	34	11	12	41	43	32	34
8 years	80	81	39	40	..	..	19	23	0	0	29	33	11	12	36	40	32	37
10 years	80	81	..	..	..	..	..	..	0	0	29	34	11	13	..	..	..	..

RELATIVE SURVIVAL (%) BY AGE AND PERIOD

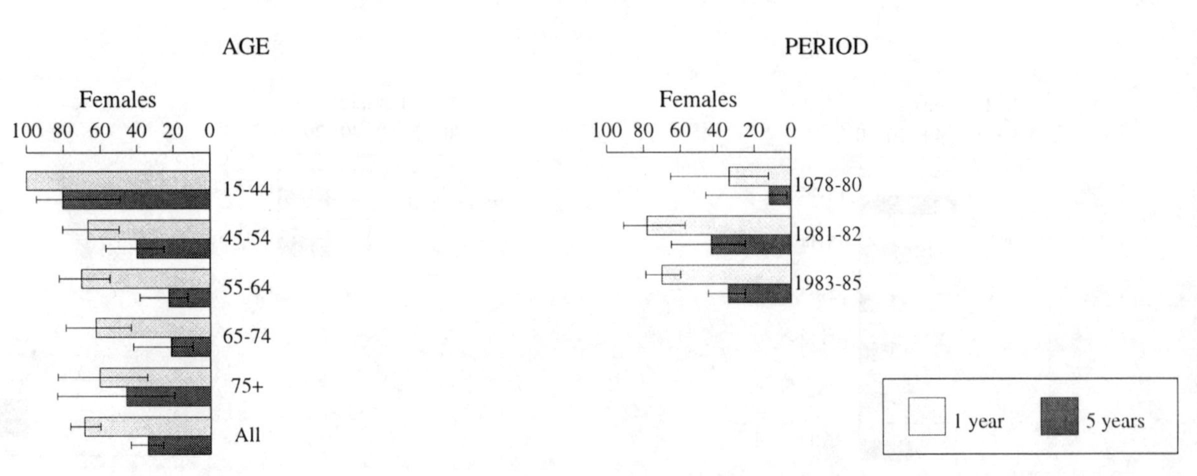

OVARY

SWISS REGISTRIES

REGISTRY	NUMBER OF CASES	PERIOD OF DIAGNOSIS
Basel	126	1981-1984
Geneva	227	1978-1984
Mean age (years)	62.7	

RELATIVE SURVIVAL (%)

Time since diagnosis (years)

OBSERVED AND RELATIVE SURVIVAL (%) BY AGE AND PERIOD
(Number of cases in parentheses)

	AGE CLASS												PERIOD					
	15-44		45-54		55-64		65-74		75+		All		1978-80		1981-82		1983-85	
	obs	rel	obs	rel	obs	rel	obs	rel	obs	rel	obs	rel	obs	rel	obs	rel	obs	rel
Females	(39)		(70)		(74)		(89)		(81)		(353)		(93)		(123)		(137)	
1 year	90	90	81	81	69	69	57	58	28	31	61	63	65	66	65	66	56	58
3 years	70	71	53	54	35	36	37	39	15	19	38	41	37	40	42	45	36	39
5 years	65	65	45	45	32	33	30	34	15	23	34	38	34	39	36	40	31	36
8 years	65	66	45	46	32	34	26	32	..	..	32	40	..	..	35	42	..	..
10 years	..	..	..	..	..	..	..	..	..	..	..	..	..	..	..	..	..	..

RELATIVE SURVIVAL (%) BY AGE AND PERIOD

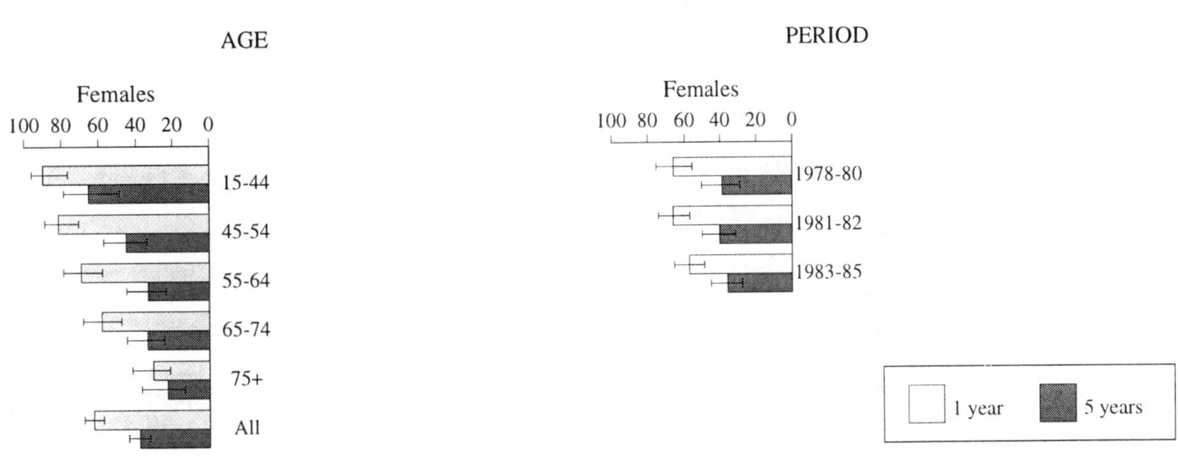

OVARY

EUROPEAN REGISTRIES

Weighted analysis

REGISTRY	WEIGHTS (Yearly expected cases in the country)
DENMARK	569
DUTCH REGISTRIES	1217
ENGLISH REGISTRIES	6112
ESTONIA	136
FINLAND	333
FRENCH REGISTRIES	3974
GERMAN REGISTRIES	7356
ITALIAN REGISTRIES	3248
POLISH REGISTRIES	2655
SCOTLAND	428
SPANISH REGISTRIES	1106
SWISS REGISTRIES	532

RELATIVE SURVIVAL (%)
(Age-standardized)

OBSERVED AND RELATIVE SURVIVAL (%) BY AGE AND PERIOD

	AGE CLASS												PERIOD					
	15-44		45-54		55-64		65-74		75+		All		1978-80		1981-82		1983-85	
	obs	rel	obs	rel	obs	rel	obs	rel	obs	rel	obs	rel	obs	rel	obs	rel	obs	rel
Females																		
1 year	83	83	72	73	61	62	46	47	33	36	58	59	53	54	60	61	60	62
3 years	65	65	45	45	34	35	25	27	17	22	35	37	31	33	37	39	37	39
5 years	59	60	36	37	27	28	18	21	13	20	28	32	25	28	29	32	30	34
8 years	56	56	31	32	22	24	15	19	9	19	24	29	21	26	25	30	24	30
10 years	52	53	30	32	19	22	13	20	5	15	22	29	20	26	20	26	..	..

RELATIVE SURVIVAL (%) BY AGE AND PERIOD

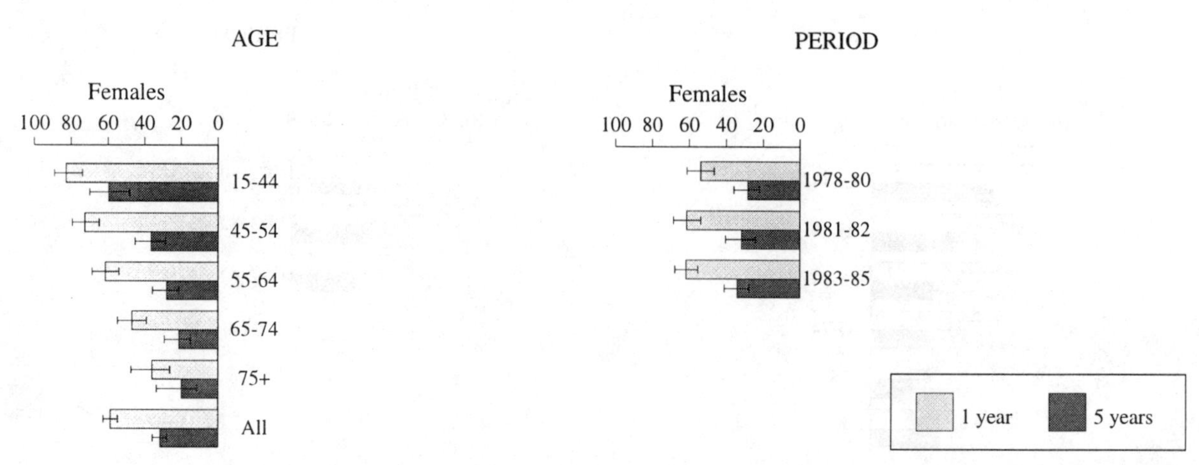

VAGINA & VULVA

DENMARK

REGISTRY	NUMBER OF CASES	PERIOD OF DIAGNOSIS
Denmark	829	1978-1984
Mean age (years)	69.4	

RELATIVE SURVIVAL (%)

Time since diagnosis (years)

OBSERVED AND RELATIVE SURVIVAL (%) BY AGE AND PERIOD
(Number of cases in parentheses)

	AGE CLASS												PERIOD					
	15-44		45-54		55-64		65-74		75+		All		1978-80		1981-82		1983-85	
	obs	rel	obs	rel	obs	rel	obs	rel	obs	rel	obs	rel	obs	rel	obs	rel	obs	rel
Females	(47)		(73)		(130)		(243)		(336)		(829)		(353)		(231)		(245)	
1 year	89	89	85	85	87	88	79	81	61	67	74	78	75	78	72	75	75	78
3 years	83	83	71	72	66	68	60	65	36	48	54	62	51	58	54	62	58	66
5 years	81	82	67	69	60	63	53	61	27	45	46	59	44	55	46	59	50	64
8 years	76	77	64	67	59	66	44	58	15	37	39	58	37	54	40	61	..	..
10 years	76	78	61	66	49	57	33	48	8	28	31	53	29	49	..	..	..	..

RELATIVE SURVIVAL (%) BY AGE AND PERIOD

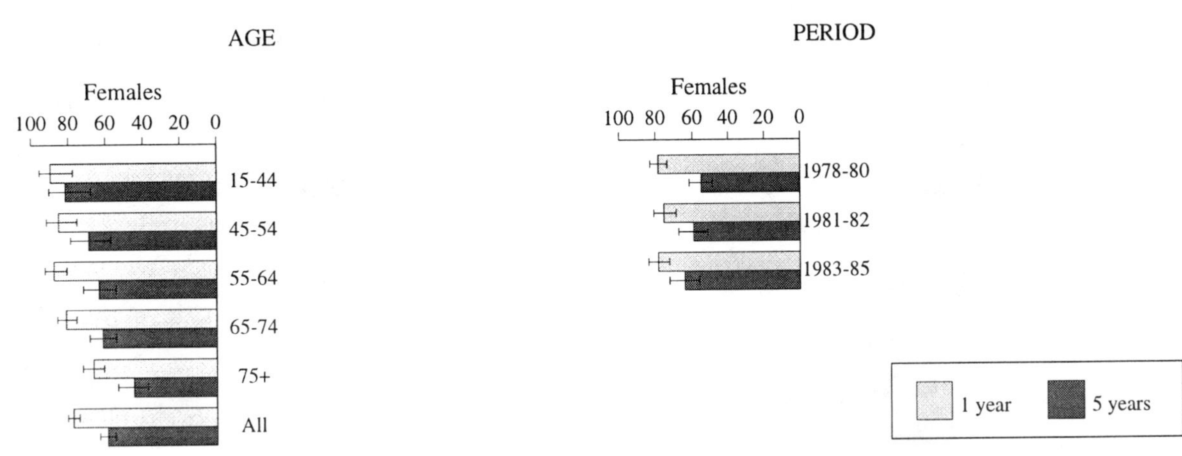

VAGINA & VULVA

ENGLISH REGISTRIES

REGISTRY	NUMBER OF CASES	PERIOD OF DIAGNOSIS
East Anglia	274	1979-1984
Mersey	268	1978-1984
South Thames	828	1978-1984
Wessex	124	1983-1984
West Midlands	548	1979-1984
Yorkshire	498	1978-1984
Mean age (years)	71.4	

RELATIVE SURVIVAL (%)

100
80
60
40
20
0
0 1 2 3 4 5
Time since diagnosis (years)

OBSERVED AND RELATIVE SURVIVAL (%) BY AGE AND PERIOD
(Number of cases in parentheses)

	AGE CLASS												PERIOD					
	15-44		45-54		55-64		65-74		75+		All		1978-80		1981-82		1983-85	
	obs	rel	obs	rel	obs	rel	obs	rel	obs	rel	obs	rel	obs	rel	obs	rel	obs	rel
Females	(97)		(159)		(374)		(757)		(1153)		(2540)		(1001)		(727)		(812)	
1 year	88	88	81	81	78	78	69	71	54	60	65	69	65	69	65	69	66	69
3 years	70	70	70	71	60	62	52	57	32	44	46	55	46	54	46	55	46	54
5 years	70	71	67	68	55	58	46	54	23	42	39	53	39	52	39	52	40	54
8 years	65	66	60	62	49	55	39	52	16	45	33	53	32	52	33	54	30	48
10 years	65	66	59	62	45	52	32	47	12	44	27	51	28	50	25	48	..	..

RELATIVE SURVIVAL (%) BY AGE AND PERIOD

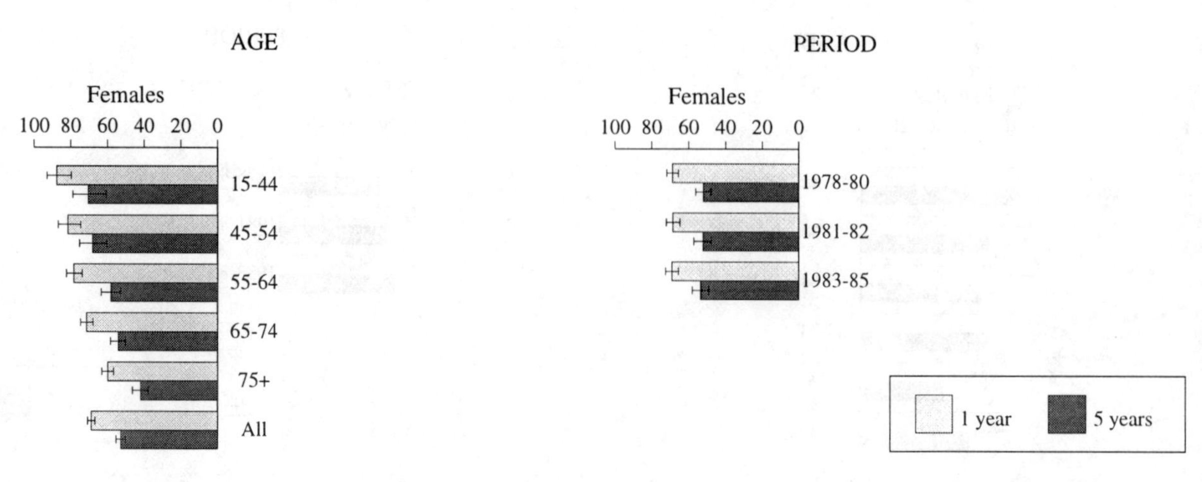

VAGINA & VULVA

ESTONIA

REGISTRY	NUMBER OF CASES	PERIOD OF DIAGNOSIS
Estonia	184	1978-1984
Mean age (years)	70.6	

RELATIVE SURVIVAL (%)

OBSERVED AND RELATIVE SURVIVAL (%) BY AGE AND PERIOD
(Number of cases in parentheses)

	AGE CLASS												PERIOD					
	15-44		45-54		55-64		65-74		75+		All		1978-80		1981-82		1983-85	
	obs	rel	obs	rel	obs	rel	obs	rel	obs	rel	obs	rel	obs	rel	obs	rel	obs	rel
Females	(5)		(15)		(27)		(62)		(75)		(184)		(102)		(37)		(45)	
1 year	80	80	93	94	74	75	56	58	56	63	63	66	63	67	70	73	56	59
3 years	60	60	73	75	52	54	35	39	24	35	37	44	33	40	49	56	36	44
5 years	60	61	73	75	48	51	27	33	19	36	32	43	28	39	43	55	29	42
8 years	60	61	51	54	48	55	14	21	14	45	23	39	21	35	32	50	..	..
10 years	36	37	51	55	39	47	14	25	14	69	21	42	19	37	..	..	..	..

RELATIVE SURVIVAL (%) BY AGE AND PERIOD

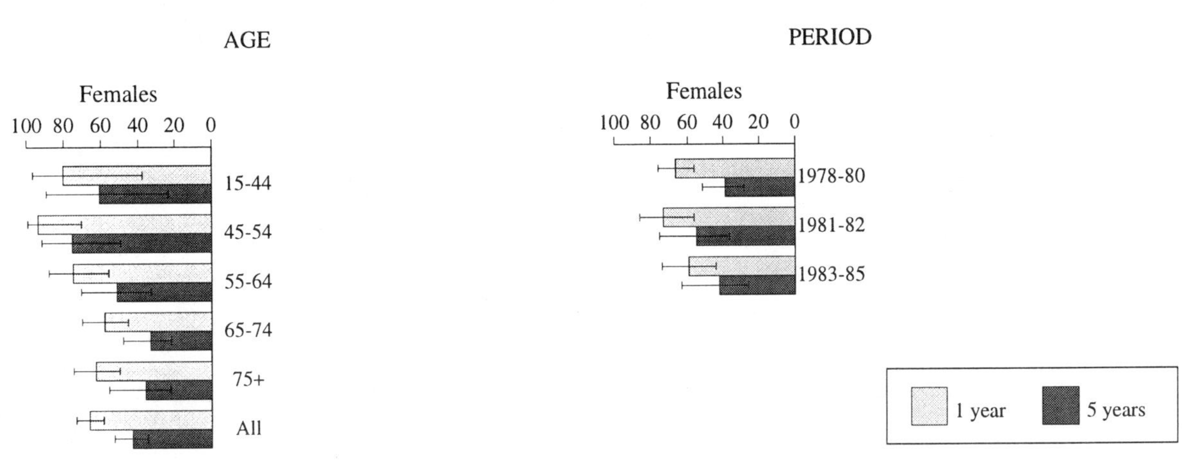

VAGINA & VULVA

FINLAND

REGISTRY	NUMBER OF CASES	PERIOD OF DIAGNOSIS
Finland	510	1978-1984
Mean age (years)	69.3	

RELATIVE SURVIVAL (%)

Time since diagnosis (years)

OBSERVED AND RELATIVE SURVIVAL (%) BY AGE AND PERIOD
(Number of cases in parentheses)

	AGE CLASS												PERIOD					
	15-44		45-54		55-64		65-74		75+		All		1978-80		1981-82		1983-85	
	obs	rel	obs	rel	obs	rel	obs	rel	obs	rel	obs	rel	obs	rel	obs	rel	obs	rel
Females	(34)		(34)		(80)		(173)		(189)		(510)		(202)		(142)		(166)	
1 year	94	94	82	83	85	86	68	70	60	66	70	74	69	73	70	73	72	76
3 years	91	91	68	68	68	69	50	54	33	46	50	58	53	61	49	57	48	55
5 years	91	92	65	66	66	70	43	51	23	41	44	56	47	60	41	53	43	55
8 years	84	85	61	63	56	61	32	43	15	40	35	52	38	57	32	49	34	50
10 years	84	85	61	64	51	58	28	42	12	46	31	53	34	58	31	53	..	..

RELATIVE SURVIVAL (%) BY AGE AND PERIOD

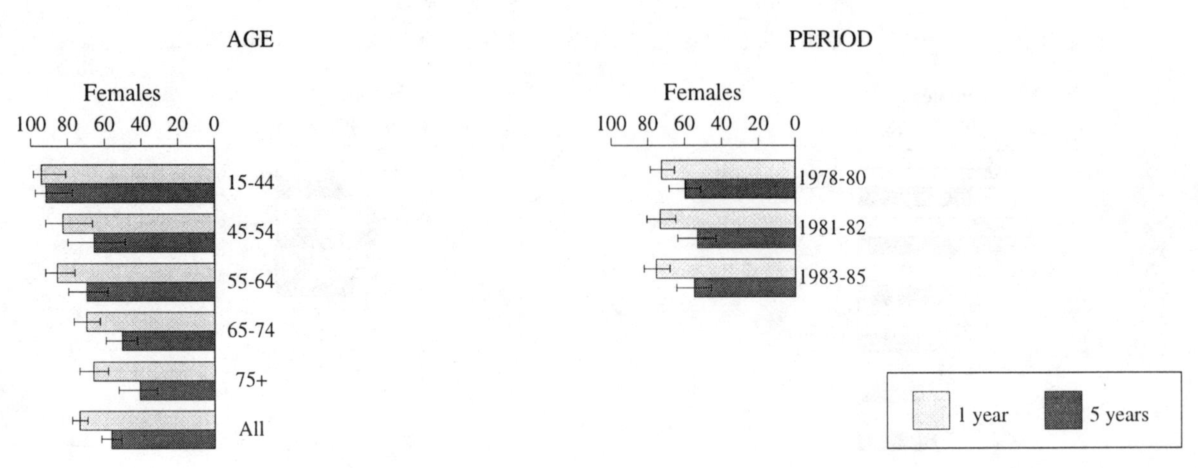

VAGINA & VULVA

GERMAN REGISTRIES

REGISTRY	NUMBER OF CASES	PERIOD OF DIAGNOSIS	RELATIVE SURVIVAL (%)
Saarland	139	1978-1984	
Mean age (years)	70.2		

OBSERVED AND RELATIVE SURVIVAL (%) BY AGE AND PERIOD
(Number of cases in parentheses)

	AGE CLASS												PERIOD					
	15-44		45-54		55-64		65-74		75+		All		1978-80		1981-82		1983-85	
	obs	rel	obs	rel	obs	rel	obs	rel	obs	rel	obs	rel	obs	rel	obs	rel	obs	rel
Females	(6)		(12)		(25)		(38)		(58)		(139)		(58)		(40)		(41)	
1 year	83	83	83	84	76	77	63	65	48	53	62	65	55	58	65	69	68	72
3 years	67	67	50	51	52	54	42	47	21	28	37	43	36	42	38	45	37	42
5 years	67	67	25	26	44	46	32	38	17	30	29	37	33	42	28	37	24	31
8 years	67	68	25	26	39	43	23	32	14	34	24	37	28	42	28	44	..	..
10 years	67	68	25	26	39	45	23	36	14	45	24	42	28	47	..	..	..	..

RELATIVE SURVIVAL (%) BY AGE AND PERIOD

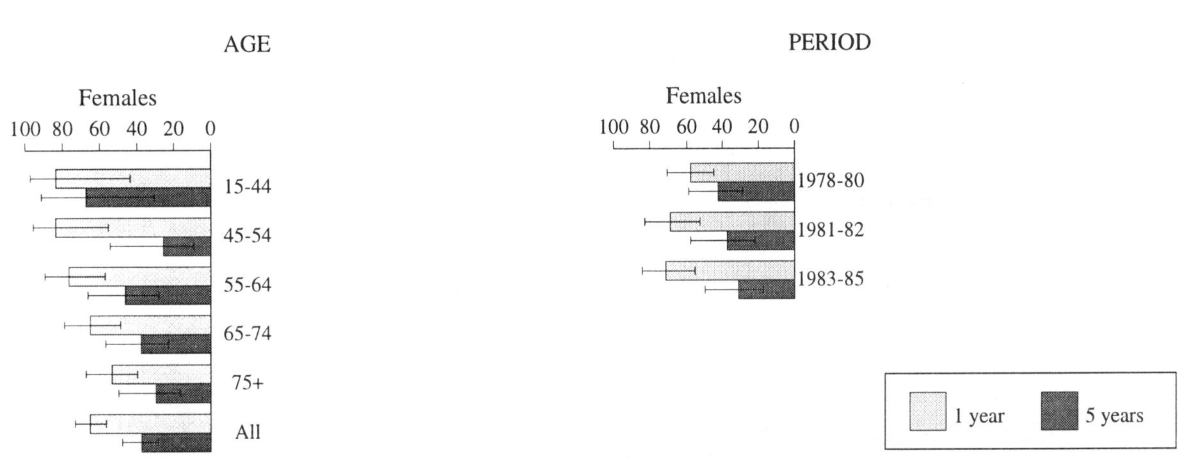

VAGINA & VULVA

ITALIAN REGISTRIES

REGISTRY	NUMBER OF CASES	PERIOD OF DIAGNOSIS
Latina	7	1983-1984
Ragusa	11	1981-1984
Varese	108	1978-1984
Mean age (years)	68.4	

RELATIVE SURVIVAL (%)

Time since diagnosis (years)

OBSERVED AND RELATIVE SURVIVAL (%) BY AGE AND PERIOD
(Number of cases in parentheses)

	AGE CLASS												PERIOD					
	15-44		45-54		55-64		65-74		75+		All		1978-80		1981-82		1983-85	
	obs	rel	obs	rel	obs	rel	obs	rel	obs	rel	obs	rel	obs	rel	obs	rel	obs	rel
Females	(6)		(9)		(29)		(34)		(48)		(126)		(41)		(43)		(42)	
1 year	100	100	56	56	76	76	79	81	44	47	64	67	61	64	56	58	76	79
3 years	100	100	44	45	48	49	62	67	23	29	44	50	37	43	42	46	55	61
5 years	100	100	44	45	45	47	47	54	17	26	37	46	32	42	35	41	45	54
8 years	100	100	33	35	41	45	35	45	12	27	31	44	29	47	28	36	37	50
10 years	100	100	33	35	41	46	30	44	8	24	28	45	24	45	28	39	..	..

RELATIVE SURVIVAL (%) BY AGE AND PERIOD

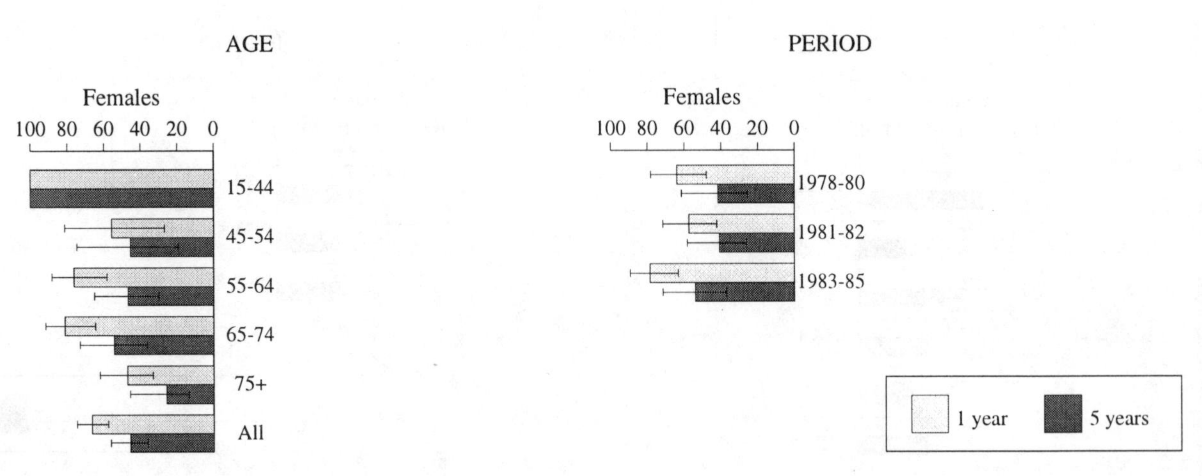

VAGINA & VULVA

SCOTLAND

REGISTRY	NUMBER OF CASES	PERIOD OF DIAGNOSIS
Scotland	495	1978-1982
Mean age (years)	70.8	

RELATIVE SURVIVAL (%)

100, 80, 60, 40, 20, 0

0 1 2 3 4 5

Time since diagnosis (years)

OBSERVED AND RELATIVE SURVIVAL (%) BY AGE AND PERIOD
(Number of cases in parentheses)

	AGE CLASS												PERIOD					
	15-44		45-54		55-64		65-74		75+		All		1978-80		1981-82		1983-85	
	obs	rel	obs	rel	obs	rel	obs	rel	obs	rel	obs	rel	obs	rel	obs	rel	obs	rel
Females	(21)		(42)		(62)		(146)		(224)		(495)		(295)		(200)		(0)	
1 year	95	95	79	79	69	70	67	69	58	65	66	70	67	71	64	67	..	..
3 years	57	57	55	56	55	57	47	52	33	46	43	51	42	51	44	52	..	..
5 years	57	58	48	49	48	52	42	50	21	36	34	46	32	44	37	49	..	..
8 years	57	58	39	42	45	51	31	44	11	30	26	42	24	40	..	..	..	..
10 years	..	..	39	43	45	53	28	43	11	41	25	47	24	45	..	..	..	..

RELATIVE SURVIVAL (%) BY AGE AND PERIOD

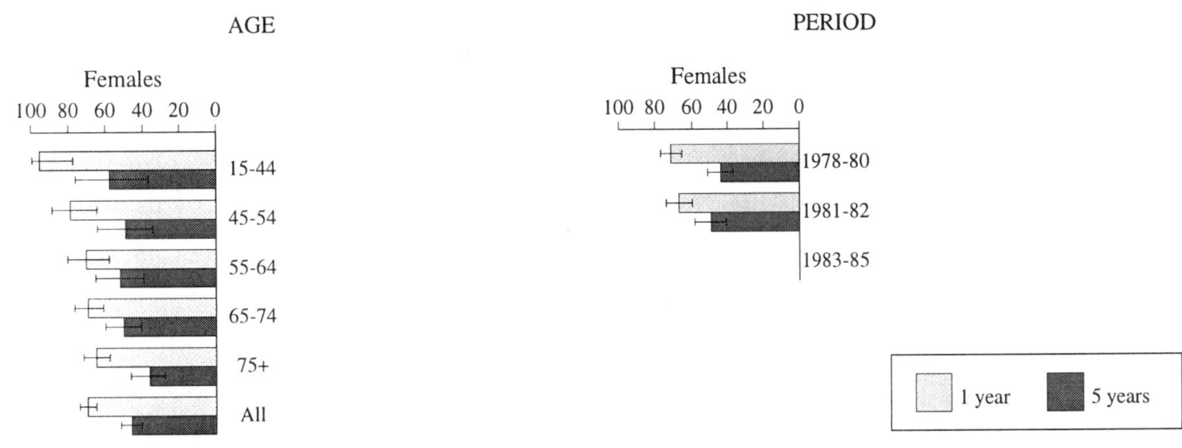

VAGINA & VULVA

DUTCH REGISTRIES

REGISTRY	NUMBER OF CASES	PERIOD OF DIAGNOSIS
Eindhoven	70	1978-1985
Mean age (years)	68.5	

RELATIVE SURVIVAL (%)

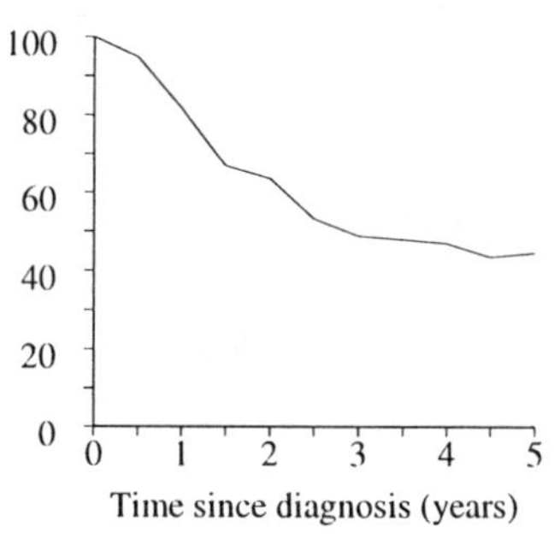

OBSERVED AND RELATIVE SURVIVAL (%) BY PERIOD
(Number of cases in parentheses)

	PERIOD							
	1978-80		1981-82		1983-85		All	
	obs	rel	obs	rel	obs	rel	obs	rel
N. Cases	(30)		(15)		(25)		(70)	
1 year	80	83	67	70	84	87	79	82
3 years	47	53	33	40	44	48	43	49
5 years	37	46	27	36	44	52	36	45
8 years	29	41	..	..	..	..	29	43
10 years	29	47	..	..	..	..	29	49

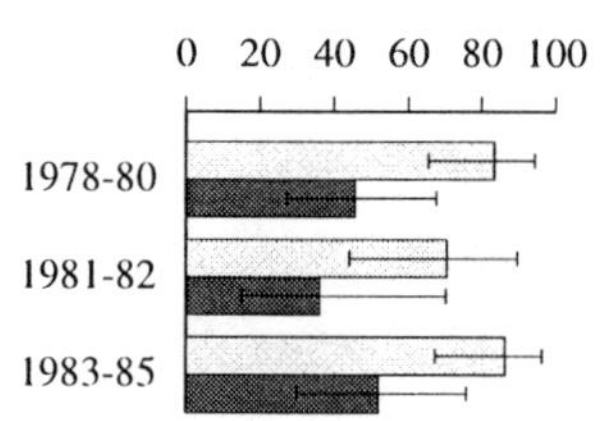

FRENCH REGISTRIES

REGISTRY	NUMBER OF CASES	PERIOD OF DIAGNOSIS
Amiens	19	1983-1984
Doubs	74	1978-1985
Mean age (years)	71.0	

RELATIVE SURVIVAL (%)

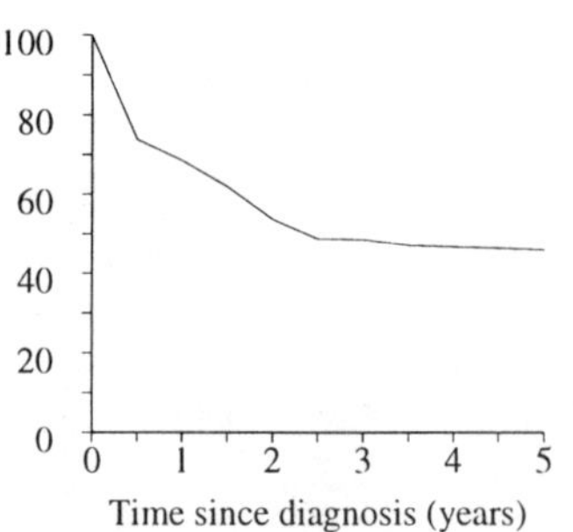

OBSERVED AND RELATIVE SURVIVAL (%) BY PERIOD
(Number of cases in parentheses)

	PERIOD							
	1978-80		1981-82		1983-85		All	
	obs	rel	obs	rel	obs	rel	obs	rel
N. Cases	(32)		(25)		(36)		(93)	
1 year	59	63	68	71	69	71	65	69
3 years	31	37	40	46	54	61	42	49
5 years	28	37	36	46	44	54	36	46
8 years	25	38	27	41	..	..	28	41
10 years	18	31	..	..	..	..	18	30

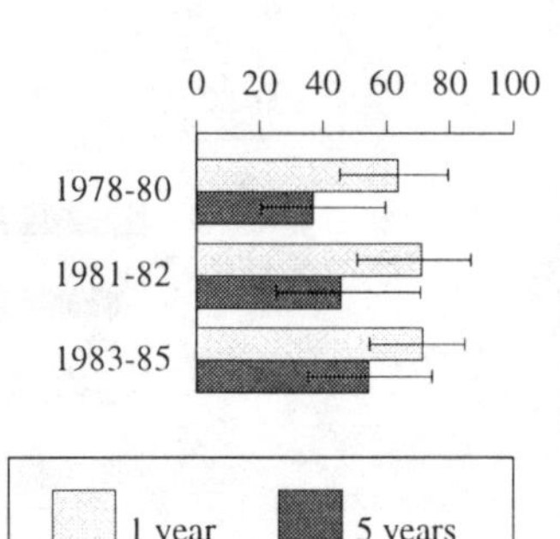

VAGINA & VULVA

POLISH REGISTRIES

REGISTRY	NUMBER OF CASES	PERIOD OF DIAGNOSIS
Cracow	65	1978-1984
Mean age (years)	69.1	

RELATIVE SURVIVAL (%)

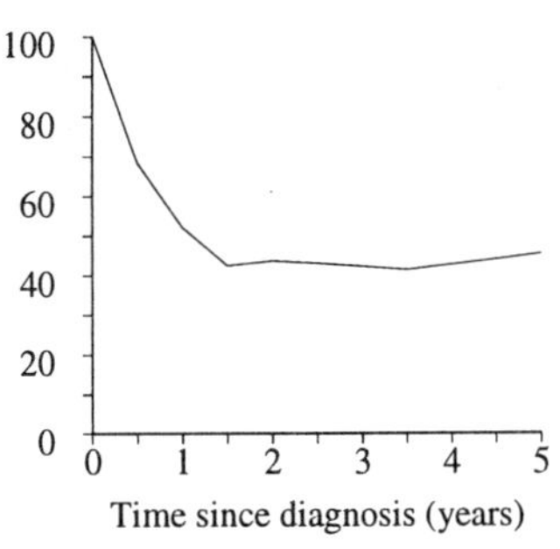

OBSERVED AND RELATIVE SURVIVAL (%) BY PERIOD
(Number of cases in parentheses)

	PERIOD						All	
	1978-80		1981-82		1983-85			
	obs	rel	obs	rel	obs	rel	obs	rel
N. Cases	(24)		(19)		(22)		(65)	
1 year	61	65	31	32	51	54	49	52
3 years	53	62	24	29	26	31	36	42
5 years	53	70	18	24	26	35	34	45
8 years	38	59	18	29	21	34	26	42
10 years	32	57	18	32	..	..	22	41

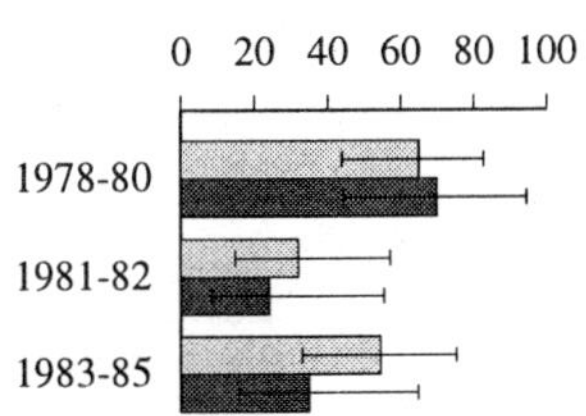

SPANISH REGISTRIES

REGISTRY	NUMBER OF CASES	PERIOD OF DIAGNOSIS
Girona	27	1980-1985
Tarragona	13	1985-1985
Mean age (years)	70.6	

RELATIVE SURVIVAL (%)

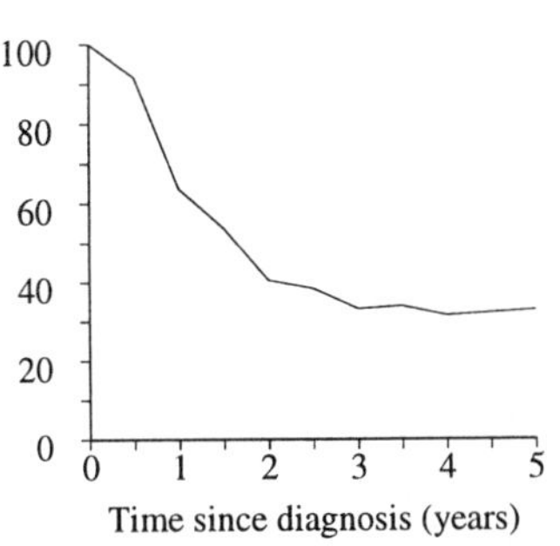

OBSERVED AND RELATIVE SURVIVAL (%) BY PERIOD
(Number of cases in parentheses)

	PERIOD						All	
	1978-80		1981-82		1983-85			
	obs	rel	obs	rel	obs	rel	obs	rel
N. Cases	(6)		(4)		(30)		(40)	
1 year	58	60	50	53	63	66	61	64
3 years	0	0	50	60	30	34	29	33
5 years	0	0	50	69	27	32	27	33
8 years	0	0	50	85	..	..	21	32
10 years	0	0	50	97	..	..	21	37

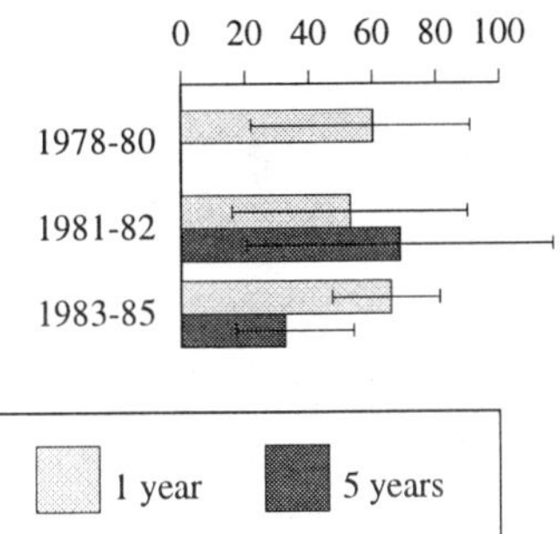

VAGINA & VULVA

SWISS REGISTRIES

REGISTRY	NUMBER OF CASES	PERIOD OF DIAGNOSIS
Basel	35	1981-1984
Geneva	45	1978-1984
Mean age (years)	68.4	

RELATIVE SURVIVAL (%)

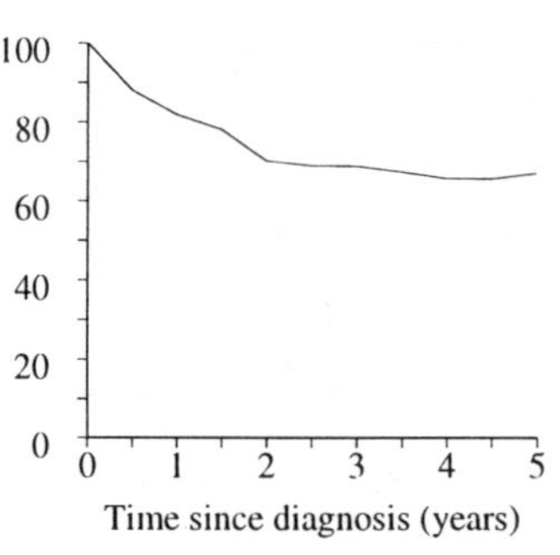

OBSERVED AND RELATIVE SURVIVAL (%) BY PERIOD
(Number of cases in parentheses)

	PERIOD							
	1978-80		1981-82		1983-85		All	
	obs	rel	obs	rel	obs	rel	obs	rel
N. Cases	(16)		(27)		(37)		(80)	
1 year	81	85	70	73	84	87	79	82
3 years	50	58	56	63	70	78	61	69
5 years	50	63	52	64	59	71	55	67
8 years	..	..	45	66	..	..	51	73
10 years	..	..	..	..	..	..	..	..

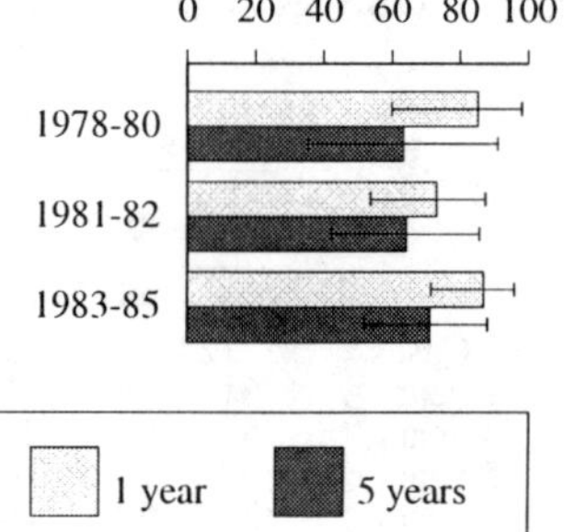

VAGINA & VULVA

EUROPEAN REGISTRIES

Unweighted analysis

REGISTRY	CASES
DENMARK	829
DUTCH REGISTRIES	70
ENGLISH REGISTRIES	2540
ESTONIA	184
FINLAND	510
FRENCH REGISTRIES	93
GERMAN REGISTRIES	139
ITALIAN REGISTRIES	126
POLISH REGISTRIES	65
SCOTLAND	495
SPANISH REGISTRIES	40
SWISS REGISTRIES	80
Mean age (years)	70.6

RELATIVE SURVIVAL (%)
(Age-standardized)

Females
100 80 60 40 20 0
DK
ENG
EST
FIN
D
I
SCO
EUR

OBSERVED AND RELATIVE SURVIVAL (%) BY AGE AND PERIOD
(Number of cases in parentheses)

	AGE CLASS												PERIOD					
	15-44		45-54		55-64		65-74		75+		All		1978-80		1981-82		1983-85	
	obs	rel	obs	rel	obs	rel	obs	rel	obs	rel	obs	rel	obs	rel	obs	rel	obs	rel
Females	(233)		(367)		(791)		(1569)		(2211)		(5171)		(2160)		(1510)		(1501)	
1 year	89	89	82	83	79	80	70	72	56	62	67	71	67	71	66	69	69	72
3 years	75	75	67	68	61	63	51	56	32	44	47	55	46	54	47	55	48	56
5 years	74	75	63	64	56	59	45	53	23	41	40	52	39	51	39	52	42	54
8 years	70	71	56	58	51	56	36	49	15	41	32	51	32	50	33	53	32	48
10 years	68	70	54	58	46	53	30	45	11	42	28	50	27	49	27	49	..	..

RELATIVE SURVIVAL (%) BY AGE AND PERIOD

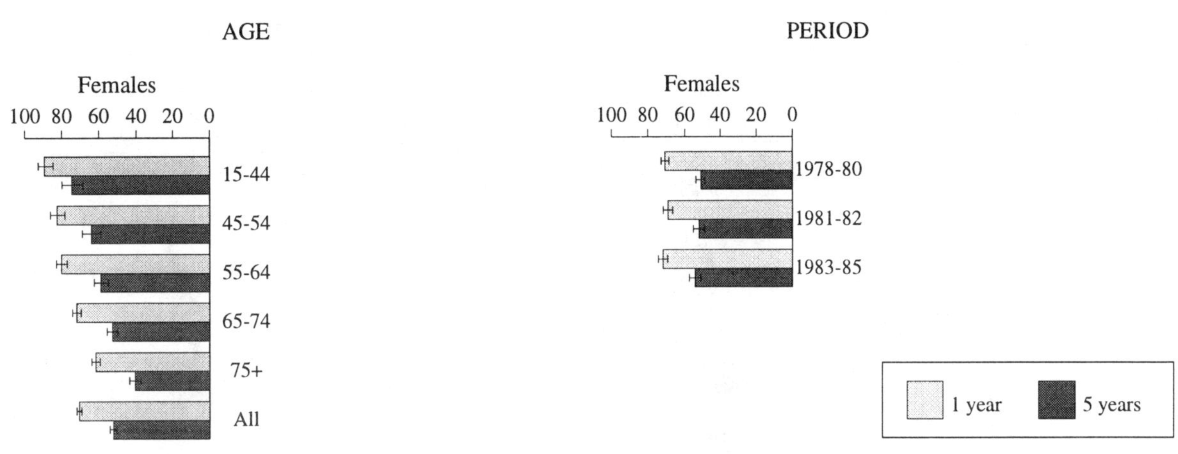

TESTIS

DENMARK

REGISTRY	NUMBER OF CASES	PERIOD OF DIAGNOSIS
Denmark	1580	1978-1984
Mean age (years)	37.4	

RELATIVE SURVIVAL (%)

Time since diagnosis (years)

OBSERVED AND RELATIVE SURVIVAL (%) BY AGE AND PERIOD
(Number of cases in parentheses)

	AGE CLASS												PERIOD					
	15-44		45-54		55-64		65-74		75+		All		1978-80		1981-82		1983-85	
	obs	rel	obs	rel	obs	rel	obs	rel	obs	rel	obs	rel	obs	rel	obs	rel	obs	rel
Males	(1202)		(185)		(94)		(66)		(33)		(1580)		(688)		(428)		(464)	
1 year	96	96	95	95	83	84	74	77	58	65	94	94	94	95	93	94	93	94
3 years	91	91	93	95	77	81	64	73	21	31	88	90	88	90	86	88	89	90
5 years	90	91	89	92	69	76	52	66	18	36	85	89	86	89	82	86	87	90
8 years	89	90	85	91	57	69	42	66	14	44	83	89	84	89	77	84	..	..
10 years	87	89	77	85	52	67	30	57	7	32	80	87	81	88	..	..	..	..

RELATIVE SURVIVAL (%) BY AGE AND PERIOD

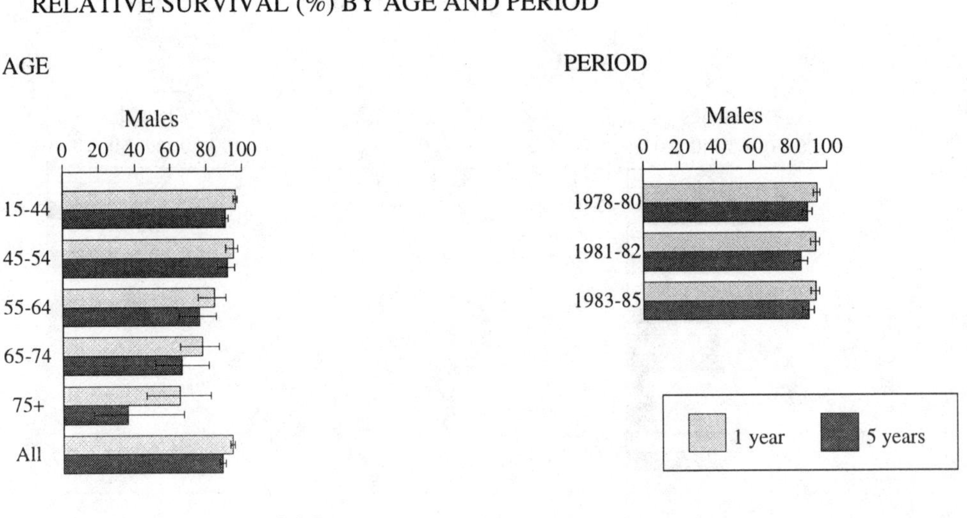

TESTIS

DUTCH REGISTRIES

REGISTRY	NUMBER OF CASES	PERIOD OF DIAGNOSIS
Eindhoven	112	1978-1985
Mean age (years)	38.3	

RELATIVE SURVIVAL (%)

Time since diagnosis (years)

OBSERVED AND RELATIVE SURVIVAL (%) BY AGE AND PERIOD
(Number of cases in parentheses)

	AGE CLASS												PERIOD					
	15-44		45-54		55-64		65-74		75+		All		1978-80		1981-82		1983-85	
	obs	rel	obs	rel	obs	rel	obs	rel	obs	rel	obs	rel	obs	rel	obs	rel	obs	rel
Males	(78)		(14)		(14)		(2)		(4)		(112)		(41)		(26)		(45)	
1 year	99	99	86	86	79	80	100	100	50	55	93	93	88	88	88	89	100	100
3 years	96	96	86	87	64	67	100	100	50	69	89	91	88	90	81	83	96	98
5 years	91	92	86	88	64	70	100	100	25	45	85	88	83	86	81	85	87	91
8 years	88	89	86	90	39	45	100	100	..	..	80	86	78	82	..	..	..	..
10 years	84	85	86	91	39	48	..	..	..	..	77	84	74	80	..	..	..	..

RELATIVE SURVIVAL (%) BY AGE AND PERIOD

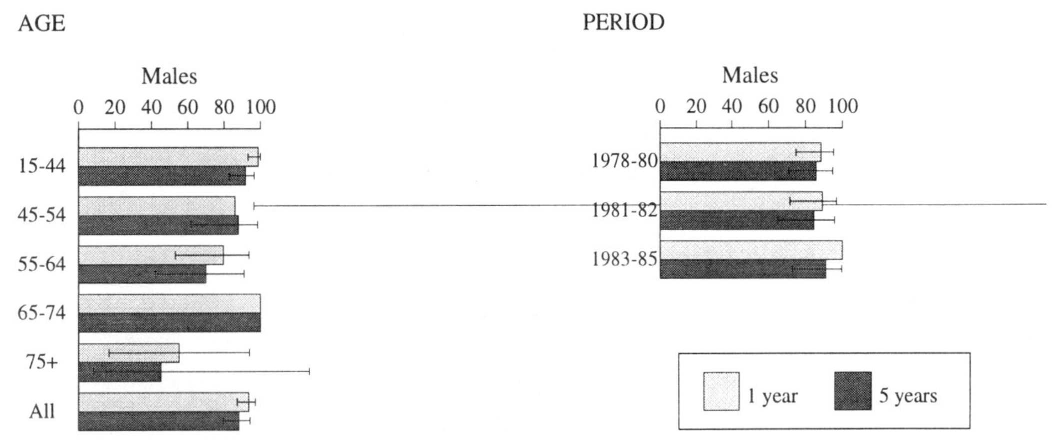

TESTIS

ENGLISH REGISTRIES

REGISTRY	NUMBER OF CASES	PERIOD OF DIAGNOSIS
East Anglia	270	1979-1984
Mersey	319	1978-1984
South Thames	721	1978-1984
Wessex	105	1983-1984
West Midlands	507	1979-1984
Yorkshire	470	1978-1984
Mean age (years)	36.6	

RELATIVE SURVIVAL (%)

OBSERVED AND RELATIVE SURVIVAL (%) BY AGE AND PERIOD
(Number of cases in parentheses)

	AGE CLASS												PERIOD					
	15-44		45-54		55-64		65-74		75+		All		1978-80		1981-82		1983-85	
	obs	rel	obs	rel	obs	rel	obs	rel	obs	rel	obs	rel	obs	rel	obs	rel	obs	rel
Males	(1877)		(257)		(151)		(62)		(45)		(2392)		(893)		(731)		(768)	
1 year	94	94	93	94	86	88	69	73	38	43	92	93	90	90	94	95	93	93
3 years	88	89	88	90	78	83	61	71	22	33	86	87	83	84	88	89	87	89
5 years	87	87	86	89	74	81	44	56	20	40	83	86	81	83	86	88	84	87
8 years	86	87	82	87	71	86	37	60	16	51	82	86	79	83	84	88	81	86
10 years	81	83	76	84	64	82	32	60	16	75	77	83	76	81	77	83	..	..

RELATIVE SURVIVAL (%) BY AGE AND PERIOD

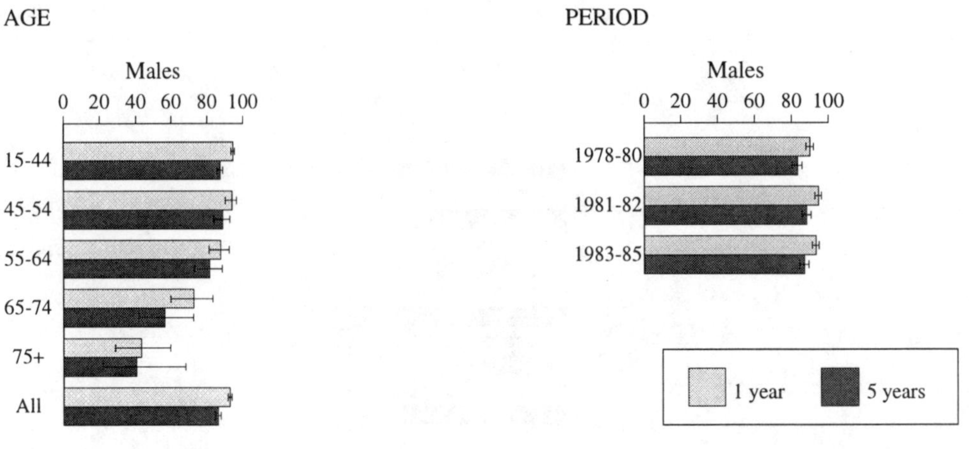

TESTIS

FINLAND

REGISTRY	NUMBER OF CASES	PERIOD OF DIAGNOSIS
Finland	284	1978-1984
Mean age (years)	36.0	

RELATIVE SURVIVAL (%)

100
80
60
40
20
0
0 1 2 3 4 5
Time since diagnosis (years)

OBSERVED AND RELATIVE SURVIVAL (%) BY AGE AND PERIOD

(Number of cases in parentheses)

	AGE CLASS												PERIOD					
	15-44		45-54		55-64		65-74		75+		All		1978-80		1981-82		1983-85	
	obs	rel	obs	rel	obs	rel	obs	rel	obs	rel	obs	rel	obs	rel	obs	rel	obs	rel
Males	(229)		(25)		(10)		(15)		(5)		(284)		(112)		(79)		(93)	
1 year	87	88	92	93	90	92	67	70	60	68	86	87	88	88	85	86	86	87
3 years	79	80	84	86	80	85	47	55	40	59	77	79	71	73	78	80	83	85
5 years	77	78	84	88	80	90	40	53	20	39	75	78	71	73	73	77	82	85
8 years	74	76	84	92	70	86	40	65	20	64	72	77	68	72	71	76	77	82
10 years	74	76	84	94	70	92	40	77	..	..	72	78	68	74	71	77	..	..

RELATIVE SURVIVAL (%) BY AGE AND PERIOD

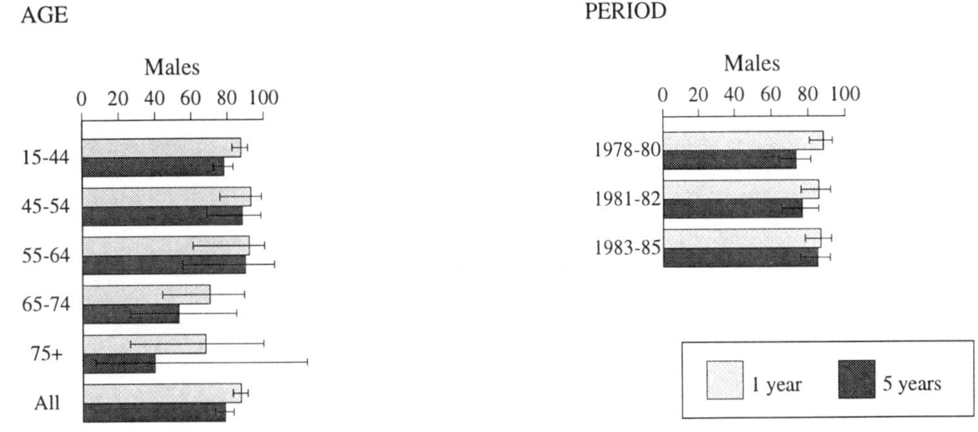

TESTIS

FRENCH REGISTRIES

REGISTRY	NUMBER OF CASES	PERIOD OF DIAGNOSIS
Amiens	21	1983-1984
Doubs	79	1978-1985
Mean age (years)	38.6	

RELATIVE SURVIVAL (%)

100 80 60 40 20 0

0 1 2 3 4 5

Time since diagnosis (years)

OBSERVED AND RELATIVE SURVIVAL (%) BY AGE AND PERIOD
(Number of cases in parentheses)

	AGE CLASS												PERIOD					
	15-44		45-54		55-64		65-74		75+		All		1978-80		1981-82		1983-85	
	obs	rel	obs	rel	obs	rel	obs	rel	obs	rel	obs	rel	obs	rel	obs	rel	obs	rel
Males	(71)		(14)		(6)		(4)		(5)		(100)		(33)		(14)		(53)	
1 year	93	93	93	93	83	85	75	78	20	27	88	89	85	85	86	87	90	93
3 years	81	81	93	95	67	71	25	28	20	42	76	79	76	77	79	81	75	80
5 years	81	81	86	89	67	74	25	32	20	62	75	80	73	75	79	83	75	83
8 years	81	82	70	75	33	40	..	..	20	100	70	77	69	73	79	86	0	0
10 years	73	75	70	77	33	42	..	..	20	100	64	72	64	68	..	..	0	0

RELATIVE SURVIVAL (%) BY AGE AND PERIOD

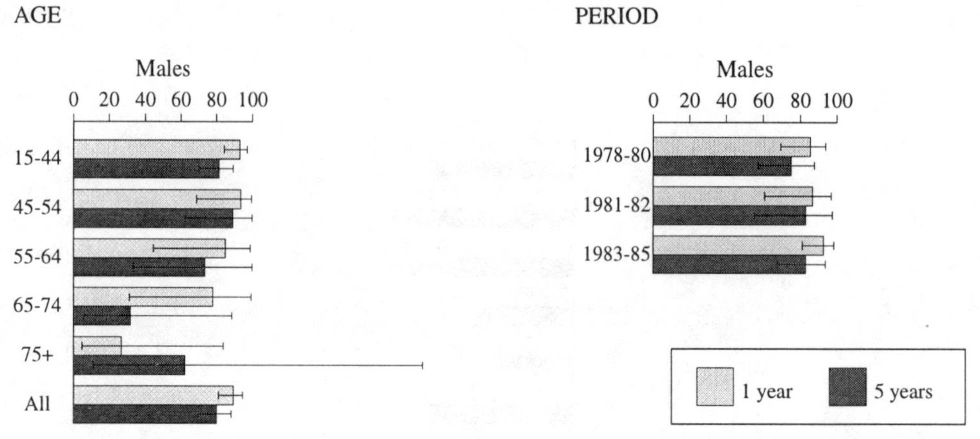

TESTIS

GERMAN REGISTRIES

REGISTRY	NUMBER OF CASES	PERIOD OF DIAGNOSIS
Saarland	200	1978-1984
Mean age (years)	32.5	

RELATIVE SURVIVAL (%)

100
80
60
40
20
0
0 1 2 3 4 5
Time since diagnosis (years)

OBSERVED AND RELATIVE SURVIVAL (%) BY AGE AND PERIOD
(Number of cases in parentheses)

	AGE CLASS												PERIOD					
	15-44		45-54		55-64		65-74		75+		All		1978-80		1981-82		1983-85	
	obs	rel	obs	rel	obs	rel	obs	rel	obs	rel	obs	rel	obs	rel	obs	rel	obs	rel
Males	(175)		(15)		(8)		(1)		(1)		(200)		(78)		(55)		(67)	
1 year	91	92	93	94	88	89	100	100	0	0	91	91	88	89	93	93	93	93
3 years	83	84	80	82	88	93	0	0	0	0	83	83	82	83	84	84	82	83
5 years	79	80	73	76	75	83	0	0	0	0	78	79	72	73	80	81	82	84
8 years	77	78	64	69	63	76	0	0	0	0	74	77	72	75	72	74	..	..
10 years	75	77	21	24	63	81	0	0	0	0	71	74	69	72	..	..	..	..

RELATIVE SURVIVAL (%) BY AGE AND PERIOD

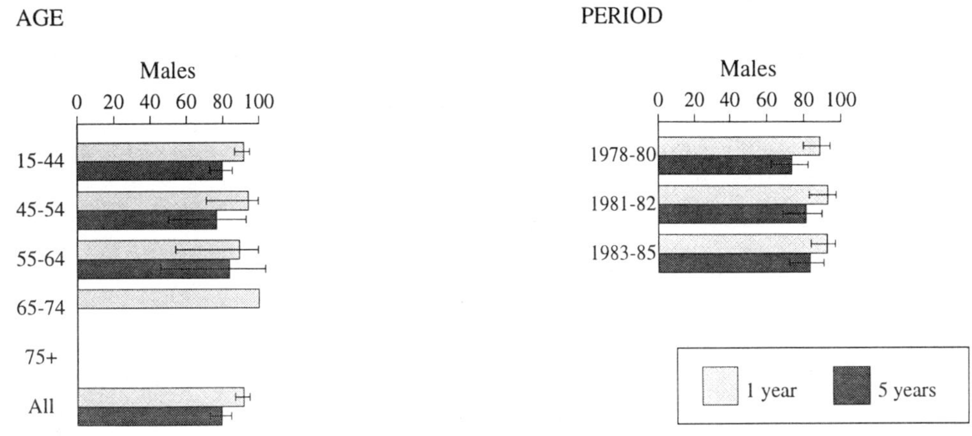

TESTIS

ITALIAN REGISTRIES

REGISTRY	NUMBER OF CASES	PERIOD OF DIAGNOSIS
Latina	5	1983-1984
Ragusa	10	1981-1984
Varese	98	1978-1984
Mean age (years)	38.4	

RELATIVE SURVIVAL (%)

100
80
60
40
20
0
0 1 2 3 4 5
Time since diagnosis (years)

OBSERVED AND RELATIVE SURVIVAL (%) BY AGE AND PERIOD
(Number of cases in parentheses)

	AGE CLASS												PERIOD					
	15-44		45-54		55-64		65-74		75+		All		1978-80		1981-82		1983-85	
	obs	rel	obs	rel	obs	rel	obs	rel	obs	rel	obs	rel	obs	rel	obs	rel	obs	rel
Males	(79)		(14)		(10)		(5)		(5)		(113)		(37)		(40)		(36)	
1 year	95	95	86	86	100	100	60	63	60	66	91	92	92	93	93	93	89	90
3 years	90	90	86	87	100	100	60	68	60	80	88	90	92	95	90	92	81	83
5 years	89	89	79	81	100	100	40	51	40	67	84	88	86	91	90	93	75	79
8 years	89	90	71	76	89	100	20	30	40	100	81	87	84	90	85	90	75	83
10 years	84	86	71	78	72	88	..	..	..	..	76	84	78	86	81	87	..	..

RELATIVE SURVIVAL (%) BY AGE AND PERIOD

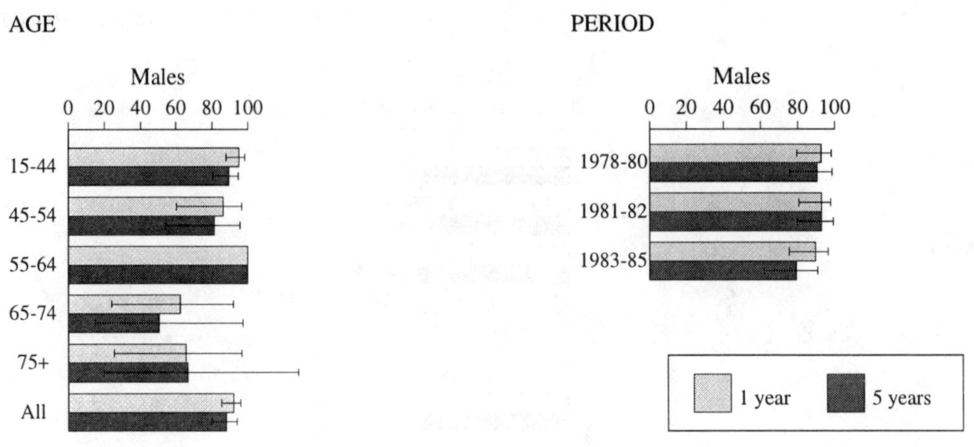

TESTIS

SCOTLAND

REGISTRY	NUMBER OF CASES	PERIOD OF DIAGNOSIS
Scotland	562	1978-1982
Mean age (years)	35.3	

RELATIVE SURVIVAL (%)

Time since diagnosis (years)

OBSERVED AND RELATIVE SURVIVAL (%) BY AGE AND PERIOD
(Number of cases in parentheses)

	AGE CLASS												PERIOD					
	15-44		45-54		55-64		65-74		75+		All		1978-80		1981-82		1983-85	
	obs	rel	obs	rel	obs	rel	obs	rel	obs	rel	obs	rel	obs	rel	obs	rel	obs	rel
Males	(467)		(57)		(20)		(12)		(6)		(562)		(321)		(241)		(0)	
1 year	92	92	88	88	85	87	100	100	67	77	91	92	89	89	95	95	..	..
3 years	83	83	81	83	80	86	67	79	33	53	81	83	79	80	85	86	..	..
5 years	81	82	75	79	80	90	58	79	0	0	79	82	76	79	84	85	..	..
8 years	80	81	73	79	62	78	58	99	0	0	77	81	74	78	..	..	..	..
10 years	79	81	73	81	62	84	58	100	0	0	77	82	73	79	..	..	..	..

RELATIVE SURVIVAL (%) BY AGE AND PERIOD

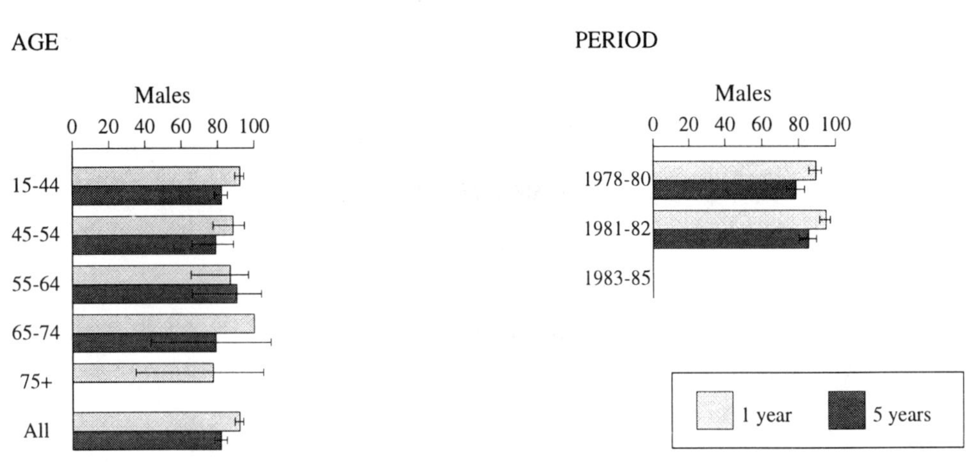

TESTIS

SWISS REGISTRIES

REGISTRY	NUMBER OF CASES	PERIOD OF DIAGNOSIS	RELATIVE SURVIVAL (%)
Basel	64	1981-1984	
Geneva	74	1978-1984	
Mean age (years)	34.8		

OBSERVED AND RELATIVE SURVIVAL (%) BY AGE AND PERIOD
(Number of cases in parentheses)

	AGE CLASS												PERIOD					
	15-44		45-54		55-64		65-74		75+		All		1978-80		1981-82		1983-85	
	obs	rel	obs	rel	obs	rel	obs	rel	obs	rel	obs	rel	obs	rel	obs	rel	obs	rel
Males	(116)		(16)		(1)		(4)		(1)		(138)		(24)		(66)		(48)	
1 year	97	98	94	94	0	0	75	78	100	100	96	96	92	92	97	97	96	96
3 years	90	91	94	95	0	0	50	57	0	0	88	89	83	84	91	91	88	89
5 years	90	90	94	97	0	0	50	63	0	0	88	89	79	81	91	92	88	90
8 years	90	91	94	99	0	0	..	..	0	0	88	90	..	..	91	93	..	..
10 years	..	..	..	..	0	0	..	..	0	0	..	..	..	..	..	..	..	..

RELATIVE SURVIVAL (%) BY AGE AND PERIOD

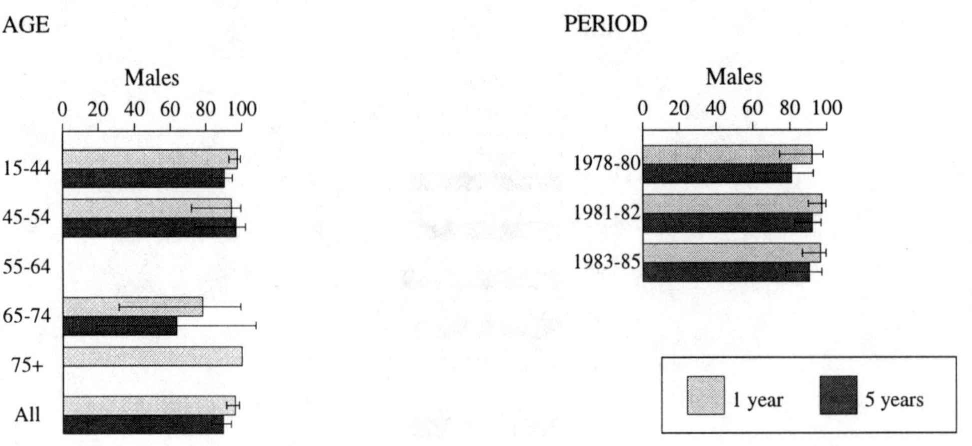

TESTIS

ESTONIA

REGISTRY	NUMBER OF CASES	PERIOD OF DIAGNOSIS
Estonia	64	1978-1984
Mean age (years)	41.7	

RELATIVE SURVIVAL (%)

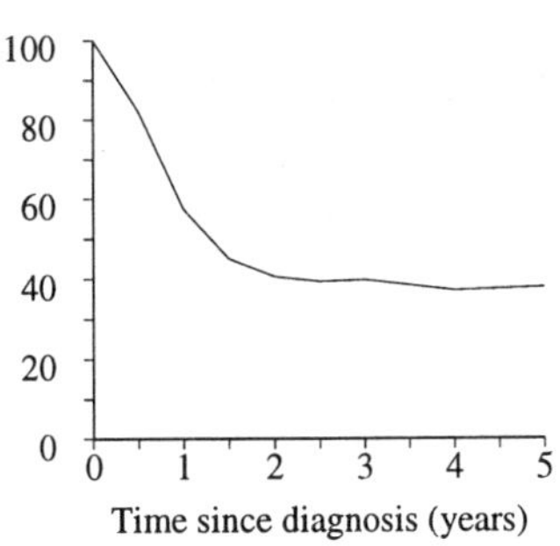

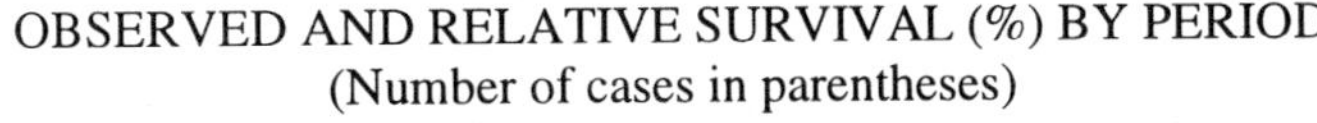

OBSERVED AND RELATIVE SURVIVAL (%) BY PERIOD
(Number of cases in parentheses)

	PERIOD							
	1978-80		1981-82		1983-85		All	
	obs	rel	obs	rel	obs	rel	obs	rel
N. Cases	(25)		(17)		(22)		(64)	
1 year	56	57	29	30	77	79	56	57
3 years	28	30	29	32	55	58	38	40
5 years	24	26	29	33	50	55	34	38
8 years	16	19	29	34	..	..	27	31
10 years	16	19	..	..	..	..	27	32

0 20 40 60 80 100

1978-80

1981-82

1983-85

POLISH REGISTRIES

REGISTRY	NUMBER OF CASES	PERIOD OF DIAGNOSIS
Cracow	68	1978-1984
Mean age (years)	35.9	

RELATIVE SURVIVAL (%)

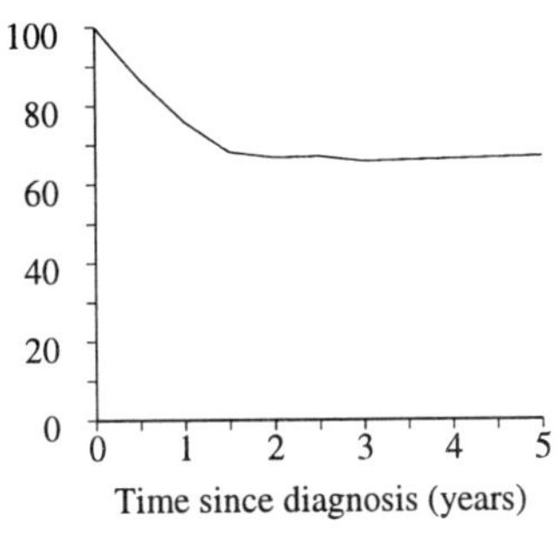

OBSERVED AND RELATIVE SURVIVAL (%) BY PERIOD
(Number of cases in parentheses)

	PERIOD							
	1978-80		1981-82		1983-85		All	
	obs	rel	obs	rel	obs	rel	obs	rel
N. Cases	(31)		(17)		(20)		(68)	
1 year	76	77	75	76	74	74	75	76
3 years	62	64	55	57	74	75	64	66
5 years	62	65	55	58	74	77	64	67
8 years	62	68	47	53	74	78	62	67
10 years	62	69	47	54	..	..	62	69

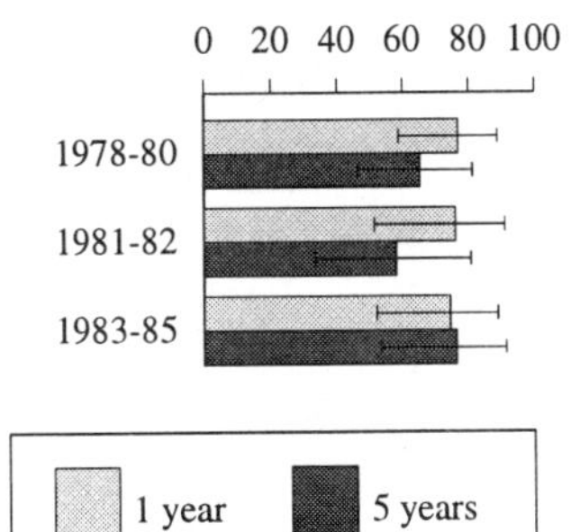

TESTIS

SPANISH REGISTRIES

REGISTRY	NUMBER OF CASES	PERIOD OF DIAGNOSIS
Tarragona	2	1985-1985
Mean age (years)	36.5	

Not enough cases for reliable estimation

TESTIS

EUROPEAN REGISTRIES

Unweighted analysis

REGISTRY	CASES
DENMARK	1580
DUTCH REGISTRIES	112
ENGLISH REGISTRIES	2392
ESTONIA	64
FINLAND	284
FRENCH REGISTRIES	100
GERMAN REGISTRIES	200
ITALIAN REGISTRIES	113
POLISH REGISTRIES	68
SCOTLAND	562
SWISS REGISTRIES	138
Mean age (years)	36.6

RELATIVE SURVIVAL (%)

(Age-standardized)

Males

0 20 40 60 80 100

DK
NL
ENG
FIN
F
D
I
SCO
CH
EUR

OBSERVED AND RELATIVE SURVIVAL (%) BY AGE AND PERIOD

(Number of cases in parentheses)

	AGE CLASS												PERIOD					
	15-44		45-54		55-64		65-74		75+		All		1978-80		1981-82		1983-85	
	obs	rel	obs	rel	obs	rel	obs	rel	obs	rel	obs	rel	obs	rel	obs	rel	obs	rel
Males	(4394)		(608)		(323)		(180)		(110)		(5615)		(2283)		(1714)		(1618)	
1 year	94	94	93	93	84	85	73	76	46	53	91	92	90	91	93	93	92	93
3 years	87	88	88	90	76	81	59	68	25	37	84	86	82	84	85	87	86	88
5 years	86	86	84	88	72	79	47	61	18	36	82	85	80	83	83	86	84	87
8 years	84	86	81	86	64	78	39	62	15	50	80	85	78	83	81	86	81	86
10 years	81	83	75	82	58	75	32	61	12	61	76	82	75	81	75	81	..	..

RELATIVE SURVIVAL (%) BY AGE AND PERIOD

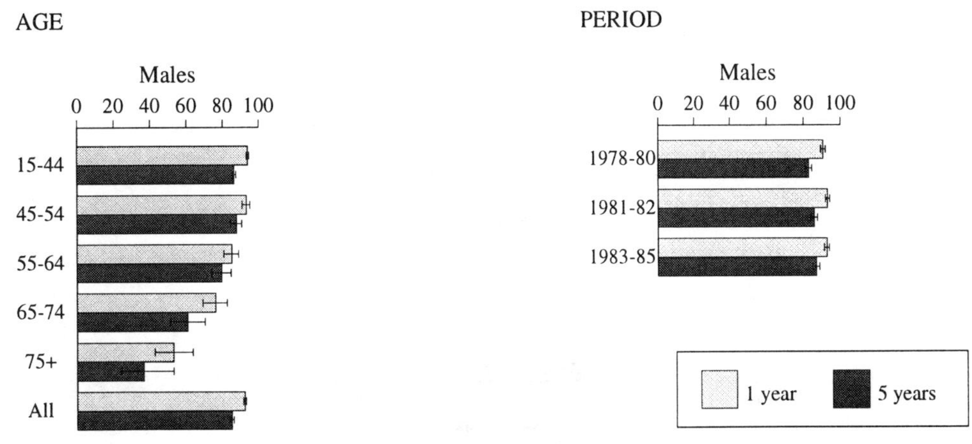

PENIS

DENMARK

REGISTRY	NUMBER OF CASES	PERIOD OF DIAGNOSIS
Denmark	314	1978-1984
Mean age (years)	66.5	

RELATIVE SURVIVAL (%)

100
80
60
40
20
0
0 1 2 3 4 5
Time since diagnosis (years)

OBSERVED AND RELATIVE SURVIVAL (%) BY AGE AND PERIOD
(Number of cases in parentheses)

	AGE CLASS												PERIOD					
	15-44		45-54		55-64		65-74		75+		All		1978-80		1981-82		1983-85	
	obs	rel	obs	rel	obs	rel	obs	rel	obs	rel	obs	rel	obs	rel	obs	rel	obs	rel
Males	(25)		(37)		(60)		(92)		(100)		(314)		(129)		(97)		(88)	
1 year	96	96	92	93	92	93	85	89	63	71	81	85	79	84	79	84	85	90
3 years	92	93	84	86	78	83	62	72	47	69	65	77	65	77	68	80	63	74
5 years	88	89	78	82	73	81	46	60	36	70	55	74	57	76	59	77	49	66
8 years	80	81	74	80	58	70	38	61	14	45	41	67	44	71	44	70	..	..
10 years	48	49	64	72	58	75	26	50	6	30	32	60	34	64	..	..	..	..

RELATIVE SURVIVAL (%) BY AGE AND PERIOD

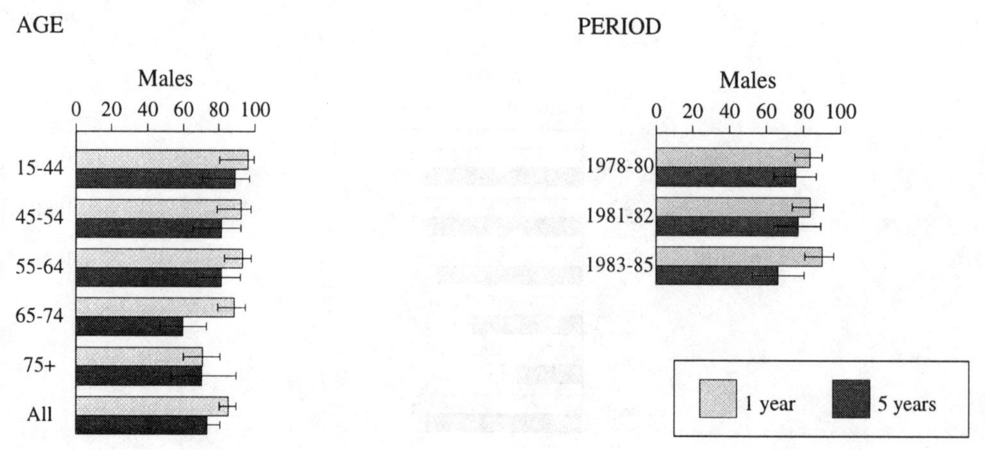

PENIS

ENGLISH REGISTRIES

REGISTRY	NUMBER OF CASES	PERIOD OF DIAGNOSIS
East Anglia	81	1979-1984
Mersey	128	1978-1984
South Thames	222	1978-1984
Wessex	36	1983-1984
West Midlands	232	1979-1984
Yorkshire	185	1978-1984
Mean age (years)	66.4	

RELATIVE SURVIVAL (%)

Time since diagnosis (years)

OBSERVED AND RELATIVE SURVIVAL (%) BY AGE AND PERIOD
(Number of cases in parentheses)

	AGE CLASS												PERIOD					
	15-44		45-54		55-64		65-74		75+		All		1978-80		1981-82		1983-85	
	obs	rel	obs	rel	obs	rel	obs	rel	obs	rel	obs	rel	obs	rel	obs	rel	obs	rel
Males	(62)		(81)		(186)		(323)		(232)		(884)		(337)		(283)		(264)	
1 year	90	90	91	92	83	85	77	81	60	69	76	81	78	82	77	82	73	78
3 years	79	79	81	83	66	70	57	67	33	50	56	67	56	66	60	71	53	64
5 years	74	75	76	79	62	69	47	63	23	48	48	65	49	64	51	68	45	62
8 years	69	70	71	76	56	68	35	58	17	61	40	65	40	63	41	67	39	65
10 years	66	68	67	75	46	60	31	63	10	54	34	63	34	61	37	67	..	..

RELATIVE SURVIVAL (%) BY AGE AND PERIOD

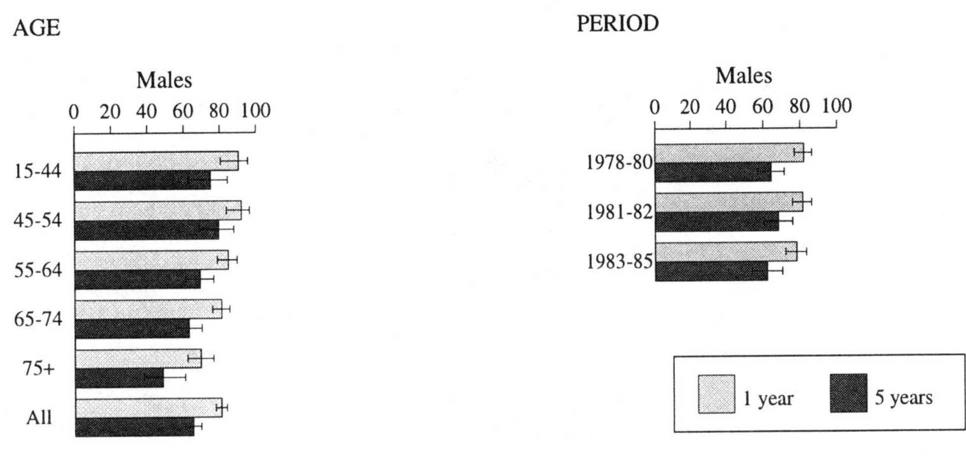

PENIS

SCOTLAND

REGISTRY	NUMBER OF CASES	PERIOD OF DIAGNOSIS
Scotland	164	1978-1982
Mean age (years)	65.8	

RELATIVE SURVIVAL (%)

100
80
60
40
20
0
0 1 2 3 4 5
Time since diagnosis (years)

OBSERVED AND RELATIVE SURVIVAL (%) BY AGE AND PERIOD
(Number of cases in parentheses)

	AGE CLASS												PERIOD					
	15-44		45-54		55-64		65-74		75+		All		1978-80		1981-82		1983-85	
	obs	rel	obs	rel	obs	rel	obs	rel	obs	rel	obs	rel	obs	rel	obs	rel	obs	rel
Males	(11)		(19)		(37)		(57)		(40)		(164)		(99)		(65)		(0)	
1 year	73	73	100	100	92	94	82	87	60	69	80	85	83	88	77	81	..	..
3 years	73	73	89	92	78	85	58	70	40	61	63	75	69	82	54	64	..	..
5 years	73	74	89	95	57	65	39	54	33	67	49	67	55	74	42	56	..	..
8 years	73	75	89	99	53	68	30	53	19	65	43	70	46	75	..	..	..	..
10 years	73	76	44	51	53	74	30	65	19	97	35	67	38	72	..	..	..	..

RELATIVE SURVIVAL (%) BY AGE AND PERIOD

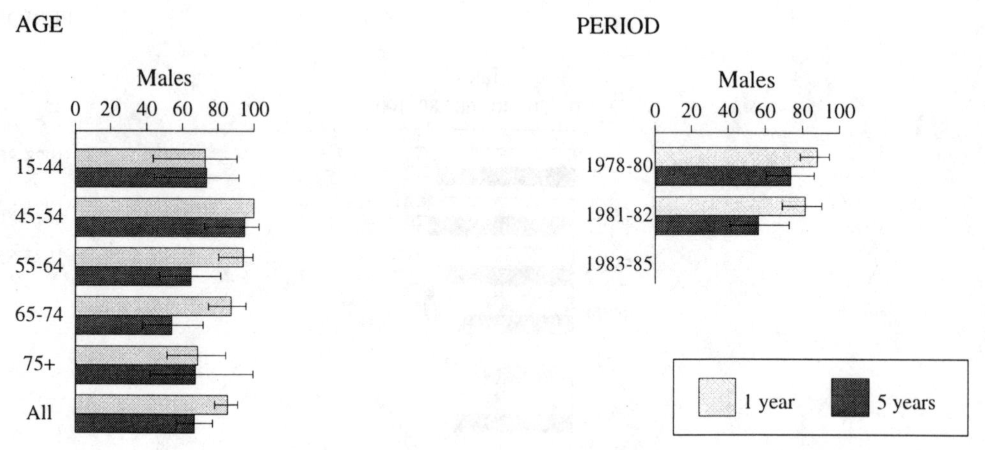

PENIS

DUTCH REGISTRIES

REGISTRY	NUMBER OF CASES	PERIOD OF DIAGNOSIS
Eindhoven	26	1978-1985
Mean age (years)	70.4	

RELATIVE SURVIVAL (%)

Time since diagnosis (years)

OBSERVED AND RELATIVE SURVIVAL (%) BY PERIOD
(Number of cases in parentheses)

	1978-80 obs	1978-80 rel	1981-82 obs	1981-82 rel	1983-85 obs	1983-85 rel	All obs	All rel
N. Cases	(7)		(9)		(10)		(26)	
1 year	71	76	67	70	80	86	73	78
3 years	71	88	67	79	59	76	65	81
5 years	71	100	67	91	..	..	65	95
8 years	57	100	..	..	..	..	54	100
10 years	..	..	..	..	..	..	..	..

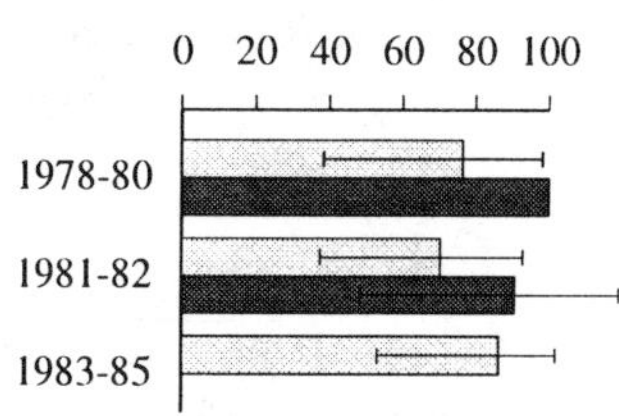

ESTONIA

REGISTRY	NUMBER OF CASES	PERIOD OF DIAGNOSIS
Estonia	37	1978-1984
Mean age (years)	62.4	

RELATIVE SURVIVAL (%)

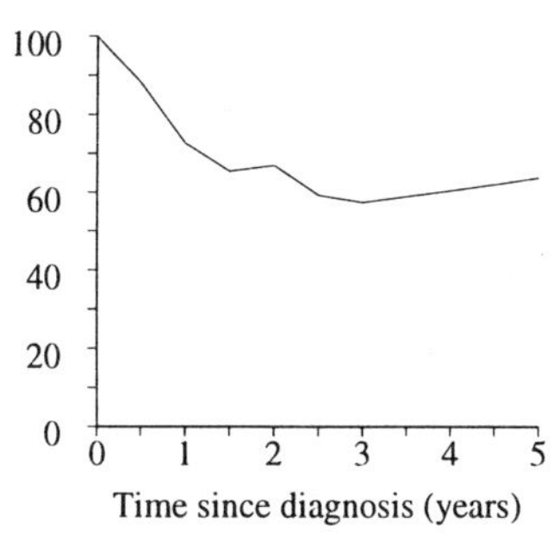

OBSERVED AND RELATIVE SURVIVAL (%) BY PERIOD
(Number of cases in parentheses)

	1978-80 obs	1978-80 rel	1981-82 obs	1981-82 rel	1983-85 obs	1983-85 rel	All obs	All rel
N. Cases	(15)		(11)		(11)		(37)	
1 year	57	61	91	95	64	66	70	73
3 years	43	51	64	72	45	51	50	57
5 years	43	58	64	79	45	56	50	64
8 years	36	60	53	77	..	..	42	64
10 years	18	36	..	..	..	..	21	38

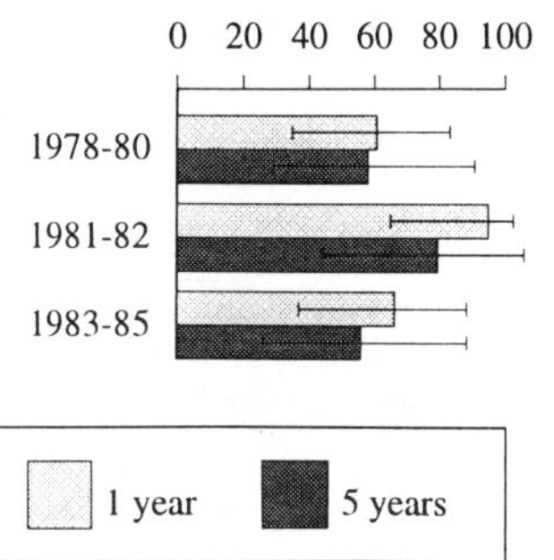

PENIS

FINLAND

REGISTRY	NUMBER OF CASES	PERIOD OF DIAGNOSIS
Finland	96	1978-1984
Mean age (years)	61.6	

RELATIVE SURVIVAL (%)

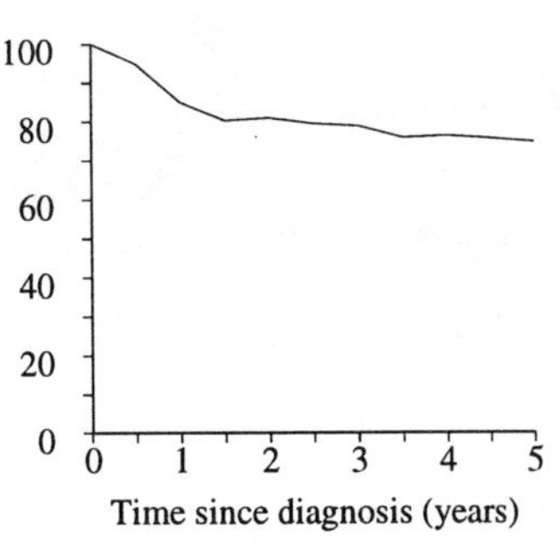

OBSERVED AND RELATIVE SURVIVAL (%) BY PERIOD
(Number of cases in parentheses)

	PERIOD						All	
	1978-80		1981-82		1983-85			
	obs	rel	obs	rel	obs	rel	obs	rel
N. Cases	(43)		(19)		(34)		(96)	
1 year	81	85	79	83	82	86	81	85
3 years	67	77	68	80	71	81	69	79
5 years	60	75	68	89	53	66	59	75
8 years	49	70	47	71	47	68	46	67
10 years	47	74	47	78	..	..	44	71

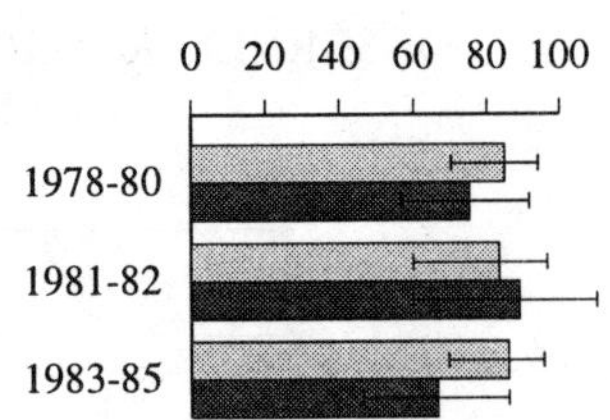

FRENCH REGISTRIES

REGISTRY	NUMBER OF CASES	PERIOD OF DIAGNOSIS
Amiens	9	1983-1984
Doubs	18	1978-1985
Mean age (years)	62.0	

RELATIVE SURVIVAL (%)

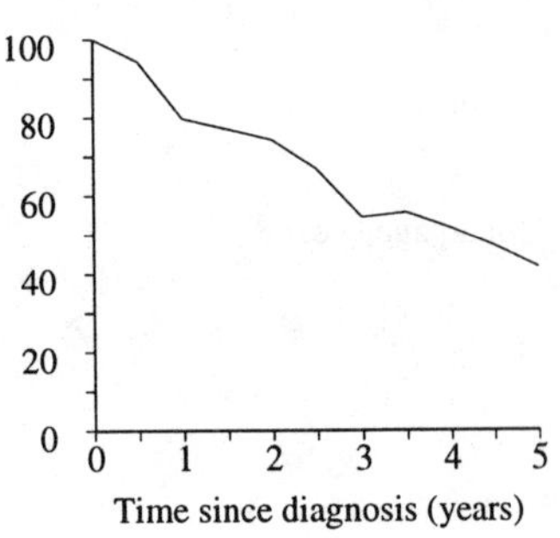

OBSERVED AND RELATIVE SURVIVAL (%) BY PERIOD
(Number of cases in parentheses)

	PERIOD						All	
	1978-80		1981-82		1983-85			
	obs	rel	obs	rel	obs	rel	obs	rel
N. Cases	(8)		(3)		(16)		(27)	
1 year	63	63	67	69	87	91	77	80
3 years	50	52	0	0	58	68	48	55
5 years	38	41	0	0	38	51	34	42
8 years	38	44	0	0	..	..	34	47
10 years	38	46	0	0	..	..	34	50

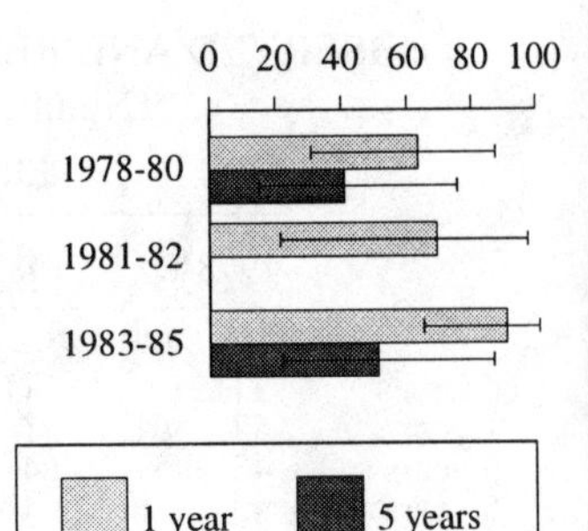

PENIS

GERMAN REGISTRIES

REGISTRY	NUMBER OF CASES	PERIOD OF DIAGNOSIS
Saarland	42	1978-1984
Mean age (years)	64.7	

RELATIVE SURVIVAL (%)

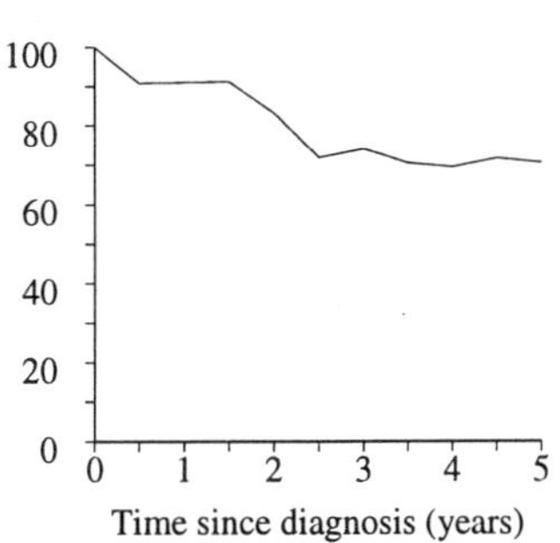

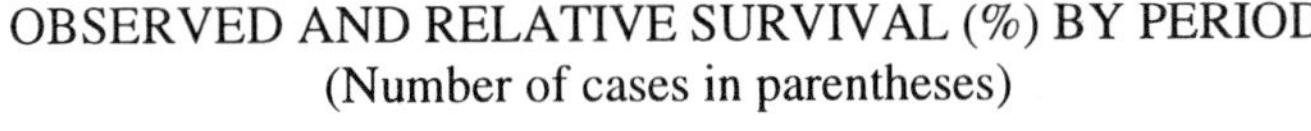

OBSERVED AND RELATIVE SURVIVAL (%) BY PERIOD
(Number of cases in parentheses)

	PERIOD							
	1978-80		1981-82		1983-85		All	
	obs	rel	obs	rel	obs	rel	obs	rel
N. Cases	(13)		(18)		(11)		(42)	
1 year	92	97	89	96	73	75	86	91
3 years	69	82	56	71	64	70	62	74
5 years	69	91	39	58	55	65	52	71
8 years	62	96	28	52	..	..	42	69
10 years	46	80	..	..	..	..	32	58

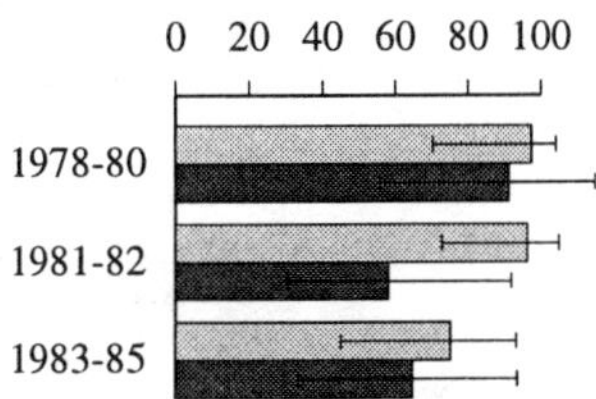

ITALIAN REGISTRIES

REGISTRY	NUMBER OF CASES	PERIOD OF DIAGNOSIS
Latina	6	1983-1984
Ragusa	7	1981-1984
Varese	30	1978-1984
Mean age (years)	61.4	

RELATIVE SURVIVAL (%)

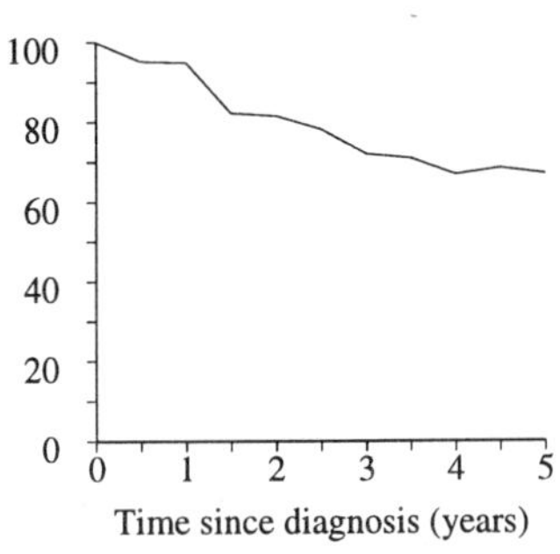

OBSERVED AND RELATIVE SURVIVAL (%) BY PERIOD
(Number of cases in parentheses)

	PERIOD							
	1978-80		1981-82		1983-85		All	
	obs	rel	obs	rel	obs	rel	obs	rel
N. Cases	(11)		(11)		(21)		(43)	
1 year	82	86	91	97	95	99	91	95
3 years	73	84	45	55	67	74	63	72
5 years	55	70	36	50	62	74	53	67
8 years	45	68	27	46	62	80	47	69
10 years	45	77	27	56	..	..	47	78

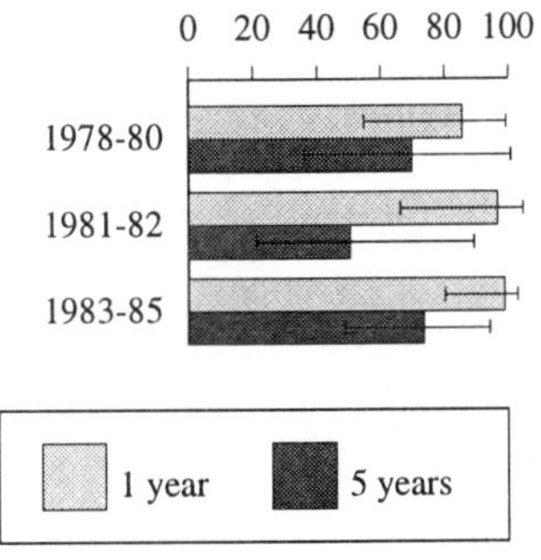

PENIS

POLISH REGISTRIES

REGISTRY	NUMBER OF CASES	PERIOD OF DIAGNOSIS
Cracow	9	1978-1983
Mean age (years)	58.1	

RELATIVE SURVIVAL (%)

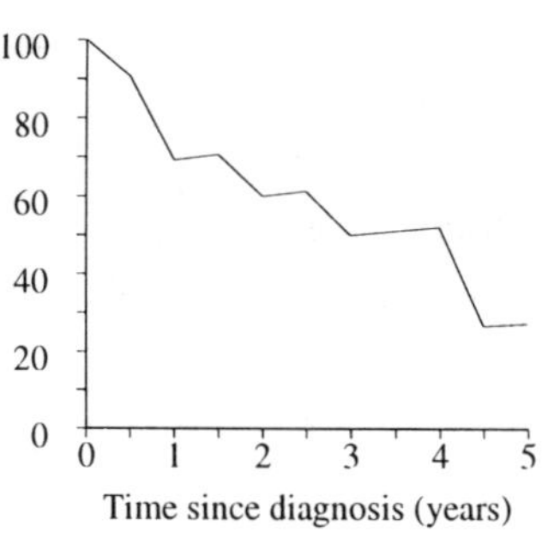

OBSERVED AND RELATIVE SURVIVAL (%) BY PERIOD
(Number of cases in parentheses)

	1978-80		1981-82		1983-85		All	
	obs	rel	obs	rel	obs	rel	obs	rel
N. Cases	(2)		(4)		(3)		(9)	
1 year	0	0	75	77	100	100	67	69
3 years	0	0	50	53	67	74	44	50
5 years	0	0	25	28	33	40	22	27
8 years	0	0	25	30	0	0	11	16
10 years	0	0	..	..	0	0	..	..

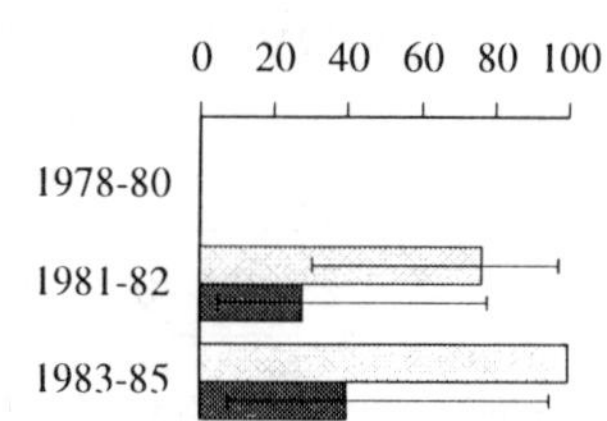

SPANISH REGISTRIES

REGISTRY	NUMBER OF CASES	PERIOD OF DIAGNOSIS
Tarragona	7	1985-1985
Mean age (years)	66.7	

RELATIVE SURVIVAL (%)

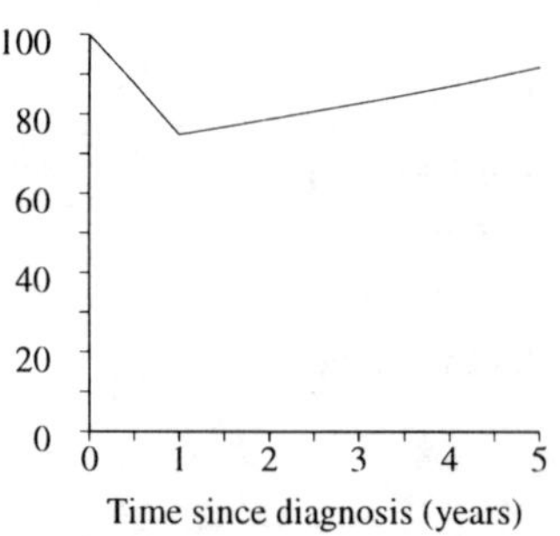

OBSERVED AND RELATIVE SURVIVAL (%) BY PERIOD
(Number of cases in parentheses)

	1978-80		1981-82		1983-85		All	
	obs	rel	obs	rel	obs	rel	obs	rel
N. Cases	(0)		(0)		(7)		(7)	
1 year	..	..	..	..	71	75	71	75
3 years	..	..	..	..	71	83	71	83
5 years	..	..	..	..	71	92	71	92
8 years	..	..	..	..	..	..	..	..
10 years	..	..	..	..	..	..	..	..

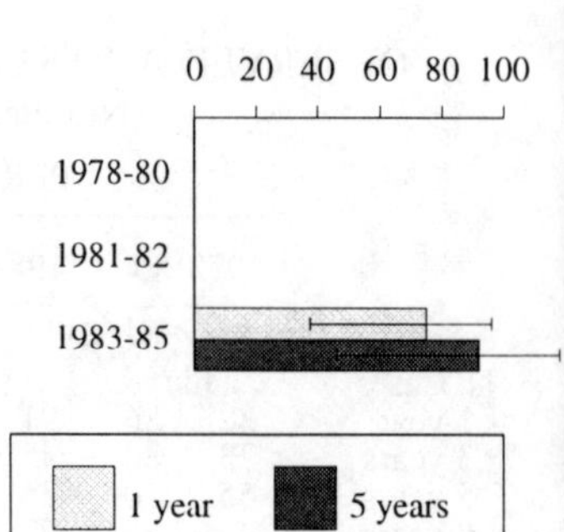

PENIS

SWISS REGISTRIES

REGISTRY	NUMBER OF CASES	PERIOD OF DIAGNOSIS
Basel	13	1981-1984
Geneva	8	1978-1983
Mean age (years)	63.3	

RELATIVE SURVIVAL (%)

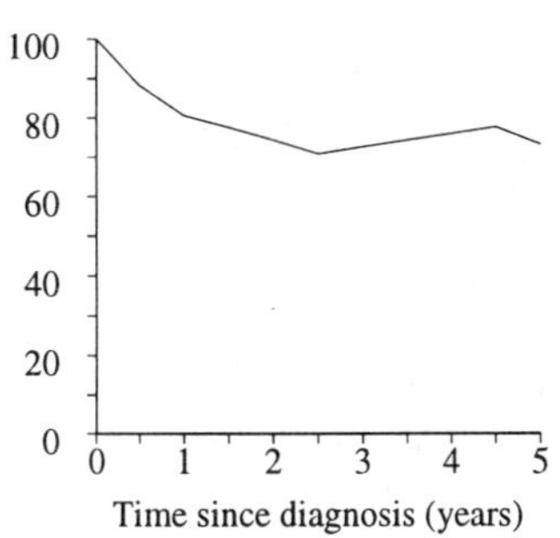

OBSERVED AND RELATIVE SURVIVAL (%) BY PERIOD
(Number of cases in parentheses)

	PERIOD							
	1978-80		1981-82		1983-85		All	
	obs	rel	obs	rel	obs	rel	obs	rel
N. Cases	(5)		(8)		(8)		(21)	
1 year	60	64	63	69	100	100	76	81
3 years	60	72	50	66	75	79	62	73
5 years	60	81	50	75	63	68	57	73
8 years	..	..	50	90	..	..	57	86
10 years	..	..	..	..	..	..	..	..

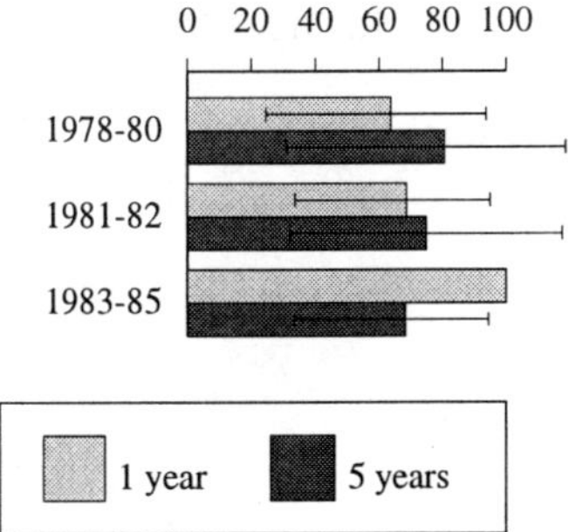

PENIS

EUROPEAN REGISTRIES

Unweighted analysis

REGISTRY	CASES
DENMARK	314
DUTCH REGISTRIES	26
ENGLISH REGISTRIES	884
ESTONIA	37
FINLAND	96
FRENCH REGISTRIES	27
GERMAN REGISTRIES	42
ITALIAN REGISTRIES	43
POLISH REGISTRIES	9
SCOTLAND	164
SPANISH REGISTRIES	7
SWISS REGISTRIES	21
Mean age (years)	65.7

RELATIVE SURVIVAL (%)

(Age-standardized)

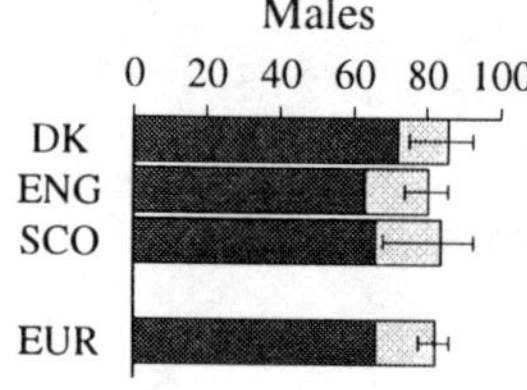

OBSERVED AND RELATIVE SURVIVAL (%) BY AGE AND PERIOD

(Number of cases in parentheses)

	AGE CLASS												PERIOD					
	15-44		45-54		55-64		65-74		75+		All		1978-80		1981-82		1983-85	
	obs	rel	obs	rel	obs	rel	obs	rel	obs	rel	obs	rel	obs	rel	obs	rel	obs	rel
Males	(137)		(186)		(347)		(554)		(446)		(1670)		(669)		(528)		(473)	
1 year	91	91	90	90	86	88	79	83	62	70	78	83	78	83	78	83	78	83
3 years	80	81	80	82	69	74	59	70	38	57	60	71	60	71	60	72	58	69
5 years	76	77	75	78	62	70	48	64	28	57	51	68	52	69	51	69	48	64
8 years	71	73	70	77	53	66	36	61	17	60	42	66	43	68	40	65	42	67
10 years	65	67	62	70	47	61	32	64	11	57	35	64	36	65	37	67	..	..

RELATIVE SURVIVAL (%) BY AGE AND PERIOD

AGE

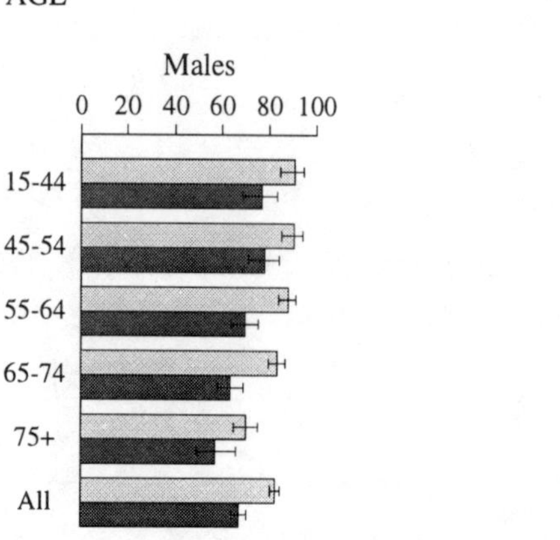

PERIOD

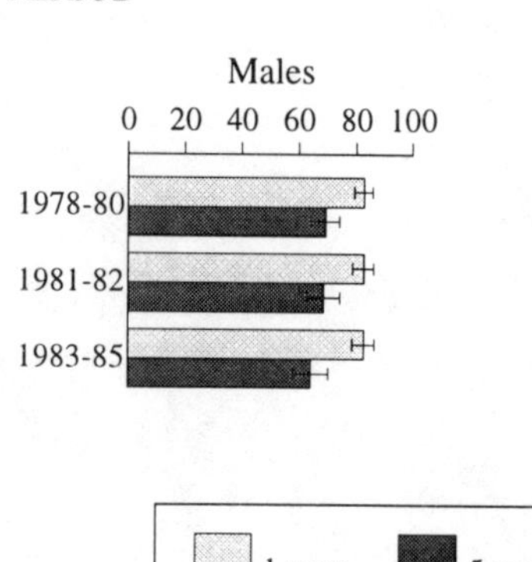

1 year 5 years

KIDNEY

DENMARK

REGISTRY	NUMBER OF CASES			PERIOD OF DIAGNOSIS
	Males	Females	All	
Denmark	1922	1626	3548	1978-1984
Mean age (years)	65.3	66.8	66.0	

RELATIVE SURVIVAL (%)

100
80
60
40
20
0
Males
Females
0 1 2 3 4 5
Time since diagnosis (years)

OBSERVED AND RELATIVE SURVIVAL (%) BY AGE AND PERIOD
(Number of cases in parentheses)

	AGE CLASS												PERIOD					
	15-44		45-54		55-64		65-74		75+		All		1978-80		1981-82		1983-85	
	obs	rel	obs	rel	obs	rel	obs	rel	obs	rel	obs	rel	obs	rel	obs	rel	obs	rel
Males	(111)		(213)		(522)		(652)		(424)		(1922)		(746)		(582)		(594)	
1 year	69	70	62	63	57	58	48	50	37	41	51	53	52	54	52	54	48	50
3 years	53	54	43	44	38	41	29	33	17	24	32	37	32	37	32	37	30	35
5 years	49	50	39	41	33	36	21	28	11	20	26	33	27	34	26	34	23	29
8 years	41	42	33	36	23	28	12	19	7	20	18	27	19	28	18	27	..	..
10 years	41	42	28	31	19	25	6	11	2	9	13	22	14	24	..	..	..	..
Females	(57)		(171)		(423)		(547)		(428)		(1626)		(691)		(441)		(494)	
1 year	56	56	58	58	53	54	54	55	33	35	49	50	46	47	49	51	53	54
3 years	53	53	43	43	36	37	38	41	19	24	33	37	30	33	34	37	38	42
5 years	53	53	34	35	30	31	29	34	11	18	26	31	24	28	26	31	29	35
8 years	53	54	30	31	22	25	21	28	7	16	20	27	19	25	19	26	..	..
10 years	44	45	29	31	22	25	17	24	5	15	17	26	16	24	..	..	..	..
Overall	(168)		(384)		(945)		(1199)		(852)		(3548)		(1437)		(1023)		(1088)	
1 year	65	65	60	61	55	56	51	52	35	38	50	52	49	51	50	52	50	52
3 years	53	53	43	44	37	39	33	37	18	24	33	37	31	35	33	37	34	38
5 years	50	51	37	38	31	34	25	31	11	19	26	32	26	31	26	32	26	32
8 years	45	46	32	34	23	26	16	23	7	18	19	27	19	27	18	26	..	..
10 years	41	43	28	31	20	25	11	18	3	11	15	24	15	24	..	..	..	..

RELATIVE SURVIVAL (%) BY AGE AND PERIOD

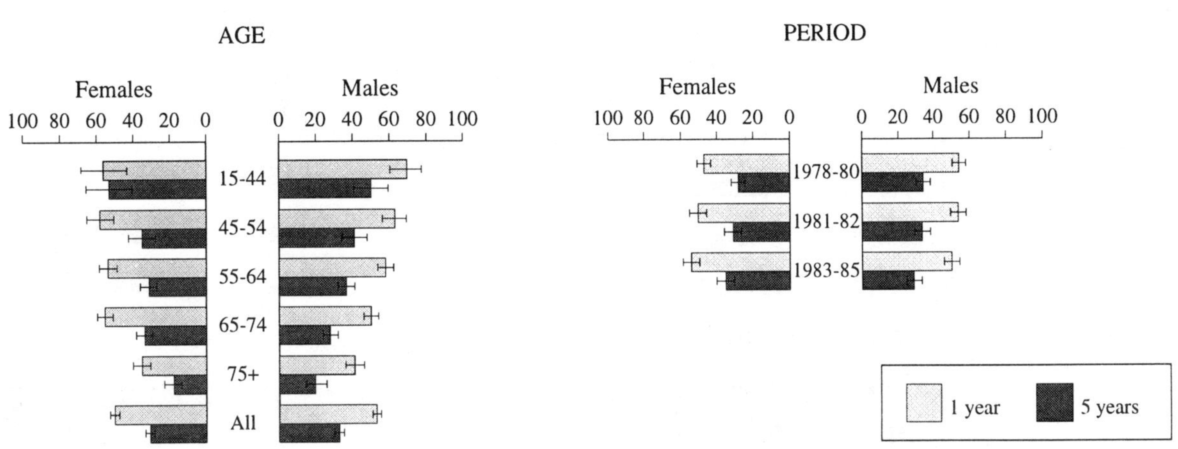

KIDNEY

DUTCH REGISTRIES

REGISTRY	NUMBER OF CASES			PERIOD OF DIAGNOSIS
	Males	Females	All	
Eindhoven	268	184	452	1978-1985
Mean age (years)	64.1	65.8	64.8	

RELATIVE SURVIVAL (%)

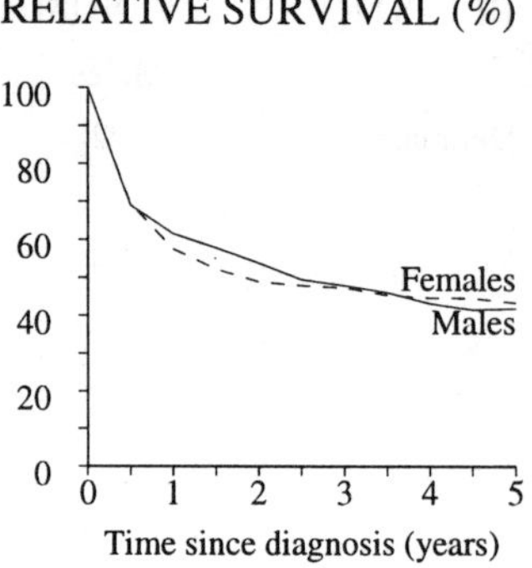

OBSERVED AND RELATIVE SURVIVAL (%) BY AGE AND PERIOD
(Number of cases in parentheses)

	AGE CLASS												PERIOD					
	15-44		45-54		55-64		65-74		75+		All		1978-80		1981-82		1983-85	
	obs	rel	obs	rel	obs	rel	obs	rel	obs	rel	obs	rel	obs	rel	obs	rel	obs	rel
Males	(14)		(46)		(75)		(75)		(58)		(268)		(98)		(79)		(91)	
1 year	64	64	70	70	72	73	51	53	43	49	59	62	59	62	47	49	69	72
3 years	50	50	54	55	58	61	34	40	19	28	42	48	40	45	33	37	52	60
5 years	42	42	49	51	47	52	23	30	13	27	33	42	30	37	29	36	43	55
8 years	..	..	41	44	29	35	13	21	4	13	20	31	18	27	..	..	..	..
10 years	..	..	41	46	29	37	9	17	..	..	19	32	17	28	..	..	..	..
Females	(7)		(28)		(48)		(51)		(50)		(184)		(62)		(46)		(76)	
1 year	71	72	86	86	56	57	53	54	40	43	56	58	58	60	54	56	55	57
3 years	57	57	64	64	46	47	43	46	28	36	43	47	44	48	39	43	46	50
5 years	57	58	54	55	43	45	38	43	19	29	37	43	35	42	37	43	34	39
8 years	57	58	54	55	43	47	33	43	14	30	35	46	34	45	..	..	..	..
10 years	..	..	32	34	..	..	33	47	..	..	21	30	20	29	..	..	..	..
Overall	(21)		(74)		(123)		(126)		(108)		(452)		(160)		(125)		(167)	
1 year	67	67	76	76	66	67	52	53	42	46	58	60	59	61	50	51	63	65
3 years	52	53	58	59	53	56	38	42	23	32	43	48	41	46	35	39	49	55
5 years	47	47	51	52	46	49	29	36	16	28	35	43	32	39	32	39	37	46
8 years	40	40	45	48	35	41	20	30	7	19	26	37	24	34	..	..	..	..
10 years	..	..	30	33	30	37	17	28	..	..	20	32	18	29	..	..	..	..

RELATIVE SURVIVAL (%) BY AGE AND PERIOD

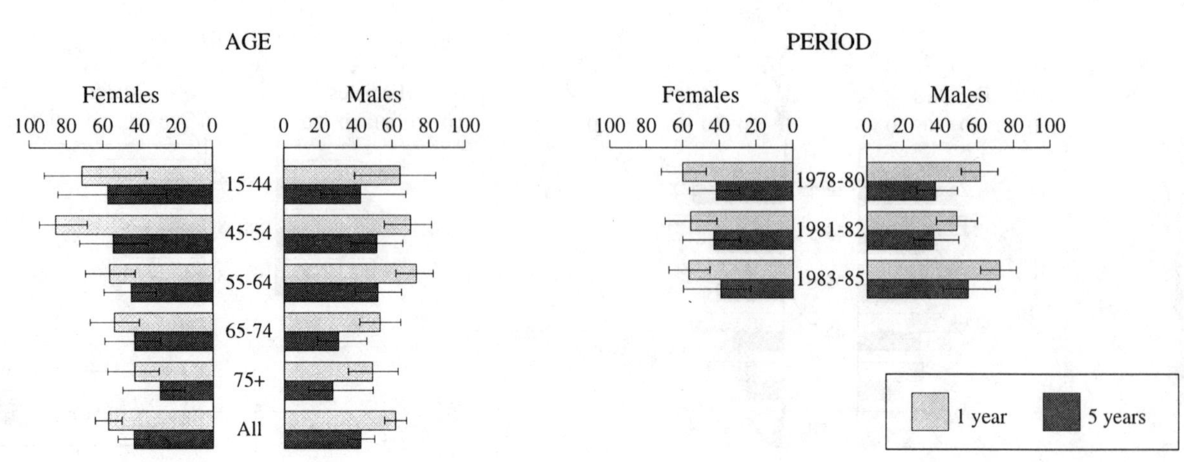

KIDNEY

ENGLISH REGISTRIES

REGISTRY	NUMBER OF CASES			PERIOD OF DIAGNOSIS
	Males	Females	All	
East Anglia	503	256	759	1979-1984
Mersey	513	298	811	1978-1984
South Thames	1563	964	2527	1978-1984
Wessex	218	138	356	1983-1984
West Midlands	963	492	1455	1979-1984
Yorkshire	822	596	1418	1978-1984
Mean age (years)	63.8	66.3	64.7	

RELATIVE SURVIVAL (%)

100
80
60
40
20
0
Males
Females
0 1 2 3 4 5
Time since diagnosis (years)

OBSERVED AND RELATIVE SURVIVAL (%) BY AGE AND PERIOD
(Number of cases in parentheses)

	AGE CLASS												PERIOD					
	15-44		45-54		55-64		65-74		75+		All		1978-80		1981-82		1983-85	
	obs	rel	obs	rel	obs	rel	obs	rel	obs	rel	obs	rel	obs	rel	obs	rel	obs	rel
Males	(266)		(693)		(1281)		(1531)		(811)		(4582)		(1648)		(1349)		(1585)	
1 year	70	70	61	62	56	57	48	50	37	41	51	54	50	53	51	53	53	55
3 years	54	55	49	50	41	44	33	38	21	30	37	42	35	40	38	44	37	42
5 years	51	51	42	43	35	39	26	34	14	26	30	37	28	36	32	39	30	37
8 years	43	44	35	38	27	33	18	29	8	25	23	33	22	33	23	34	22	32
10 years	40	41	31	34	23	30	15	29	5	22	19	31	19	31	19	31	..	..
Females	(168)		(273)		(674)		(850)		(779)		(2744)		(992)		(760)		(992)	
1 year	68	68	59	59	56	57	46	47	33	36	47	49	44	46	49	51	49	51
3 years	56	56	45	46	41	43	31	34	19	25	33	37	32	36	32	36	35	39
5 years	51	52	40	41	36	38	26	30	13	21	28	34	26	31	27	33	30	36
8 years	47	47	32	33	31	35	19	26	10	23	23	31	20	28	22	30	27	36
10 years	43	44	31	33	30	35	17	25	8	25	21	31	18	28	21	32	..	..
Overall	(434)		(966)		(1955)		(2381)		(1590)		(7326)		(2640)		(2109)		(2577)	
1 year	69	69	61	61	56	57	47	49	35	39	50	52	48	50	50	52	51	53
3 years	55	55	48	49	41	43	32	37	20	27	35	40	34	38	36	41	36	41
5 years	51	51	41	43	35	39	26	33	13	23	29	36	28	34	30	37	30	37
8 years	44	45	34	37	29	34	19	28	9	24	23	32	22	31	23	32	24	34
10 years	41	42	31	34	25	32	16	28	6	23	20	31	19	30	20	31	..	..

RELATIVE SURVIVAL (%) BY AGE AND PERIOD

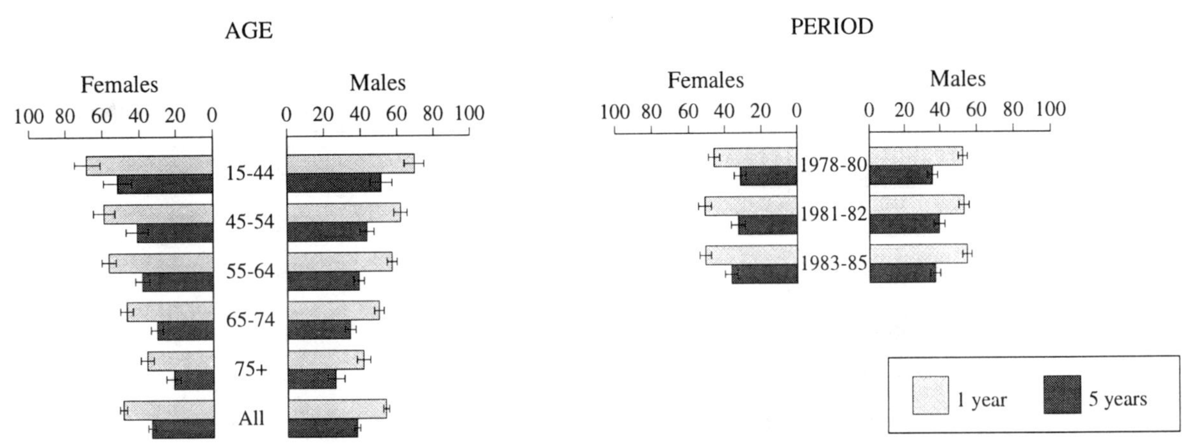

KIDNEY

ESTONIA

REGISTRY	NUMBER OF CASES			PERIOD OF DIAGNOSIS
	Males	Females	All	
Estonia	317	276	593	1978-1984
Mean age (years)	59.1	62.8	60.8	

RELATIVE SURVIVAL (%)

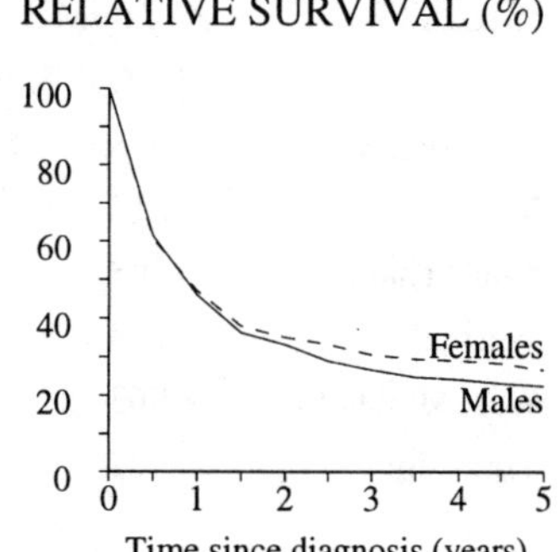

OBSERVED AND RELATIVE SURVIVAL (%) BY AGE AND PERIOD
(Number of cases in parentheses)

	AGE CLASS												PERIOD					
	15-44		45-54		55-64		65-74		75+		All		1978-80		1981-82		1983-85	
	obs	rel	obs	rel	obs	rel	obs	rel	obs	rel	obs	rel	obs	rel	obs	rel	obs	rel
Males	(30)		(79)		(97)		(87)		(24)		(317)		(145)		(89)		(83)	
1 year	50	50	57	58	40	41	41	44	25	28	44	46	43	44	46	48	46	47
3 years	33	34	34	36	19	20	20	23	17	24	24	27	21	24	26	29	27	29
5 years	23	24	26	29	15	18	17	24	4	8	19	23	15	18	21	26	22	26
8 years	23	25	20	23	13	17	11	20	4	14	15	21	10	14	20	28	..	..
10 years	23	26	17	20	10	15	11	24	4	22	13	20	9	14	..	..	..	..
Females	(18)		(45)		(80)		(94)		(39)		(276)		(108)		(82)		(86)	
1 year	56	56	60	60	43	43	46	47	33	36	46	47	49	50	46	48	42	43
3 years	39	39	40	41	30	31	24	27	15	20	28	31	32	35	28	31	23	25
5 years	33	34	35	36	24	25	21	26	8	13	23	27	27	31	23	27	19	21
8 years	28	28	23	25	22	25	21	31	3	7	20	26	23	30	18	24	..	..
10 years	28	29	23	25	19	23	19	32	3	10	18	26	21	30	..	..	..	..
Overall	(48)		(124)		(177)		(181)		(63)		(593)		(253)		(171)		(169)	
1 year	52	52	58	59	41	42	44	45	30	33	45	47	45	47	46	48	44	45
3 years	35	36	36	38	24	25	22	25	16	22	26	29	26	29	27	30	25	27
5 years	27	28	30	31	19	21	19	25	6	11	21	25	20	24	22	26	20	24
8 years	25	26	21	24	17	21	16	26	3	9	17	23	15	21	19	26	..	..
10 years	25	27	19	22	14	19	15	29	3	13	15	23	14	21	..	..	..	..

RELATIVE SURVIVAL (%) BY AGE AND PERIOD

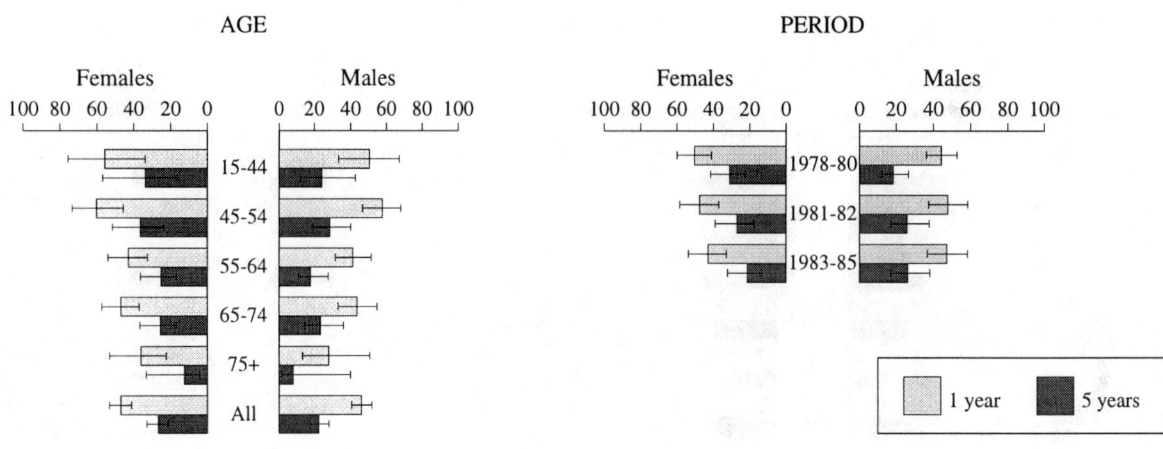

KIDNEY

FINLAND

REGISTRY	NUMBER OF CASES			PERIOD OF DIAGNOSIS
	Males	Females	All	
Finland	1406	1180	2586	1978-1984
Mean age (years)	62.5	65.2	63.7	

RELATIVE SURVIVAL (%)

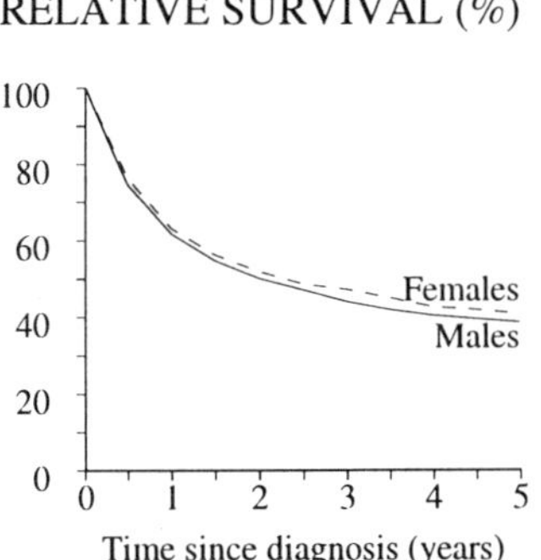

OBSERVED AND RELATIVE SURVIVAL (%) BY AGE AND PERIOD
(Number of cases in parentheses)

	AGE CLASS												PERIOD					
	15-44		45-54		55-64		65-74		75+		All		1978-80		1981-82		1983-85	
	obs	rel	obs	rel	obs	rel	obs	rel	obs	rel	obs	rel	obs	rel	obs	rel	obs	rel
Males	(90)		(263)		(417)		(423)		(213)		(1406)		(537)		(423)		(446)	
1 year	71	71	73	74	61	62	56	58	41	46	59	62	59	62	59	61	60	62
3 years	48	48	55	57	41	45	33	39	22	32	39	44	39	45	39	44	39	44
5 years	46	46	49	51	34	38	24	31	14	27	31	39	30	37	31	39	33	40
8 years	38	39	36	39	27	34	16	26	6	20	23	33	22	32	23	32	23	33
10 years	35	36	33	38	23	30	13	25	2	10	19	30	18	28	21	32	..	..
Females	(66)		(133)		(322)		(389)		(270)		(1180)		(444)		(339)		(397)	
1 year	80	80	78	78	64	65	57	59	51	55	61	63	61	62	65	67	58	60
3 years	71	71	62	62	48	49	40	43	28	36	43	47	43	46	47	51	41	46
5 years	61	61	52	53	41	43	30	35	20	32	35	41	35	40	37	43	34	40
8 years	59	60	42	44	36	39	24	31	13	29	28	37	28	36	30	40	28	37
10 years	59	60	42	44	32	37	20	29	8	25	25	36	24	33	30	42	..	..
Overall	(156)		(396)		(739)		(812)		(483)		(2586)		(981)		(762)		(843)	
1 year	75	75	75	75	62	63	56	59	47	51	60	62	60	62	62	64	59	61
3 years	58	58	57	59	44	46	36	41	25	34	41	46	41	45	42	47	40	45
5 years	52	53	50	52	37	40	27	33	18	30	33	40	32	38	34	41	33	40
8 years	47	48	38	41	31	36	20	29	10	26	25	35	25	34	26	36	25	35
10 years	45	47	36	40	27	33	16	27	6	20	22	33	21	31	25	37	..	..

RELATIVE SURVIVAL (%) BY AGE AND PERIOD

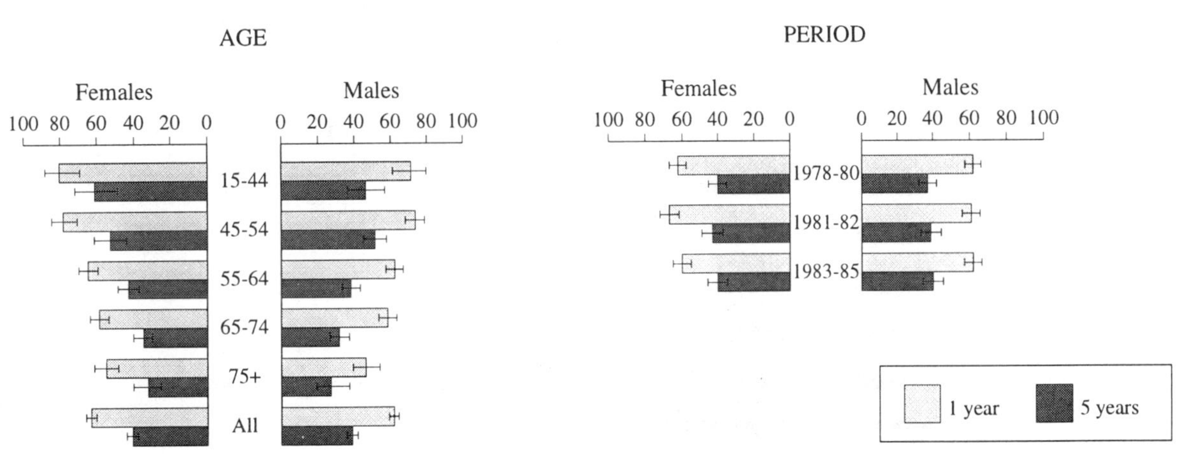

KIDNEY

FRENCH REGISTRIES

REGISTRY	NUMBER OF CASES			PERIOD OF DIAGNOSIS
	Males	Females	All	
Amiens	59	26	85	1983-1984
Doubs	134	80	214	1978-1985
Mean age (years)	63.1	65.5	63.9	

RELATIVE SURVIVAL (%)

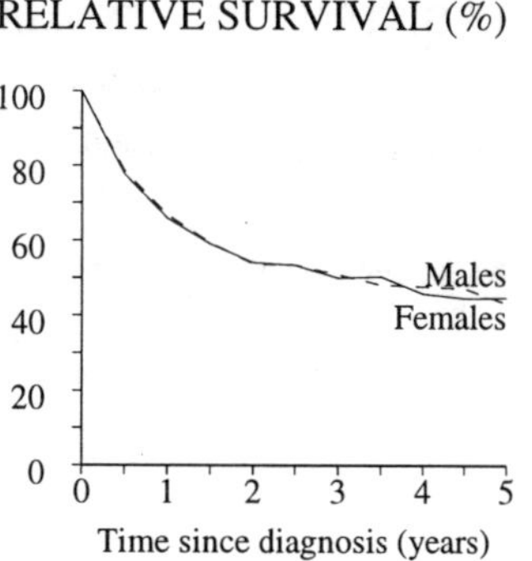

OBSERVED AND RELATIVE SURVIVAL (%) BY AGE AND PERIOD
(Number of cases in parentheses)

	AGE CLASS												PERIOD					
	15-44		45-54		55-64		65-74		75+		All		1978-80		1981-82		1983-85	
	obs	rel	obs	rel	obs	rel	obs	rel	obs	rel	obs	rel	obs	rel	obs	rel	obs	rel
Males	(16)		(38)		(40)		(65)		(34)		(193)		(53)		(33)		(107)	
1 year	75	75	75	75	64	65	61	63	50	56	63	66	69	71	73	75	58	60
3 years	56	57	57	59	50	53	41	46	25	36	44	50	50	55	45	50	41	47
5 years	50	51	57	60	47	52	26	33	13	24	37	45	38	45	39	47	35	44
8 years	50	51	40	43	40	47	22	34	..	..	30	41	31	40	36	49	..	..
10 years	50	52	..	..	0	0	17	29	..	..	22	33	24	35	..	..	..	..
Females	(10)		(14)		(20)		(35)		(27)		(106)		(22)		(15)		(69)	
1 year	78	78	93	93	69	69	61	62	43	50	64	67	51	53	73	76	65	69
3 years	78	78	57	58	46	47	43	46	31	47	45	51	36	39	53	60	46	53
5 years	52	52	57	58	37	38	33	37	22	43	36	43	31	36	40	48	37	45
8 years	37	37	29	29	37	39	25	30	..	..	24	32	18	24	25	33	..	..
10 years	..	..	..	..	37	40	..	..	..	..	24	35	18	26	..	..	..	..
Overall	(26)		(52)		(60)		(100)		(61)		(299)		(75)		(48)		(176)	
1 year	76	76	80	80	65	66	61	63	47	54	63	66	64	65	73	76	61	64
3 years	63	64	57	59	49	51	41	46	28	41	45	50	46	51	48	53	43	49
5 years	50	51	57	60	45	48	29	35	17	33	36	44	36	42	40	47	36	45
8 years	44	45	38	40	39	44	22	31	..	..	28	38	27	35	32	44	..	..
10 years	44	45	..	..	19	23	18	28	..	..	22	33	23	32	..	..	..	..

RELATIVE SURVIVAL (%) BY AGE AND PERIOD

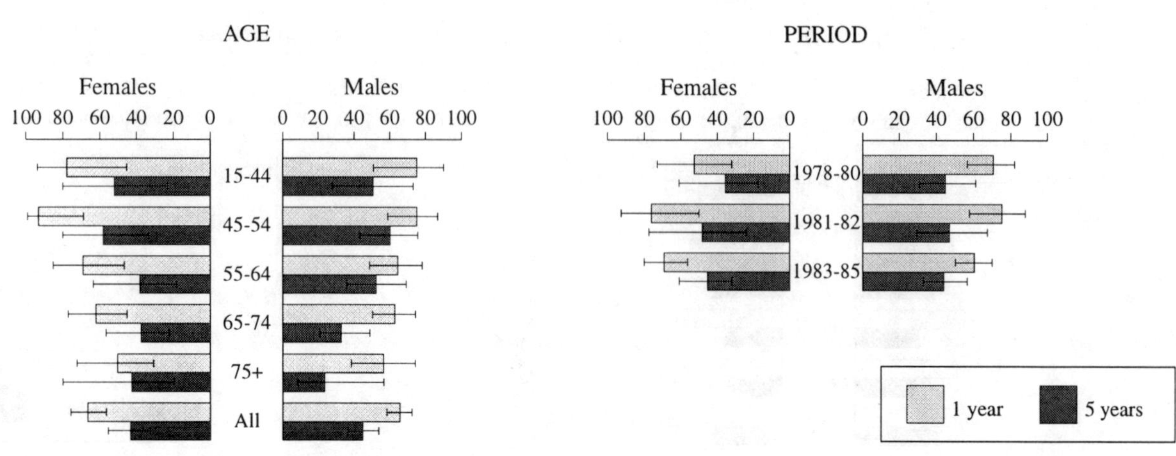

KIDNEY

GERMAN REGISTRIES

REGISTRY	NUMBER OF CASES			PERIOD OF DIAGNOSIS
	Males	Females	All	
Saarland	416	270	686	1978-1984
Mean age (years)	60.8	63.7	61.9	

RELATIVE SURVIVAL (%)

OBSERVED AND RELATIVE SURVIVAL (%) BY AGE AND PERIOD
(Number of cases in parentheses)

	AGE CLASS												PERIOD					
	15-44		45-54		55-64		65-74		75+		All		1978-80		1981-82		1983-85	
	obs	rel	obs	rel	obs	rel	obs	rel	obs	rel	obs	rel	obs	rel	obs	rel	obs	rel
Males	(39)		(79)		(134)		(115)		(49)		(416)		(160)		(129)		(127)	
1 year	77	77	66	66	73	75	56	59	57	64	65	68	64	66	66	68	67	69
3 years	62	62	54	56	57	61	43	52	39	56	51	57	49	55	53	60	51	57
5 years	59	60	49	52	47	53	37	51	29	55	44	53	44	53	44	53	43	52
8 years	59	61	43	47	42	51	25	43	13	40	35	49	35	48	39	53	..	..
10 years	59	62	39	43	38	51	22	44	13	58	33	49	33	49	..	..	..	..
Females	(21)		(34)		(76)		(91)		(48)		(270)		(91)		(83)		(96)	
1 year	76	76	85	86	76	77	66	68	63	67	71	73	64	65	76	78	75	77
3 years	62	62	74	74	66	68	47	52	42	52	56	60	46	50	63	68	59	64
5 years	57	58	74	75	53	55	38	45	31	47	47	54	40	45	55	64	47	53
8 years	52	53	61	64	43	48	25	34	23	46	36	46	30	37	45	58	..	..
10 years	52	54	54	57	43	49	25	37	23	59	35	48	30	40	..	..	..	..
Overall	(60)		(113)		(210)		(206)		(97)		(686)		(251)		(212)		(223)	
1 year	77	77	72	72	74	75	60	63	60	66	68	70	64	66	70	72	70	73
3 years	62	62	60	61	60	64	45	52	40	54	53	59	48	53	57	63	55	60
5 years	58	59	57	59	49	54	38	48	30	50	45	53	42	50	49	58	45	53
8 years	57	58	48	52	42	50	25	38	18	43	36	48	33	44	42	55	..	..
10 years	57	59	43	47	40	50	23	40	18	58	34	48	31	46	..	..	..	..

RELATIVE SURVIVAL (%) BY AGE AND PERIOD

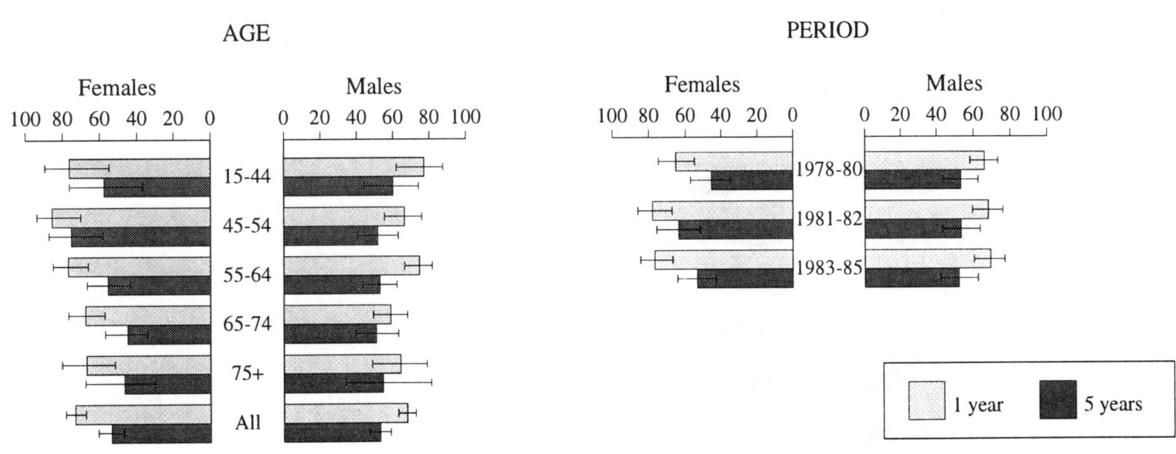

KIDNEY

ITALIAN REGISTRIES

REGISTRY	NUMBER OF CASES			PERIOD OF DIAGNOSIS
	Males	Females	All	
Latina	24	11	35	1983-1984
Ragusa	15	8	23	1981-1984
Varese	277	138	415	1978-1984
Mean age (years)	61.9	65.3	63.0	

RELATIVE SURVIVAL (%)

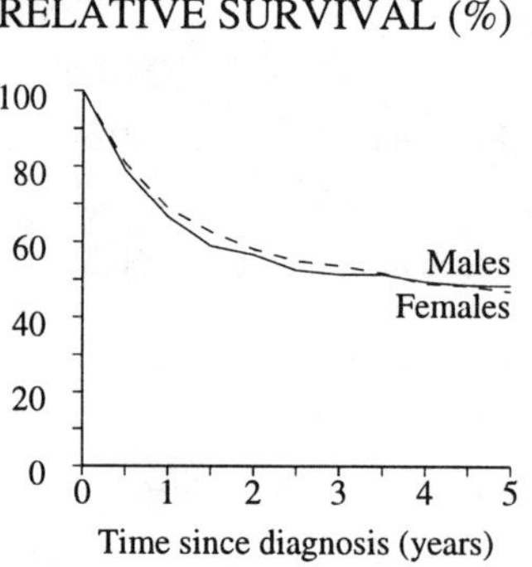

OBSERVED AND RELATIVE SURVIVAL (%) BY AGE AND PERIOD
(Number of cases in parentheses)

	AGE CLASS												PERIOD					
	15-44		45-54		55-64		65-74		75+		All		1978-80		1981-82		1983-85	
	obs	rel	obs	rel	obs	rel	obs	rel	obs	rel	obs	rel	obs	rel	obs	rel	obs	rel
Males	(24)		(56)		(97)		(87)		(52)		(316)		(100)		(87)		(129)	
1 year	88	88	70	70	70	71	57	60	48	53	64	67	66	68	62	64	64	67
3 years	67	67	55	57	48	52	43	49	27	37	46	51	47	52	41	46	48	54
5 years	67	67	46	49	44	50	33	44	23	41	40	48	40	48	38	46	41	51
8 years	67	68	38	41	36	44	20	32	7	19	30	42	29	39	29	40	35	49
10 years	67	69	34	39	32	42	13	25	0	0	25	37	24	35	24	37	..	..
Females	(11)		(18)		(37)		(50)		(41)		(157)		(51)		(47)		(59)	
1 year	82	82	78	78	78	79	62	63	54	58	67	69	71	73	77	79	56	57
3 years	55	55	78	79	54	55	50	54	29	38	49	54	51	55	53	59	44	48
5 years	45	46	67	68	51	54	38	43	20	30	40	47	41	47	43	51	37	43
8 years	36	37	55	57	40	43	26	33	7	16	28	37	29	37	30	41	30	38
10 years	36	37	55	57	33	37	26	36	..	..	27	38	29	40	24	37	..	..
Overall	(35)		(74)		(134)		(137)		(93)		(473)		(151)		(134)		(188)	
1 year	86	86	72	72	72	74	59	61	51	55	65	67	68	70	67	70	62	64
3 years	63	63	61	62	50	53	45	51	28	37	47	52	48	53	46	51	47	52
5 years	60	61	51	53	46	51	35	44	22	36	40	48	40	48	40	48	40	48
8 years	57	58	42	45	37	44	22	33	8	20	30	40	29	38	29	40	34	45
10 years	57	59	40	44	33	41	18	30	..	..	26	38	26	37	25	37	..	..

RELATIVE SURVIVAL (%) BY AGE AND PERIOD

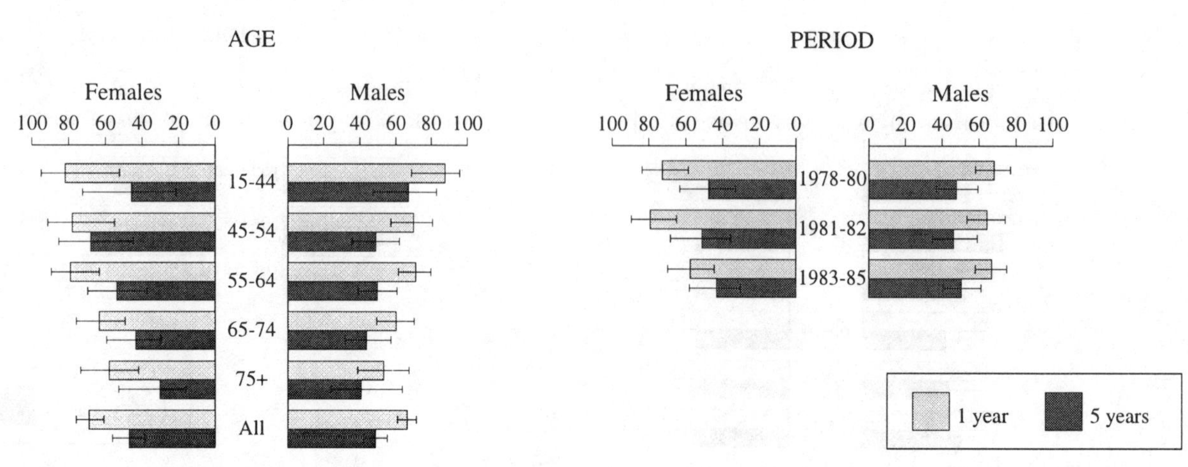

KIDNEY

POLISH REGISTRIES

REGISTRY	NUMBER OF CASES Males	Females	All	PERIOD OF DIAGNOSIS
Cracow	162	111	273	1978-1984
Mean age (years)	59.3	61.5	60.2	

RELATIVE SURVIVAL (%)

OBSERVED AND RELATIVE SURVIVAL (%) BY AGE AND PERIOD
(Number of cases in parentheses)

	AGE CLASS 15-44 obs	rel	45-54 obs	rel	55-64 obs	rel	65-74 obs	rel	75+ obs	rel	All obs	rel	PERIOD 1978-80 obs	rel	1981-82 obs	rel	1983-85 obs	rel
Males	(13)		(41)		(58)		(33)		(17)		(162)		(71)		(33)		(58)	
1 year	60	60	47	47	40	41	30	32	32	36	40	42	44	45	44	46	33	34
3 years	51	52	37	38	22	24	15	18	16	23	26	29	28	31	25	28	24	26
5 years	34	35	34	36	21	24	12	17	0	0	21	26	20	25	25	31	20	24
8 years	..	..	23	25	19	24	6	11	0	0	15	21	11	15	25	35	..	..
10 years	..	..	23	27	19	26	6	13	0	0	15	23	11	17	25	39	..	..
Females	(7)		(26)		(26)		(38)		(14)		(111)		(52)		(28)		(31)	
1 year	36	36	69	70	42	43	44	45	43	46	49	50	49	50	43	44	54	55
3 years	18	18	61	62	35	36	33	36	29	36	39	42	44	46	32	34	37	40
5 years	18	18	53	55	27	29	25	29	14	22	30	34	36	40	18	20	33	39
8 years	18	18	43	46	27	30	25	35	14	32	28	35	34	42	14	18	33	45
10 years	18	18	35	37	27	31	25	40	0	0	24	33	28	38	..	..	..	..
Overall	(20)		(67)		(84)		(71)		(31)		(273)		(123)		(61)		(89)	
1 year	52	52	56	56	40	41	37	39	37	41	44	45	46	48	44	45	40	42
3 years	40	41	47	48	26	28	24	28	22	30	31	34	34	38	29	31	28	31
5 years	29	29	42	44	23	25	19	24	7	13	25	29	27	32	22	26	25	29
8 years	16	17	31	34	21	25	16	25	7	19	20	27	20	27	20	27	22	30
10 years	16	17	28	31	21	27	16	29	0	0	19	27	18	26	20	29	..	..

RELATIVE SURVIVAL (%) BY AGE AND PERIOD

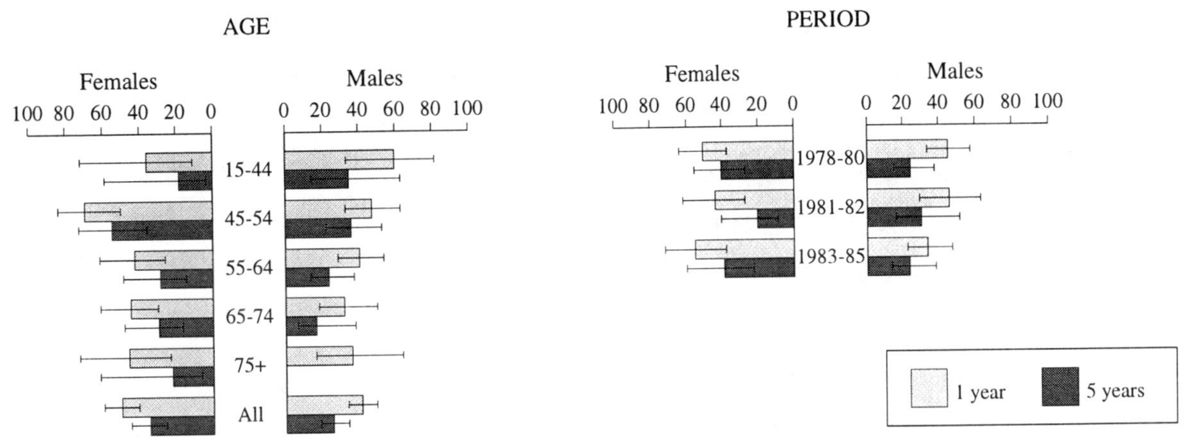

KIDNEY

SCOTLAND

REGISTRY	NUMBER OF CASES			PERIOD OF DIAGNOSIS
	Males	Females	All	
Scotland	995	673	1668	1978-1982
Mean age (years)	64.0	66.8	65.1	

RELATIVE SURVIVAL (%)

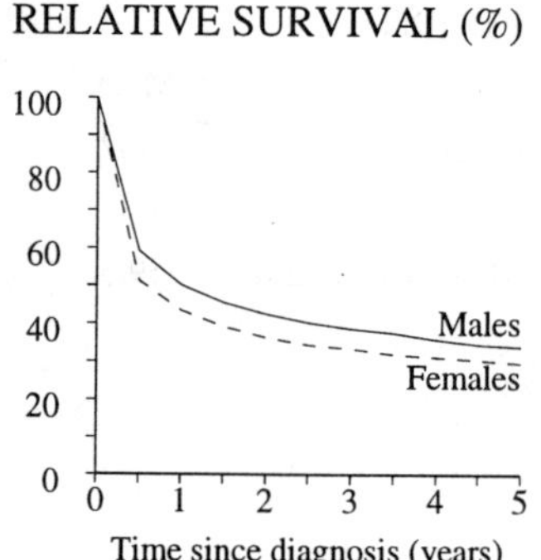

OBSERVED AND RELATIVE SURVIVAL (%) BY AGE AND PERIOD
(Number of cases in parentheses)

	AGE CLASS												PERIOD					
	15-44		45-54		55-64		65-74		75+		All		1978-80		1981-82		1983-85	
	obs	rel	obs	rel	obs	rel	obs	rel	obs	rel	obs	rel	obs	rel	obs	rel	obs	rel
Males	(63)		(143)		(264)		(342)		(183)		(995)		(565)		(430)		(0)	
1 year	70	70	67	68	53	54	42	45	28	32	48	50	48	50	48	50	..	..
3 years	60	61	51	53	37	40	28	34	14	21	33	39	32	38	35	40	..	..
5 years	57	58	43	46	28	32	20	27	11	23	26	34	25	33	28	36	..	..
8 years	55	57	38	42	19	24	13	24	2	7	19	29	17	27	..	..	..	..
10 years	42	43	32	37	19	26	12	25	..	..	16	29	15	27	..	..	..	..
Females	(31)		(66)		(173)		(214)		(189)		(673)		(401)		(272)		(0)	
1 year	68	68	50	50	49	49	43	45	26	29	42	43	42	44	41	43	..	..
3 years	65	65	38	39	35	36	29	32	16	22	30	33	31	35	27	31	..	..
5 years	58	59	35	36	32	35	21	26	10	17	24	30	26	32	22	27	..	..
8 years	58	59	32	34	25	29	16	22	6	15	19	27	21	30	..	..	..	..
10 years	58	59	32	35	24	28	16	25	6	20	19	30	21	32	..	..	..	..
Overall	(94)		(209)		(437)		(556)		(372)		(1668)		(966)		(702)		(0)	
1 year	69	69	62	62	51	52	43	45	27	30	45	47	45	48	45	47	..	..
3 years	62	62	47	48	36	38	29	33	15	22	32	37	32	37	32	36	..	..
5 years	57	58	41	43	30	33	20	26	11	20	25	32	25	32	25	32	..	..
8 years	56	58	36	39	22	26	15	23	4	11	19	28	19	28	..	..	..	..
10 years	49	50	33	37	21	27	13	25	4	15	18	29	17	29	..	..	..	..

RELATIVE SURVIVAL (%) BY AGE AND PERIOD

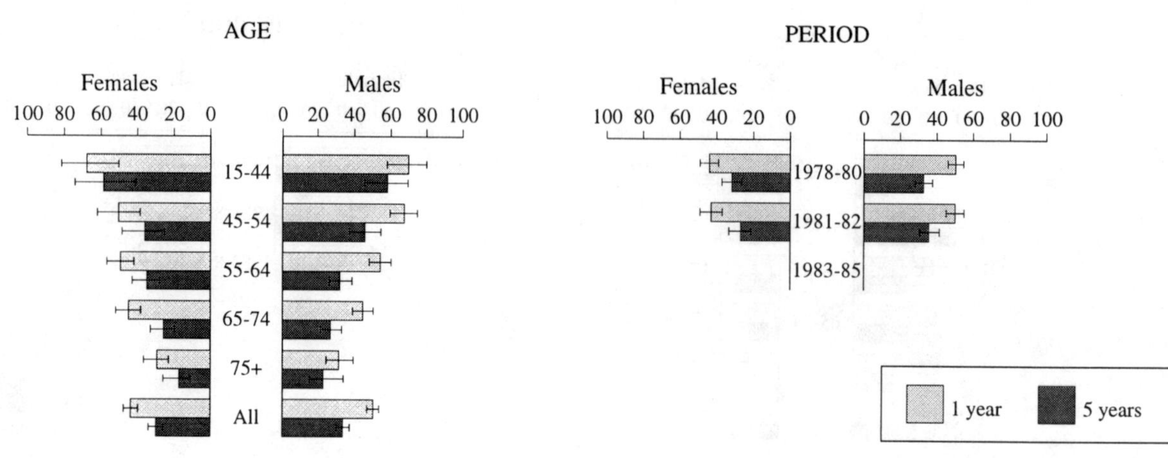

KIDNEY

SPANISH REGISTRIES

REGISTRY	NUMBER OF CASES Males	Females	All	PERIOD OF DIAGNOSIS
Tarragona	7	3	10	1985-1985
Mean age (years)	65.3	70.3	66.8	

RELATIVE SURVIVAL (%)

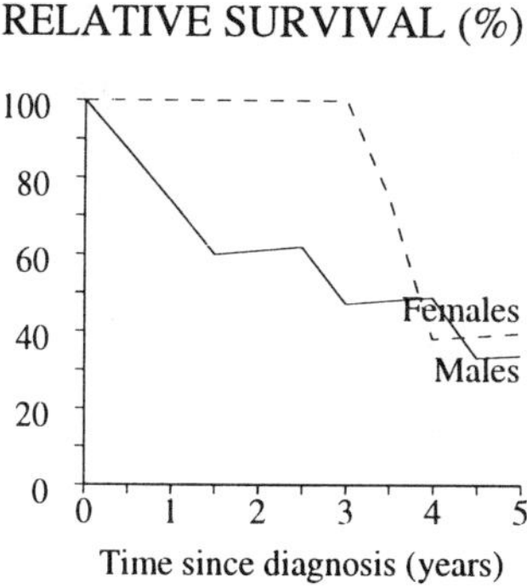

OBSERVED AND RELATIVE SURVIVAL (%) BY AGE AND PERIOD
(Number of cases in parentheses)

	AGE CLASS 15-44 obs	rel	45-54 obs	rel	55-64 obs	rel	65-74 obs	rel	75+ obs	rel	All obs	rel	PERIOD 1978-80 obs	rel	1981-82 obs	rel	1983-85 obs	rel
Males	(1)		(0)		(1)		(4)		(1)		(7)		(0)		(0)		(7)	
1 year	100	100	..	..	100	100	75	77	0	0	71	74	..	..	..	..	71	74
3 years	0	0	..	..	0	0	75	82	0	0	43	47	..	..	..	..	43	47
5 years	0	0	..	..	0	0	50	59	0	0	29	34	..	..	..	..	29	34
8 years	0	0	..	..	0	0	..	..	0	0	..	..	..	..	..	..	..	..
10 years	0	0	..	..	0	0	..	..	0	0	..	..	..	..	..	..	..	..
Females	(0)		(0)		(1)		(1)		(1)		(3)		(0)		(0)		(3)	
1 year	..	..	..	..	100	100	100	100	100	100	100	100	..	..	..	..	100	100
3 years	..	..	..	..	100	100	100	100	100	100	100	100	..	..	..	..	100	100
5 years	..	..	..	..	0	0	100	100	0	0	33	40	..	..	..	..	33	40
8 years	..	..	..	..	0	0	..	..	0	0	..	..	..	..	..	..	..	..
10 years	..	..	..	..	0	0	..	..	0	0	..	..	..	..	..	..	..	..
Overall	(1)		(0)		(2)		(5)		(2)		(10)		(0)		(0)		(10)	
1 year	100	100	..	..	100	100	80	82	50	54	80	83	..	..	..	..	80	83
3 years	0	0	..	..	50	52	80	87	50	65	60	66	..	..	..	..	60	66
5 years	0	0	..	..	0	0	60	70	0	0	30	36	..	..	..	..	30	36
8 years	0	0	..	..	0	0	..	..	0	0	..	..	..	..	..	..	..	..
10 years	0	0	..	..	0	0	..	..	0	0	..	..	..	..	..	..	..	..

RELATIVE SURVIVAL (%) BY AGE AND PERIOD

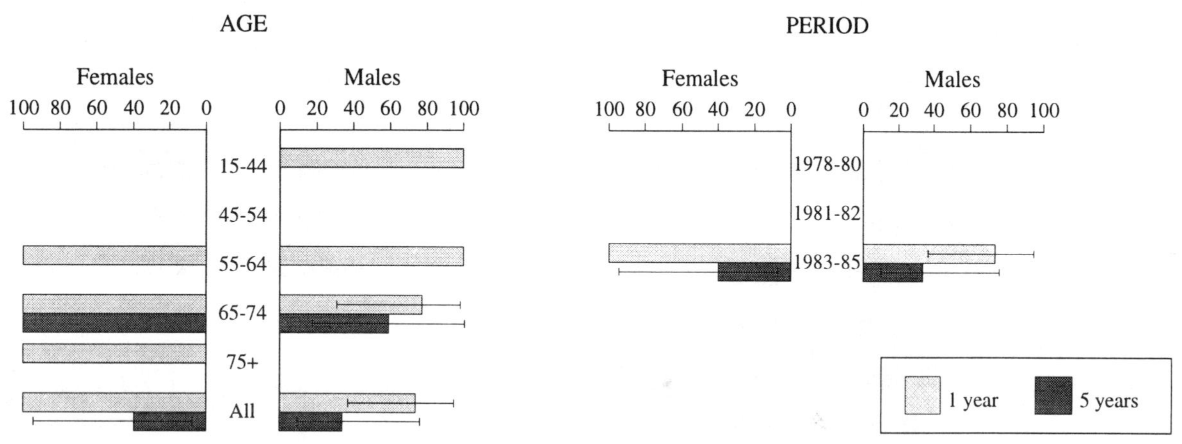

KIDNEY

SWISS REGISTRIES

REGISTRY	NUMBER OF CASES			PERIOD OF DIAGNOSIS
	Males	Females	All	
Basel	77	70	147	1981-1984
Geneva	109	76	185	1978-1984
Mean age (years)	66.3	67.6	66.9	

RELATIVE SURVIVAL (%)

100 80 60 40 20 0
Males
Females
0 1 2 3 4 5
Time since diagnosis (years)

OBSERVED AND RELATIVE SURVIVAL (%) BY AGE AND PERIOD
(Number of cases in parentheses)

	AGE CLASS												PERIOD					
	15-44		45-54		55-64		65-74		75+		All		1978-80		1981-82		1983-85	
	obs	rel	obs	rel	obs	rel	obs	rel	obs	rel	obs	rel	obs	rel	obs	rel	obs	rel
Males	(8)		(28)		(42)		(51)		(57)		(186)		(35)		(65)		(86)	
1 year	88	88	89	90	71	72	55	57	46	50	62	65	63	66	63	66	62	64
3 years	63	63	71	73	50	52	41	46	25	34	44	50	51	60	35	40	47	53
5 years	63	63	61	63	45	49	35	44	19	34	38	47	46	59	31	38	39	50
8 years	63	64	49	52	31	36	30	45	19	52	31	46	..	..	28	41	..	..
10 years	..	..	..	..	..	..	..	..	..	..	..	..	..	..	..	..	..	..
Females	(6)		(16)		(32)		(51)		(41)		(146)		(31)		(54)		(61)	
1 year	50	50	69	69	66	66	59	60	54	58	60	61	68	69	44	46	69	71
3 years	33	33	56	57	56	57	33	35	37	47	42	46	52	56	30	33	48	52
5 years	17	17	56	57	53	55	25	28	32	49	36	42	48	55	24	29	41	47
8 years	..	..	..	..	53	57	25	31	26	57	34	46	..	..	24	33	..	..
10 years	..	..	..	..	..	..	..	..	..	..	..	..	..	..	..	..	..	..
Overall	(14)		(44)		(74)		(102)		(98)		(332)		(66)		(119)		(147)	
1 year	71	72	82	82	69	70	57	58	49	54	61	63	65	68	55	57	65	67
3 years	50	50	66	67	53	55	37	41	30	39	43	48	52	58	33	37	47	53
5 years	42	42	59	61	49	52	30	36	24	41	37	45	47	57	28	34	40	49
8 years	42	42	50	53	40	45	28	38	22	54	32	46	..	..	26	37	..	..
10 years	..	..	..	..	..	..	..	..	..	..	..	..	..	..	..	..	..	..

RELATIVE SURVIVAL (%) BY AGE AND PERIOD

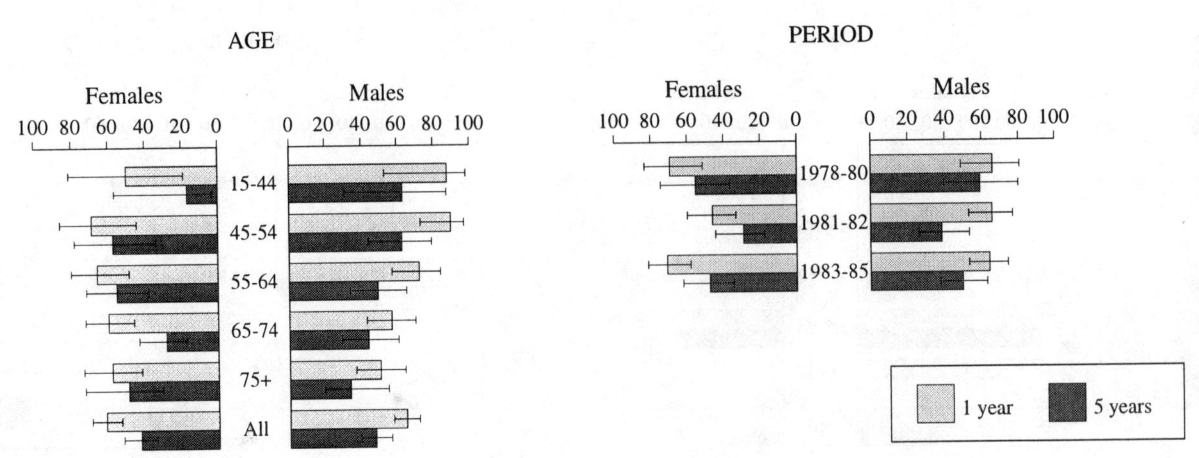

KIDNEY

EUROPEAN REGISTRIES
Weighted analysis

REGISTRY	WEIGHTS (Yearly expected cases in the country) Males	Females	All
DENMARK	304	249	553
DUTCH REGISTRIES	778	518	1296
ENGLISH REGISTRIES	2493	1499	3992
ESTONIA	46	41	87
FINLAND	205	171	376
FRENCH REGISTRIES	2935	1810	4745
GERMAN REGISTRIES	5099	3509	8608
ITALIAN REGISTRIES	2681	1392	4073
POLISH REGISTRIES	1003	708	1711
SCOTLAND	202	139	341
SPANISH REGISTRIES	849	505	1354
SWISS REGISTRIES	358	274	632

RELATIVE SURVIVAL (%)
(Age-standardized)

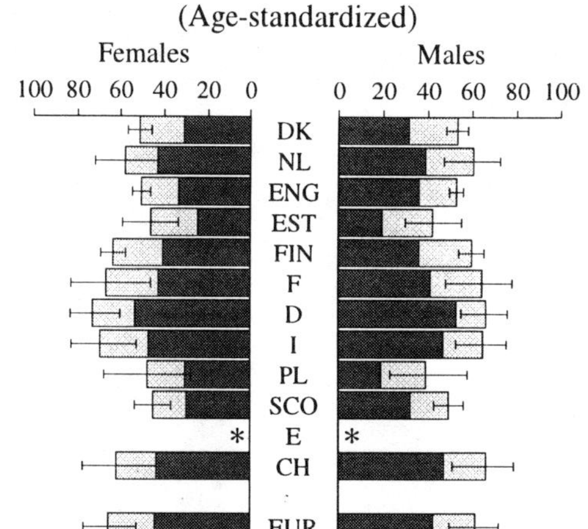

* Not enough cases for reliable estimation

OBSERVED AND RELATIVE SURVIVAL (%) BY AGE AND PERIOD

	AGE CLASS 15-44 obs	rel	45-54 obs	rel	55-64 obs	rel	65-74 obs	rel	75+ obs	rel	All obs	rel	PERIOD 1978-80 obs	rel	1981-82 obs	rel	1983-85 obs	rel
Males																		
1 year	77	77	67	67	67	68	55	57	45	51	61	63	61	63	61	64	60	63
3 years	56	56	53	55	46	49	40	46	26	38	44	49	44	50	44	49	44	50
5 years	52	53	48	50	40	45	31	40	18	34	36	45	37	45	37	45	37	45
8 years	52	53	39	42	33	41	20	33	9	26	29	40	28	39	32	45	29	41
10 years	51	53	35	39	24	32	16	31	6	28	25	38	24	37	23	35	..	..
Females																		
1 year	72	72	79	79	69	69	60	62	52	56	64	66	58	59	66	68	65	67
3 years	59	59	64	65	54	56	45	48	35	44	49	53	42	46	50	54	50	55
5 years	50	50	60	61	42	44	37	42	22	34	38	45	35	41	41	48	39	45
8 years	44	45	47	49	36	40	24	32	15	31	30	38	26	34	32	42	29	39
10 years	44	45	45	48	34	39	24	35	14	37	28	39	25	34	23	35	..	..
Overall																		
1 year	75	75	72	72	68	69	57	59	48	53	62	64	60	62	63	65	62	64
3 years	57	57	57	58	50	52	42	47	30	40	46	51	43	48	46	51	47	52
5 years	51	52	53	55	41	44	33	41	19	34	37	45	36	43	39	47	37	45
8 years	49	50	42	45	34	40	22	33	11	28	29	40	27	37	32	43	29	40
10 years	48	50	39	42	28	34	19	33	9	32	26	38	25	36	23	35	..	..

RELATIVE SURVIVAL (%) BY AGE AND PERIOD

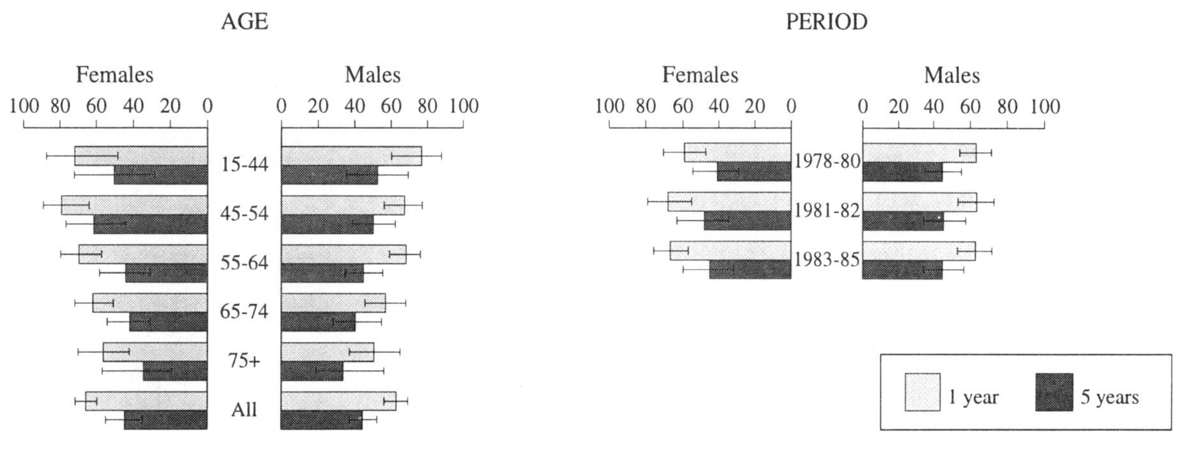

BRAIN

DENMARK

REGISTRY	NUMBER OF CASES			PERIOD OF DIAGNOSIS
	Males	Females	All	
Denmark	1173	910	2083	1978-1984
Mean age (years)	55.4	57.0	56.1	

RELATIVE SURVIVAL (%)

OBSERVED AND RELATIVE SURVIVAL (%) BY AGE AND PERIOD
(Number of cases in parentheses)

	AGE CLASS												PERIOD					
	15-44		45-54		55-64		65-74		75+		All		1978-80		1981-82		1983-85	
	obs	rel	obs	rel	obs	rel	obs	rel	obs	rel	obs	rel	obs	rel	obs	rel	obs	rel
Males	(269)		(207)		(334)		(273)		(90)		(1173)		(498)		(338)		(337)	
1 year	67	67	36	36	18	18	5	5	3	4	28	29	29	30	29	29	26	27
3 years	45	46	14	15	5	6	1	1	1	1	15	16	16	17	14	15	14	15
5 years	33	33	11	11	3	4	1	1	1	2	11	12	11	12	11	12	10	11
8 years	25	25	7	8	2	2	0	0	0	0	7	9	8	10	4	5	..	..
10 years	22	23	6	6	..	..	0	0	0	0	7	9	7	10	..	..	..	..
Females	(192)		(143)		(257)		(227)		(91)		(910)		(412)		(231)		(267)	
1 year	63	63	30	30	18	18	8	8	3	4	25	26	25	25	24	25	27	28
3 years	42	42	13	13	6	6	3	3	1	1	13	14	11	11	13	13	17	18
5 years	32	33	9	9	3	4	1	1	1	2	10	11	7	8	9	9	14	16
8 years	27	28	7	8	1	1	1	1	0	0	7	9	6	7	7	8	..	..
10 years	26	26	..	..	..	..	..	..	0	0	6	7	5	6	..	..	..	..
Overall	(461)		(350)		(591)		(500)		(181)		(2083)		(910)		(569)		(604)	
1 year	65	65	34	34	18	18	6	7	3	4	27	28	27	28	27	27	27	27
3 years	44	44	14	14	6	6	2	2	1	1	14	15	14	14	13	14	15	16
5 years	33	33	10	10	3	4	1	1	1	2	10	11	9	10	10	11	12	13
8 years	25	26	7	8	2	2	0	0	0	0	7	9	7	9	5	6	..	..
10 years	23	24	4	4	..	..	..	..	0	0	6	8	6	8	..	..	..	..

RELATIVE SURVIVAL (%) BY AGE AND PERIOD

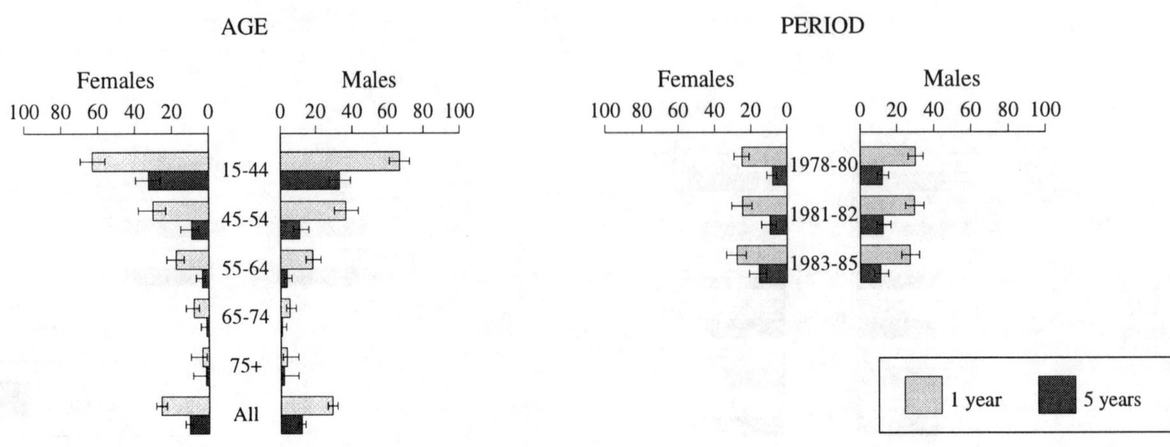

BRAIN

DUTCH REGISTRIES

REGISTRY	NUMBER OF CASES			PERIOD OF DIAGNOSIS
	Males	Females	All	
Eindhoven	150	92	242	1978-1985
Mean age (years)	50.5	50.7	50.6	

RELATIVE SURVIVAL (%)

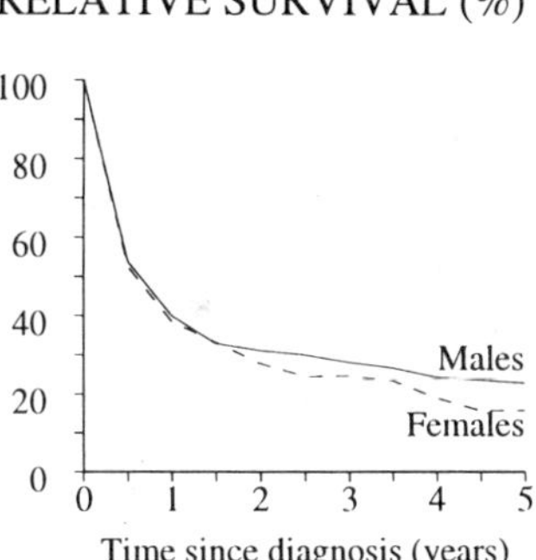

OBSERVED AND RELATIVE SURVIVAL (%) BY AGE AND PERIOD
(Number of cases in parentheses)

	AGE CLASS												PERIOD					
	15-44		45-54		55-64		65-74		75+		All		1978-80		1981-82		1983-85	
	obs	rel	obs	rel	obs	rel	obs	rel	obs	rel	obs	rel	obs	rel	obs	rel	obs	rel
Males	(55)		(24)		(34)		(32)		(5)		(150)		(50)		(47)		(53)	
1 year	73	73	38	38	18	18	9	10	20	22	39	40	36	37	38	39	43	44
3 years	54	55	25	25	9	9	3	4	0	0	27	28	24	25	28	29	28	30
5 years	45	46	14	15	6	6	3	4	0	0	21	23	16	18	26	28	21	23
8 years	41	42	0	0	..	..	3	5	0	0	17	20	14	17	..	..	..	..
10 years	0	0	0	0	..	..	..	..	0	0	0	0	0	0	..	..	..	..
Females	(38)		(14)		(17)		(15)		(8)		(92)		(29)		(28)		(35)	
1 year	61	61	36	36	18	18	20	20	13	13	38	38	31	31	43	44	40	40
3 years	47	47	7	7	6	6	7	7	13	16	24	25	17	18	25	26	29	30
5 years	35	36	7	7	0	0	0	0	0	0	15	16	10	11	18	19	14	15
8 years	35	36	0	0	0	0	0	0	0	0	13	14	10	11	..	..	..	..
10 years	0	0	0	0	0	0	0	0	0	0	0	0	0	0	..	..	..	..
Overall	(93)		(38)		(51)		(47)		(13)		(242)		(79)		(75)		(88)	
1 year	68	68	37	37	18	18	13	13	15	17	39	39	34	35	40	41	42	43
3 years	51	51	18	19	8	8	4	5	8	10	25	27	22	22	27	28	28	30
5 years	41	42	12	12	4	4	2	3	0	0	19	20	14	15	23	25	18	20
8 years	39	39	0	0	..	..	2	3	0	0	15	18	13	15	..	..	..	..
10 years	0	0	0	0	..	..	..	..	0	0	0	0	0	0	..	..	..	..

RELATIVE SURVIVAL (%) BY AGE AND PERIOD

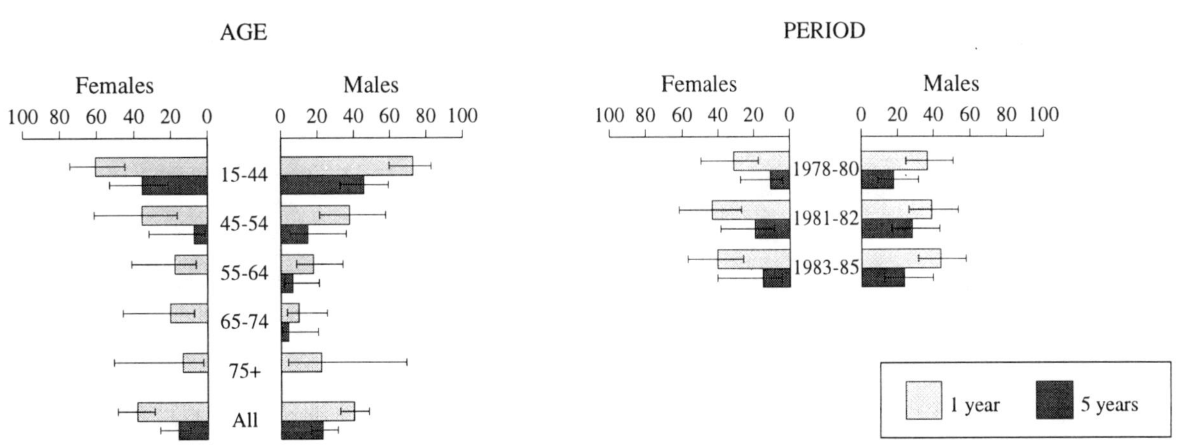

BRAIN

ENGLISH REGISTRIES

REGISTRY	NUMBER OF CASES			PERIOD OF DIAGNOSIS
	Males	Females	All	
East Anglia	363	254	617	1979-1984
Mersey	386	300	686	1978-1984
South Thames	1407	1026	2433	1978-1984
Wessex	179	131	310	1983-1984
West Midlands	728	490	1218	1979-1984
Yorkshire	621	587	1208	1978-1984
Mean age (years)	55.5	56.6	56.0	

RELATIVE SURVIVAL (%)

OBSERVED AND RELATIVE SURVIVAL (%) BY AGE AND PERIOD
(Number of cases in parentheses)

	AGE CLASS												PERIOD					
	15-44		45-54		55-64		65-74		75+		All		1978-80		1981-82		1983-85	
	obs	rel	obs	rel	obs	rel	obs	rel	obs	rel	obs	rel	obs	rel	obs	rel	obs	rel
Males	(799)		(693)		(1040)		(933)		(219)		(3684)		(1400)		(1088)		(1196)	
1 year	64	64	32	32	16	16	9	9	2	2	27	27	27	27	26	27	27	28
3 years	43	43	14	14	5	6	3	3	1	1	14	16	14	16	13	14	16	17
5 years	34	34	10	10	4	4	2	3	0	1	11	12	11	12	10	11	12	14
8 years	25	25	7	8	2	3	2	3	0	0	8	10	8	10	7	9	8	10
10 years	20	20	6	7	2	3	2	4	0	0	7	9	7	9	4	6	..	..
Females	(567)		(497)		(749)		(721)		(254)		(2788)		(1046)		(826)		(916)	
1 year	66	66	32	32	17	17	8	9	7	7	27	27	26	27	27	28	26	27
3 years	46	46	18	18	8	8	4	4	2	3	16	17	16	16	16	17	16	17
5 years	38	38	12	13	6	6	3	3	1	2	12	13	12	14	12	13	12	13
8 years	28	28	9	10	4	5	2	3	1	2	9	11	10	12	9	10	9	10
10 years	24	25	7	7	4	4	2	3	1	3	8	10	8	10	8	10	..	..
Overall	(1366)		(1190)		(1789)		(1654)		(473)		(6472)		(2446)		(1914)		(2112)	
1 year	65	65	32	32	17	17	9	9	4	5	27	27	26	27	27	27	27	27
3 years	44	44	16	16	6	7	3	4	2	2	15	16	15	16	14	15	16	17
5 years	35	36	11	11	5	5	2	3	1	1	11	13	12	13	11	12	12	13
8 years	26	27	8	9	3	4	2	3	1	1	8	10	9	11	8	9	9	10
10 years	22	22	7	7	3	3	2	3	1	2	7	9	8	10	6	8	..	..

RELATIVE SURVIVAL (%) BY AGE AND PERIOD

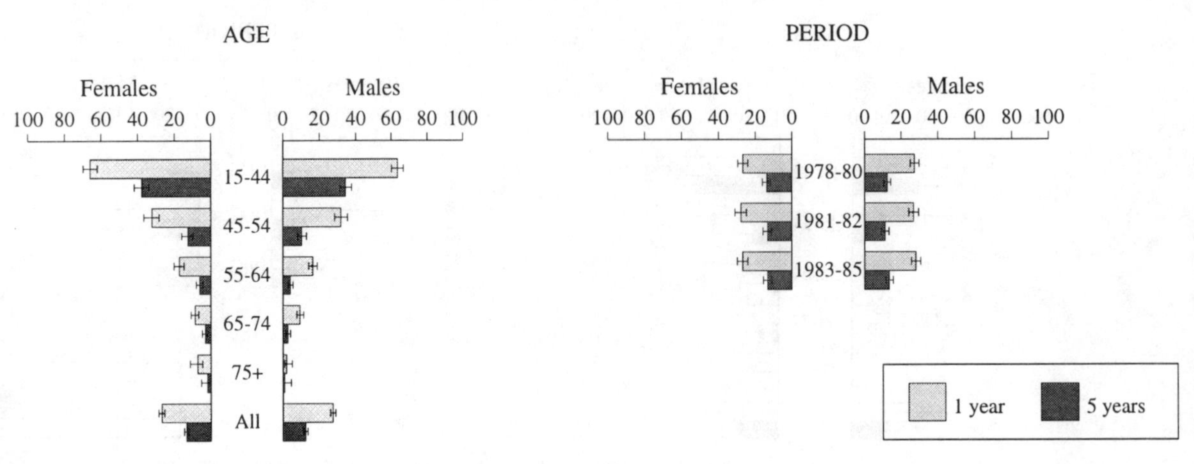

BRAIN

ESTONIA

REGISTRY	NUMBER OF CASES			PERIOD OF DIAGNOSIS
	Males	Females	All	
Estonia	129	146	275	1978-1984
Mean age (years)	49.1	52.1	50.7	

RELATIVE SURVIVAL (%)

100 80 60 40 20 0

0 1 2 3 4 5

Females

Males

Time since diagnosis (years)

OBSERVED AND RELATIVE SURVIVAL (%) BY AGE AND PERIOD
(Number of cases in parentheses)

	AGE CLASS												PERIOD					
	15-44		45-54		55-64		65-74		75+		All		1978-80		1981-82		1983-85	
	obs	rel	obs	rel	obs	rel	obs	rel	obs	rel	obs	rel	obs	rel	obs	rel	obs	rel
Males	(42)		(40)		(27)		(18)		(2)		(129)		(46)		(38)		(45)	
1 year	48	48	18	18	11	11	11	12	0	0	25	25	22	22	26	27	27	27
3 years	33	34	10	10	11	12	6	7	0	0	17	18	17	18	18	20	16	17
5 years	24	25	10	11	4	4	6	7	0	0	12	14	13	14	16	18	9	10
8 years	21	22	7	8	4	5	..	..	0	0	10	13	11	13	13	15	..	..
10 years	21	23	7	8	..	..	..	..	0	0	10	13	11	14	..	..	..	..
Females	(38)		(33)		(49)		(23)		(3)		(146)		(65)		(39)		(42)	
1 year	55	55	39	40	20	21	17	18	33	36	34	34	32	33	41	41	29	29
3 years	29	29	24	25	14	15	9	9	0	0	19	20	22	22	23	24	12	12
5 years	24	24	18	19	10	11	4	5	0	0	14	15	17	18	15	16	10	10
8 years	24	24	18	19	6	7	..	..	0	0	13	14	14	15	15	17	..	..
10 years	24	24	18	19	6	7	..	..	0	0	13	15	14	16	..	..	..	..
Overall	(80)		(73)		(76)		(41)		(5)		(275)		(111)		(77)		(87)	
1 year	51	51	27	28	17	17	15	15	20	22	29	30	28	28	34	34	28	28
3 years	31	32	16	17	13	14	7	8	0	0	18	19	20	21	21	22	14	15
5 years	24	24	14	14	8	9	5	6	0	0	13	15	15	16	16	17	9	10
8 years	22	23	12	13	5	6	..	..	0	0	12	14	13	14	14	16	..	..
10 years	22	23	12	13	5	7	..	..	0	0	12	14	13	15	..	..	..	..

RELATIVE SURVIVAL (%) BY AGE AND PERIOD

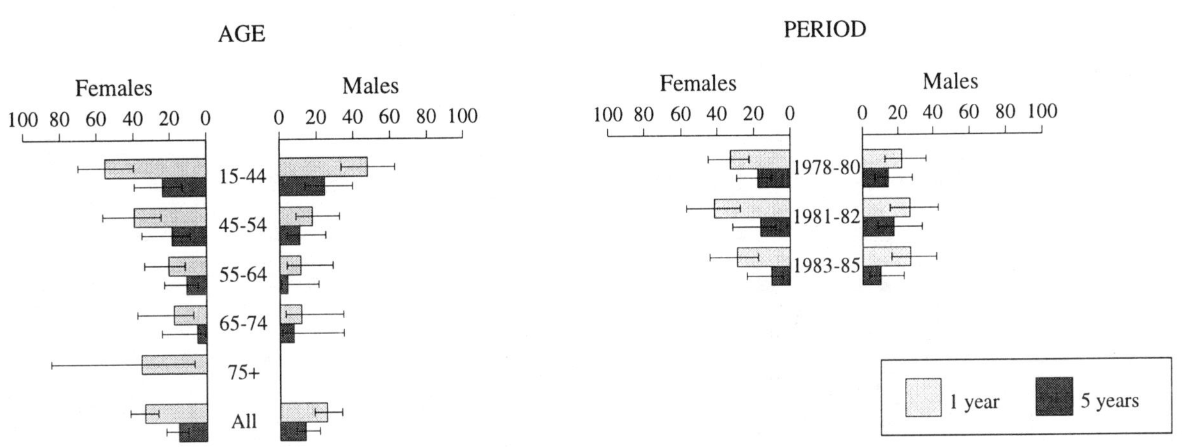

BRAIN

FINLAND

REGISTRY	NUMBER OF CASES			PERIOD OF DIAGNOSIS
	Males	Females	All	
Finland	864	842	1706	1978-1984
Mean age (years)	48.5	52.6	50.5	

RELATIVE SURVIVAL (%)

100
80
60
40
20
0
Females
Males
0 1 2 3 4 5
Time since diagnosis (years)

OBSERVED AND RELATIVE SURVIVAL (%) BY AGE AND PERIOD
(Number of cases in parentheses)

	AGE CLASS												PERIOD					
	15-44		45-54		55-64		65-74		75+		All		1978-80		1981-82		1983-85	
	obs	rel	obs	rel	obs	rel	obs	rel	obs	rel	obs	rel	obs	rel	obs	rel	obs	rel
Males	(340)		(165)		(202)		(122)		(35)		(864)		(359)		(240)		(265)	
1 year	81	81	56	56	43	43	24	25	17	19	56	57	52	53	60	61	59	60
3 years	62	63	31	32	16	17	9	11	6	8	36	38	31	33	40	42	38	40
5 years	50	51	25	26	12	14	4	5	6	10	28	31	25	28	32	35	29	32
8 years	40	41	19	21	7	9	2	3	0	0	21	25	19	22	24	28	23	27
10 years	36	37	17	20	6	8	..	..	0	0	19	23	16	20	23	27	..	..
Females	(275)		(126)		(198)		(183)		(60)		(842)		(353)		(232)		(257)	
1 year	85	86	66	66	41	42	33	34	23	25	56	57	61	62	55	55	51	52
3 years	68	68	47	47	21	21	14	15	18	23	38	40	44	45	35	37	33	35
5 years	57	58	36	36	19	20	10	12	10	15	31	34	37	39	30	32	26	28
8 years	46	46	26	27	16	17	10	13	5	10	25	28	30	33	25	28	20	23
10 years	38	39	20	21	15	17	8	12	5	13	21	25	25	28	23	27	..	..
Overall	(615)		(291)		(400)		(305)		(95)		(1706)		(712)		(472)		(522)	
1 year	83	83	60	61	42	43	30	31	21	23	56	57	57	57	57	58	55	56
3 years	65	65	38	39	19	19	12	13	14	18	37	39	38	39	38	40	36	38
5 years	53	54	30	31	16	17	8	10	8	13	30	32	31	33	31	34	27	30
8 years	43	43	22	24	12	13	6	9	3	7	23	27	24	28	25	28	21	25
10 years	37	37	18	20	11	13	5	8	3	9	20	24	20	24	23	27	..	..

RELATIVE SURVIVAL (%) BY AGE AND PERIOD

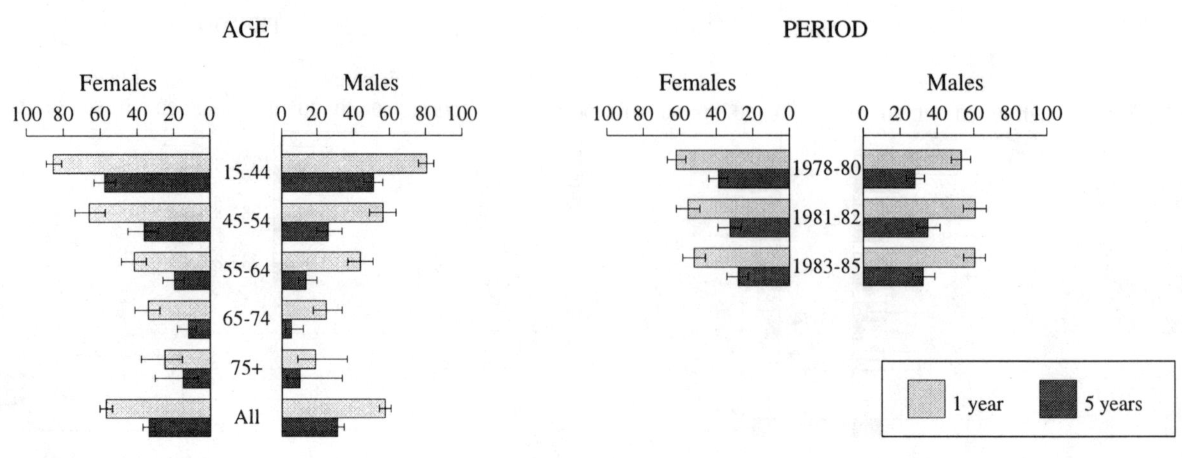

BRAIN

FRENCH REGISTRIES

REGISTRY	NUMBER OF CASES Males	Females	All	PERIOD OF DIAGNOSIS
Amiens	33	30	63	1983-1984
Doubs	100	76	176	1978-1985
Mean age (years)	53.0	54.6	53.7	

RELATIVE SURVIVAL (%)

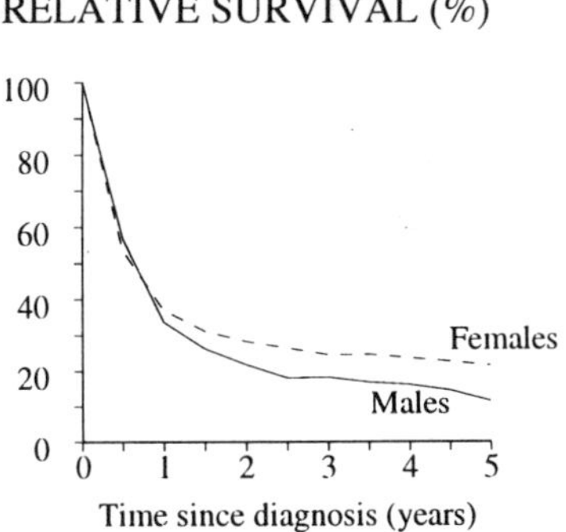

OBSERVED AND RELATIVE SURVIVAL (%) BY AGE AND PERIOD
(Number of cases in parentheses)

	AGE CLASS 15-44 obs	rel	45-54 obs	rel	55-64 obs	rel	65-74 obs	rel	75+ obs	rel	All obs	rel	PERIOD 1978-80 obs	rel	1981-82 obs	rel	1983-85 obs	rel
Males	(36)		(31)		(31)		(29)		(6)		(133)		(33)		(30)		(70)	
1 year	67	67	32	33	16	16	17	18	0	0	33	34	42	43	30	30	30	31
3 years	47	48	13	13	3	3	3	4	0	0	17	18	18	19	23	25	14	15
5 years	28	29	6	7	..	..	3	4	0	0	10	12	15	17	10	11	9	9
8 years	24	25	3	4	..	..	3	5	0	0	8	9	15	18	5	6	..	..
10 years	24	25	..	..	..	..	3	6	0	0	8	10	15	20	..	..	..	..
Females	(25)		(20)		(30)		(22)		(9)		(106)		(28)		(24)		(54)	
1 year	76	76	45	45	21	21	6	6	22	25	36	37	47	49	38	38	30	31
3 years	56	56	25	25	7	7	6	6	22	29	24	25	31	33	13	13	25	26
5 years	47	47	25	25	0	0	6	7	22	32	20	22	24	26	13	13	22	24
8 years	42	42	9	9	0	0	6	7	22	41	16	17	24	27	4	5	17	18
10 years	30	30	9	9	0	0	6	8	22	49	13	15	20	23	..	..	..	..
Overall	(61)		(51)		(61)		(51)		(15)		(239)		(61)		(54)		(124)	
1 year	70	71	37	37	19	19	13	13	13	15	35	35	45	46	33	34	30	31
3 years	51	51	18	18	5	5	4	5	13	17	20	21	24	26	19	19	19	20
5 years	36	36	14	14	..	..	4	5	13	20	15	16	19	21	11	12	15	16
8 years	31	32	5	5	..	..	4	6	13	27	11	13	19	22	5	6	10	12
10 years	27	27	5	6	..	..	4	7	13	36	10	12	17	21	..	..	..	..

RELATIVE SURVIVAL (%) BY AGE AND PERIOD

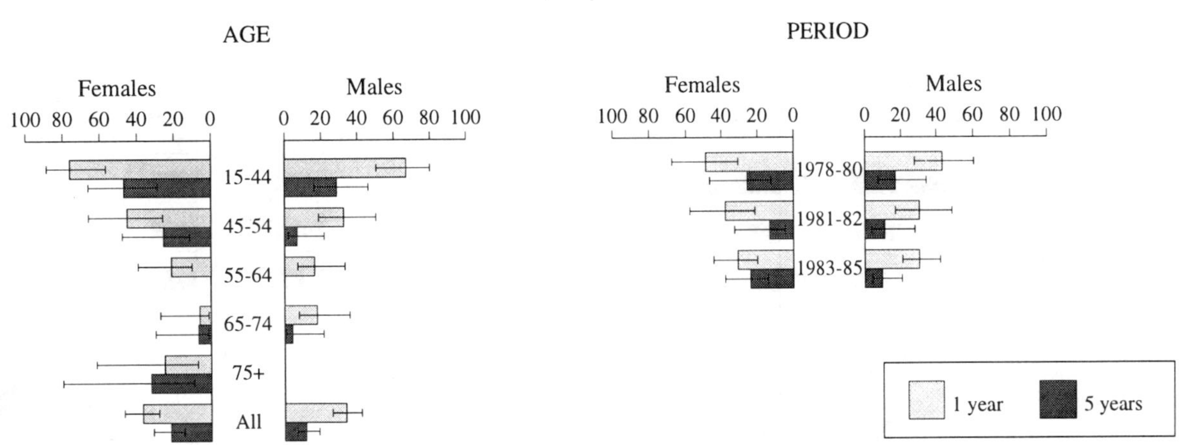

BRAIN

GERMAN REGISTRIES

REGISTRY	NUMBER OF CASES			PERIOD OF DIAGNOSIS
	Males	Females	All	
Saarland	195	160	355	1978-1984
Mean age (years)	50.4	53.6	51.9	

RELATIVE SURVIVAL (%)

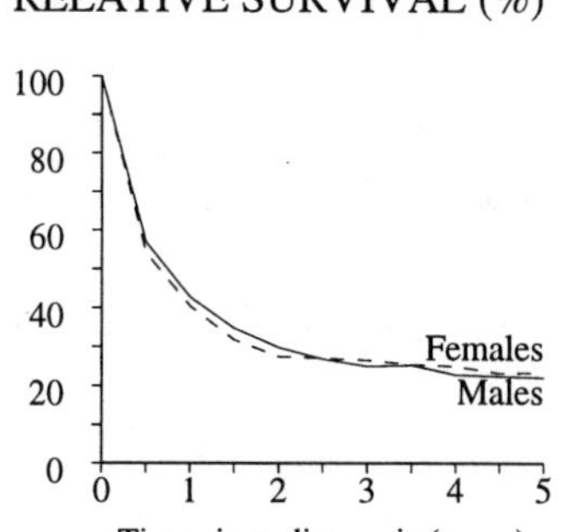

OBSERVED AND RELATIVE SURVIVAL (%) BY AGE AND PERIOD
(Number of cases in parentheses)

	AGE CLASS												PERIOD					
	15-44		45-54		55-64		65-74		75+		All		1978-80		1981-82		1983-85	
	obs	rel	obs	rel	obs	rel	obs	rel	obs	rel	obs	rel	obs	rel	obs	rel	obs	rel
Males	(65)		(42)		(44)		(40)		(4)		(195)		(91)		(49)		(55)	
1 year	66	66	38	38	41	42	13	13	0	0	42	43	37	38	39	40	53	54
3 years	48	48	17	17	14	14	5	6	0	0	24	25	25	27	24	26	20	21
5 years	40	40	17	17	11	13	3	3	0	0	20	22	21	23	22	25	16	18
8 years	24	24	14	15	11	14	0	0	0	0	13	16	14	17	16	20	..	..
10 years	16	17	14	15	11	15	0	0	0	0	11	14	12	15	..	..	..	..
Females	(37)		(41)		(39)		(35)		(8)		(160)		(70)		(54)		(36)	
1 year	68	68	46	47	33	34	17	18	13	13	40	40	37	38	44	45	39	39
3 years	65	65	27	27	10	11	3	3	13	15	26	27	24	25	31	33	19	20
5 years	54	54	27	27	8	8	3	3	0	0	22	23	20	21	28	30	17	18
8 years	51	52	22	23	3	3	3	4	0	0	18	21	19	21	24	27	..	..
10 years	51	52	22	23	..	..	3	4	0	0	18	21	19	22	..	..	..	..
Overall	(102)		(83)		(83)		(75)		(12)		(355)		(161)		(103)		(91)	
1 year	67	67	42	42	37	38	15	15	8	9	41	42	37	38	42	42	47	48
3 years	54	54	22	22	12	13	4	5	8	11	25	26	25	26	28	30	20	21
5 years	45	46	22	22	10	10	3	3	0	0	21	23	20	22	25	28	16	18
8 years	34	34	18	19	7	8	1	2	0	0	16	18	16	19	20	23	..	..
10 years	28	29	18	19	7	8	1	2	0	0	14	17	15	18	..	..	..	..

RELATIVE SURVIVAL (%) BY AGE AND PERIOD

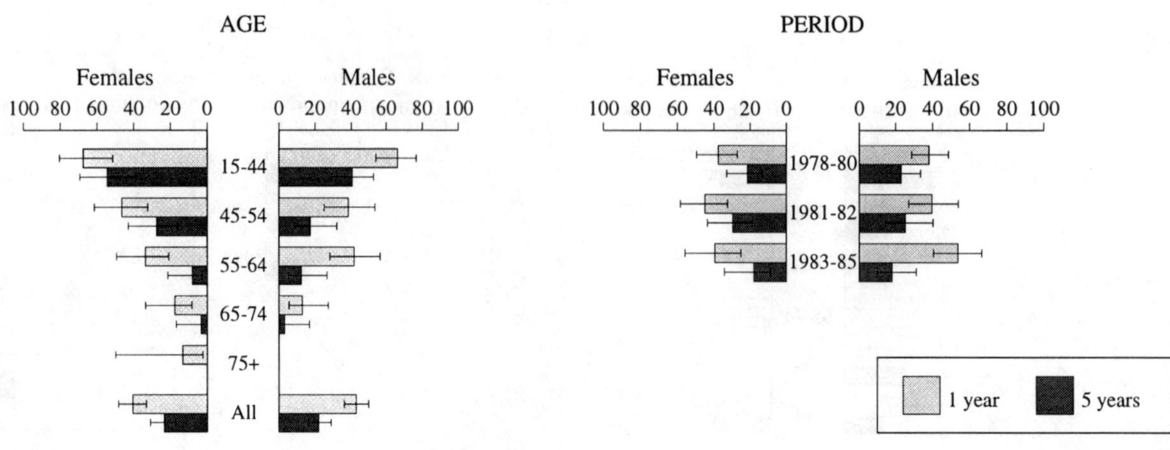

BRAIN

ITALIAN REGISTRIES

REGISTRY	NUMBER OF CASES			PERIOD OF DIAGNOSIS
	Males	Females	All	
Latina	26	9	35	1983-1984
Ragusa	27	11	38	1981-1984
Varese	139	134	273	1978-1984
Mean age (years)	55.0	56.1	55.5	

RELATIVE SURVIVAL (%)

100
80
60
40
20
0
Females
Males
0 1 2 3 4 5
Time since diagnosis (years)

OBSERVED AND RELATIVE SURVIVAL (%) BY AGE AND PERIOD
(Number of cases in parentheses)

	AGE CLASS												PERIOD					
	15-44		45-54		55-64		65-74		75+		All		1978-80		1981-82		1983-85	
	obs	rel	obs	rel	obs	rel	obs	rel	obs	rel	obs	rel	obs	rel	obs	rel	obs	rel
Males	(43)		(39)		(50)		(44)		(16)		(192)		(52)		(60)		(80)	
1 year	63	63	26	26	28	29	23	24	13	14	33	34	29	29	33	34	35	36
3 years	51	51	13	13	8	8	2	3	6	8	17	19	12	12	17	18	21	23
5 years	35	35	5	5	8	9	2	3	0	0	11	13	10	11	10	12	14	15
8 years	28	28	0	0	8	10	..	..	0	0	8	10	10	12	5	7	11	13
10 years	18	18	0	0	8	10	..	..	0	0	6	8	8	10	0	0	..	..
Females	(33)		(27)		(36)		(44)		(14)		(154)		(49)		(44)		(61)	
1 year	79	79	44	45	28	28	9	9	14	15	35	36	27	27	32	32	44	45
3 years	61	61	11	11	14	14	0	0	7	9	19	20	14	15	11	12	28	29
5 years	42	43	11	11	11	12	0	0	7	11	14	16	10	11	9	10	21	23
8 years	36	37	0	0	11	12	0	0	..	..	10	11	6	7	5	5	21	24
10 years	29	29	0	0	..	..	0	0	..	..	8	9	4	5	..	..	..	..
Overall	(76)		(66)		(86)		(88)		(30)		(346)		(101)		(104)		(141)	
1 year	70	70	33	34	28	28	16	16	13	15	34	35	28	28	33	33	39	40
3 years	55	55	12	12	10	11	1	1	7	9	18	19	13	14	14	16	24	26
5 years	38	38	8	8	9	10	1	1	3	5	13	14	10	11	10	11	17	19
8 years	32	32	0	0	9	11	..	..	..	..	9	11	8	9	5	6	16	18
10 years	22	22	0	0	9	11	..	..	..	..	7	8	6	7	0	0	..	..

RELATIVE SURVIVAL (%) BY AGE AND PERIOD

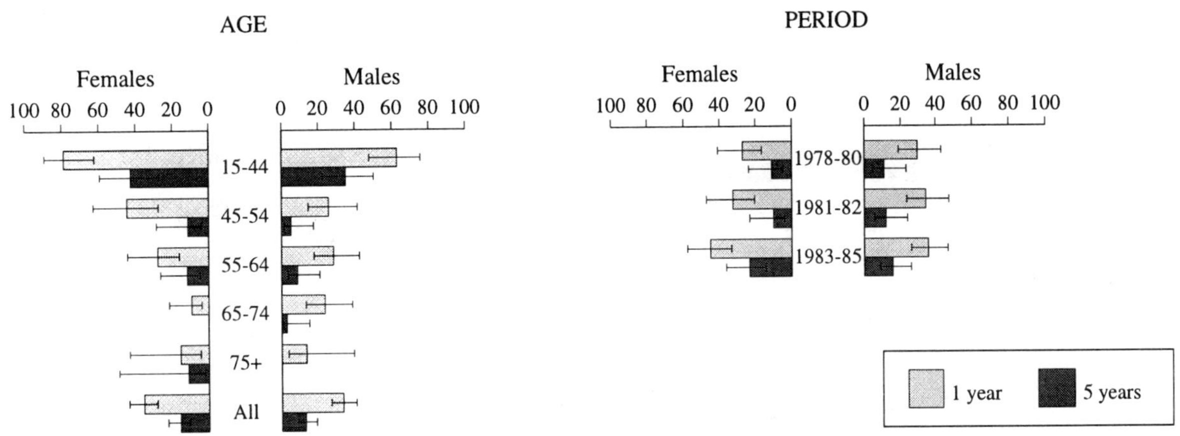

BRAIN

POLISH REGISTRIES

REGISTRY	NUMBER OF CASES			PERIOD OF DIAGNOSIS
	Males	Females	All	
Cracow	121	74	195	1978-1984
Mean age (years)	50.9	49.4	50.3	

RELATIVE SURVIVAL (%)

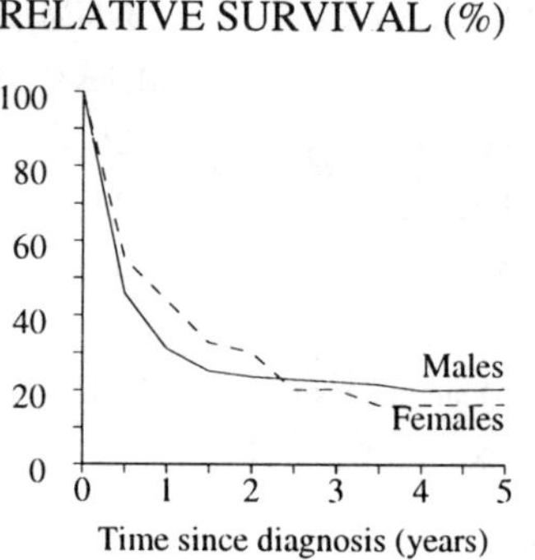

OBSERVED AND RELATIVE SURVIVAL (%) BY AGE AND PERIOD
(Number of cases in parentheses)

	AGE CLASS												PERIOD					
	15-44		45-54		55-64		65-74		75+		All		1978-80		1981-82		1983-85	
	obs	rel	obs	rel	obs	rel	obs	rel	obs	rel	obs	rel	obs	rel	obs	rel	obs	rel
Males	(37)		(26)		(33)		(22)		(3)		(121)		(57)		(33)		(31)	
1 year	50	51	29	29	26	26	10	11	0	0	31	31	32	32	29	29	30	31
3 years	36	37	12	13	19	21	10	12	0	0	21	22	24	26	16	17	20	22
5 years	34	34	8	9	19	22	5	7	0	0	18	21	22	25	16	18	14	15
8 years	22	23	0	0	19	25	..	..	0	0	13	16	19	23	6	8	..	..
10 years	15	15	0	0	19	27	..	..	0	0	10	13	14	19	..	..	..	..
Females	(31)		(14)		(12)		(14)		(3)		(74)		(34)		(19)		(21)	
1 year	74	74	36	36	10	10	21	22	0	0	44	44	41	42	45	46	46	47
3 years	40	40	7	7	0	0	7	8	0	0	20	20	26	27	17	18	10	11
5 years	30	30	7	7	0	0	7	8	0	0	15	16	21	22	11	12	10	11
8 years	23	23	7	7	0	0	7	10	0	0	12	14	15	16	11	13	10	12
10 years	23	23	7	8	0	0	7	11	0	0	12	14	15	17	11	13	..	..
Overall	(68)		(40)		(45)		(36)		(6)		(195)		(91)		(52)		(52)	
1 year	61	61	31	31	22	22	15	15	0	0	36	36	35	36	35	35	37	37
3 years	38	38	10	11	14	15	9	10	0	0	20	22	25	26	16	17	16	17
5 years	32	32	8	8	14	16	6	8	0	0	17	19	22	24	14	16	12	13
8 years	22	23	3	3	14	18	6	9	0	0	13	15	17	20	8	10	10	12
10 years	18	18	3	3	14	19	6	11	0	0	11	14	15	18	8	10	..	..

RELATIVE SURVIVAL (%) BY AGE AND PERIOD

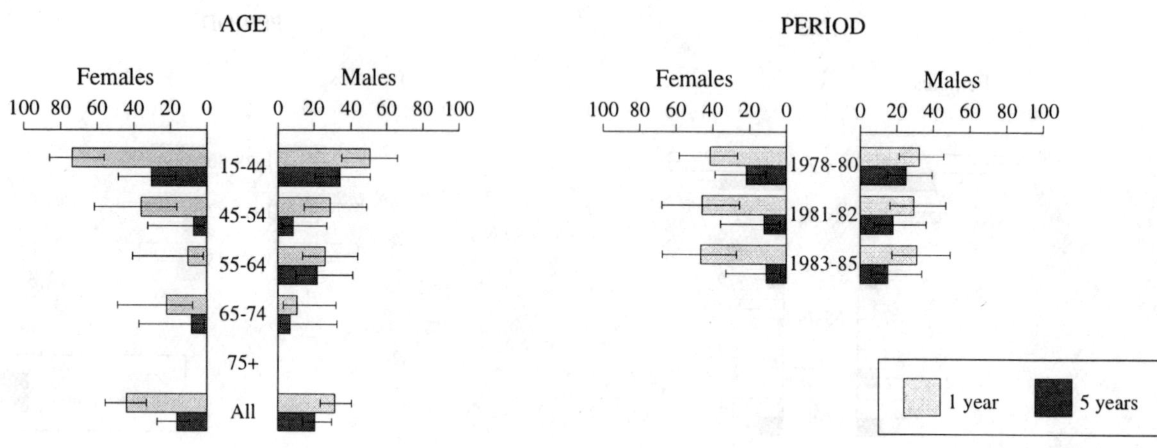

BRAIN

SCOTLAND

REGISTRY	NUMBER OF CASES			PERIOD OF DIAGNOSIS
	Males	Females	All	
Scotland	672	505	1177	1978-1982
Mean age (years)	54.5	55.9	55.1	

RELATIVE SURVIVAL (%)

100
80
60
40
20
0
Females
Males
0 1 2 3 4 5
Time since diagnosis (years)

OBSERVED AND RELATIVE SURVIVAL (%) BY AGE AND PERIOD
(Number of cases in parentheses)

	AGE CLASS												PERIOD					
	15-44		45-54		55-64		65-74		75+		All		1978-80		1981-82		1983-85	
	obs	rel	obs	rel	obs	rel	obs	rel	obs	rel	obs	rel	obs	rel	obs	rel	obs	rel
Males	(160)		(133)		(187)		(144)		(48)		(672)		(404)		(268)		(0)	
1 year	51	51	20	20	13	14	6	7	2	2	21	22	23	23	19	20	..	..
3 years	35	35	8	8	4	5	3	3	2	3	12	13	13	14	10	11	..	..
5 years	28	28	6	6	3	4	2	3	2	4	9	11	10	12	8	9	..	..
8 years	18	18	3	4	1	2	1	2	2	6	6	7	6	8	..	..	..	..
10 years	16	16	3	4	..	..	..	..	..	..	5	7	6	8	..	..	..	..
Females	(106)		(96)		(129)		(134)		(40)		(505)		(282)		(223)		(0)	
1 year	54	54	30	30	18	18	2	2	5	5	23	23	22	22	24	24	..	..
3 years	37	37	15	15	7	7	2	2	5	6	13	14	12	13	14	15	..	..
5 years	29	29	10	11	5	6	1	2	5	8	10	11	10	10	11	12	..	..
8 years	22	22	9	10	4	4	..	..	..	..	8	9	7	8	..	..	..	..
10 years	22	22	9	10	..	..	..	..	..	..	8	9	7	9	..	..	..	..
Overall	(266)		(229)		(316)		(278)		(88)		(1177)		(686)		(491)		(0)	
1 year	52	52	24	24	15	15	4	4	3	4	22	22	22	23	21	22	..	..
3 years	36	36	10	11	5	6	3	3	3	5	12	13	13	14	12	13	..	..
5 years	29	29	8	8	4	5	2	2	3	6	10	11	10	11	9	11	..	..
8 years	19	20	5	6	2	3	1	2	3	9	6	8	7	8	..	..	..	..
10 years	18	18	5	6	..	..	..	..	..	..	6	8	6	8	..	..	..	..

RELATIVE SURVIVAL (%) BY AGE AND PERIOD

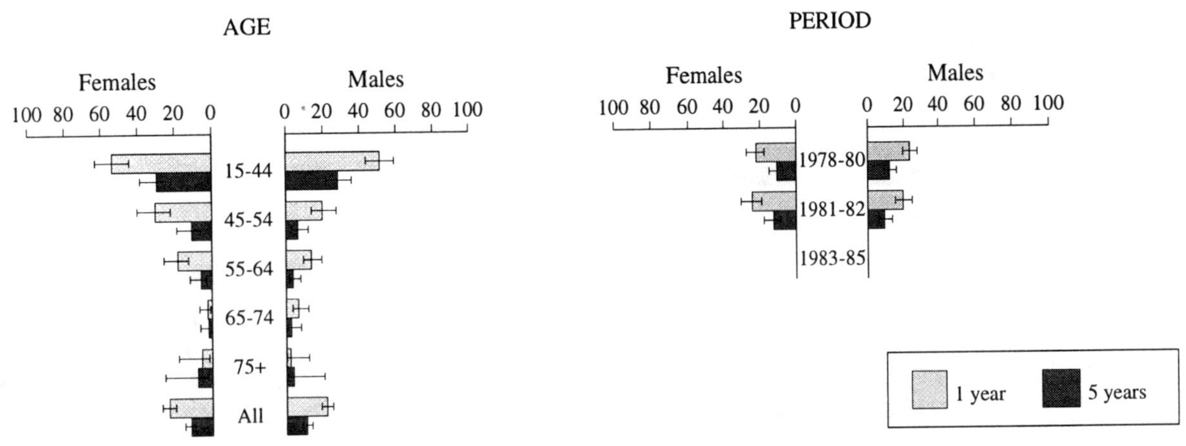

BRAIN

SPANISH REGISTRIES

REGISTRY	NUMBER OF CASES			PERIOD OF DIAGNOSIS
	Males	Females	All	
Tarragona	9	16	25	1985-1985
Mean age (years)	60.8	51.4	54.8	

RELATIVE SURVIVAL (%)

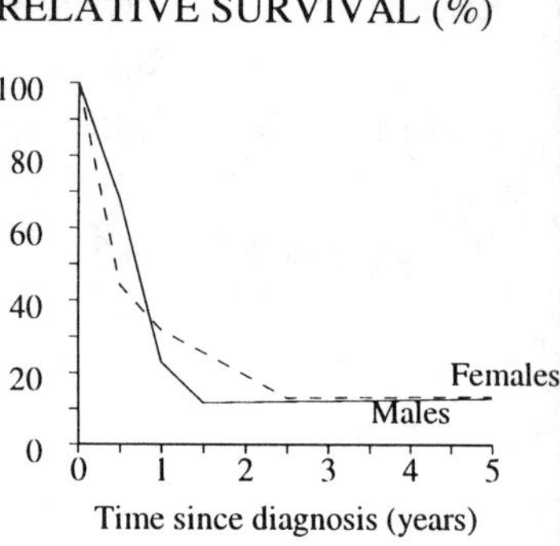

OBSERVED AND RELATIVE SURVIVAL (%) BY AGE AND PERIOD
(Number of cases in parentheses)

	AGE CLASS												PERIOD					
	15-44		45-54		55-64		65-74		75+		All		1978-80		1981-82		1983-85	
	obs	rel	obs	rel	obs	rel	obs	rel	obs	rel	obs	rel	obs	rel	obs	rel	obs	rel
Males	(2)		(1)		(2)		(3)		(1)		(9)		(0)		(0)		(9)	
1 year	50	50	0	0	0	0	33	35	0	0	22	23	..	..	..	..	22	23
3 years	50	50	0	0	0	0	0	0	0	0	11	12	..	..	..	..	11	12
5 years	50	50	0	0	0	0	0	0	0	0	11	13	..	..	..	..	11	13
8 years	..	..	0	0	0	0	0	0	0	0	..	..	..	..	..	..	..	..
10 years	..	..	0	0	0	0	0	0	0	0	..	..	..	..	..	..	..	..
Females	(6)		(2)		(3)		(3)		(2)		(16)		(0)		(0)		(16)	
1 year	33	33	100	100	0	0	0	0	50	56	31	32	..	..	..	..	31	32
3 years	33	33	0	0	0	0	0	0	0	0	13	13	..	..	..	..	13	13
5 years	33	33	0	0	0	0	0	0	0	0	13	14	..	..	..	..	13	14
8 years	..	..	0	0	0	0	0	0	0	0	..	..	..	..	..	..	..	..
10 years	..	..	0	0	0	0	0	0	0	0	..	..	..	..	..	..	..	..
Overall	(8)		(3)		(5)		(6)		(3)		(25)		(0)		(0)		(25)	
1 year	38	38	67	67	0	0	17	17	33	38	28	29	..	..	..	..	28	29
3 years	38	38	0	0	0	0	0	0	0	0	12	13	..	..	..	..	12	13
5 years	38	38	0	0	0	0	0	0	0	0	12	13	..	..	..	..	12	13
8 years	..	..	0	0	0	0	0	0	0	0	..	..	..	..	..	..	..	..
10 years	..	..	0	0	0	0	0	0	0	0	..	..	..	..	..	..	..	..

RELATIVE SURVIVAL (%) BY AGE AND PERIOD

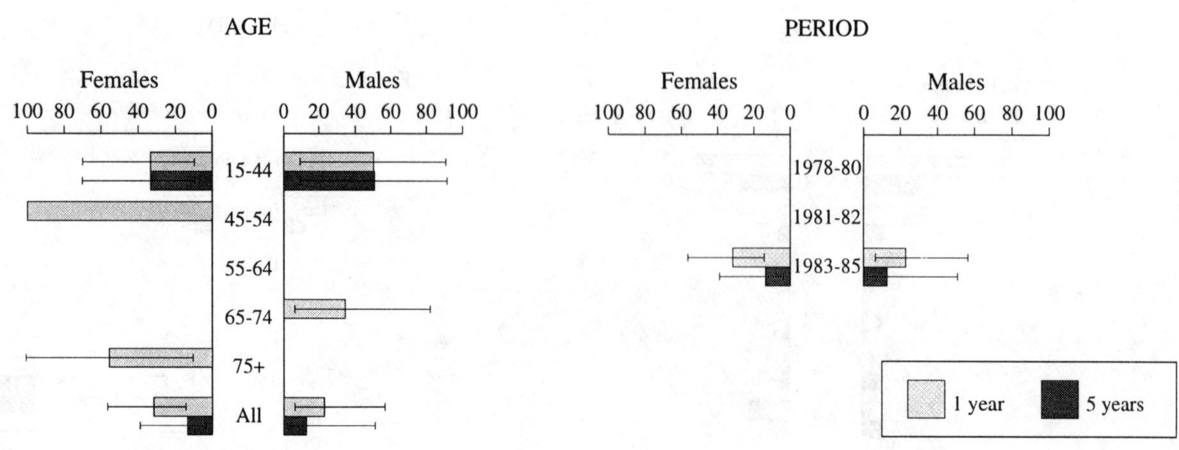

BRAIN

SWISS REGISTRIES

REGISTRY	NUMBER OF CASES Males	Females	All	PERIOD OF DIAGNOSIS
Basel	45	31	76	1981-1984
Geneva	61	66	127	1978-1984
Mean age (years)	53.9	59.6	56.7	

RELATIVE SURVIVAL (%)

100, 80, 60, 40, 20, 0 — Males, Females — 0, 1, 2, 3, 4, 5 — Time since diagnosis (years)

OBSERVED AND RELATIVE SURVIVAL (%) BY AGE AND PERIOD
(Number of cases in parentheses)

	AGE CLASS												PERIOD					
	15-44		45-54		55-64		65-74		75+		All		1978-80		1981-82		1983-85	
	obs	rel	obs	rel	obs	rel	obs	rel	obs	rel	obs	rel	obs	rel	obs	rel	obs	rel
Males	(29)		(20)		(30)		(18)		(9)		(106)		(23)		(32)		(51)	
1 year	79	79	55	55	26	26	11	12	0	0	41	42	39	40	47	48	39	39
3 years	57	57	10	10	4	4	0	0	0	0	19	20	24	26	22	23	14	15
5 years	46	46	10	10	0	0	0	0	0	0	15	16	18	21	19	21	10	11
8 years	38	39	10	11	0	0	0	0	0	0	13	15	..	..	14	17	..	..
10 years	..	..	..	..	0	0	0	0	0	0	..	..	..	..	..	..	..	..
Females	(16)		(17)		(19)		(30)		(15)		(97)		(22)		(35)		(40)	
1 year	75	75	24	24	37	37	10	10	0	0	27	27	23	23	14	15	40	40
3 years	44	44	6	6	5	5	0	0	0	0	9	10	9	10	3	3	15	16
5 years	38	38	0	0	0	0	0	0	0	0	6	7	5	5	3	3	10	11
8 years	..	..	0	0	0	0	0	0	0	0	..	..	..	..	..	..	..	..
10 years	..	..	0	0	0	0	0	0	0	0	..	..	..	..	..	..	..	..
Overall	(45)		(37)		(49)		(48)		(24)		(203)		(45)		(67)		(91)	
1 year	78	78	41	41	30	30	10	11	0	0	34	35	31	32	30	30	39	40
3 years	52	52	8	8	4	4	0	0	0	0	14	15	16	18	12	13	15	15
5 years	43	43	5	6	0	0	0	0	0	0	10	12	11	12	10	12	10	11
8 years	34	34	5	6	0	0	0	0	0	0	9	10	..	..	8	9	..	..
10 years	..	..	..	..	0	0	0	0	0	0	..	..	..	..	..	..	..	..

RELATIVE SURVIVAL (%) BY AGE AND PERIOD

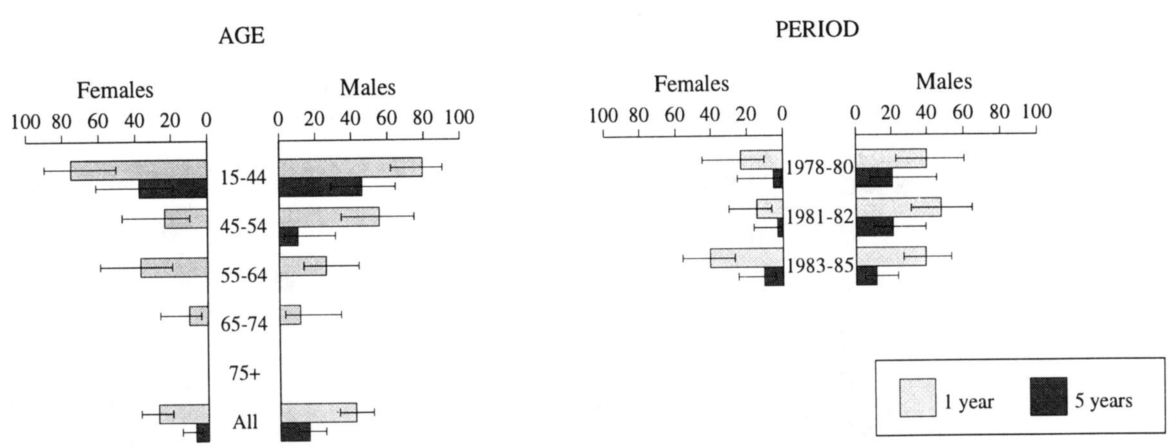

BRAIN

EUROPEAN REGISTRIES
Weighted analysis

REGISTRY	WEIGHTS (Yearly expected cases in the country) Males	Females	All
DENMARK	199	160	359
DUTCH REGISTRIES	605	627	1232
ENGLISH REGISTRIES	2514	3106	5620
ESTONIA	20	24	44
FINLAND	141	136	277
FRENCH REGISTRIES	1857	2125	3982
GERMAN REGISTRIES	2142	3134	5276
ITALIAN REGISTRIES	3069	3864	6933
POLISH REGISTRIES	1392	1069	2461
SCOTLAND	145	113	258
SPANISH REGISTRIES	1939	2406	4345
SWISS REGISTRIES	207	176	383

RELATIVE SURVIVAL (%)
(Age-standardized)

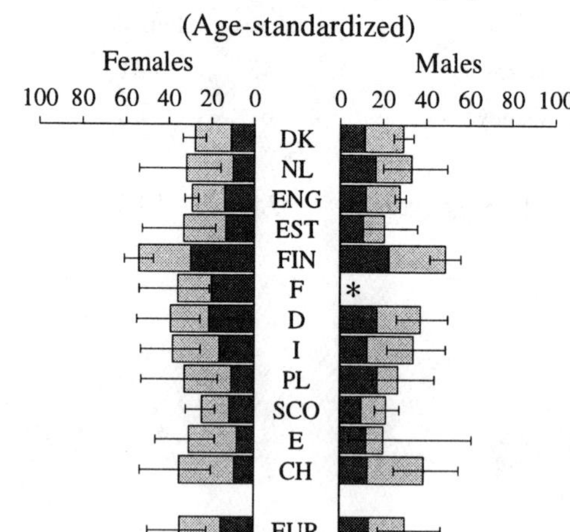

* Not enough cases for reliable estimation

OBSERVED AND RELATIVE SURVIVAL (%) BY AGE AND PERIOD

	AGE CLASS 15-44 obs	rel	45-54 obs	rel	55-64 obs	rel	65-74 obs	rel	75+ obs	rel	All obs	rel	PERIOD 1978-80 obs	rel	1981-82 obs	rel	1983-85 obs	rel
Males																		
1 year	62	62	28	28	22	22	17	18	4	5	32	33	33	34	32	33	34	35
3 years	47	47	12	13	8	8	3	4	2	2	18	19	18	19	19	20	18	19
5 years	37	38	8	9	7	8	2	3	0	0	14	15	15	17	14	16	13	15
8 years	26	27	4	5	7	9	1	2	0	0	10	12	12	15	8	10	10	12
10 years	18	18	4	5	7	10	1	2	..	..	8	10	10	13	3	3	..	..
Females																		
1 year	66	66	49	49	21	21	10	10	17	19	35	35	33	34	36	36	36	37
3 years	52	52	15	15	8	8	3	3	8	10	19	20	20	21	18	19	20	21
5 years	42	42	14	14	5	5	2	3	5	7	16	17	16	17	15	16	16	18
8 years	37	38	8	8	4	4	2	3	4	7	13	15	13	15	11	12	15	18
10 years	31	32	7	8	1	2	2	3	4	9	11	13	11	13	9	11	..	..
Overall																		
1 year	64	64	39	40	21	21	13	14	11	12	33	34	33	34	34	35	35	36
3 years	50	50	14	14	8	8	3	4	5	6	19	20	19	20	18	19	19	20
5 years	40	40	11	12	6	7	2	3	3	4	15	16	15	17	14	16	15	16
8 years	32	33	6	6	5	6	2	3	2	4	12	14	13	15	9	11	13	15
10 years	25	26	6	6	4	5	2	3	2	5	9	12	11	13	6	8	..	..

RELATIVE SURVIVAL (%) BY AGE AND PERIOD

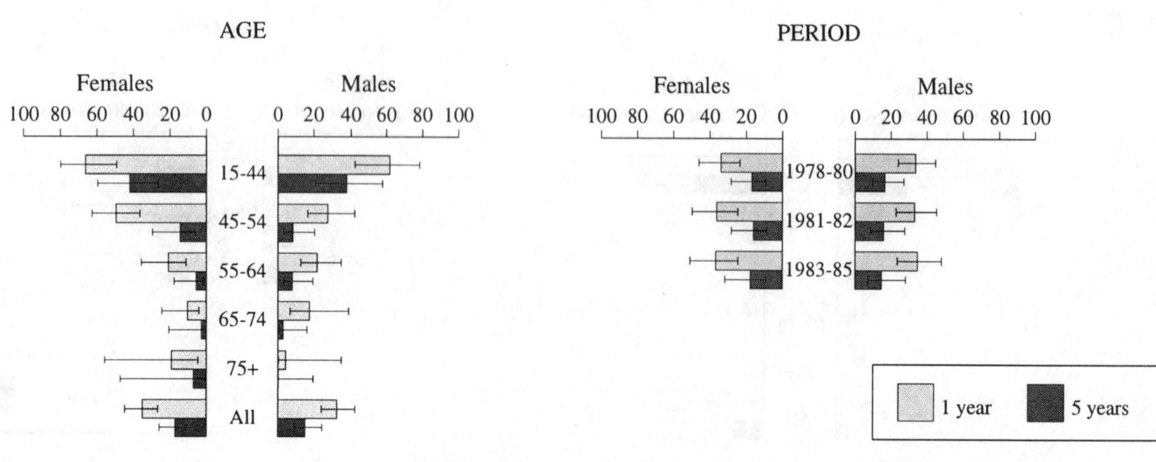

HODGKIN'S DISEASE

DENMARK

REGISTRY	NUMBER OF CASES			PERIOD OF DIAGNOSIS
	Males	Females	All	
Denmark	505	316	821	1978-1984
Mean age (years)	45.5	45.6	45.5	

RELATIVE SURVIVAL (%)

100
80
60
40
20
0
— Males
-- Females
0 1 2 3 4 5
Time since diagnosis (years)

OBSERVED AND RELATIVE SURVIVAL (%) BY AGE AND PERIOD
(Number of cases in parentheses)

	AGE CLASS												PERIOD					
	15-44		45-54		55-64		65-74		75+		All		1978-80		1981-82		1983-85	
	obs	rel	obs	rel	obs	rel	obs	rel	obs	rel	obs	rel	obs	rel	obs	rel	obs	rel
Males	(257)		(66)		(73)		(64)		(45)		(505)		(217)		(154)		(134)	
1 year	97	97	95	96	77	78	55	57	31	35	83	84	80	81	84	86	85	86
3 years	86	87	77	79	53	57	34	39	22	31	68	72	65	69	68	72	73	77
5 years	80	80	68	71	47	52	22	27	13	23	60	66	59	65	58	64	65	71
8 years	75	76	56	61	31	37	14	21	10	30	52	61	50	59	52	62	..	..
10 years	73	74	34	38	31	40	14	25	10	43	48	60	47	58	..	..	..	..
Females	(161)		(34)		(39)		(53)		(29)		(316)		(136)		(96)		(84)	
1 year	96	96	100	100	82	83	57	58	59	64	84	86	83	84	88	89	83	85
3 years	90	90	88	89	72	74	28	30	34	46	72	75	69	72	78	82	70	74
5 years	87	87	82	84	59	62	21	23	13	22	65	70	59	62	73	79	67	72
8 years	86	87	74	77	34	38	14	17	..	..	59	67	54	59	64	74	..	..
10 years	86	87	74	79	34	40	9	13	..	..	58	68	53	60	..	..	..	..
Overall	(418)		(100)		(112)		(117)		(74)		(821)		(353)		(250)		(218)	
1 year	96	97	97	98	79	80	56	57	42	46	83	85	81	82	86	87	84	86
3 years	88	88	81	83	60	63	32	35	27	37	70	73	67	70	72	75	72	76
5 years	82	83	73	75	51	56	21	25	13	22	62	67	59	64	64	70	66	71
8 years	79	80	63	67	32	38	14	19	9	25	55	63	52	59	57	67	..	..
10 years	78	79	50	55	32	40	11	17	9	34	52	63	49	59	..	..	..	..

RELATIVE SURVIVAL (%) BY AGE AND PERIOD

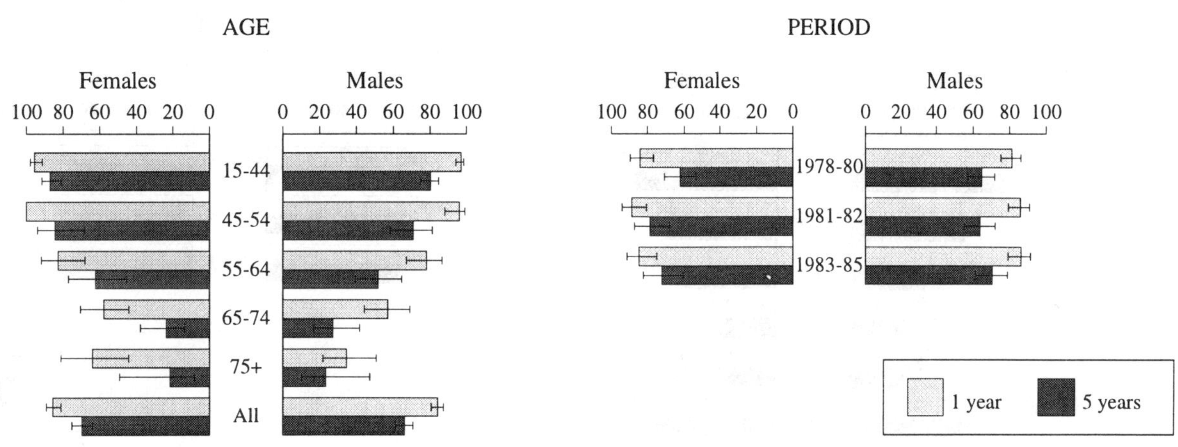

HODGKIN'S DISEASE

ENGLISH REGISTRIES

REGISTRY	NUMBER OF CASES			PERIOD OF DIAGNOSIS
	Males	Females	All	
East Anglia	179	138	317	1979-1984
Mersey	225	160	385	1978-1984
South Thames	663	440	1103	1978-1984
Wessex	72	48	120	1983-1984
West Midlands	445	275	720	1979-1984
Yorkshire	378	254	632	1978-1984
Mean age (years)	42.8	45.7	43.9	

RELATIVE SURVIVAL (%)

— Males
- - Females

Time since diagnosis (years)

OBSERVED AND RELATIVE SURVIVAL (%) BY AGE AND PERIOD
(Number of cases in parentheses)

	AGE CLASS												PERIOD					
	15-44		45-54		55-64		65-74		75+		All		1978-80		1981-82		1983-85	
	obs	rel	obs	rel	obs	rel	obs	rel	obs	rel	obs	rel	obs	rel	obs	rel	obs	rel
Males	(1127)		(236)		(257)		(238)		(104)		(1962)		(768)		(601)		(593)	
1 year	94	94	83	84	71	73	49	51	46	52	82	83	78	80	81	82	87	88
3 years	84	85	69	70	54	57	32	37	25	36	69	72	65	68	67	70	77	79
5 years	78	78	61	63	47	52	24	31	21	39	62	67	58	63	60	65	69	74
8 years	73	74	50	54	36	43	15	24	16	47	55	63	51	59	53	60	65	71
10 years	68	69	44	48	26	34	10	20	16	67	50	58	46	55	47	56	..	..
Females	(693)		(107)		(173)		(176)		(166)		(1315)		(545)		(381)		(389)	
1 year	95	95	79	80	72	72	60	61	46	50	80	81	76	77	81	83	83	84
3 years	88	88	70	71	57	59	36	39	26	34	67	71	61	65	69	73	74	77
5 years	85	86	63	64	50	53	26	30	19	31	63	68	57	62	65	70	69	73
8 years	78	79	57	60	39	44	16	21	12	28	55	63	50	58	56	65	60	66
10 years	72	72	57	61	36	41	11	16	11	34	50	60	46	55	51	62	..	..
Overall	(1820)		(343)		(430)		(414)		(270)		(3277)		(1313)		(982)		(982)	
1 year	94	94	82	83	71	72	54	56	46	51	81	82	77	79	81	82	85	86
3 years	86	86	69	71	55	58	33	38	26	34	68	72	63	67	68	71	76	78
5 years	81	81	61	64	48	53	24	30	20	34	62	67	57	63	62	67	69	73
8 years	75	76	53	56	37	44	15	22	13	34	55	63	50	58	54	62	63	69
10 years	69	70	48	52	30	37	11	18	13	45	50	59	46	55	49	58	..	..

RELATIVE SURVIVAL (%) BY AGE AND PERIOD

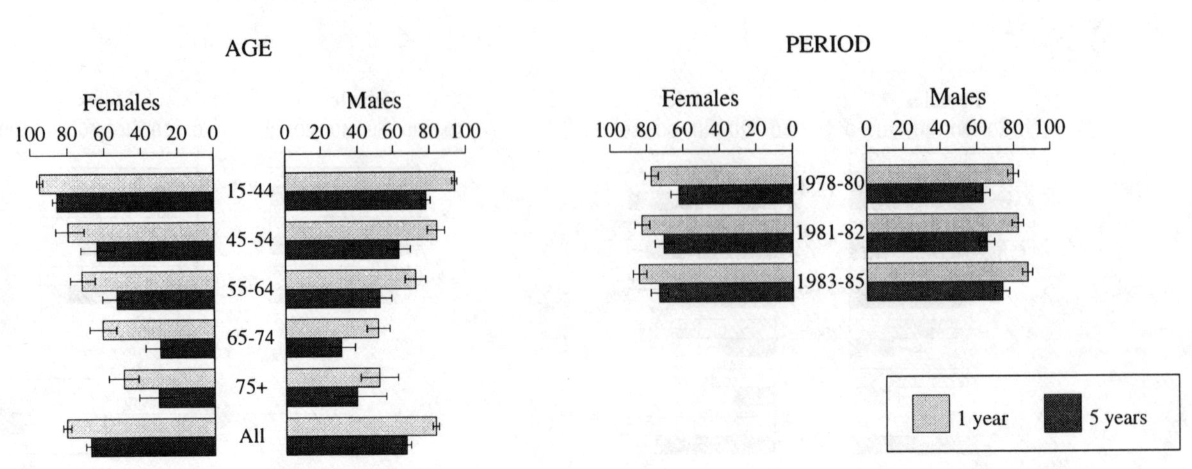

HODGKIN'S DISEASE

ESTONIA

REGISTRY	NUMBER OF CASES			PERIOD OF DIAGNOSIS
	Males	Females	All	
Estonia	92	110	202	1978-1984
Mean age (years)	42.2	46.5	44.5	

RELATIVE SURVIVAL (%)

100
80
60
40
20
0
— Males
- - Females
0 1 2 3 4 5
Time since diagnosis (years)

OBSERVED AND RELATIVE SURVIVAL (%) BY AGE AND PERIOD
(Number of cases in parentheses)

	AGE CLASS												PERIOD					
	15-44		45-54		55-64		65-74		75+		All		1978-80		1981-82		1983-85	
	obs	rel	obs	rel	obs	rel	obs	rel	obs	rel	obs	rel	obs	rel	obs	rel	obs	rel
Males	(53)		(12)		(13)		(10)		(4)		(92)		(36)		(29)		(27)	
1 year	87	87	75	76	38	39	50	53	0	0	71	72	72	74	72	73	67	68
3 years	68	68	75	78	23	25	30	36	0	0	55	59	52	57	55	57	59	62
5 years	58	59	75	81	23	27	30	42	0	0	50	55	46	54	45	47	59	65
8 years	55	57	66	75	15	20	30	55	0	0	45	54	41	52	45	49	..	..
10 years	55	58	66	79	15	23	30	68	0	0	45	57	41	56	..	..	..	..
Females	(57)		(9)		(9)		(21)		(14)		(110)		(46)		(26)		(38)	
1 year	91	91	78	78	78	79	52	54	50	54	76	78	72	73	77	78	82	83
3 years	77	77	78	79	44	46	29	32	29	38	59	62	61	64	53	56	61	65
5 years	62	63	67	69	33	35	24	29	21	36	48	53	54	59	40	45	45	51
8 years	55	55	67	70	22	25	14	20	11	29	40	47	45	52	36	43	..	..
10 years	47	48	0	0	11	13	7	12	11	44	29	36	32	38	..	..	..	..
Overall	(110)		(21)		(22)		(31)		(18)		(202)		(82)		(55)		(65)	
1 year	89	89	76	77	55	56	52	54	39	43	74	75	72	73	75	76	75	77
3 years	72	73	76	79	32	34	29	33	22	30	57	61	57	61	54	56	60	64
5 years	60	61	71	76	27	31	26	33	17	29	49	54	51	57	43	46	51	56
8 years	55	56	65	72	18	22	19	30	8	24	42	50	43	52	41	47	..	..
10 years	50	52	43	49	12	15	13	24	8	37	36	44	36	45	..	..	..	..

RELATIVE SURVIVAL (%) BY AGE AND PERIOD

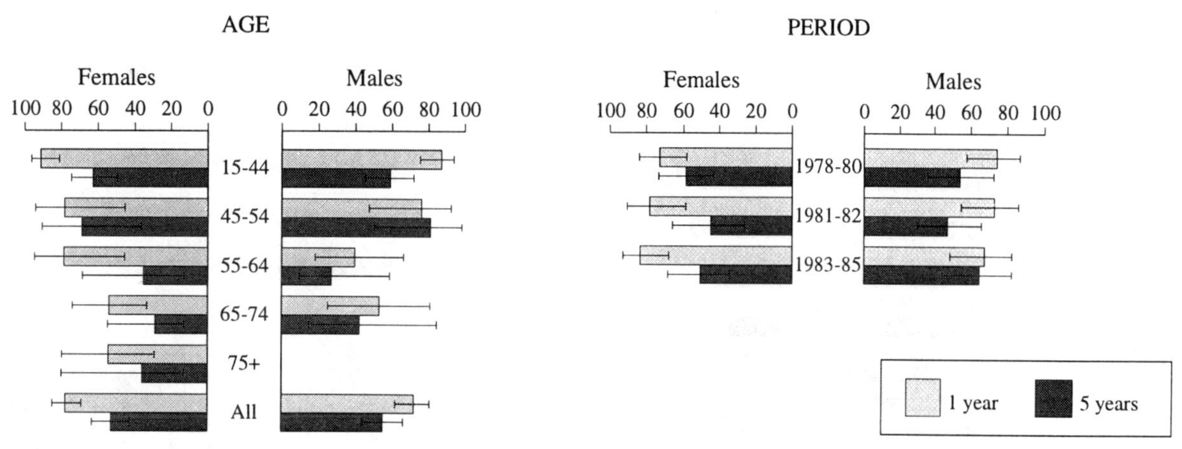

HODGKIN'S DISEASE

FINLAND

REGISTRY	NUMBER OF CASES			PERIOD OF DIAGNOSIS
	Males	Females	All	
Finland	453	328	781	1978-1984
Mean age (years)	44.4	49.5	46.5	

RELATIVE SURVIVAL (%)

100
80
60
40
20
0
— Males
- - Females
0 1 2 3 4 5
Time since diagnosis (years)

OBSERVED AND RELATIVE SURVIVAL (%) BY AGE AND PERIOD
(Number of cases in parentheses)

	AGE CLASS												PERIOD					
	15-44		45-54		55-64		65-74		75+		All		1978-80		1981-82		1983-85	
	obs	rel	obs	rel	obs	rel	obs	rel	obs	rel	obs	rel	obs	rel	obs	rel	obs	rel
Males	(259)		(48)		(57)		(65)		(24)		(453)		(200)		(138)		(115)	
1 year	92	92	73	74	74	75	51	53	29	33	79	80	77	78	76	77	85	87
3 years	82	83	60	62	54	58	31	36	8	13	65	69	63	67	62	65	72	77
5 years	77	78	52	55	37	42	25	33	4	9	58	64	56	62	54	58	66	74
8 years	68	70	48	52	27	34	12	20	..	..	49	57	50	58	47	53	51	60
10 years	65	67	41	46	24	32	7	14	..	..	46	55	45	55	47	55	..	..
Females	(153)		(25)		(46)		(63)		(41)		(328)		(143)		(101)		(84)	
1 year	97	97	92	92	63	64	68	70	34	37	79	80	76	77	84	85	77	79
3 years	92	92	80	81	48	49	52	57	10	13	67	71	64	67	73	77	65	70
5 years	87	87	72	73	46	48	41	48	5	8	61	67	58	64	69	75	56	62
8 years	83	84	63	65	41	44	33	44	..	..	56	65	54	63	62	71	55	64
10 years	80	81	57	60	37	42	24	37	..	..	52	63	50	62	53	62	..	..
Overall	(412)		(73)		(103)		(128)		(65)		(781)		(343)		(239)		(199)	
1 year	94	94	79	80	69	70	59	62	32	36	79	80	76	78	79	81	82	84
3 years	86	86	67	69	51	54	41	47	9	13	66	70	63	67	67	70	69	74
5 years	81	81	59	61	41	45	33	41	5	8	59	65	57	63	60	65	62	69
8 years	74	75	53	57	33	39	22	33	..	..	52	61	51	60	54	61	53	62
10 years	71	72	46	51	29	37	16	27	..	..	48	58	47	57	49	57	..	..

RELATIVE SURVIVAL (%) BY AGE AND PERIOD

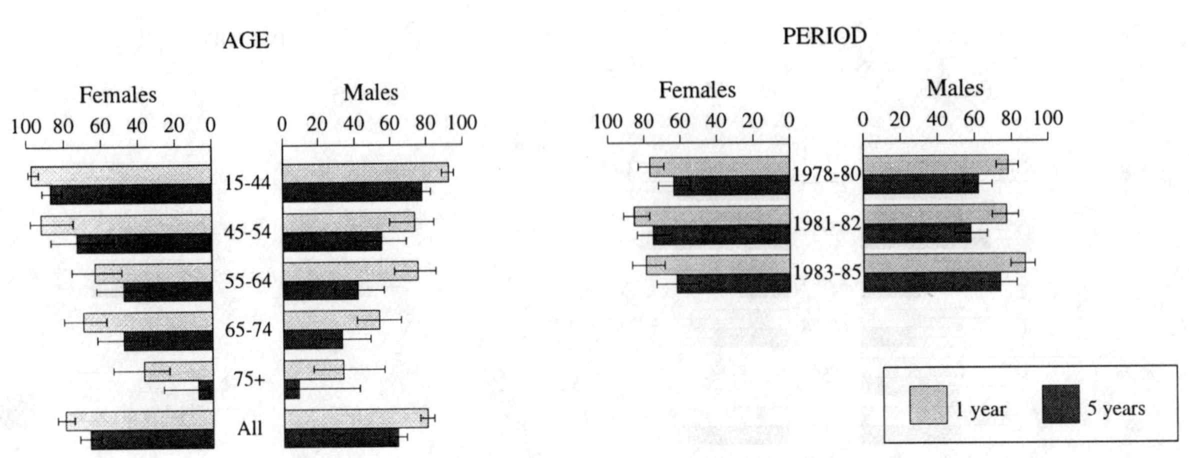

HODGKIN'S DISEASE

ITALIAN REGISTRIES

REGISTRY	NUMBER OF CASES Males	Females	All	PERIOD OF DIAGNOSIS
Latina	5	5	10	1983-1984
Ragusa	18	11	29	1981-1984
Varese	120	76	196	1978-1984
Mean age (years)	45.9	41.2	44.1	

RELATIVE SURVIVAL (%)

100
80
60
40
20
0
— Males
- - Females
0 1 2 3 4 5
Time since diagnosis (years)

OBSERVED AND RELATIVE SURVIVAL (%) BY AGE AND PERIOD
(Number of cases in parentheses)

	AGE CLASS 15-44 obs	rel	45-54 obs	rel	55-64 obs	rel	65-74 obs	rel	75+ obs	rel	All obs	rel	PERIOD 1978-80 obs	rel	1981-82 obs	rel	1983-85 obs	rel
Males	(68)		(26)		(21)		(20)		(8)		(143)		(54)		(46)		(43)	
1 year	93	93	85	85	67	68	65	68	50	56	81	82	76	77	87	88	81	83
3 years	84	84	58	59	52	56	30	34	25	35	64	67	67	71	63	66	60	64
5 years	81	82	54	56	48	53	15	19	0	0	57	62	63	69	59	63	49	53
8 years	76	77	50	54	48	58	10	15	0	0	54	62	57	67	57	64	45	51
10 years	74	75	50	56	20	26	..	..	0	0	47	56	48	59	57	65	..	..
Females	(60)		(9)		(7)		(11)		(5)		(92)		(36)		(28)		(28)	
1 year	92	92	78	78	71	72	73	74	80	84	86	86	86	87	82	83	89	90
3 years	82	82	56	56	29	29	36	39	40	47	67	69	69	71	57	59	75	77
5 years	77	77	56	56	29	30	18	21	0	0	60	62	61	63	54	56	64	67
8 years	75	75	56	57	29	32	0	0	0	0	57	60	58	62	54	58	57	61
10 years	72	73	56	58	0	0	0	0	0	0	52	57	53	57	54	58	..	..
Overall	(128)		(35)		(28)		(31)		(13)		(235)		(90)		(74)		(71)	
1 year	92	92	83	83	68	69	68	70	62	67	83	84	80	81	85	86	85	86
3 years	83	83	57	58	46	49	32	36	31	40	65	68	68	71	61	63	66	69
5 years	79	79	54	56	43	47	16	20	0	0	58	62	62	67	57	60	55	59
8 years	76	76	51	55	43	51	6	9	0	0	55	61	58	65	55	61	50	55
10 years	73	74	51	56	15	19	..	..	0	0	49	57	50	58	55	63	..	..

RELATIVE SURVIVAL (%) BY AGE AND PERIOD

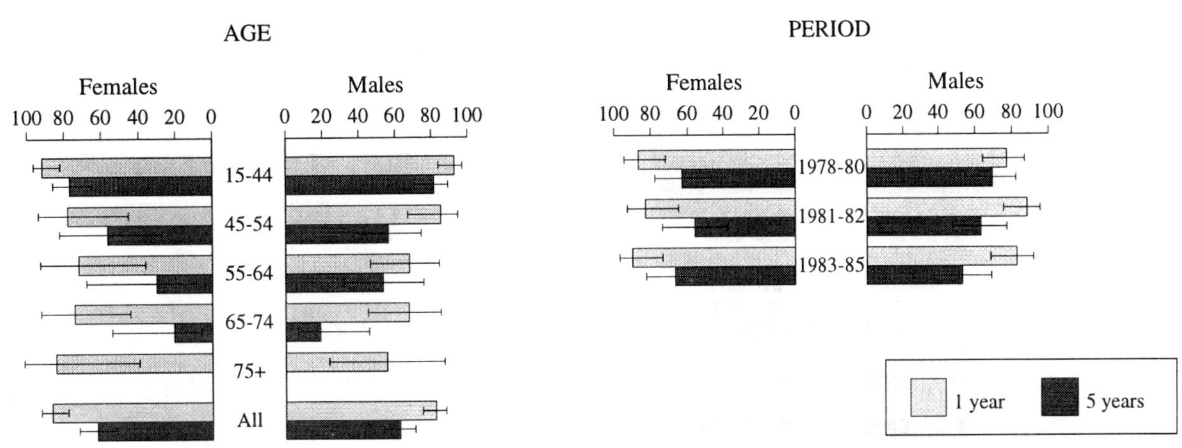

HODGKIN'S DISEASE

SCOTLAND

REGISTRY	NUMBER OF CASES			PERIOD OF DIAGNOSIS
	Males	Females	All	
Scotland	396	303	699	1978-1982
Mean age (years)	43.0	48.5	45.4	

RELATIVE SURVIVAL (%)

100
80
60
40
20
0
— Males
- - Females
0 1 2 3 4 5
Time since diagnosis (years)

OBSERVED AND RELATIVE SURVIVAL (%) BY AGE AND PERIOD
(Number of cases in parentheses)

	AGE CLASS												PERIOD					
	15-44		45-54		55-64		65-74		75+		All		1978-80		1981-82		1983-85	
	obs	rel	obs	rel	obs	rel	obs	rel	obs	rel	obs	rel	obs	rel	obs	rel	obs	rel
Males	(229)		(53)		(41)		(39)		(34)		(396)		(249)		(147)		(0)	
1 year	92	92	66	67	66	67	49	51	26	30	76	77	73	75	80	81	..	..
3 years	81	81	51	52	51	55	26	30	18	27	63	67	60	64	68	72	..	..
5 years	76	77	47	49	41	47	21	28	9	19	57	63	55	61	62	68	..	..
8 years	74	75	45	49	32	39	11	19	4	16	54	63	51	60	..	..	..	..
10 years	72	74	41	46	32	43	..	..	..	..	51	64	48	60	..	..	..	..
Females	(144)		(22)		(33)		(63)		(41)		(303)		(180)		(123)		(0)	
1 year	94	94	82	82	67	68	44	46	32	35	71	73	68	69	76	78	..	..
3 years	83	83	73	74	52	54	33	37	17	23	59	63	57	60	63	68	..	..
5 years	76	77	68	70	39	42	22	26	15	25	52	58	48	54	58	65	..	..
8 years	71	72	51	54	24	27	17	23	15	37	46	55	42	50	..	..	..	..
10 years	71	72	..	..	24	28	14	21	10	32	43	55	40	50	..	..	..	..
Overall	(373)		(75)		(74)		(102)		(75)		(699)		(429)		(270)		(0)	
1 year	92	93	71	71	66	67	46	48	29	33	74	75	71	73	78	80	..	..
3 years	82	82	57	59	51	54	30	34	17	25	61	65	59	62	66	70	..	..
5 years	76	77	53	56	41	45	22	27	12	23	55	61	52	58	60	66	..	..
8 years	73	74	49	53	28	34	15	22	11	31	50	59	47	56	..	..	..	..
10 years	72	73	45	50	28	36	11	18	8	30	48	60	45	56	..	..	..	..

RELATIVE SURVIVAL (%) BY AGE AND PERIOD

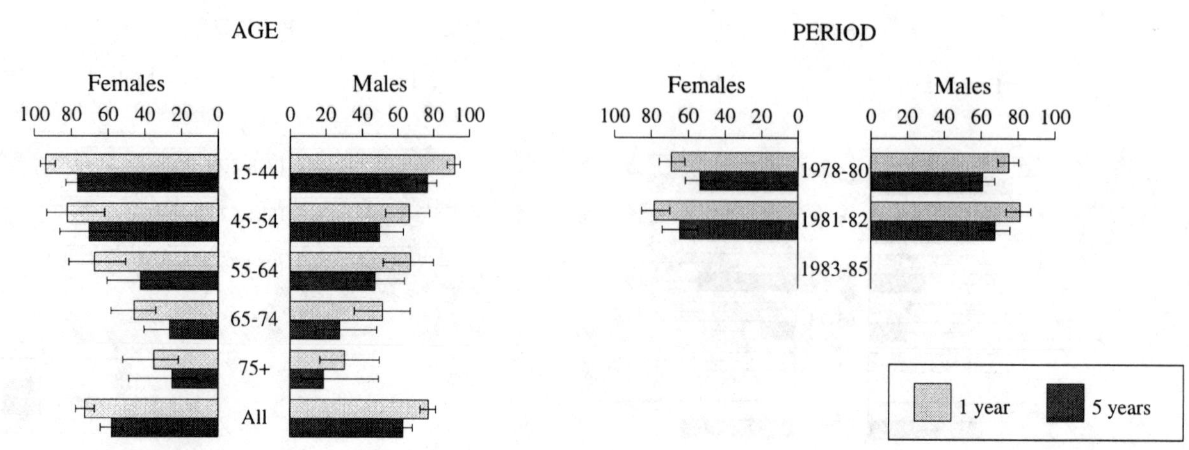

HODGKIN'S DISEASE

DUTCH REGISTRIES

REGISTRY	NUMBER OF CASES			PERIOD OF DIAGNOSIS
	Males	Females	All	
Eindhoven	80	57	137	1978-1985
Mean age (years)	39.3	39.8	39.5	

RELATIVE SURVIVAL (%)
(Both sexes)

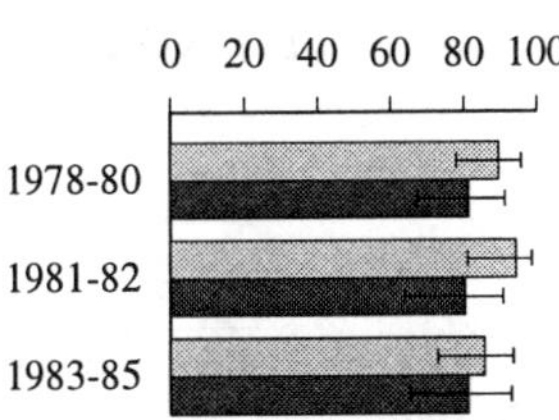

OBSERVED AND RELATIVE SURVIVAL (%) BY PERIOD AND SEX
(Number of cases in parentheses)

	PERIOD						SEX					
	1978-80		1981-82		1983-85		Males		Females		All	
	obs	rel	obs	rel	obs	rel	obs	rel	obs	rel	obs	rel
N. Cases	(53)		(34)		(50)		(80)		(57)		(137)	
1 year	89	90	94	94	84	86	89	90	88	89	88	89
3 years	83	86	82	83	73	77	80	83	78	81	79	82
5 years	77	81	79	80	73	81	74	78	78	83	75	80
8 years	67	73	..	..	..	..	66	73	68	73	66	73
10 years	67	76	..	..	..	..	66	76	68	75	66	76

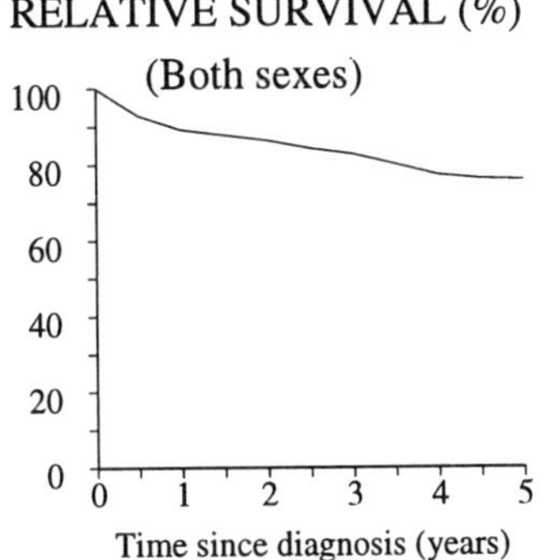

FRENCH REGISTRIES

REGISTRY	NUMBER OF CASES			PERIOD OF DIAGNOSIS
	Males	Females	All	
Amiens	14	17	31	1983-1984
Côte-d'Or	33	22	55	1980-1984
Doubs	47	42	89	1978-1985
Mean age (years)	39.0	37.9	38.5	

RELATIVE SURVIVAL (%)
(Both sexes)

100
80
60
40
20
0
0 1 2 3 4 5
Time since diagnosis (years)

OBSERVED AND RELATIVE SURVIVAL (%) BY PERIOD AND SEX
(Number of cases in parentheses)

	PERIOD						SEX					
	1978-80		1981-82		1983-85		Males		Females		All	
	obs	rel	obs	rel	obs	rel	obs	rel	obs	rel	obs	rel
N. Cases	(50)		(40)		(85)		(94)		(81)		(175)	
1 year	88	89	90	91	88	88	86	87	91	92	88	89
3 years	86	89	79	82	78	79	79	82	82	84	81	83
5 years	76	80	74	78	70	72	73	77	72	75	72	76
8 years	64	71	63	69	..	..	62	68	62	66	62	67
10 years	51	58	..	..	..	..	59	67	34	37	50	56

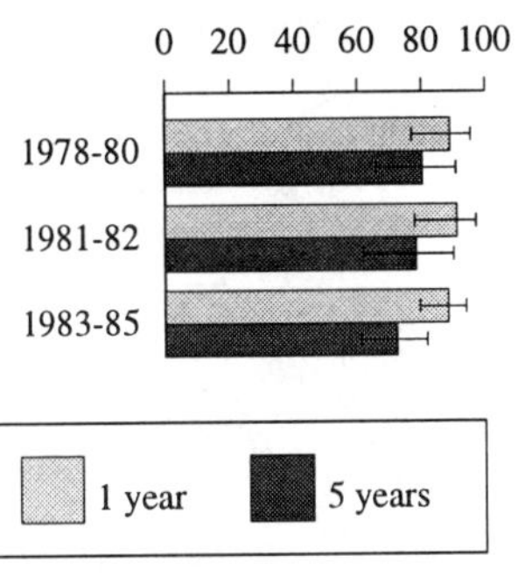

HODGKIN'S DISEASE

GERMAN REGISTRIES

REGISTRY	NUMBER OF CASES			PERIOD OF DIAGNOSIS
	Males	Females	All	
Saarland	95	70	165	1978-1984
Mean age (years)	44.3	46.9	45.4	

RELATIVE SURVIVAL (%)
(Both sexes)

Time since diagnosis (years)

OBSERVED AND RELATIVE SURVIVAL (%) BY PERIOD AND SEX
(Number of cases in parentheses)

	PERIOD						SEX					
	1978-80		1981-82		1983-85		Males		Females		All	
	obs	rel	obs	rel	obs	rel	obs	rel	obs	rel	obs	rel
N. Cases	(74)		(38)		(53)		(95)		(70)		(165)	
1 year	76	77	87	88	79	81	80	81	79	80	79	81
3 years	59	63	74	78	64	68	64	68	64	68	64	68
5 years	54	59	66	72	60	66	57	62	61	68	59	64
8 years	45	52	50	57	..	..	43	50	55	64	48	56
10 years	39	47	..	..	..	..	39	47	47	57	42	51

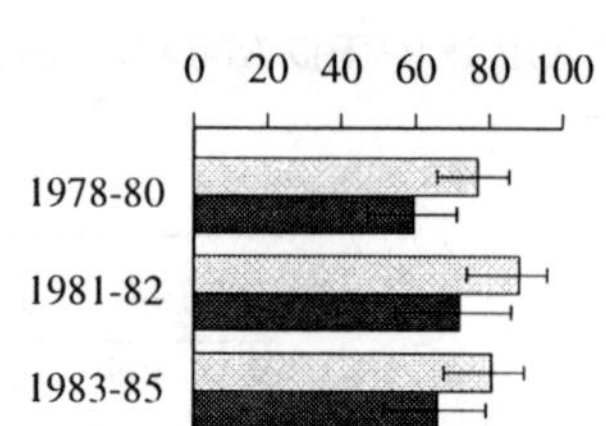

POLISH REGISTRIES

REGISTRY	NUMBER OF CASES			PERIOD OF DIAGNOSIS
	Males	Females	All	
Cracow	67	58	125	1978-1984
Mean age (years)	42.1	42.5	42.3	

RELATIVE SURVIVAL (%)
(Both sexes)

Time since diagnosis (years)

OBSERVED AND RELATIVE SURVIVAL (%) BY PERIOD AND SEX
(Number of cases in parentheses)

	PERIOD						SEX					
	1978-80		1981-82		1983-85		Males		Females		All	
	obs	rel	obs	rel	obs	rel	obs	rel	obs	rel	obs	rel
N. Cases	(43)		(38)		(44)		(67)		(58)		(125)	
1 year	77	78	89	90	81	81	81	82	83	83	82	83
3 years	64	66	83	86	60	62	66	69	71	73	68	71
5 years	58	63	73	78	55	58	61	66	63	66	62	66
8 years	45	51	70	78	48	54	48	55	60	67	54	60
10 years	39	46	67	76	..	..	42	50	57	65	49	56

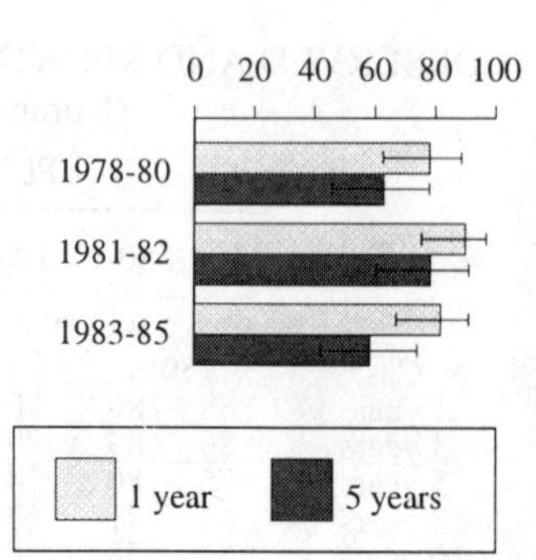

HODGKIN'S DISEASE

SPANISH REGISTRIES

REGISTRY	NUMBER OF CASES Males	Females	All	PERIOD OF DIAGNOSIS
Tarragona	8	4	12	1985-1985
Mean age (years)	44.8	60.3	49.9	

RELATIVE SURVIVAL (%)

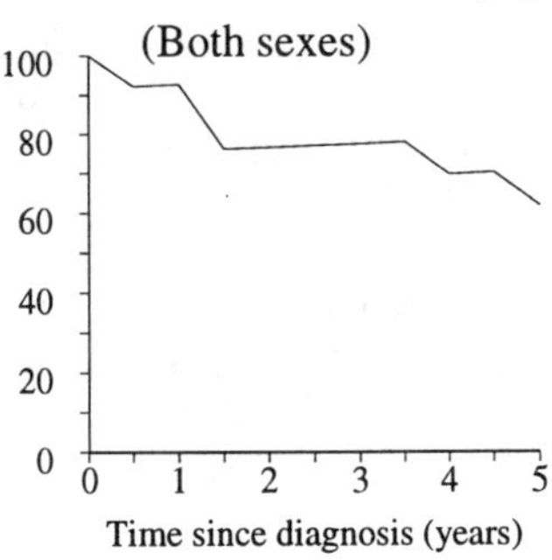

OBSERVED AND RELATIVE SURVIVAL (%) BY PERIOD AND SEX
(Number of cases in parentheses)

	PERIOD 1978-80 obs	rel	1981-82 obs	rel	1983-85 obs	rel	SEX Males obs	rel	Females obs	rel	All obs	rel
N. Cases	(0)		(0)		(12)		(8)		(4)		(12)	
1 year	..	..	..	..	92	93	100	100	75	77	92	93
3 years	..	..	..	..	75	78	88	89	50	53	75	78
5 years	..	..	..	..	58	62	75	78	25	28	58	62
8 years	..	..	..	..	..	..	..	..	..	..	..	..
10 years	..	..	..	..	..	..	..	..	..	..	..	..

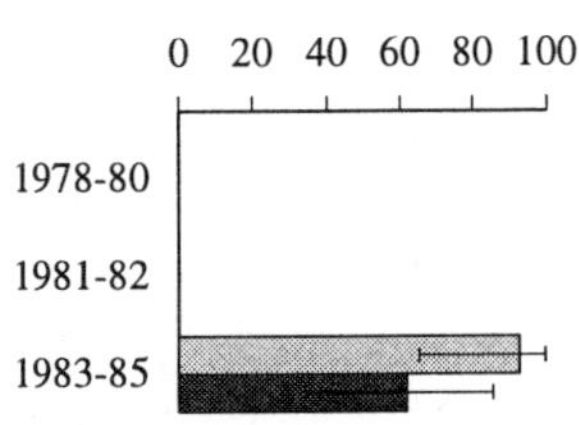

SWISS REGISTRIES

REGISTRY	NUMBER OF CASES Males	Females	All	PERIOD OF DIAGNOSIS
Basel	20	16	36	1981-1984
Geneva	38	25	63	1978-1984
Mean age (years)	44.3	42.8	43.7	

RELATIVE SURVIVAL (%)

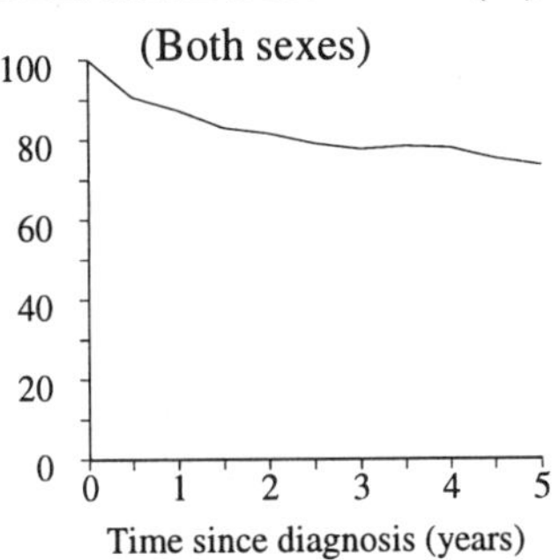

OBSERVED AND RELATIVE SURVIVAL (%) BY PERIOD AND SEX
(Number of cases in parentheses)

	PERIOD 1978-80 obs	rel	1981-82 obs	rel	1983-85 obs	rel	SEX Males obs	rel	Females obs	rel	All obs	rel
N. Cases	(33)		(31)		(35)		(58)		(41)		(99)	
1 year	88	90	77	79	91	92	84	86	88	89	86	87
3 years	76	82	64	69	79	82	68	73	80	84	73	78
5 years	73	82	54	61	74	77	65	72	70	76	67	74
8 years	..	..	54	66	..	..	57	69	70	83	63	75
10 years	..	..	..	..	..	..	..	..	..	..	..	..

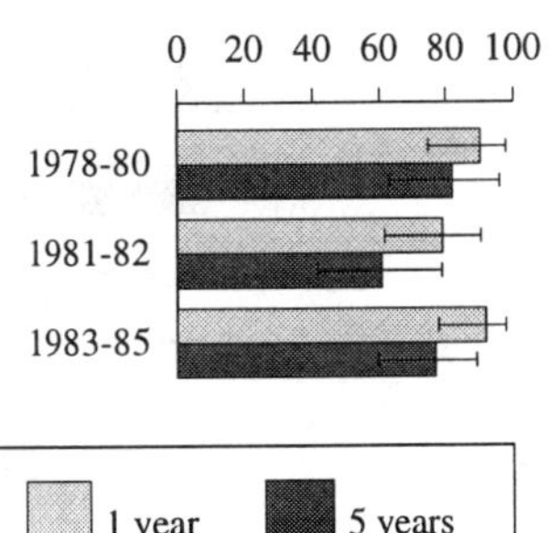

HODGKIN'S DISEASE

EUROPEAN REGISTRIES

Unweighted analysis

REGISTRY	CASES Males	Females	All
DENMARK	505	316	821
DUTCH REGISTRIES	80	57	137
ENGLISH REGISTRIES	1962	1315	3277
ESTONIA	92	110	202
FINLAND	453	328	781
FRENCH REGISTRIES	94	81	175
GERMAN REGISTRIES	95	70	165
ITALIAN REGISTRIES	143	92	235
POLISH REGISTRIES	67	58	125
SCOTLAND	396	303	699
SPANISH REGISTRIES	8	4	12
SWISS REGISTRIES	58	41	99
Mean age (years)	43.3	45.9	44.4

RELATIVE SURVIVAL (%)
(Age-standardized)

Females / Males

100 80 60 40 20 0 / 0 20 40 60 80 100

DK
ENG
EST
FIN
I
SCO
EUR

OBSERVED AND RELATIVE SURVIVAL (%) BY AGE AND PERIOD
(Number of cases in parentheses)

	AGE CLASS 15-44 obs	rel	45-54 obs	rel	55-64 obs	rel	65-74 obs	rel	75+ obs	rel	All obs	rel	PERIOD 1978-80 obs	rel	1981-82 obs	rel	1983-85 obs	rel
Males	(2242)		(493)		(502)		(473)		(243)		(3953)		(1676)		(1219)		(1058)	
1 year	93	93	83	83	71	73	52	54	37	42	81	82	78	79	81	83	85	86
3 years	84	84	66	68	54	57	32	37	20	29	68	71	64	68	67	70	74	77
5 years	78	78	59	61	45	51	23	30	14	26	61	66	58	63	60	65	67	72
8 years	73	74	50	54	33	41	13	21	10	30	54	62	51	59	53	61	60	67
10 years	68	70	43	48	25	33	9	17	10	44	49	58	46	56	49	58	..	..
Females	(1452)		(245)		(344)		(409)		(325)		(2775)		(1187)		(832)		(756)	
1 year	95	95	85	85	72	73	58	59	44	48	80	81	76	78	82	84	83	84
3 years	87	88	73	74	56	58	38	41	24	32	67	71	63	67	70	73	72	75
5 years	84	84	66	68	48	51	28	32	16	26	61	67	57	62	64	70	65	70
8 years	78	79	61	63	37	41	18	25	10	24	55	63	51	58	57	66	58	65
10 years	73	74	56	59	33	38	12	18	9	28	50	59	46	55	52	63	..	..
Overall	(3694)		(738)		(846)		(882)		(568)		(6728)		(2863)		(2051)		(1814)	
1 year	94	94	83	84	72	73	55	57	41	45	80	82	77	79	82	83	84	85
3 years	85	86	69	70	55	58	34	39	22	31	68	71	64	67	68	71	73	76
5 years	80	81	61	64	46	51	25	31	15	26	61	66	57	63	62	67	66	71
8 years	75	76	53	57	35	41	16	23	10	26	54	62	51	59	55	63	59	66
10 years	70	71	47	52	28	35	10	18	9	34	49	59	46	55	50	60	..	..

RELATIVE SURVIVAL (%) BY AGE AND PERIOD

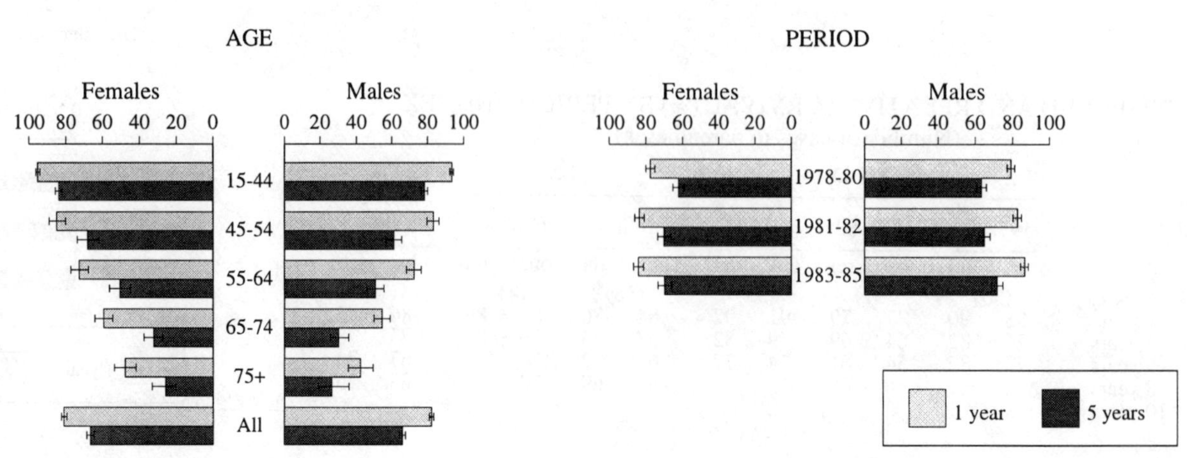

ACUTE LYMPHATIC LEUKAEMIA

DENMARK

REGISTRY	NUMBER OF CASES			PERIOD OF DIAGNOSIS
	Males	Females	All	
Denmark	105	69	174	1978-1984
Mean age (years)	44.3	46.6	45.2	

RELATIVE SURVIVAL (%)

— Males
- - Females

Time since diagnosis (years)

OBSERVED AND RELATIVE SURVIVAL (%) BY AGE AND PERIOD
(Number of cases in parentheses)

	AGE CLASS												PERIOD					
	15-44		45-54		55-64		65-74		75+		All		1978-80		1981-82		1983-85	
	obs	rel	obs	rel	obs	rel	obs	rel	obs	rel	obs	rel	obs	rel	obs	rel	obs	rel
Males	(57)		(5)		(14)		(14)		(15)		(105)		(37)		(30)		(38)	
1 year	63	63	40	40	36	36	21	22	7	7	45	46	54	55	40	41	39	41
3 years	30	30	0	0	14	15	14	16	0	0	20	21	24	26	17	18	18	20
5 years	28	28	0	0	7	8	14	18	0	0	18	20	22	24	17	18	16	18
8 years	18	18	0	0	..	..	..	..	0	0	12	14	11	13	17	19	..	..
10 years	18	18	0	0	..	..	..	..	0	0	12	14	11	13	..	..	..	..
Females	(34)		(5)		(12)		(9)		(9)		(69)		(26)		(14)		(29)	
1 year	68	68	80	80	25	25	33	34	33	35	52	53	58	58	57	58	45	45
3 years	32	32	20	20	8	9	11	12	11	13	22	23	23	24	29	30	17	18
5 years	20	20	20	21	8	9	11	13	0	0	14	15	15	16	21	24	10	10
8 years	20	21	0	0	..	..	..	..	0	0	12	14	12	13	21	26	..	..
10 years	20	21	0	0	..	..	..	..	0	0	12	14	12	13	..	..	..	..
Overall	(91)		(10)		(26)		(23)		(24)		(174)		(63)		(44)		(67)	
1 year	65	65	60	60	31	31	26	27	17	18	48	49	56	57	45	46	42	43
3 years	31	31	10	10	12	12	13	15	4	6	21	22	24	25	20	22	18	19
5 years	25	25	10	10	8	8	13	16	0	0	17	18	19	21	18	20	13	15
8 years	19	19	0	0	..	..	..	..	0	0	12	14	11	13	18	21	..	..
10 years	19	19	0	0	..	..	..	..	0	0	12	15	11	13	..	..	..	..

RELATIVE SURVIVAL (%) BY AGE AND PERIOD

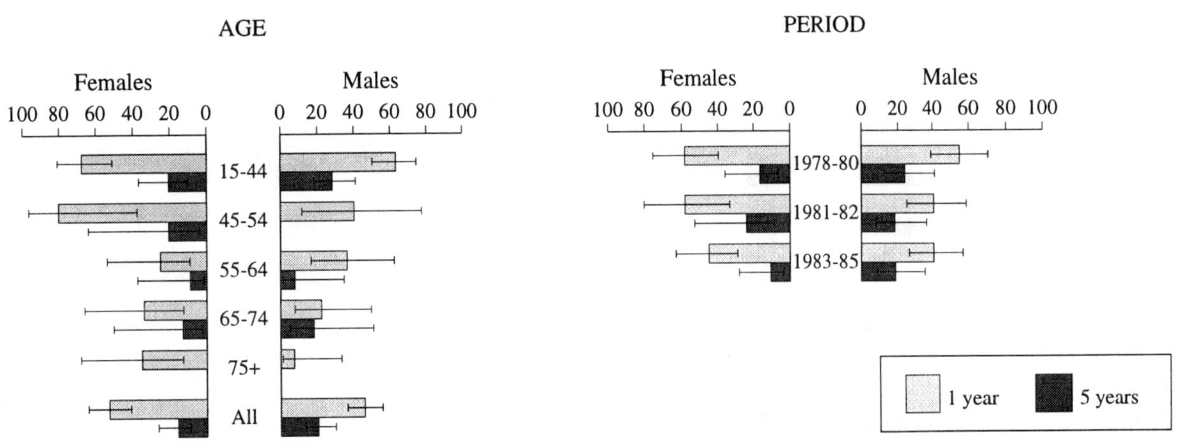

ACUTE LYMPHATIC LEUKAEMIA

ENGLISH REGISTRIES

REGISTRY	NUMBER OF CASES Males	Females	All	PERIOD OF DIAGNOSIS
East Anglia	36	15	51	1979-1984
South Thames	104	102	206	1978-1984
Wessex	24	29	53	1983-1984
West Midlands	95	74	169	1979-1984
Yorkshire	72	60	132	1978-1984
Mean age (years)	46.3	51.1	48.5	

RELATIVE SURVIVAL (%)

— Males
- - Females

Time since diagnosis (years)

OBSERVED AND RELATIVE SURVIVAL (%) BY AGE AND PERIOD
(Number of cases in parentheses)

	AGE CLASS 15-44 obs	rel	45-54 obs	rel	55-64 obs	rel	65-74 obs	rel	75+ obs	rel	All obs	rel	PERIOD 1978-80 obs	rel	1981-82 obs	rel	1983-85 obs	rel
Males	(164)		(26)		(36)		(59)		(46)		(331)		(120)		(92)		(119)	
1 year	70	70	58	58	23	24	17	18	2	2	45	47	52	53	43	45	39	41
3 years	34	34	19	20	9	9	5	6	0	0	20	22	18	19	18	20	24	26
5 years	23	23	19	20	3	3	5	7	0	0	14	16	13	14	10	11	19	23
8 years	20	20	..	..	..	..	3	6	0	0	12	15	10	12	10	12	15	20
10 years	19	19	..	..	..	..	3	7	0	0	11	15	9	12	..	..	..	..
Females	(117)		(16)		(36)		(49)		(62)		(280)		(102)		(67)		(111)	
1 year	74	74	56	56	42	42	22	23	13	14	46	47	47	49	45	46	46	47
3 years	44	44	36	36	16	16	10	11	6	9	26	28	24	27	27	29	26	28
5 years	35	36	29	29	12	13	8	9	5	9	21	24	19	22	22	25	21	24
8 years	34	34	20	21	12	14	8	11	..	..	18	23	18	23	17	21	21	25
10 years	34	34	..	..	12	14	..	..	..	..	18	24	18	25	..	..	..	..
Overall	(281)		(42)		(72)		(108)		(108)		(611)		(222)		(159)		(230)	
1 year	72	72	57	57	33	33	19	20	8	9	46	47	50	51	44	45	43	44
3 years	38	38	25	26	12	13	7	8	4	5	23	25	21	22	22	24	25	27
5 years	28	28	23	24	8	8	6	8	3	5	17	20	16	18	15	17	20	23
8 years	26	26	17	18	8	9	6	8	..	..	15	19	14	17	13	16	18	22
10 years	25	25	..	..	8	9	6	10	..	..	14	19	13	17	..	..	..	..

RELATIVE SURVIVAL (%) BY AGE AND PERIOD

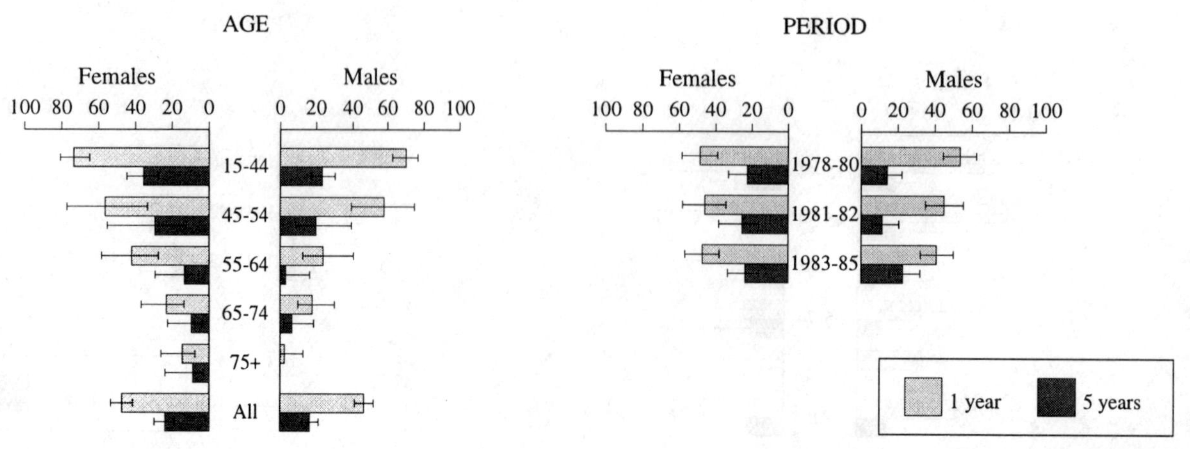

ACUTE LYMPHATIC LEUKAEMIA

FINLAND

REGISTRY	NUMBER OF CASES			PERIOD OF DIAGNOSIS
	Males	Females	All	
Finland	101	80	181	1978-1984
Mean age (years)	40.2	48.8	44.0	

RELATIVE SURVIVAL (%)

— Males
- - Females

100 80 60 40 20 0

0 1 2 3 4 5

Time since diagnosis (years)

OBSERVED AND RELATIVE SURVIVAL (%) BY AGE AND PERIOD
(Number of cases in parentheses)

	AGE CLASS												PERIOD					
	15-44		45-54		55-64		65-74		75+		All		1978-80		1981-82		1983-85	
	obs	rel	obs	rel	obs	rel	obs	rel	obs	rel	obs	rel	obs	rel	obs	rel	obs	rel
Males	(62)		(6)		(13)		(10)		(10)		(101)		(42)		(33)		(26)	
1 year	66	66	67	67	23	24	50	53	0	0	52	54	52	53	48	50	58	59
3 years	24	24	17	17	0	0	0	0	0	0	16	17	10	10	15	17	27	28
5 years	16	16	17	18	0	0	0	0	0	0	11	12	7	8	12	14	15	17
8 years	11	11	17	18	0	0	0	0	0	0	8	9	2	3	12	16	12	13
10 years	11	11	0	0	0	0	0	0	0	0	6	8	2	3	9	12	..	..
Females	(37)		(3)		(16)		(17)		(7)		(80)		(38)		(22)		(20)	
1 year	65	65	33	33	44	44	47	48	29	31	52	53	55	56	55	55	45	45
3 years	30	30	0	0	13	13	18	19	0	0	20	21	16	16	18	19	30	31
5 years	24	24	0	0	6	7	0	0	0	0	13	13	5	6	18	20	20	21
8 years	14	14	0	0	..	..	0	0	0	0	7	8	5	6	9	10	10	11
10 years	14	14	0	0	..	..	0	0	0	0	7	9	5	6	9	11	..	..
Overall	(99)		(9)		(29)		(27)		(17)		(181)		(80)		(55)		(46)	
1 year	66	66	56	56	34	35	48	50	12	13	52	53	54	54	51	52	52	53
3 years	26	26	11	11	7	7	11	12	0	0	18	19	13	13	16	18	28	30
5 years	19	19	11	12	3	4	0	0	0	0	12	13	6	7	15	16	17	19
8 years	12	12	11	12	..	..	0	0	0	0	8	9	4	4	11	13	11	12
10 years	12	12	0	0	..	..	0	0	0	0	7	8	4	4	9	11	..	..

RELATIVE SURVIVAL (%) BY AGE AND PERIOD

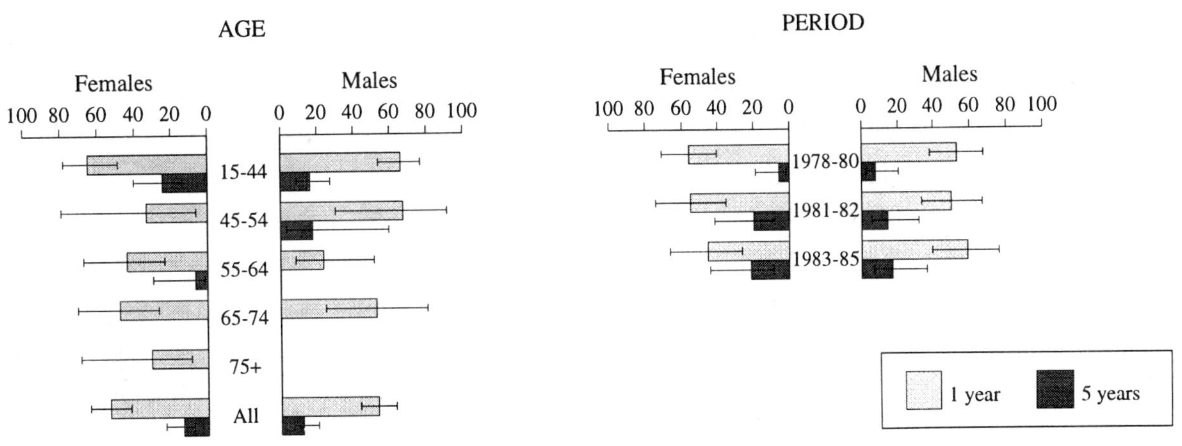

ACUTE LYMPHATIC LEUKAEMIA

DUTCH REGISTRIES

REGISTRY	NUMBER OF CASES Males	Females	All	PERIOD OF DIAGNOSIS
Eindhoven	11	9	20	1978-1985
Mean age (years)	41.1	44.1	42.5	

RELATIVE SURVIVAL (%)
(Both sexes)

100
80
60
40
20
0
0 1 2 3 4 5
Time since diagnosis (years)

OBSERVED AND RELATIVE SURVIVAL (%) BY PERIOD AND SEX
(Number of cases in parentheses)

	PERIOD						SEX					
	1978-80		1981-82		1983-85		Males		Females		All	
	obs	rel	obs	rel	obs	rel	obs	rel	obs	rel	obs	rel
N. Cases	(9)		(4)		(7)		(11)		(9)		(20)	
1 year	67	67	75	76	57	58	64	65	67	67	65	66
3 years	41	42	50	53	41	43	42	44	43	45	43	45
5 years	27	29	50	55	..	..	42	46	26	28	35	38
8 years	27	30	..	..	..	..	42	49	26	29	35	40
10 years	..	..	..	..	..	..	..	..	..	..	..	..

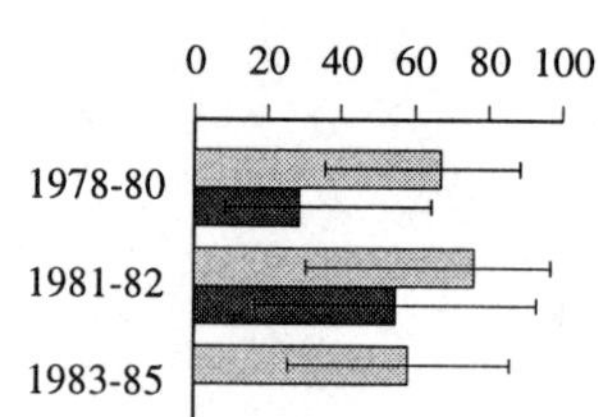

ESTONIA

REGISTRY	NUMBER OF CASES Males	Females	All	PERIOD OF DIAGNOSIS
Estonia	12	19	31	1978-1984
Mean age (years)	54.9	52.6	53.5	

RELATIVE SURVIVAL (%)
(Both sexes)

100
80
60
40
20
0
0 1 2 3 4 5
Time since diagnosis (years)

OBSERVED AND RELATIVE SURVIVAL (%) BY PERIOD AND SEX
(Number of cases in parentheses)

	PERIOD						SEX					
	1978-80		1981-82		1983-85		Males		Females		All	
	obs	rel	obs	rel	obs	rel	obs	rel	obs	rel	obs	rel
N. Cases	(15)		(3)		(13)		(12)		(19)		(31)	
1 year	20	20	67	69	31	32	17	17	37	37	29	30
3 years	0	0	0	0	8	9	0	0	5	6	3	3
5 years	0	0	0	0	0	0	0	0	0	0	0	0
8 years	0	0	0	0	0	0	0	0	0	0	0	0
10 years	0	0	0	0	0	0	0	0	0	0	0	0

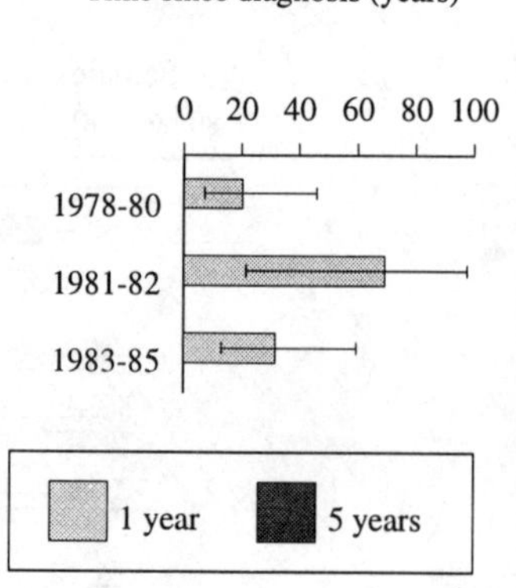

ACUTE LYMPHATIC LEUKAEMIA

FRENCH REGISTRIES

REGISTRY	NUMBER OF CASES			PERIOD OF DIAGNOSIS
	Males	Females	All	
Côte-d'Or	9	7	16	1980-1984
Mean age (years)	44.9	43.1	44.1	

RELATIVE SURVIVAL (%)
(Both sexes)

Time since diagnosis (years)

OBSERVED AND RELATIVE SURVIVAL (%) BY PERIOD AND SEX
(Number of cases in parentheses)

	PERIOD						SEX					
	1978-80		1981-82		1983-85		Males		Females		All	
	obs	rel	obs	rel	obs	rel	obs	rel	obs	rel	obs	rel
N. Cases	(3)		(5)		(8)		(9)		(7)		(16)	
1 year	67	67	80	80	63	65	56	57	86	86	69	70
3 years	33	34	40	40	38	42	33	36	43	44	38	40
5 years	33	34	20	20	38	45	33	39	29	30	31	34
8 years	0	0	0	0	..	..	..	..	0	0	..	..
10 years	0	0	0	0	..	..	..	..	0	0	..	..

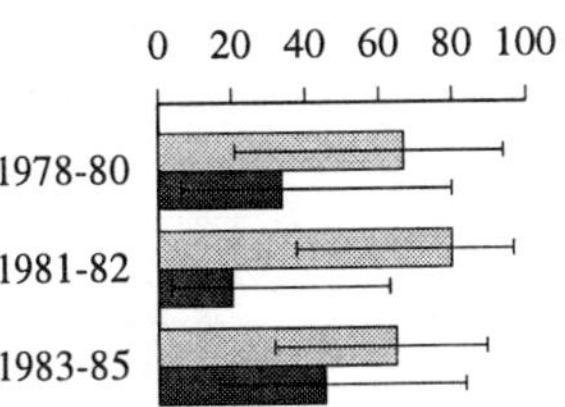

GERMAN REGISTRIES

REGISTRY	NUMBER OF CASES			PERIOD OF DIAGNOSIS
	Males	Females	All	
Saarland	18	8	26	1978-1984
Mean age (years)	49.6	49.0	49.4	

RELATIVE SURVIVAL (%)
(Both sexes)

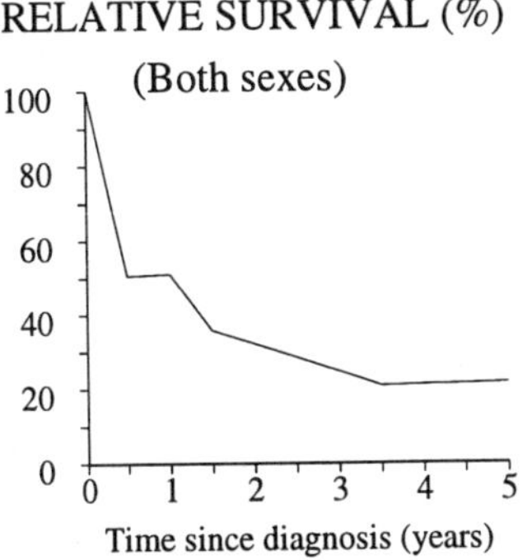

OBSERVED AND RELATIVE SURVIVAL (%) BY PERIOD AND SEX
(Number of cases in parentheses)

	PERIOD						SEX					
	1978-80		1981-82		1983-85		Males		Females		All	
	obs	rel	obs	rel	obs	rel	obs	rel	obs	rel	obs	rel
N. Cases	(11)		(8)		(7)		(18)		(8)		(26)	
1 year	55	56	38	38	57	58	50	51	50	51	50	51
3 years	27	30	13	13	29	30	22	24	25	26	23	25
5 years	18	21	13	14	29	31	17	19	25	27	19	22
8 years	0	0	..	..	..	..	..	..	0	0	..	..
10 years	0	0	..	..	..	..	..	..	0	0	..	..

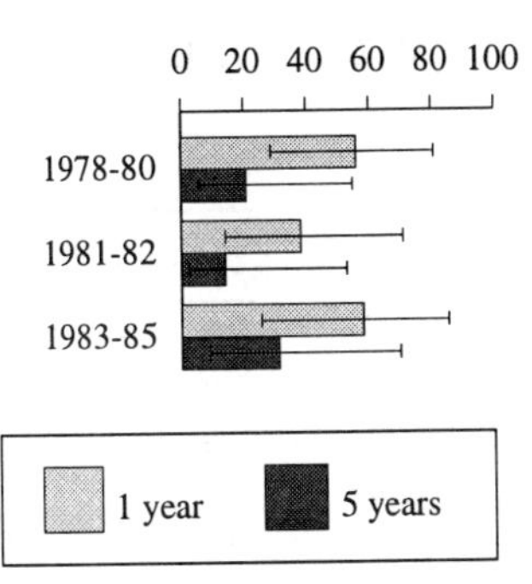

ACUTE LYMPHATIC LEUKAEMIA

ITALIAN REGISTRIES

REGISTRY	NUMBER OF CASES Males	Females	All	PERIOD OF DIAGNOSIS
Latina	4	4	8	1983-1984
Ragusa	5	6	11	1981-1984
Varese	21	13	34	1978-1984
Mean age (years)	46.5	52.5	49.1	

RELATIVE SURVIVAL (%)
(Both sexes)

100 80 60 40 20 0

0 1 2 3 4 5

Time since diagnosis (years)

OBSERVED AND RELATIVE SURVIVAL (%) BY PERIOD AND SEX
(Number of cases in parentheses)

	PERIOD						SEX					
	1978-80		1981-82		1983-85		Males		Females		All	
	obs	rel	obs	rel	obs	rel	obs	rel	obs	rel	obs	rel
N. Cases	(6)		(19)		(28)		(30)		(23)		(53)	
1 year	67	68	53	54	46	48	50	51	52	54	51	52
3 years	17	18	16	17	32	35	23	25	26	29	25	27
5 years	17	19	11	12	25	29	20	23	17	21	19	22
8 years	17	21	5	7	21	26	13	16	17	23	15	18
10 years	17	22	..	..	..	..	13	16	..	..	15	19

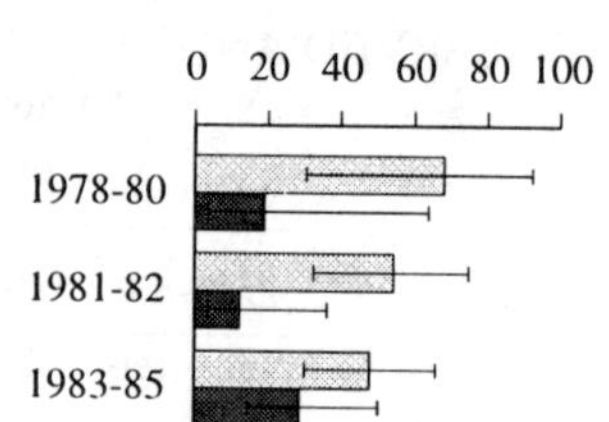

POLISH REGISTRIES

REGISTRY	NUMBER OF CASES Males	Females	All	PERIOD OF DIAGNOSIS
Cracow	11	11	22	1978-1984
Mean age (years)	48.5	40.6	44.5	

RELATIVE SURVIVAL (%)
(Both sexes)

100 80 60 40 20 0

0 1 2 3 4 5

Time since diagnosis (years)

OBSERVED AND RELATIVE SURVIVAL (%) BY PERIOD AND SEX
(Number of cases in parentheses)

	PERIOD						SEX					
	1978-80		1981-82		1983-85		Males		Females		All	
	obs	rel	obs	rel	obs	rel	obs	rel	obs	rel	obs	rel
N. Cases	(6)		(8)		(8)		(11)		(11)		(22)	
1 year	33	34	38	38	..	..	14	15	36	37	25	26
3 years	17	18	13	13	..	..	0	0	18	19	10	11
5 years	17	19	0	0	..	..	0	0	9	9	5	6
8 years	17	21	0	0	..	..	0	0	9	10	5	6
10 years	17	22	0	0	..	..	0	0	9	10	5	6

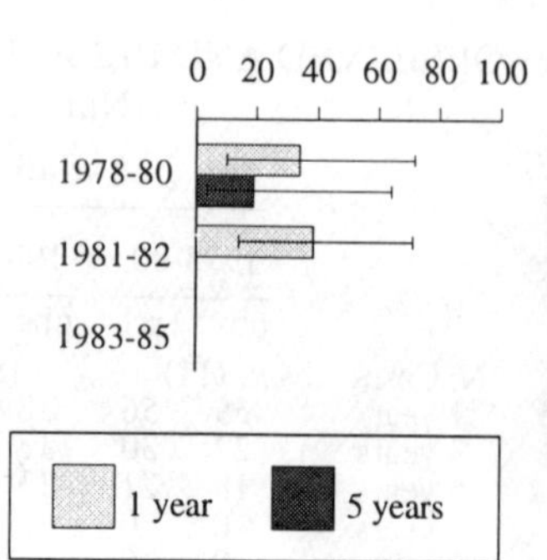

ACUTE LYMPHATIC LEUKAEMIA

SCOTLAND

REGISTRY	NUMBER OF CASES			PERIOD OF DIAGNOSIS
	Males	Females	All	
Scotland	56	31	87	1978-1982
Mean age (years)	46.7	45.6	46.3	

RELATIVE SURVIVAL (%)
(Both sexes)

100
80
60
40
20
0
0 1 2 3 4 5
Time since diagnosis (years)

OBSERVED AND RELATIVE SURVIVAL (%) BY PERIOD AND SEX
(Number of cases in parentheses)

	PERIOD						SEX					
	1978-80		1981-82		1983-85		Males		Females		All	
	obs	rel	obs	rel	obs	rel	obs	rel	obs	rel	obs	rel
N. Cases	(56)		(31)		(0)		(56)		(31)		(87)	
1 year	41	42	52	53	..	..	38	39	58	59	45	46
3 years	25	27	23	24	..	..	20	22	32	34	24	26
5 years	23	27	19	22	..	..	18	21	29	32	22	25
8 years	20	25	..	..	..	..	14	18	29	34	19	24
10 years	20	26	..	..	..	..	..	..	29	36	19	26

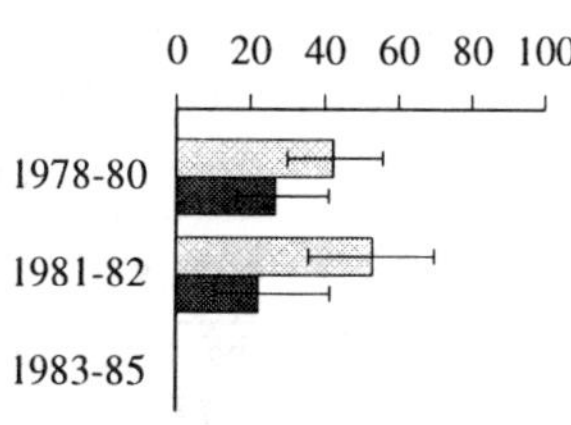

SPANISH REGISTRIES

REGISTRY	NUMBER OF CASES			PERIOD OF DIAGNOSIS
	Males	Females	All	
Tarragona	5	0	5	1985-1985
Mean age (years)	46.6	..	46.6	

RELATIVE SURVIVAL (%)

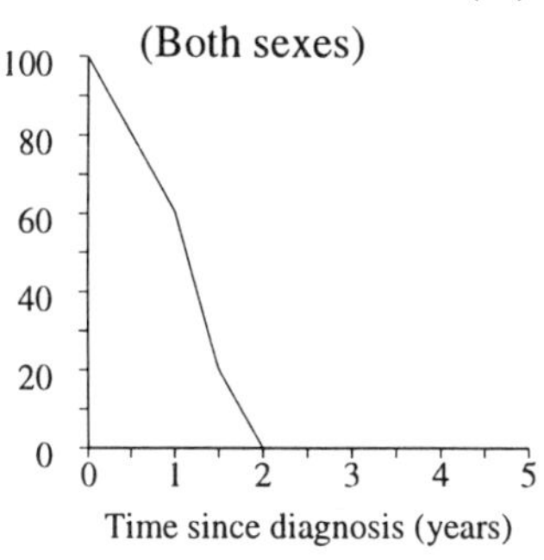

OBSERVED AND RELATIVE SURVIVAL (%) BY PERIOD AND SEX
(Number of cases in parentheses)

	PERIOD						SEX					
	1978-80		1981-82		1983-85		Males		Females		All	
	obs	rel	obs	rel	obs	rel	obs	rel	obs	rel	obs	rel
N. Cases	(0)		(0)		(5)		(5)		(0)		(5)	
1 year	..	..	..	..	60	61	60	61	..	..	60	61
3 years	..	..	..	..	0	0	0	0	..	..	0	0
5 years	..	..	..	..	0	0	0	0	..	..	0	0
8 years	..	..	..	..	0	0	0	0	..	..	0	0
10 years	..	..	..	..	0	0	0	0	..	..	0	0

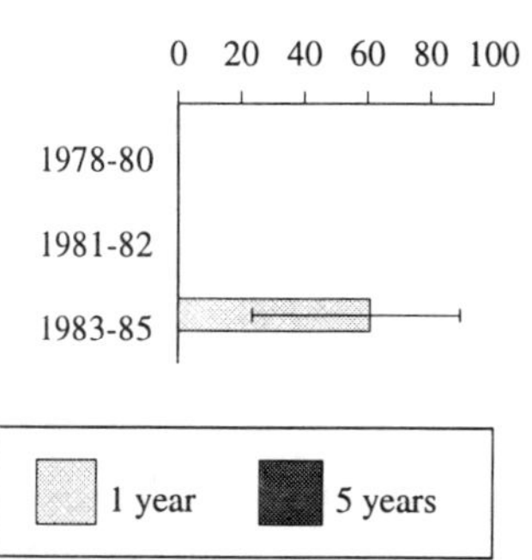

ACUTE LYMPHATIC LEUKAEMIA

SWISS REGISTRIES

REGISTRY	NUMBER OF CASES			PERIOD OF DIAGNOSIS
	Males	Females	All	
Basel	6	6	12	1981-1984
Geneva	5	4	9	1978-1984
Mean age (years)	42.5	42.1	42.3	

RELATIVE SURVIVAL (%)
(Both sexes)

Time since diagnosis (years)

OBSERVED AND RELATIVE SURVIVAL (%) BY PERIOD AND SEX
(Number of cases in parentheses)

	PERIOD						SEX					
	1978-80		1981-82		1983-85		Males		Females		All	
	obs	rel	obs	rel	obs	rel	obs	rel	obs	rel	obs	rel
N. Cases	(3)		(5)		(13)		(11)		(10)		(21)	
1 year	0	0	20	20	54	54	36	37	40	40	38	39
3 years	0	0	0	0	15	16	18	19	0	0	10	10
5 years	0	0	0	0	15	16	18	20	0	0	10	10
8 years	0	0	0	0	..	..	..	..	0	0	..	..
10 years	0	0	0	0	..	..	..	..	0	0	..	..

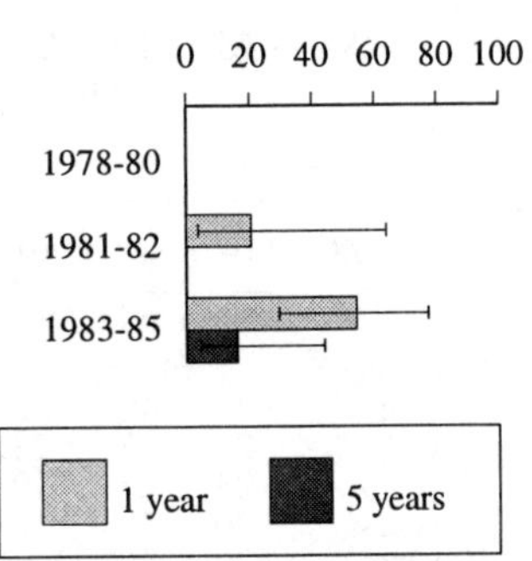

ACUTE LYMPHATIC LEUKAEMIA

EUROPEAN REGISTRIES

Unweighted analysis

REGISTRY	CASES Males	Females	All
DENMARK	105	69	174
DUTCH REGISTRIES	11	9	20
ENGLISH REGISTRIES	331	280	611
ESTONIA	12	19	31
FINLAND	101	80	181
FRENCH REGISTRIES	9	7	16
GERMAN REGISTRIES	18	8	26
ITALIAN REGISTRIES	30	23	53
POLISH REGISTRIES	11	11	22
SCOTLAND	56	31	87
SPANISH REGISTRIES	5	0	5
SWISS REGISTRIES	11	10	21
Mean age (years)	45.3	49.4	47.1

RELATIVE SURVIVAL (%)
(Age-standardized)

Females / Males

100 80 60 40 20 0 / 0 20 40 60 80 100

DK
ENG
FIN
EUR

OBSERVED AND RELATIVE SURVIVAL (%) BY AGE AND PERIOD
(Number of cases in parentheses)

	AGE CLASS 15-44 obs	rel	45-54 obs	rel	55-64 obs	rel	65-74 obs	rel	75+ obs	rel	All obs	rel	PERIOD 1978-80 obs	rel	1981-82 obs	rel	1983-85 obs	rel
Males	(360)		(53)		(82)		(113)		(92)		(700)		(266)		(199)		(235)	
1 year	66	66	49	49	31	32	22	23	4	5	45	47	49	51	43	44	42	44
3 years	30	30	15	15	11	12	8	9	0	0	19	21	18	19	17	18	23	25
5 years	23	23	15	16	7	8	7	9	0	0	15	17	14	16	12	14	19	22
8 years	18	18	11	12	7	9	4	6	0	0	11	14	10	11	11	14	14	18
10 years	17	17	0	0	..	..	4	7	0	0	10	14	9	11	10	13	..	..
Females	(244)		(33)		(77)		(98)		(95)		(547)		(208)		(142)		(197)	
1 year	73	73	58	58	36	37	28	28	18	20	49	50	50	51	52	53	46	47
3 years	40	40	26	26	11	11	12	13	5	7	24	26	22	24	25	27	24	26
5 years	31	31	23	23	8	9	6	7	3	5	18	20	16	18	20	22	18	20
8 years	27	27	13	13	8	9	6	8	..	..	15	18	14	17	14	17	17	20
10 years	27	27	..	..	8	9	..	..	..	..	15	19	14	18	14	18	..	..
Overall	(604)		(86)		(159)		(211)		(187)		(1247)		(474)		(341)		(432)	
1 year	69	69	52	53	34	34	25	26	11	12	47	48	50	51	47	48	44	45
3 years	34	34	19	20	11	12	10	11	3	4	21	23	20	21	20	22	24	26
5 years	26	26	18	19	8	9	6	8	2	3	16	18	15	17	15	17	18	21
8 years	22	22	11	12	8	9	5	7	..	..	13	16	12	14	13	16	15	19
10 years	21	21	0	0	8	10	5	8	..	..	12	16	11	14	11	15	..	..

RELATIVE SURVIVAL (%) BY AGE AND PERIOD

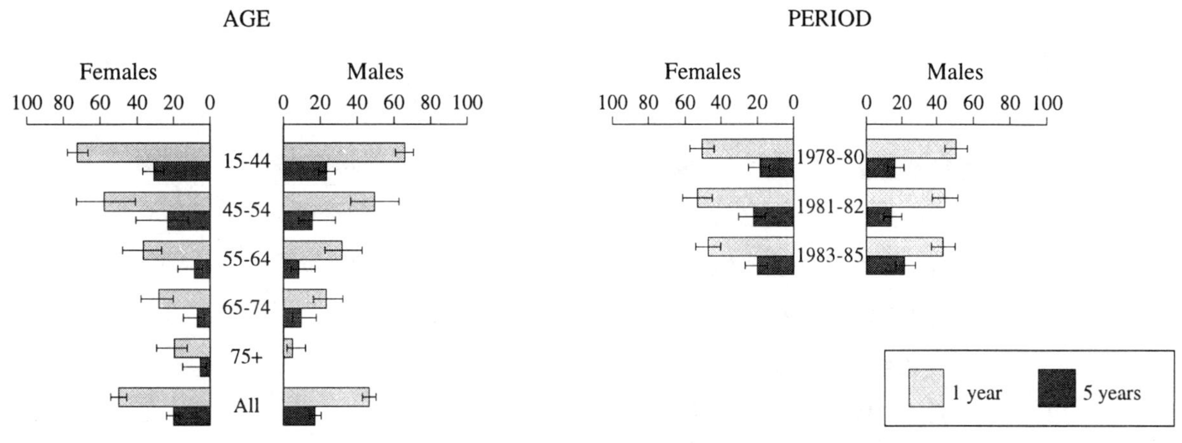

CHRONIC LYMPHATIC LEUKAEMIA

DENMARK

REGISTRY	NUMBER OF CASES			PERIOD OF DIAGNOSIS
	Males	Females	All	
Denmark	962	613	1575	1978-1984
Mean age (years)	69.6	71.5	70.3	

RELATIVE SURVIVAL (%)

— Males
- - Females

Time since diagnosis (years)

OBSERVED AND RELATIVE SURVIVAL (%) BY AGE AND PERIOD
(Number of cases in parentheses)

	AGE CLASS												PERIOD					
	15-44		45-54		55-64		65-74		75+		All		1978-80		1981-82		1983-85	
	obs	rel	obs	rel	obs	rel	obs	rel	obs	rel	obs	rel	obs	rel	obs	rel	obs	rel
Males	(17)		(64)		(192)		(376)		(313)		(962)		(390)		(271)		(301)	
1 year	94	94	94	94	83	84	67	70	52	59	68	72	65	69	69	73	69	73
3 years	76	77	77	78	67	71	47	54	26	38	47	56	43	52	50	60	49	58
5 years	64	65	64	67	49	54	28	37	10	19	29	40	26	36	32	44	33	44
8 years	64	66	30	33	24	29	15	24	4	12	15	25	14	25	11	20	..	..
10 years	64	66	7	7	15	20	10	19	3	14	9	19	9	18	..	..	..	..
Females	(10)		(32)		(104)		(210)		(257)		(613)		(245)		(170)		(198)	
1 year	100	100	94	94	87	87	80	82	56	61	72	76	71	74	74	77	72	76
3 years	90	90	81	82	75	78	64	69	34	44	54	63	54	62	55	63	54	63
5 years	70	71	72	74	58	62	50	57	21	34	41	52	38	49	44	56	40	53
8 years	..	..	42	44	38	42	27	35	10	25	23	35	22	34	17	25	..	..
10 years	..	..	42	45	27	31	14	20	7	22	15	26	15	25	..	..	..	..
Overall	(27)		(96)		(296)		(586)		(570)		(1575)		(635)		(441)		(499)	
1 year	96	96	94	94	84	85	72	75	54	60	69	73	68	71	71	75	71	74
3 years	81	82	78	80	70	73	53	60	30	41	50	59	47	56	52	61	51	60
5 years	66	67	66	69	52	57	36	45	15	26	34	45	31	41	37	49	36	48
8 years	61	62	34	37	29	34	19	28	7	19	18	30	17	28	13	22	..	..
10 years	61	62	20	23	19	24	11	20	5	18	12	22	11	21	..	..	..	..

RELATIVE SURVIVAL (%) BY AGE AND PERIOD

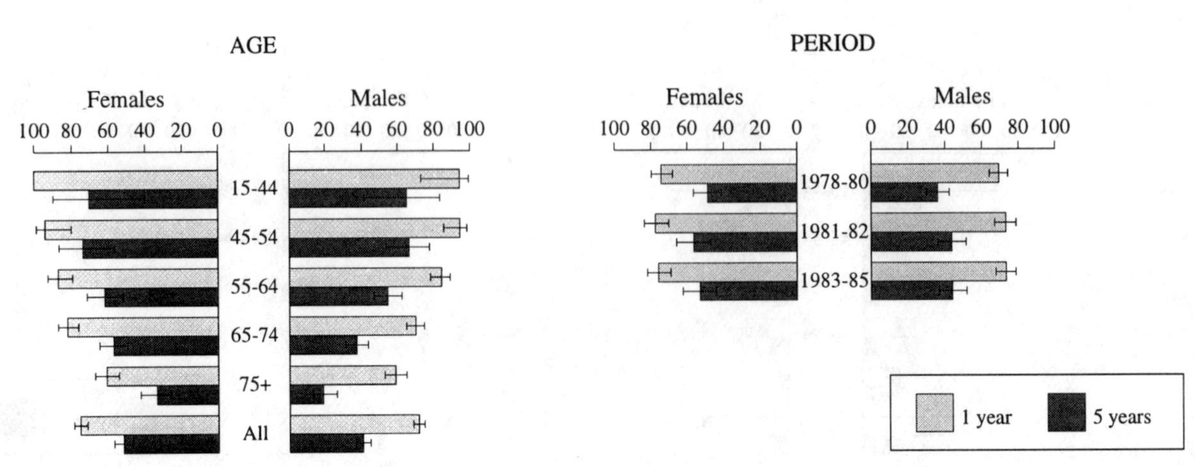

CHRONIC LYMPHATIC LEUKAEMIA

ENGLISH REGISTRIES

REGISTRY	NUMBER OF CASES			PERIOD OF DIAGNOSIS
	Males	Females	All	
East Anglia	208	126	334	1979-1984
South Thames	550	487	1037	1978-1984
Wessex	99	66	165	1983-1984
West Midlands	443	256	699	1979-1984
Yorkshire	374	288	662	1978-1984
Mean age (years)	69.8	73.7	71.4	

RELATIVE SURVIVAL (%)

100
80
60
40
20
0
— Males
- - Females
0 1 2 3 4 5
Time since diagnosis (years)

OBSERVED AND RELATIVE SURVIVAL (%) BY AGE AND PERIOD
(Number of cases in parentheses)

	AGE CLASS												PERIOD					
	15-44		45-54		55-64		65-74		75+		All		1978-80		1981-82		1983-85	
	obs	rel	obs	rel	obs	rel	obs	rel	obs	rel	obs	rel	obs	rel	obs	rel	obs	rel
Males	(22)		(120)		(354)		(589)		(589)		(1674)		(623)		(482)		(569)	
1 year	86	87	89	90	80	82	69	73	50	57	67	71	68	73	65	70	66	71
3 years	73	73	77	78	63	67	48	56	30	45	47	58	48	59	49	59	45	55
5 years	68	69	60	62	45	51	32	42	17	34	32	45	31	43	36	51	29	41
8 years	38	39	42	45	27	33	15	25	7	24	17	30	17	30	20	34	14	25
10 years	38	40	35	39	18	24	10	20	4	22	12	24	13	25	9	18	..	..
Females	(15)		(46)		(165)		(373)		(624)		(1223)		(476)		(347)		(400)	
1 year	93	93	96	96	83	84	78	80	52	58	66	70	63	67	67	71	69	73
3 years	80	80	85	86	70	72	55	60	29	41	45	55	42	51	45	55	49	59
5 years	47	47	76	78	57	61	42	49	18	32	33	46	31	43	34	46	35	48
8 years	35	36	56	59	37	41	23	31	8	22	19	32	18	31	19	32	24	41
10 years	23	24	50	54	34	40	17	26	5	20	15	30	14	28	15	29	..	..
Overall	(37)		(166)		(519)		(962)		(1213)		(2897)		(1099)		(829)		(969)	
1 year	89	89	91	92	81	82	73	76	51	58	66	71	66	70	66	70	67	72
3 years	76	76	79	81	65	69	50	57	30	43	46	56	46	56	47	57	46	57
5 years	59	60	64	67	49	54	36	45	17	33	32	45	31	43	35	49	31	44
8 years	36	37	46	49	30	36	18	28	8	23	18	31	17	30	19	33	18	30
10 years	30	31	39	43	23	29	13	23	5	20	13	26	13	27	11	22	..	..

RELATIVE SURVIVAL (%) BY AGE AND PERIOD

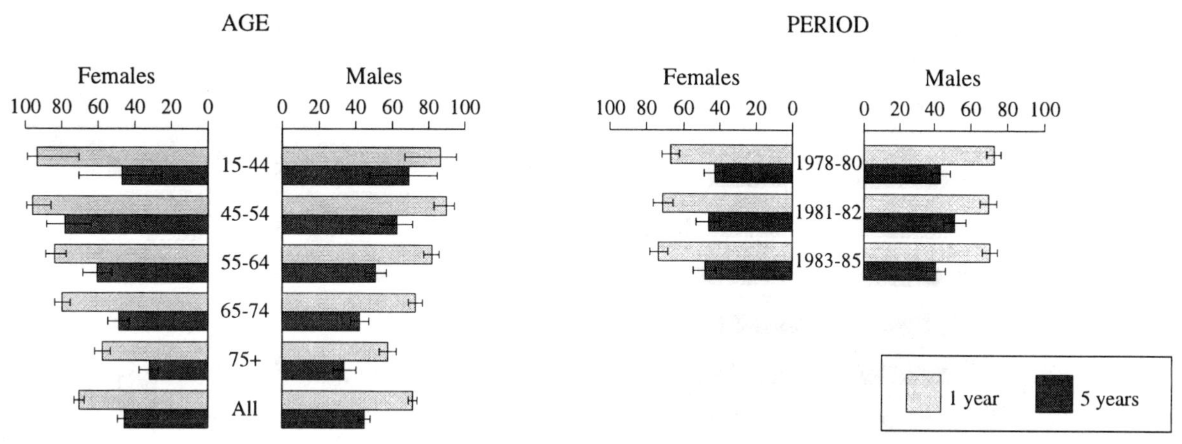

CHRONIC LYMPHATIC LEUKAEMIA

ESTONIA

REGISTRY	NUMBER OF CASES			PERIOD OF DIAGNOSIS
	Males	Females	All	
Estonia	191	177	368	1978-1984
Mean age (years)	64.2	66.1	65.1	

RELATIVE SURVIVAL (%)

100 80 60 40 20 0

— Males
- - Females

0 1 2 3 4 5

Time since diagnosis (years)

OBSERVED AND RELATIVE SURVIVAL (%) BY AGE AND PERIOD
(Number of cases in parentheses)

	AGE CLASS												PERIOD					
	15-44		45-54		55-64		65-74		75+		All		1978-80		1981-82		1983-85	
	obs	rel	obs	rel	obs	rel	obs	rel	obs	rel	obs	rel	obs	rel	obs	rel	obs	rel
Males	(9)		(31)		(56)		(58)		(37)		(191)		(68)		(49)		(74)	
1 year	78	78	94	95	89	92	78	82	57	64	80	84	79	83	80	84	80	84
3 years	67	68	87	91	77	84	55	66	32	48	63	74	62	72	63	75	63	74
5 years	41	42	70	77	46	55	34	47	24	48	42	55	39	51	44	60	43	56
8 years	41	44	45	53	33	45	20	37	13	45	28	46	23	36	36	61	..	..
10 years	41	45	36	44	19	28	20	46	..	..	20	38	16	29	..	..	..	..
Females	(6)		(26)		(37)		(66)		(42)		(177)		(75)		(46)		(56)	
1 year	83	83	92	93	84	85	76	78	52	57	75	77	76	79	70	72	77	79
3 years	67	67	85	86	70	73	59	65	43	58	62	69	68	76	52	59	61	68
5 years	50	51	73	75	68	72	47	56	31	54	51	63	60	73	36	45	52	63
8 years	..	..	53	55	59	67	45	65	13	35	40	58	46	64	29	43	..	..
10 years	..	..	45	48	59	71	35	60	..	..	33	54	37	58	..	..	..	..
Overall	(15)		(57)		(93)		(124)		(79)		(368)		(143)		(95)		(130)	
1 year	80	80	93	94	87	89	77	80	54	60	77	81	78	81	75	78	78	82
3 years	67	68	86	89	74	79	57	66	38	53	62	71	65	74	58	67	62	72
5 years	45	47	71	76	55	62	40	52	28	51	46	59	50	63	40	52	47	60
8 years	34	36	50	56	43	54	35	56	12	38	34	52	35	51	33	52	..	..
10 years	34	36	42	48	30	42	28	55	..	..	27	47	27	45	..	..	..	..

RELATIVE SURVIVAL (%) BY AGE AND PERIOD

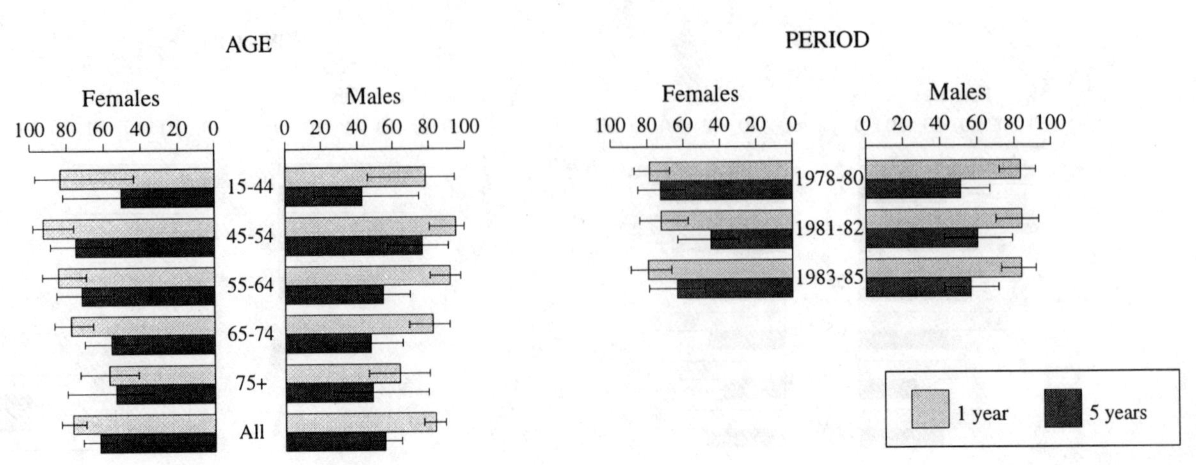

CHRONIC LYMPHATIC LEUKAEMIA

FINLAND

REGISTRY	NUMBER OF CASES			PERIOD OF DIAGNOSIS
	Males	Females	All	
Finland	444	377	821	1978-1984
Mean age (years)	68.4	71.2	69.7	

RELATIVE SURVIVAL (%)

100
80
60
40
20
0
— Males
- - Females
0 1 2 3 4 5
Time since diagnosis (years)

OBSERVED AND RELATIVE SURVIVAL (%) BY AGE AND PERIOD
(Number of cases in parentheses)

	AGE CLASS												PERIOD					
	15-44		45-54		55-64		65-74		75+		All		1978-80		1981-82		1983-85	
	obs	rel	obs	rel	obs	rel	obs	rel	obs	rel	obs	rel	obs	rel	obs	rel	obs	rel
Males	(4)		(46)		(102)		(157)		(135)		(444)		(190)		(133)		(121)	
1 year	100	100	91	92	86	88	76	80	59	67	75	80	72	76	82	87	73	77
3 years	100	100	67	70	64	68	57	67	33	49	52	63	49	60	59	71	51	62
5 years	75	77	52	55	44	50	32	43	15	30	32	44	32	45	35	49	29	39
8 years	25	26	26	29	25	32	16	27	4	14	16	27	16	27	18	31	9	15
10 years	0	0	18	21	11	14	5	10	..	..	6	12	6	13	7	13	..	..
Females	(6)		(23)		(68)		(114)		(166)		(377)		(156)		(113)		(108)	
1 year	100	100	96	96	88	89	86	88	75	82	82	87	85	89	80	83	82	87
3 years	83	84	83	83	68	70	68	73	46	61	59	69	60	70	57	65	61	71
5 years	83	84	65	66	56	59	45	52	23	38	39	51	42	55	35	45	39	51
8 years	50	51	54	56	35	38	15	21	6	16	18	28	21	32	13	21	21	32
10 years	0	0	41	42	21	24	7	11	1	3	9	15	10	18	0	0	..	..
Overall	(10)		(69)		(170)		(271)		(301)		(821)		(346)		(246)		(229)	
1 year	100	100	93	93	87	89	80	84	68	75	78	83	77	82	81	85	77	82
3 years	90	91	72	74	65	69	61	70	40	56	56	66	54	64	58	68	56	66
5 years	80	81	57	59	49	54	38	47	19	35	35	47	37	49	35	47	34	45
8 years	36	37	36	39	29	34	16	24	5	15	17	27	18	29	16	26	13	21
10 years	0	0	25	28	14	18	6	10	1	3	7	14	8	15	5	9	..	..

RELATIVE SURVIVAL (%) BY AGE AND PERIOD

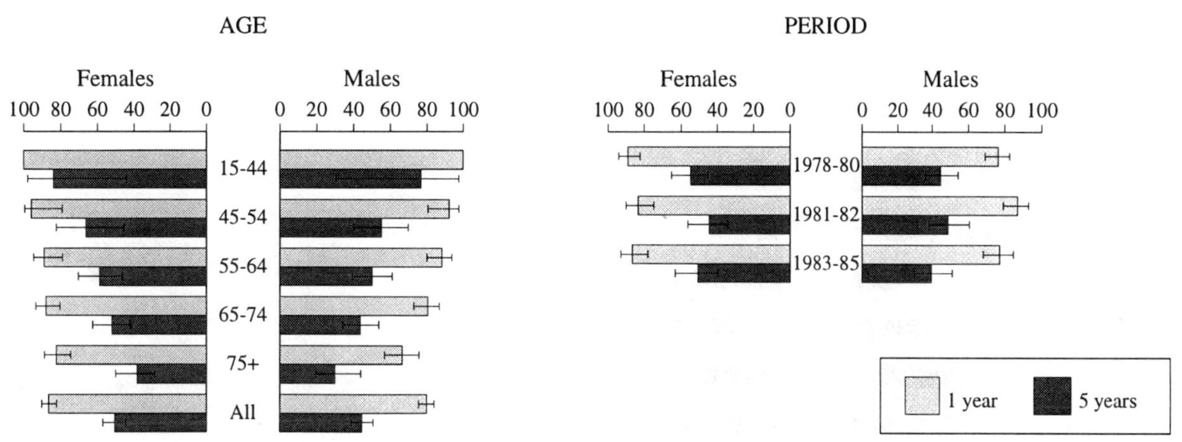

CHRONIC LYMPHATIC LEUKAEMIA

ITALIAN REGISTRIES

REGISTRY	NUMBER OF CASES Males	Females	All	PERIOD OF DIAGNOSIS
Latina	11	7	18	1983-1984
Ragusa	12	7	19	1981-1984
Varese	83	75	158	1978-1984
Mean age (years)	68.1	68.5	68.2	

RELATIVE SURVIVAL (%)

100
80
60
40
20
0
— Males
- - Females
0 1 2 3 4 5
Time since diagnosis (years)

OBSERVED AND RELATIVE SURVIVAL (%) BY AGE AND PERIOD
(Number of cases in parentheses)

	AGE CLASS 15-44 obs	rel	45-54 obs	rel	55-64 obs	rel	65-74 obs	rel	75+ obs	rel	All obs	rel	PERIOD 1978-80 obs	rel	1981-82 obs	rel	1983-85 obs	rel
Males	(4)		(8)		(21)		(46)		(27)		(106)		(29)		(35)		(42)	
1 year	100	100	88	88	90	92	85	89	59	68	80	85	83	87	83	89	76	80
3 years	100	100	75	77	67	71	57	66	33	51	56	67	48	57	57	71	60	70
5 years	100	100	38	39	57	64	46	60	22	47	43	59	34	46	49	70	45	59
8 years	50	51	..	..	47	57	32	53	12	42	30	49	24	39	31	56	20	31
10 years	0	0	..	..	47	62	22	44	6	31	20	38	14	25	28	60	..	..
Females	(2)		(9)		(16)		(34)		(28)		(89)		(36)		(23)		(30)	
1 year	100	100	78	78	81	82	88	90	64	71	79	82	83	86	91	96	63	66
3 years	50	50	78	79	69	71	59	63	39	55	56	64	64	71	65	75	40	46
5 years	50	50	78	79	50	52	44	50	36	63	46	57	56	67	48	61	33	42
8 years	50	50	53	55	44	48	32	40	18	48	32	45	44	60	30	45	19	26
10 years	50	50	53	55	44	49	32	43	7	24	29	44	42	61	10	16	..	..
Overall	(6)		(17)		(37)		(80)		(55)		(195)		(65)		(58)		(72)	
1 year	100	100	82	83	86	88	86	89	62	70	79	84	83	87	86	92	71	74
3 years	83	84	76	78	68	71	58	65	36	53	56	65	57	65	60	73	51	60
5 years	83	84	59	61	54	59	45	55	29	56	45	58	46	58	48	66	40	52
8 years	50	51	36	38	46	53	32	47	15	46	31	47	35	51	31	51	21	31
10 years	25	26	36	39	46	55	28	46	7	28	25	42	29	47	19	36	..	..

RELATIVE SURVIVAL (%) BY AGE AND PERIOD

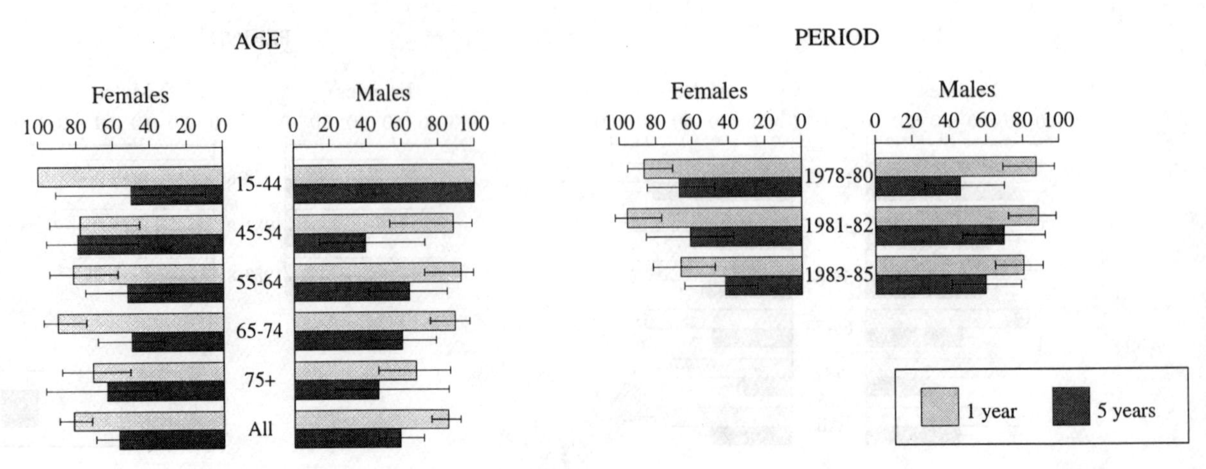

CHRONIC LYMPHATIC LEUKAEMIA

SCOTLAND

REGISTRY	NUMBER OF CASES			PERIOD OF DIAGNOSIS
	Males	Females	All	
Scotland	347	221	568	1978-1982
Mean age (years)	69.4	73.1	70.8	

RELATIVE SURVIVAL (%)

OBSERVED AND RELATIVE SURVIVAL (%) BY AGE AND PERIOD
(Number of cases in parentheses)

	AGE CLASS												PERIOD					
	15-44		45-54		55-64		65-74		75+		All		1978-80		1981-82		1983-85	
	obs	rel	obs	rel	obs	rel	obs	rel	obs	rel	obs	rel	obs	rel	obs	rel	obs	rel
Males	(5)		(27)		(64)		(136)		(115)		(347)		(205)		(142)		(0)	
1 year	100	100	100	100	83	85	60	64	57	65	67	72	65	70	70	75	..	..
3 years	60	60	78	80	72	77	40	48	26	41	44	55	39	49	52	64	..	..
5 years	60	61	78	82	52	59	26	36	12	26	31	45	28	41	35	50	..	..
8 years	40	41	61	68	39	49	12	21	2	8	17	32	15	28	..	..	..	..
10 years	..	..	39	45	..	..	12	26	0	0	14	31	12	27	..	..	..	..
Females	(4)		(6)		(29)		(78)		(104)		(221)		(125)		(96)		(0)	
1 year	75	75	83	84	90	91	76	78	50	56	66	70	65	70	67	70	..	..
3 years	75	75	67	68	76	79	63	69	33	46	51	62	50	61	52	62	..	..
5 years	75	76	67	69	69	74	47	57	19	35	38	53	39	56	36	49	..	..
8 years	..	..	67	71	50	57	29	39	5	15	22	37	23	41	..	..	..	..
10 years	..	..	..	..	..	..	18	28	5	21	16	33	17	36	..	..	..	..
Overall	(9)		(33)		(93)		(214)		(219)		(568)		(330)		(238)		(0)	
1 year	89	89	97	98	85	87	66	69	53	61	66	71	65	70	68	73	..	..
3 years	67	67	76	78	73	78	48	56	29	43	47	58	43	54	52	63	..	..
5 years	67	67	76	80	57	64	34	45	16	31	34	48	32	47	36	50	..	..
8 years	52	53	63	69	43	52	18	29	4	12	19	34	18	33	..	..	..	..
10 years	..	..	45	51	..	..	13	25	2	9	15	31	14	30	..	..	..	..

RELATIVE SURVIVAL (%) BY AGE AND PERIOD

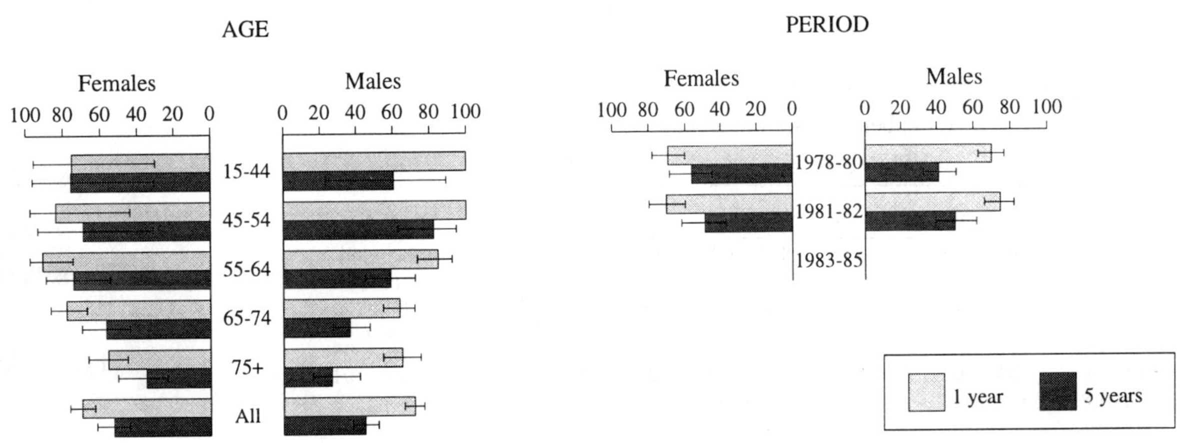

CHRONIC LYMPHATIC LEUKAEMIA

DUTCH REGISTRIES

REGISTRY	NUMBER OF CASES			PERIOD OF DIAGNOSIS
	Males	Females	All	
Eindhoven	77	45	122	1978-1985
Mean age (years)	66.8	70.4	68.2	

RELATIVE SURVIVAL (%)
(Both sexes)

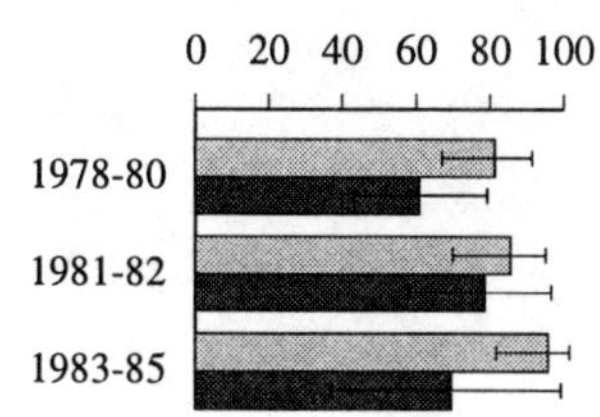

OBSERVED AND RELATIVE SURVIVAL (%) BY PERIOD AND SEX
(Number of cases in parentheses)

	PERIOD						SEX					
	1978-80		1981-82		1983-85		Males		Females		All	
	obs	rel	obs	rel	obs	rel	obs	rel	obs	rel	obs	rel
N. Cases	(48)		(38)		(36)		(77)		(45)		(122)	
1 year	77	81	82	85	92	96	84	89	80	84	83	87
3 years	60	71	71	82	81	92	66	77	76	86	70	81
5 years	46	61	61	79	54	69	49	65	64	82	55	71
8 years	31	51	..	..	..	..	35	57	44	69	38	61
10 years	0	0	..	..	..	..	0	0	0	0	0	0

FRENCH REGISTRIES

REGISTRY	NUMBER OF CASES			PERIOD OF DIAGNOSIS
	Males	Females	All	
Côte-d'Or	83	48	131	1980-1984
Mean age (years)	67.7	73.2	69.7	

RELATIVE SURVIVAL (%)
(Both sexes)

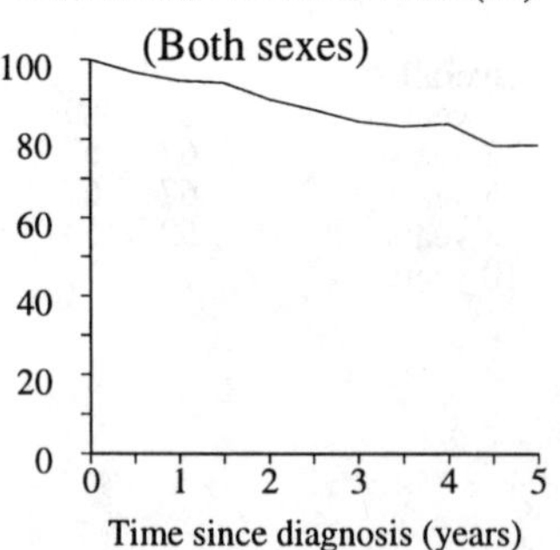

OBSERVED AND RELATIVE SURVIVAL (%) BY PERIOD AND SEX
(Number of cases in parentheses)

	PERIOD						SEX					
	1978-80		1981-82		1983-85		Males		Females		All	
	obs	rel	obs	rel	obs	rel	obs	rel	obs	rel	obs	rel
N. Cases	(20)		(59)		(52)		(83)		(48)		(131)	
1 year	85	92	90	94	90	96	90	95	87	94	89	95
3 years	60	76	71	83	75	89	73	87	66	81	71	85
5 years	45	66	59	77	63	85	60	79	55	77	58	79
8 years	34	62	36	57	..	..	36	57	39	69	37	61
10 years	..	..	..	..	..	..	..	..	..	..	..	..

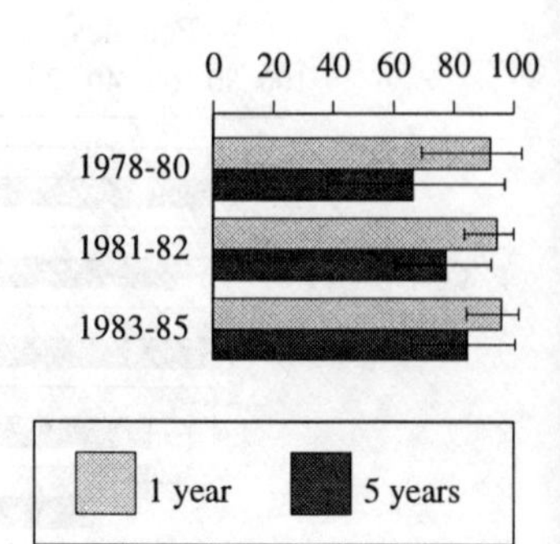

CHRONIC LYMPHATIC LEUKAEMIA

GERMAN REGISTRIES

REGISTRY	NUMBER OF CASES			PERIOD OF DIAGNOSIS
	Males	Females	All	
Saarland	92	53	145	1978-1984
Mean age (years)	66.3	70.1	67.7	

RELATIVE SURVIVAL (%)
(Both sexes)

100
80
60
40
20
0
0 1 2 3 4 5
Time since diagnosis (years)

OBSERVED AND RELATIVE SURVIVAL (%) BY PERIOD AND SEX
(Number of cases in parentheses)

	PERIOD						SEX					
	1978-80		1981-82		1983-85		Males		Females		All	
	obs	rel	obs	rel	obs	rel	obs	rel	obs	rel	obs	rel
N. Cases	(57)		(42)		(46)		(92)		(53)		(145)	
1 year	67	71	71	75	76	79	68	72	75	79	71	75
3 years	49	59	52	62	48	54	50	59	49	56	50	58
5 years	39	52	43	57	39	48	42	56	36	45	40	52
8 years	19	32	26	42	..	..	26	42	18	27	23	36
10 years	14	26	..	..	..	..	20	37	12	21	17	31

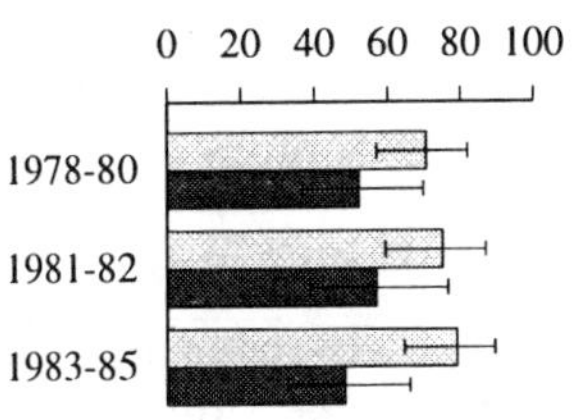

POLISH REGISTRIES

REGISTRY	NUMBER OF CASES			PERIOD OF DIAGNOSIS
	Males	Females	All	
Cracow	42	22	64	1978-1984
Mean age (years)	64.1	63.4	63.9	

RELATIVE SURVIVAL (%)
(Both sexes)

100
80
60
40
20
0
0 1 2 3 4 5
Time since diagnosis (years)

OBSERVED AND RELATIVE SURVIVAL (%) BY PERIOD AND SEX
(Number of cases in parentheses)

	PERIOD						SEX					
	1978-80		1981-82		1983-85		Males		Females		All	
	obs	rel	obs	rel	obs	rel	obs	rel	obs	rel	obs	rel
N. Cases	(29)		(15)		(20)		(42)		(22)		(64)	
1 year	62	64	38	40	50	52	52	54	55	56	53	55
3 years	31	34	23	28	40	46	27	32	41	45	32	36
5 years	17	20	15	21	20	25	12	16	27	32	18	22
8 years	7	9	8	14	..	..	3	5	11	15	6	9
10 years	7	10	..	..	..	..	3	6	11	16	6	10

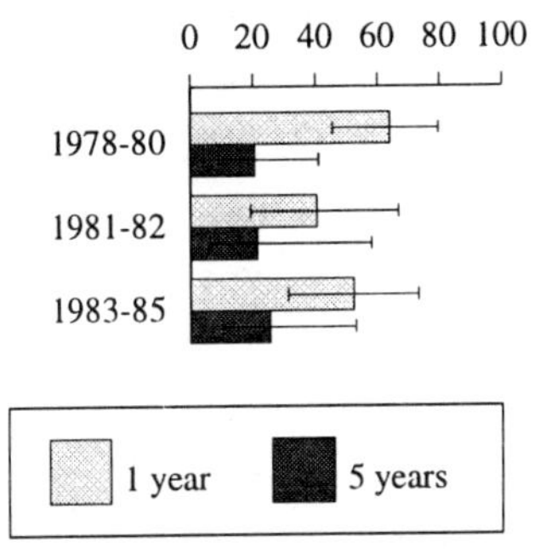

CHRONIC LYMPHATIC LEUKAEMIA

SPANISH REGISTRIES

REGISTRY	NUMBER OF CASES Males	Females	All	PERIOD OF DIAGNOSIS
Tarragona	4	2	6	1985-1985
Mean age (years)	65.0	69.5	66.5	

RELATIVE SURVIVAL (%)
(Both sexes)

Time since diagnosis (years)

OBSERVED AND RELATIVE SURVIVAL (%) BY PERIOD AND SEX
(Number of cases in parentheses)

	PERIOD						SEX					
	1978-80		1981-82		1983-85		Males		Females		All	
	obs	rel	obs	rel	obs	rel	obs	rel	obs	rel	obs	rel
N. Cases	(0)		(0)		(6)		(4)		(2)		(6)	
1 year	..	..	..	..	50	51	50	51	50	51	50	51
3 years	..	..	..	..	50	53	50	53	50	53	50	53
5 years	..	..	..	..	50	56	50	56	50	56	50	56
8 years	..	..	..	..	..	..	..	..	..	..	..	..
10 years	..	..	..	..	..	..	..	..	..	..	..	..

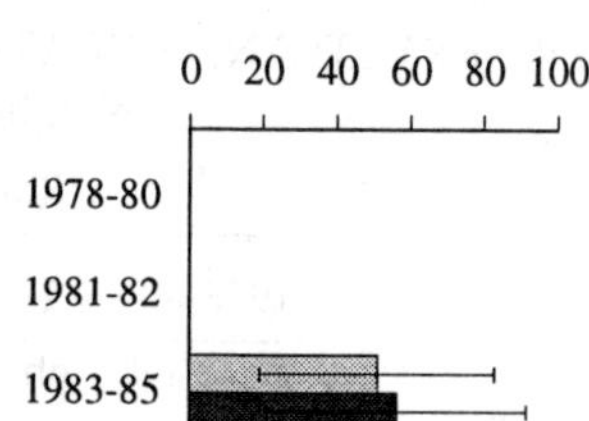

SWISS REGISTRIES

REGISTRY	NUMBER OF CASES Males	Females	All	PERIOD OF DIAGNOSIS
Basel	31	29	60	1981-1984
Geneva	51	48	99	1978-1984
Mean age (years)	68.7	71.4	70.0	

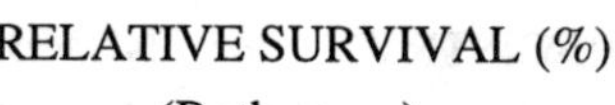

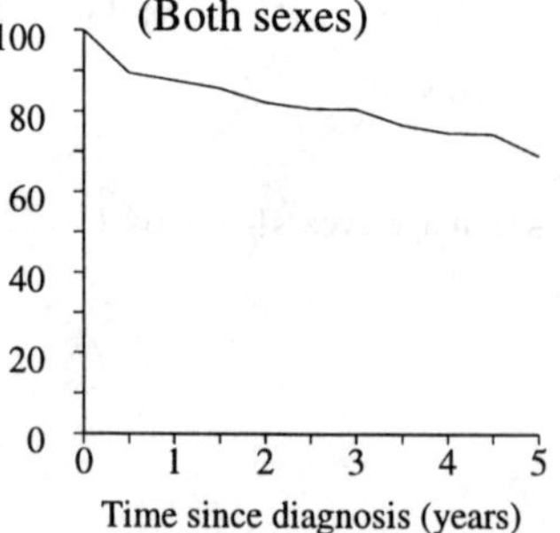

OBSERVED AND RELATIVE SURVIVAL (%) BY PERIOD AND SEX
(Number of cases in parentheses)

	PERIOD						SEX					
	1978-80		1981-82		1983-85		Males		Females		All	
	obs	rel	obs	rel	obs	rel	obs	rel	obs	rel	obs	rel
N. Cases	(30)		(60)		(69)		(82)		(77)		(159)	
1 year	83	88	80	84	87	91	85	90	82	85	84	88
3 years	73	87	56	66	80	91	72	84	67	77	70	81
5 years	57	75	41	54	63	79	57	75	50	63	54	69
8 years	..	..	33	55	..	..	37	61	41	64	39	63
10 years	..	..	..	..	..	..	0	0	..	..	..	..

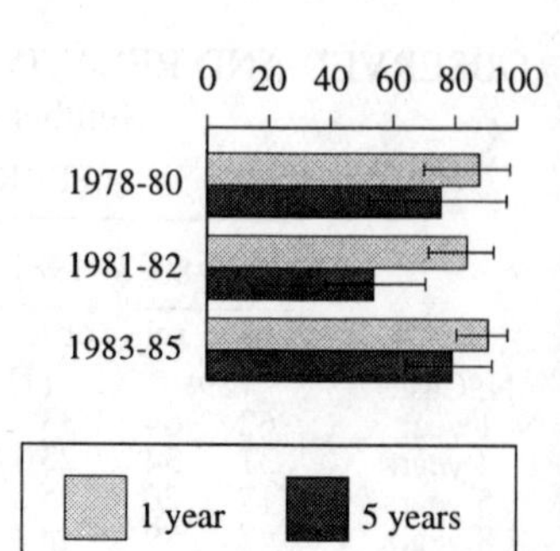

CHRONIC LYMPHATIC LEUKAEMIA

EUROPEAN REGISTRIES

Unweighted analysis

REGISTRY	CASES Males	Females	All
DENMARK	962	613	1575
DUTCH REGISTRIES	77	45	122
ENGLISH REGISTRIES	1674	1223	2897
ESTONIA	191	177	368
FINLAND	444	377	821
FRENCH REGISTRIES	83	48	131
GERMAN REGISTRIES	92	53	145
ITALIAN REGISTRIES	106	89	195
POLISH REGISTRIES	42	22	64
SCOTLAND	347	221	568
SPANISH REGISTRIES	4	2	6
SWISS REGISTRIES	82	77	159
Mean age (years)	69.0	72.0	70.2

RELATIVE SURVIVAL (%)
(Age-standardized)

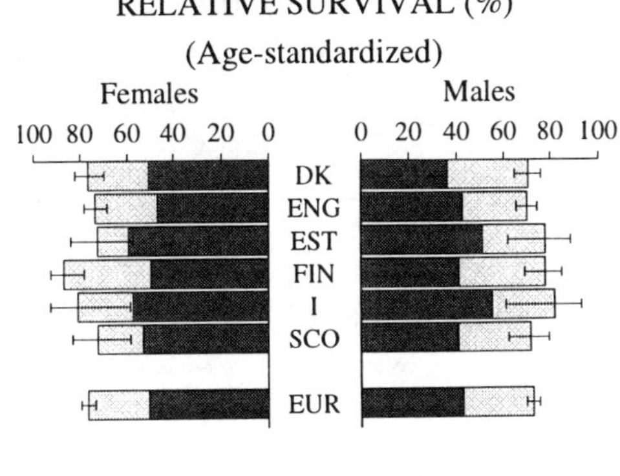

OBSERVED AND RELATIVE SURVIVAL (%) BY AGE AND PERIOD
(Number of cases in parentheses)

	AGE CLASS 15-44 obs	rel	45-54 obs	rel	55-64 obs	rel	65-74 obs	rel	75+ obs	rel	All obs	rel	PERIOD 1978-80 obs	rel	1981-82 obs	rel	1983-85 obs	rel
Males	(77)		(338)		(872)		(1501)		(1316)		(4104)		(1616)		(1239)		(1249)	
1 year	91	91	92	93	83	85	70	74	53	61	70	74	69	73	71	75	70	75
3 years	77	77	77	79	66	71	49	58	30	45	50	60	47	57	52	63	50	61
5 years	69	70	62	66	48	54	32	43	15	31	33	46	31	43	37	51	34	47
8 years	46	48	39	43	29	36	16	27	6	20	18	31	17	29	20	35	15	26
10 years	37	39	28	31	18	24	10	20	3	17	12	23	11	23	9	19	..	..
Females	(47)		(163)		(463)		(953)		(1321)		(2947)		(1186)		(882)		(879)	
1 year	94	94	93	93	85	86	80	82	57	63	71	75	69	73	72	76	73	77
3 years	77	77	83	84	71	74	60	65	35	47	52	61	51	60	52	61	54	63
5 years	60	60	73	75	59	62	46	53	21	37	38	51	38	50	39	51	39	52
8 years	41	41	53	56	39	43	27	35	9	24	22	36	23	36	21	34	26	41
10 years	23	24	47	50	32	38	19	28	5	17	16	30	17	31	11	20	..	..
Overall	(124)		(501)		(1335)		(2454)		(2637)		(7051)		(2802)		(2121)		(2128)	
1 year	92	92	92	93	84	85	74	77	55	62	70	75	69	73	71	75	72	76
3 years	77	77	79	80	68	72	54	61	32	46	51	61	49	58	52	62	52	62
5 years	65	66	66	68	52	57	38	47	18	34	36	48	34	46	37	51	36	49
8 years	44	46	44	47	32	39	20	31	8	22	20	33	19	32	21	35	19	31
10 years	31	32	34	38	23	29	14	24	4	17	14	26	13	26	10	20	..	..

RELATIVE SURVIVAL (%) BY AGE AND PERIOD

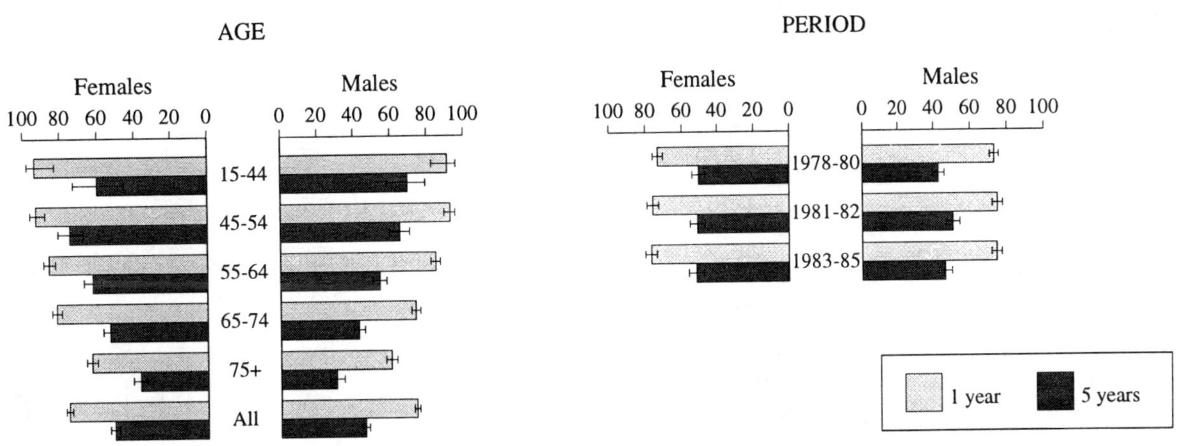

ACUTE MYELOID LEUKAEMIA

DENMARK

REGISTRY	NUMBER OF CASES Males	Females	All	PERIOD OF DIAGNOSIS
Denmark	619	578	1197	1978-1984
Mean age (years)	63.0	64.1	63.6	

RELATIVE SURVIVAL (%)

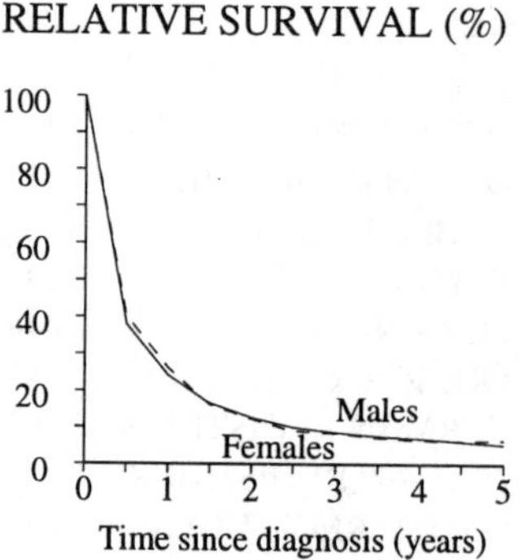

OBSERVED AND RELATIVE SURVIVAL (%) BY AGE AND PERIOD
(Number of cases in parentheses)

	AGE CLASS												PERIOD					
	15-44		45-54		55-64		65-74		75+		All		1978-80		1981-82		1983-85	
	obs	rel	obs	rel	obs	rel	obs	rel	obs	rel	obs	rel	obs	rel	obs	rel	obs	rel
Males	(95)		(55)		(118)		(188)		(163)		(619)		(281)		(151)		(187)	
1 year	51	51	22	22	25	26	21	22	9	10	23	24	21	22	26	28	24	25
3 years	21	21	11	11	8	8	5	6	1	1	7	9	5	6	10	11	9	10
5 years	13	14	5	6	5	6	3	3	0	0	4	5	4	5	4	5	5	6
8 years	8	8	5	6	5	6	1	1	0	0	3	4	3	4	2	2	..	..
10 years	..	..	..	..	0	0	..	..	0	0	..	..	..	..	..	..	..	..
Females	(76)		(56)		(102)		(183)		(161)		(578)		(241)		(165)		(172)	
1 year	51	51	46	47	29	30	21	21	9	9	25	26	21	22	29	30	28	29
3 years	20	20	11	11	11	11	6	6	1	1	8	8	6	6	10	11	8	8
5 years	16	16	7	7	10	10	3	4	0	0	6	7	4	5	7	8	6	8
8 years	16	16	..	..	3	4	3	4	0	0	4	6	3	4	5	6	..	..
10 years	16	16	..	..	3	4	2	4	0	0	3	5	2	4	..	..	..	..
Overall	(171)		(111)		(220)		(371)		(324)		(1197)		(522)		(316)		(359)	
1 year	51	51	34	34	27	28	21	21	9	10	24	25	21	22	28	29	26	27
3 years	20	21	11	11	9	10	6	6	1	1	8	8	6	6	10	11	8	9
5 years	14	14	6	7	7	8	3	4	0	0	5	6	4	5	5	7	6	7
8 years	11	12	4	4	4	5	2	3	0	0	4	5	3	4	4	5	..	..
10 years	8	8	..	..	2	3	2	3	0	0	2	4	2	3	..	..	..	..

RELATIVE SURVIVAL (%) BY AGE AND PERIOD

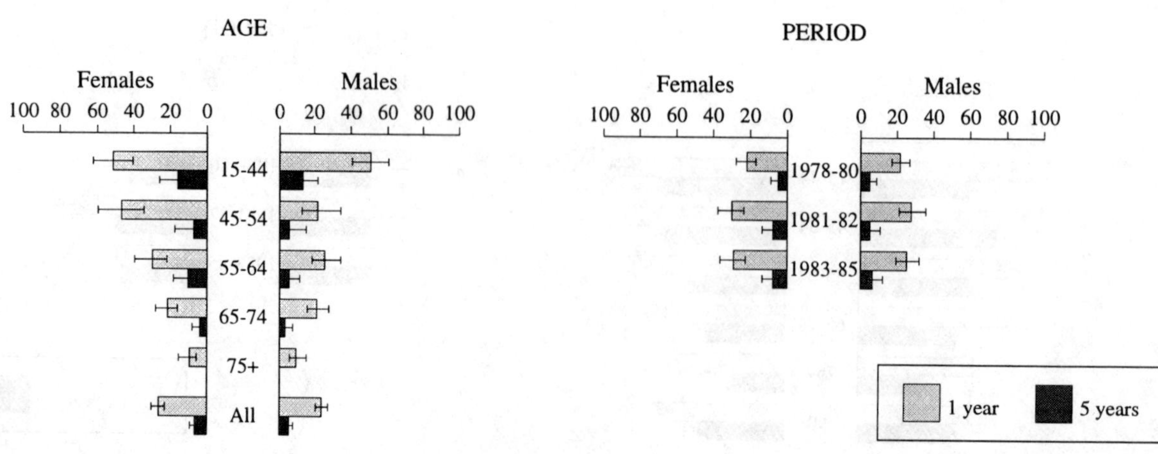

ACUTE MYELOID LEUKAEMIA

ENGLISH REGISTRIES

REGISTRY	NUMBER OF CASES Males	Females	All	PERIOD OF DIAGNOSIS
East Anglia	199	170	369	1979-1984
South Thames	553	440	993	1978-1984
Wessex	69	84	153	1983-1984
West Midlands	343	312	655	1979-1984
Yorkshire	270	248	518	1978-1984
Mean age (years)	62.4	63.1	62.7	

RELATIVE SURVIVAL (%)

100, 80, 60, 40, 20, 0
Males
Females
0 1 2 3 4 5
Time since diagnosis (years)

OBSERVED AND RELATIVE SURVIVAL (%) BY AGE AND PERIOD
(Number of cases in parentheses)

	AGE CLASS 15-44 obs	rel	45-54 obs	rel	55-64 obs	rel	65-74 obs	rel	75+ obs	rel	All obs	rel	PERIOD 1978-80 obs	rel	1981-82 obs	rel	1983-85 obs	rel
Males	(220)		(156)		(271)		(432)		(355)		(1434)		(552)		(423)		(459)	
1 year	46	46	31	31	25	25	16	17	7	8	22	23	20	21	23	24	23	24
3 years	22	22	15	15	11	11	5	5	1	2	9	10	6	8	12	14	8	10
5 years	16	16	10	11	6	7	2	2	1	2	5	7	4	5	8	10	5	7
8 years	15	15	7	8	3	4	1	2	1	3	4	6	3	5	6	8	5	7
10 years	15	15	7	8	3	4	1	2	..	..	4	7	3	5	..	..	..	..
Females	(224)		(121)		(208)		(298)		(403)		(1254)		(474)		(353)		(427)	
1 year	47	47	38	38	31	32	18	19	6	6	24	24	26	27	17	18	26	27
3 years	25	25	14	14	11	11	4	4	1	1	9	10	8	9	8	9	10	11
5 years	19	19	8	8	6	7	3	3	0	0	6	7	5	6	5	7	8	9
8 years	15	15	6	6	6	6	2	3	0	0	5	7	3	5	4	6	7	9
10 years	15	16	..	..	6	7	1	2	0	0	4	7	3	5	4	7	..	..
Overall	(444)		(277)		(479)		(730)		(758)		(2688)		(1026)		(776)		(886)	
1 year	47	47	34	34	28	28	17	18	6	7	23	24	23	24	20	21	24	25
3 years	23	23	14	15	11	11	4	5	1	1	9	10	7	9	10	11	9	10
5 years	18	18	9	10	6	7	2	3	0	1	6	7	4	5	7	8	7	8
8 years	15	15	7	7	4	5	2	2	0	1	5	7	3	5	5	7	6	8
10 years	15	15	7	7	4	5	1	2	..	..	4	7	3	5	5	8	..	..

RELATIVE SURVIVAL (%) BY AGE AND PERIOD

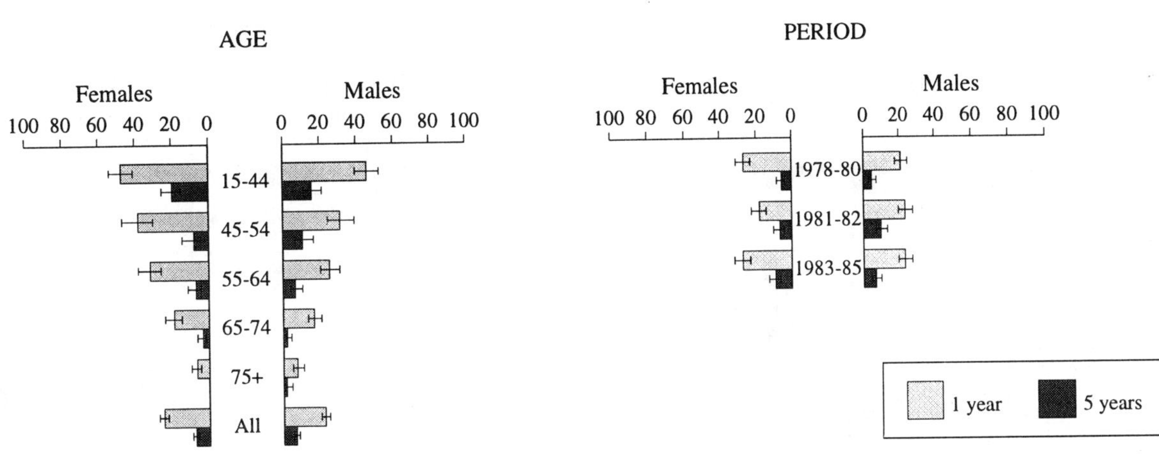

ACUTE MYELOID LEUKAEMIA

FINLAND

REGISTRY	NUMBER OF CASES			PERIOD OF DIAGNOSIS
	Males	Females	All	
Finland	370	356	726	1978-1984
Mean age (years)	59.3	62.6	60.9	

RELATIVE SURVIVAL (%)

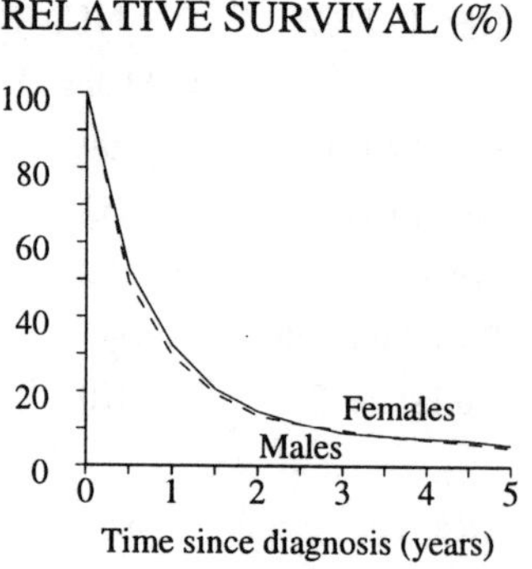

OBSERVED AND RELATIVE SURVIVAL (%) BY AGE AND PERIOD
(Number of cases in parentheses)

	AGE CLASS												PERIOD					
	15-44		45-54		55-64		65-74		75+		All		1978-80		1981-82		1983-85	
	obs	rel	obs	rel	obs	rel	obs	rel	obs	rel	obs	rel	obs	rel	obs	rel	obs	rel
Males	(71)		(52)		(62)		(119)		(66)		(370)		(155)		(110)		(105)	
1 year	46	47	48	49	32	33	24	26	12	14	31	32	32	33	30	31	31	33
3 years	13	13	13	14	10	10	5	6	2	2	8	9	6	7	8	9	10	12
5 years	6	6	10	10	6	7	3	4	0	0	5	6	3	3	5	6	8	9
8 years	6	6	6	6	5	6	1	1	0	0	3	4	0	0	4	5	7	9
10 years	..	..	..	..	..	..	..	..	0	0	..	..	0	0	..	..	..	..
Females	(62)		(34)		(57)		(104)		(99)		(356)		(138)		(123)		(95)	
1 year	55	55	41	41	47	48	21	22	5	5	29	30	25	26	35	36	25	26
3 years	23	23	9	9	14	14	5	5	1	1	9	10	8	9	7	8	12	13
5 years	15	15	3	3	4	4	2	2	1	2	4	5	4	4	4	5	5	6
8 years	13	13	3	3	4	4	0	0	1	2	3	4	3	4	2	3	5	7
10 years	8	8	..	..	4	4	0	0	1	3	3	4	2	3	..	..	..	..
Overall	(133)		(86)		(119)		(223)		(165)		(726)		(293)		(233)		(200)	
1 year	50	50	45	46	39	40	23	24	8	9	30	31	29	30	33	34	29	30
3 years	17	17	12	12	12	12	5	6	1	2	8	9	7	8	8	9	11	12
5 years	10	10	7	7	5	5	3	3	1	1	4	5	3	4	4	5	7	8
8 years	9	9	5	5	4	5	0	0	1	2	3	4	1	2	3	4	6	8
10 years	7	8	..	..	4	5	..	..	1	2	3	4	1	2	..	..	..	..

RELATIVE SURVIVAL (%) BY AGE AND PERIOD

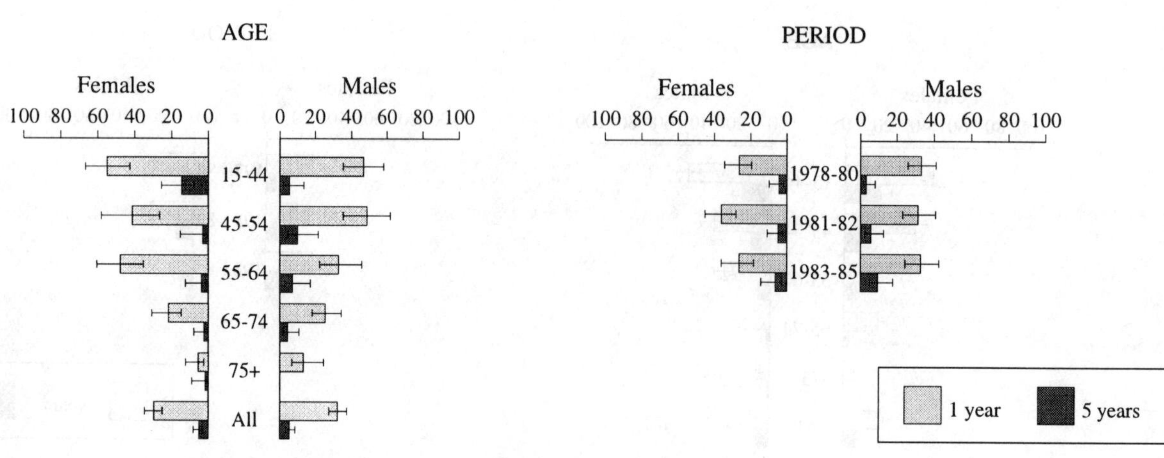

ACUTE MYELOID LEUKAEMIA

SCOTLAND

REGISTRY	NUMBER OF CASES			PERIOD OF DIAGNOSIS
	Males	Females	All	
Scotland	285	288	573	1978-1982
Mean age (years)	58.7	63.2	61.0	

RELATIVE SURVIVAL (%)

Males
Females
Time since diagnosis (years)

OBSERVED AND RELATIVE SURVIVAL (%) BY AGE AND PERIOD
(Number of cases in parentheses)

	AGE CLASS												PERIOD					
	15-44		45-54		55-64		65-74		75+		All		1978-80		1981-82		1983-85	
	obs	rel	obs	rel	obs	rel	obs	rel	obs	rel	obs	rel	obs	rel	obs	rel	obs	rel
Males	(61)		(42)		(47)		(82)		(53)		(285)		(178)		(107)		(0)	
1 year	46	46	33	34	28	28	20	21	6	6	26	27	28	29	23	25	..	..
3 years	21	21	7	7	9	9	4	4	2	3	8	10	8	10	8	10	..	..
5 years	16	17	5	5	6	7	2	3	2	4	6	8	6	7	7	10	..	..
8 years	14	15	..	..	0	0	..	..	0	0	4	5	4	5	..	..	..	..
10 years	..	..	..	..	0	0	..	..	0	0	..	..	..	..	..	..	..	..
Females	(46)		(30)		(56)		(69)		(87)		(288)		(165)		(123)		(0)	
1 year	48	48	40	40	16	16	17	18	10	11	22	23	18	19	28	29	..	..
3 years	26	26	17	17	4	4	6	6	0	0	8	9	8	9	8	9	..	..
5 years	24	24	10	10	2	2	3	3	0	0	6	7	6	8	6	7	..	..
8 years	13	13	10	11	2	2	1	2	0	0	4	6	4	5	..	..	..	..
10 years	..	..	..	..	..	..	..	..	0	0	..	..	..	..	..	..	..	..
Overall	(107)		(72)		(103)		(151)		(140)		(573)		(343)		(230)		(0)	
1 year	47	47	36	36	21	22	19	19	9	10	24	25	23	24	26	27	..	..
3 years	23	23	11	11	6	6	5	5	1	1	8	9	8	9	8	9	..	..
5 years	20	20	7	7	4	4	3	3	1	1	6	8	6	7	7	8	..	..
8 years	14	15	7	8	1	2	1	2	0	0	4	6	4	5	..	..	..	..
10 years	..	..	..	..	..	..	..	..	0	0	..	..	..	..	..	..	..	..

RELATIVE SURVIVAL (%) BY AGE AND PERIOD

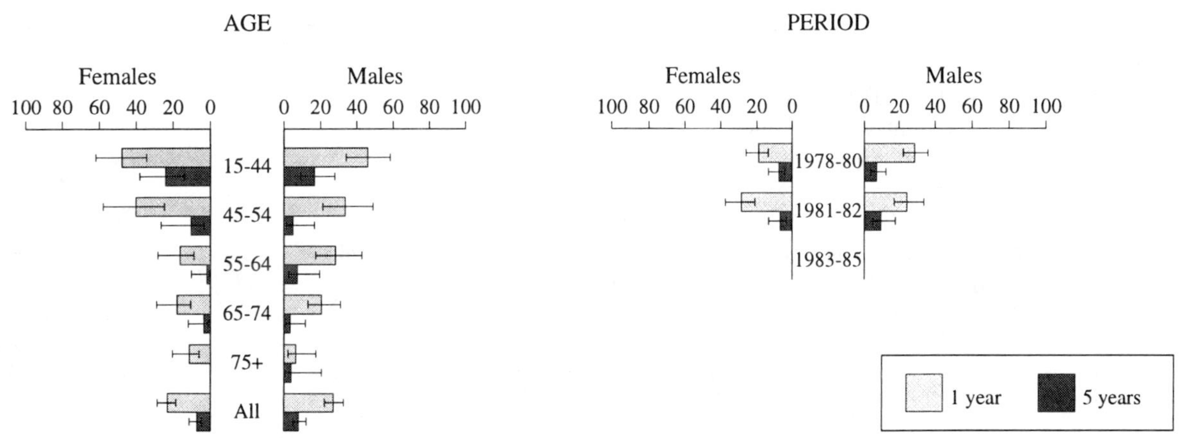

ACUTE MYELOID LEUKAEMIA

DUTCH REGISTRIES

REGISTRY	NUMBER OF CASES			PERIOD OF DIAGNOSIS
	Males	Females	All	
Eindhoven	47	46	93	1978-1985
Mean age (years)	59.6	54.6	57.2	

RELATIVE SURVIVAL (%)
(Both sexes)

100
80
60
40
20
0
0 1 2 3 4 5
Time since diagnosis (years)

OBSERVED AND RELATIVE SURVIVAL (%) BY PERIOD AND SEX
(Number of cases in parentheses)

	PERIOD						SEX					
	1978-80		1981-82		1983-85		Males		Females		All	
	obs	rel	obs	rel	obs	rel	obs	rel	obs	rel	obs	rel
N. Cases	(27)		(28)		(38)		(47)		(46)		(93)	
1 year	19	19	25	26	37	38	21	22	35	36	28	29
3 years	11	12	11	12	18	20	8	9	19	21	14	15
5 years	7	9	7	8	..	..	6	7	15	16	10	11
8 years	7	10	..	..	..	..	6	8	15	18	10	13
10 years	..	..	..	..	..	..	..	..	..	..	..	..

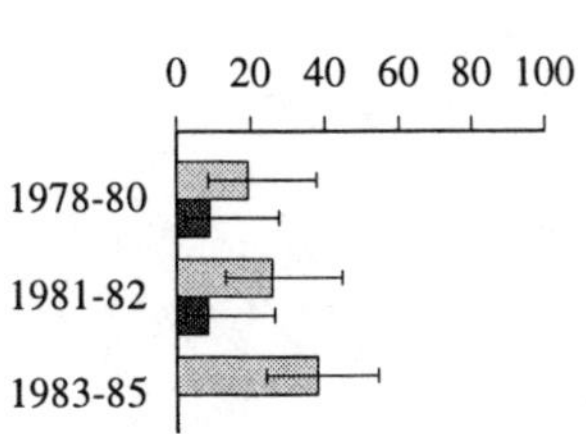

ESTONIA

REGISTRY	NUMBER OF CASES			PERIOD OF DIAGNOSIS
	Males	Females	All	
Estonia	42	60	102	1978-1984
Mean age (years)	59.2	52.2	55.1	

RELATIVE SURVIVAL (%)
(Both sexes)

100
80
60
40
20
0
0 1 2 3 4 5
Time since diagnosis (years)

OBSERVED AND RELATIVE SURVIVAL (%) BY PERIOD AND SEX
(Number of cases in parentheses)

	PERIOD						SEX					
	1978-80		1981-82		1983-85		Males		Females		All	
	obs	rel	obs	rel	obs	rel	obs	rel	obs	rel	obs	rel
N. Cases	(50)		(26)		(26)		(42)		(60)		(102)	
1 year	12	12	12	12	19	20	12	13	15	15	14	14
3 years	4	4	0	0	4	4	7	8	0	0	3	3
5 years	4	5	0	0	0	0	5	6	0	0	2	2
8 years	2	3	0	0	0	0	2	4	0	0	1	1
10 years	2	3	0	0	0	0	2	4	0	0	1	1

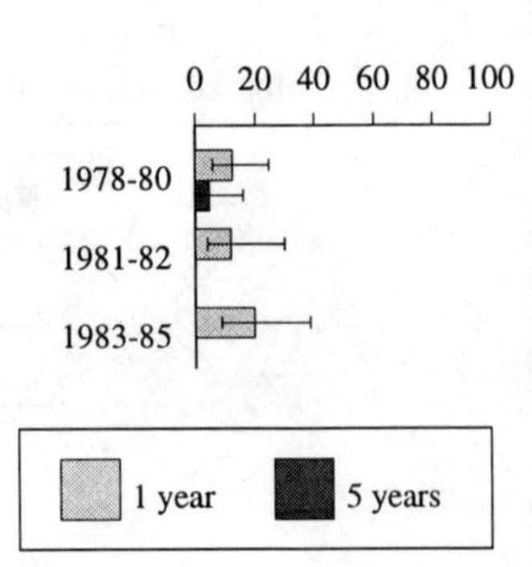

ACUTE MYELOID LEUKAEMIA

FRENCH REGISTRIES

REGISTRY	NUMBER OF CASES			PERIOD OF DIAGNOSIS
	Males	Females	All	
Côte-d'Or	31	35	66	1980-1984
Mean age (years)	64.7	66.1	65.5	

RELATIVE SURVIVAL (%)

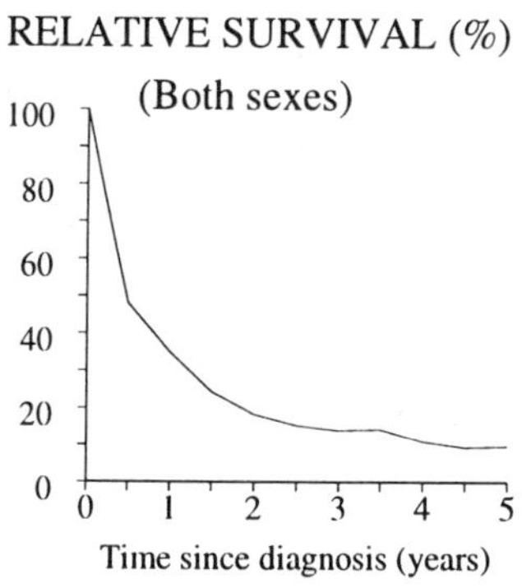

OBSERVED AND RELATIVE SURVIVAL (%) BY PERIOD AND SEX
(Number of cases in parentheses)

	PERIOD						SEX					
	1978-80		1981-82		1983-85		Males		Females		All	
	obs	rel	obs	rel	obs	rel	obs	rel	obs	rel	obs	rel
N. Cases	(15)		(19)		(32)		(31)		(35)		(66)	
1 year	13	14	47	49	34	36	35	38	31	33	33	35
3 years	0	0	16	18	16	18	23	27	3	3	12	14
5 years	0	0	5	7	13	16	13	17	3	3	8	10
8 years	0	0	0	0	..	..	0	0	..	..	0	0
10 years	0	0	0	0	..	..	0	0	..	..	0	0

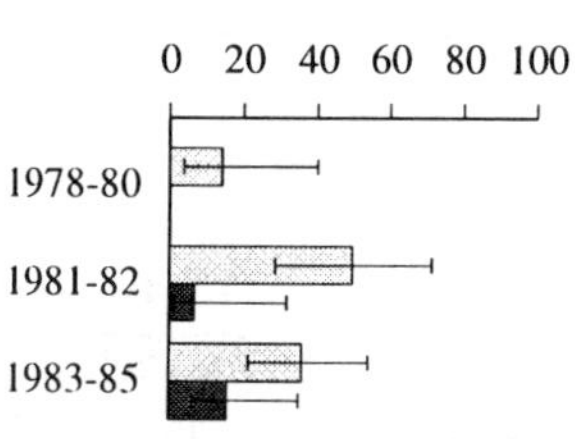

GERMAN REGISTRIES

REGISTRY	NUMBER OF CASES			PERIOD OF DIAGNOSIS
	Males	Females	All	
Saarland	27	51	78	1978-1984
Mean age (years)	58.8	55.1	56.4	

RELATIVE SURVIVAL (%)
(Both sexes)

100
80
60
40
20
0
0 1 2 3 4 5
Time since diagnosis (years)

OBSERVED AND RELATIVE SURVIVAL (%) BY PERIOD AND SEX
(Number of cases in parentheses)

	PERIOD						SEX					
	1978-80		1981-82		1983-85		Males		Females		All	
	obs	rel	obs	rel	obs	rel	obs	rel	obs	rel	obs	rel
N. Cases	(27)		(18)		(33)		(27)		(51)		(78)	
1 year	15	15	28	29	27	28	33	34	18	18	23	24
3 years	7	8	6	6	6	7	7	8	6	6	6	7
5 years	7	8	6	7	6	7	7	9	6	7	6	7
8 years	4	4	0	0	..	..	7	10	..	..	3	4
10 years	4	5	0	0	..	..	7	11	..	..	3	4

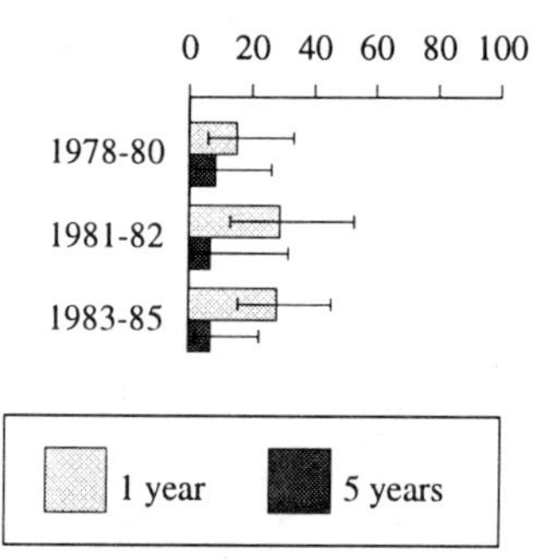

ACUTE MYELOID LEUKAEMIA

ITALIAN REGISTRIES

REGISTRY	NUMBER OF CASES			PERIOD OF DIAGNOSIS
	Males	Females	All	
Latina	13	5	18	1983-1984
Ragusa	10	6	16	1981-1984
Varese	65	55	120	1978-1984
Mean age (years)	57.5	55.3	56.6	

RELATIVE SURVIVAL (%)

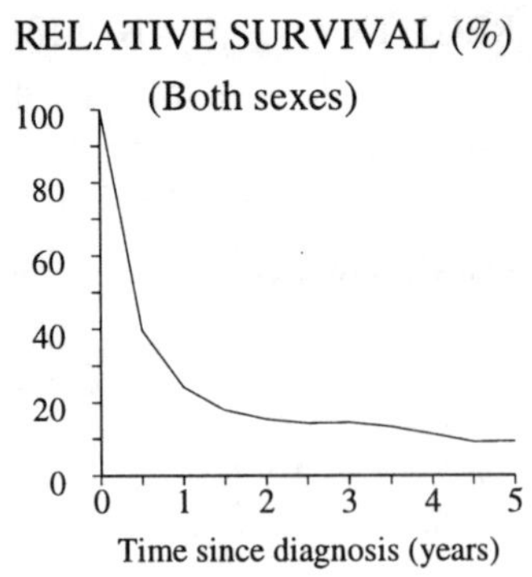

OBSERVED AND RELATIVE SURVIVAL (%) BY PERIOD AND SEX
(Number of cases in parentheses)

	PERIOD						SEX					
	1978-80		1981-82		1983-85		Males		Females		All	
	obs	rel	obs	rel	obs	rel	obs	rel	obs	rel	obs	rel
N. Cases	(46)		(51)		(57)		(88)		(66)		(154)	
1 year	17	18	25	26	26	27	23	24	24	25	23	24
3 years	9	10	14	15	16	17	13	14	14	15	13	14
5 years	2	3	8	9	12	14	9	11	6	7	8	9
8 years	2	3	6	8	..	..	6	9	6	7	6	8
10 years	2	3	..	..	..	..	6	9	..	..	6	9

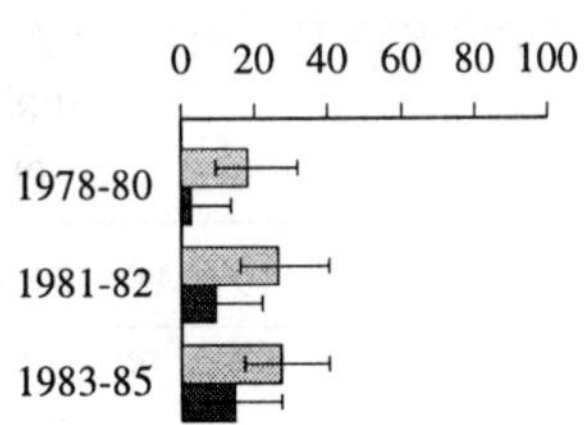

POLISH REGISTRIES

REGISTRY	NUMBER OF CASES			PERIOD OF DIAGNOSIS
	Males	Females	All	
Cracow	21	30	51	1978-1984
Mean age (years)	50.2	55.4	53.2	

RELATIVE SURVIVAL (%)
(Both sexes)

100
80
60
40
20
0
0 1 2 3 4 5
Time since diagnosis (years)

OBSERVED AND RELATIVE SURVIVAL (%) BY PERIOD AND SEX
(Number of cases in parentheses)

	PERIOD						SEX					
	1978-80		1981-82		1983-85		Males		Females		All	
	obs	rel	obs	rel	obs	rel	obs	rel	obs	rel	obs	rel
N. Cases	(20)		(15)		(16)		(21)		(30)		(51)	
1 year	13	13	7	7	19	19	6	6	17	17	13	13
3 years	0	0	7	7	6	7	0	0	7	7	4	5
5 years	0	0	7	7	6	7	0	0	7	8	4	5
8 years	0	0	7	8	6	8	0	0	7	8	4	5
10 years	0	0	..	..	..	..	0	0	..	..	..	..

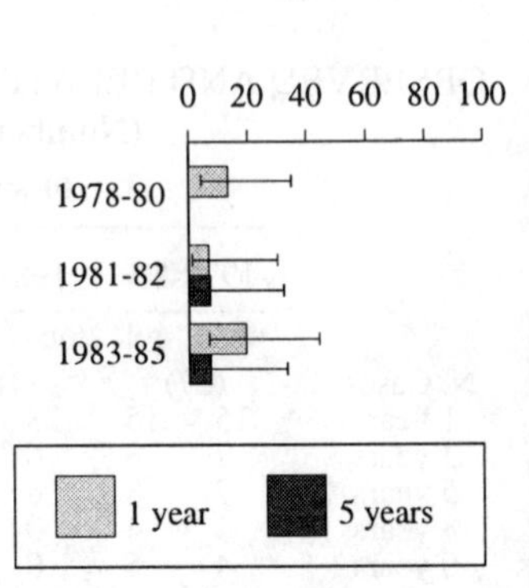

ACUTE MYELOID LEUKAEMIA

SPANISH REGISTRIES

REGISTRY	NUMBER OF CASES			PERIOD OF DIAGNOSIS
	Males	Females	All	
Tarragona	5	4	9	1985-1985
Mean age (years)	56.8	65.3	60.6	

RELATIVE SURVIVAL (%)
(Both sexes)

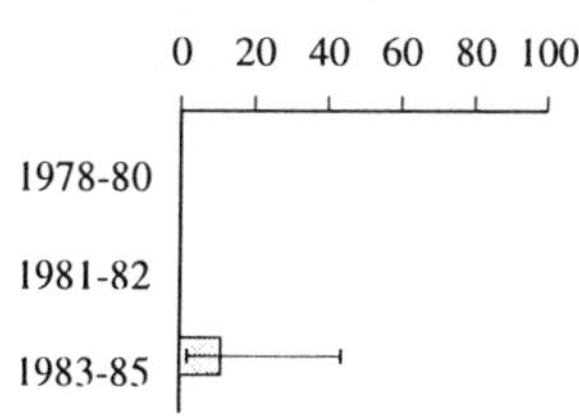

OBSERVED AND RELATIVE SURVIVAL (%) BY PERIOD AND SEX
(Number of cases in parentheses)

	PERIOD						SEX					
	1978-80		1981-82		1983-85		Males		Females		All	
	obs	rel	obs	rel	obs	rel	obs	rel	obs	rel	obs	rel
N. Cases	(0)		(0)		(9)		(5)		(4)		(9)	
1 year	..	..	..	..	11	11	20	20	0	0	11	11
3 years	..	..	..	..	0	0	0	0	0	0	0	0
5 years	..	..	..	..	0	0	0	0	0	0	0	0
8 years	..	..	..	..	0	0	0	0	0	0	0	0
10 years	..	..	..	..	0	0	0	0	0	0	0	0

SWISS REGISTRIES

REGISTRY	NUMBER OF CASES			PERIOD OF DIAGNOSIS
	Males	Females	All	
Basel	18	20	38	1981-1984
Geneva	19	28	47	1978-1984
Mean age (years)	58.5	59.3	59.0	

RELATIVE SURVIVAL (%)
(Both sexes)

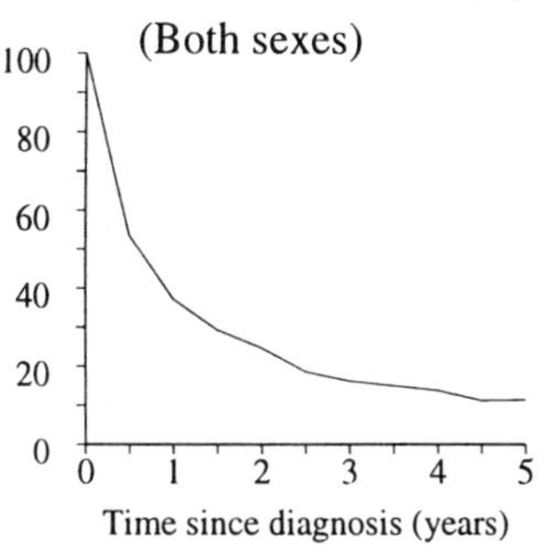

OBSERVED AND RELATIVE SURVIVAL (%) BY PERIOD AND SEX
(Number of cases in parentheses)

	PERIOD						SEX					
	1978-80		1981-82		1983-85		Males		Females		All	
	obs	rel	obs	rel	obs	rel	obs	rel	obs	rel	obs	rel
N. Cases	(20)		(31)		(34)		(37)		(48)		(85)	
1 year	25	26	42	43	38	39	43	45	31	32	36	37
3 years	0	0	23	24	17	18	16	18	14	15	15	16
5 years	0	0	16	18	10	12	11	13	10	11	10	11
8 years	0	0	16	19	..	..	11	14	10	11	10	12
10 years	0	0	..	..	..	..	..	..	..	..	..	..

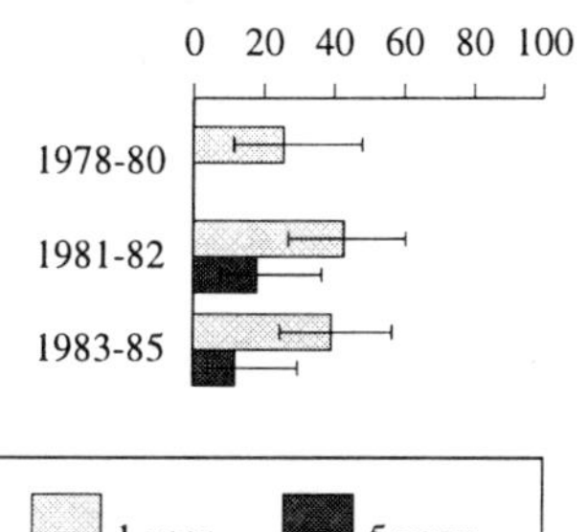

ACUTE MYELOID LEUKAEMIA

EUROPEAN REGISTRIES

Unweighted analysis

REGISTRY	CASES Males	Females	All
DENMARK	619	578	1197
DUTCH REGISTRIES	47	46	93
ENGLISH REGISTRIES	1434	1254	2688
ESTONIA	42	60	102
FINLAND	370	356	726
FRENCH REGISTRIES	31	35	66
GERMAN REGISTRIES	27	51	78
ITALIAN REGISTRIES	88	66	154
POLISH REGISTRIES	21	30	51
SCOTLAND	285	288	573
SPANISH REGISTRIES	5	4	9
SWISS REGISTRIES	37	48	85
Mean age (years)	61.4	62.4	61.9

RELATIVE SURVIVAL (%)
(Age-standardized)

Females: 100 80 60 40 20 0 — Males: 0 20 40 60 80 100

DK
ENG
FIN
SCO
EUR

OBSERVED AND RELATIVE SURVIVAL (%) BY AGE AND PERIOD
(Number of cases in parentheses)

	AGE CLASS 15-44 obs	15-44 rel	45-54 obs	45-54 rel	55-64 obs	55-64 rel	65-74 obs	65-74 rel	75+ obs	75+ rel	All obs	All rel	PERIOD 1978-80 obs	1978-80 rel	1981-82 obs	1981-82 rel	1983-85 obs	1983-85 rel
Males	(514)		(354)		(546)		(894)		(698)		(3006)		(1255)		(878)		(873)	
1 year	47	47	33	34	26	26	18	19	7	8	24	25	23	24	25	26	25	26
3 years	21	21	13	13	9	10	5	6	1	2	9	10	7	8	11	12	9	11
5 years	15	15	9	9	6	6	2	3	1	1	5	7	4	5	7	8	6	8
8 years	13	13	6	7	3	4	1	2	1	2	4	6	3	4	5	7	5	7
10 years	12	12	5	6	3	4	1	2	..	..	4	6	2	4	..	..	..	..
Females	(499)		(296)		(477)		(729)		(815)		(2816)		(1134)		(865)		(817)	
1 year	48	48	39	39	30	31	19	19	7	7	24	25	22	23	25	26	27	28
3 years	22	22	12	12	10	10	5	5	1	1	8	9	7	8	9	10	10	11
5 years	17	17	7	8	6	7	3	3	0	0	6	7	4	5	6	7	7	9
8 years	14	14	6	6	5	6	2	3	0	1	4	6	3	4	4	6	7	9
10 years	13	13	..	..	5	6	1	2	0	1	4	6	3	4	4	6	..	..
Overall	(1013)		(650)		(1023)		(1623)		(1513)		(5822)		(2389)		(1743)		(1690)	
1 year	47	47	36	36	28	28	19	19	7	8	24	25	22	23	25	26	26	27
3 years	22	22	13	13	10	10	5	6	1	1	8	10	7	8	10	11	10	11
5 years	16	16	8	8	6	7	2	3	0	1	5	7	4	5	6	8	7	8
8 years	13	13	6	6	4	5	1	2	0	1	4	6	3	4	4	6	6	8
10 years	12	13	6	6	4	5	1	2	0	1	4	6	3	4	4	7	..	..

RELATIVE SURVIVAL (%) BY AGE AND PERIOD

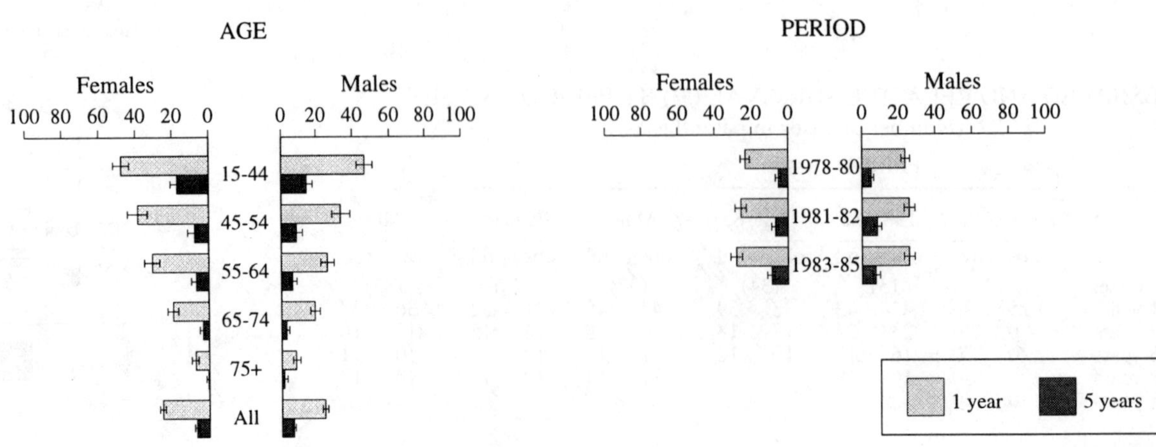

CHRONIC MYELOID LEUKAEMIA

DENMARK

REGISTRY	NUMBER OF CASES			PERIOD OF DIAGNOSIS
	Males	Females	All	
Denmark	243	185	428	1978-1984
Mean age (years)	61.1	63.4	62.1	

RELATIVE SURVIVAL (%)

100, 80, 60, 40, 20, 0

— Males
- - Females

0 1 2 3 4 5

Time since diagnosis (years)

OBSERVED AND RELATIVE SURVIVAL (%) BY AGE AND PERIOD
(Number of cases in parentheses)

	AGE CLASS												PERIOD					
	15-44		45-54		55-64		65-74		75+		All		1978-80		1981-82		1983-85	
	obs	rel	obs	rel	obs	rel	obs	rel	obs	rel	obs	rel	obs	rel	obs	rel	obs	rel
Males	(47)		(31)		(45)		(61)		(59)		(243)		(88)		(79)		(76)	
1 year	87	87	68	68	67	68	43	45	29	32	56	58	58	61	57	59	51	53
3 years	64	64	35	36	27	28	21	25	10	15	30	34	35	41	28	32	25	28
5 years	27	27	23	23	18	20	5	6	7	13	14	18	23	29	13	16	6	7
8 years	16	16	11	12	4	5	5	8	0	0	7	10	10	15	7	10	..	..
10 years	8	8	11	12	4	6	..	..	0	0	5	8	7	12	..	..	..	..
Females	(28)		(21)		(35)		(45)		(56)		(185)		(77)		(57)		(51)	
1 year	100	100	76	77	71	72	64	66	36	39	64	66	68	70	63	65	59	61
3 years	61	61	43	43	37	38	38	41	20	26	36	40	36	40	40	44	31	35
5 years	35	36	29	29	20	21	16	18	0	0	16	19	16	19	14	17	20	23
8 years	11	11	8	8	13	14	7	9	0	0	6	9	6	9	0	0	..	..
10 years	0	0	0	0	0	0	7	10	0	0	2	3	2	3	0	0	..	..
Overall	(75)		(52)		(80)		(106)		(115)		(428)		(165)		(136)		(127)	
1 year	92	92	71	72	69	70	52	54	32	36	59	61	62	65	60	62	54	56
3 years	63	63	38	39	31	33	28	32	15	20	32	37	36	41	33	37	28	31
5 years	30	30	25	26	19	20	9	12	3	6	15	18	19	24	13	16	11	14
8 years	14	14	10	10	7	8	6	9	0	0	6	9	8	12	4	6	..	..
10 years	6	6	5	5	3	4	6	10	0	0	3	5	4	7	..	..	..	..

RELATIVE SURVIVAL (%) BY AGE AND PERIOD

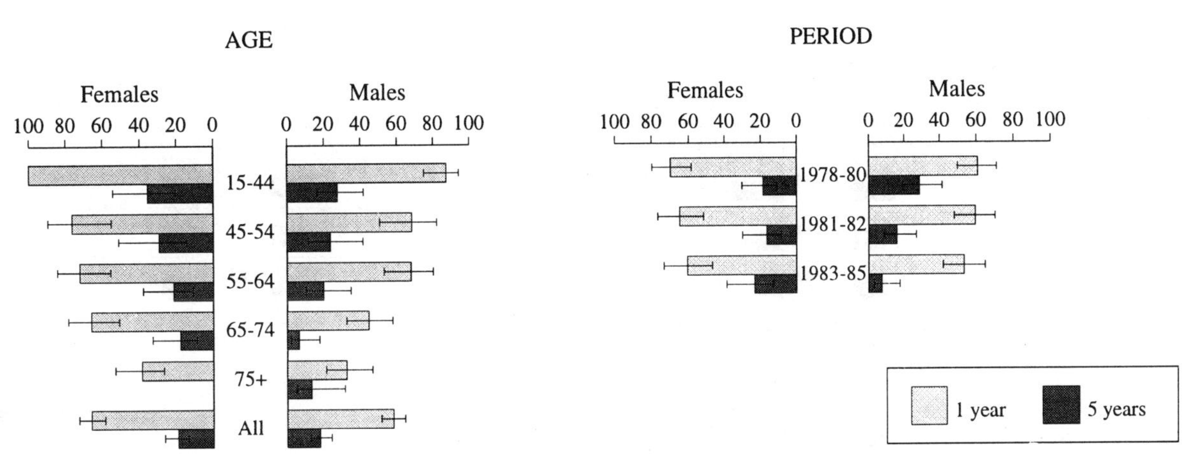

CHRONIC MYELOID LEUKAEMIA

ENGLISH REGISTRIES

REGISTRY	NUMBER OF CASES			PERIOD OF DIAGNOSIS
	Males	Females	All	
East Anglia	74	52	126	1979-1984
South Thames	237	211	448	1978-1984
Wessex	33	41	74	1983-1984
West Midlands	182	166	348	1979-1984
Yorkshire	185	144	329	1978-1984
Mean age (years)	63.0	67.5	65.1	

RELATIVE SURVIVAL (%)

OBSERVED AND RELATIVE SURVIVAL (%) BY AGE AND PERIOD
(Number of cases in parentheses)

	AGE CLASS												PERIOD					
	15-44		45-54		55-64		65-74		75+		All		1978-80		1981-82		1983-85	
	obs	rel	obs	rel	obs	rel	obs	rel	obs	rel	obs	rel	obs	rel	obs	rel	obs	rel
Males	(109)		(83)		(117)		(218)		(184)		(711)		(291)		(196)		(224)	
1 year	82	82	75	75	62	64	54	57	31	35	56	59	53	56	60	63	58	60
3 years	46	46	37	38	28	30	24	28	10	16	26	30	22	26	27	32	30	35
5 years	28	28	18	19	15	16	11	14	5	10	13	17	11	15	14	18	15	19
8 years	14	14	7	8	6	8	3	5	3	9	6	9	4	6	7	11	6	9
10 years	14	14	7	8	0	0	..	..	0	0	4	7	3	6	..	..	0	0
Females	(54)		(59)		(107)		(163)		(231)		(614)		(222)		(167)		(225)	
1 year	85	85	73	73	69	70	56	57	29	32	52	55	49	52	54	57	54	56
3 years	53	53	36	36	34	35	26	29	11	15	25	29	22	25	28	33	26	30
5 years	23	23	17	17	18	19	14	17	6	11	13	16	10	13	16	20	13	17
8 years	15	15	4	4	4	5	5	7	2	5	4	7	3	5	5	8	6	10
10 years	7	7	..	..	..	..	..	..	..	..	1	2	0	1	5	8	..	..
Overall	(163)		(142)		(224)		(381)		(415)		(1325)		(513)		(363)		(449)	
1 year	83	83	74	74	66	67	55	57	30	33	54	57	51	54	57	60	56	58
3 years	48	48	37	37	31	32	25	28	11	15	26	30	22	26	28	32	28	32
5 years	26	26	18	18	16	17	12	15	6	10	13	17	11	14	15	19	14	18
8 years	14	15	6	6	5	6	4	6	2	7	5	8	4	6	6	9	6	8
10 years	12	12	6	6	0	0	..	..	..	..	3	5	2	3	5	9	0	0

RELATIVE SURVIVAL (%) BY AGE AND PERIOD

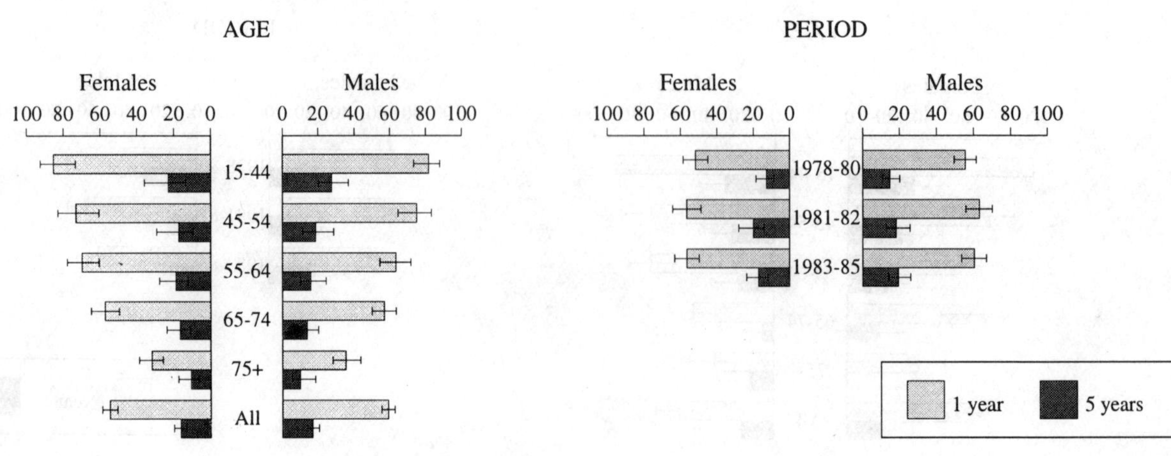

CHRONIC MYELOID LEUKAEMIA

FINLAND

REGISTRY	NUMBER OF CASES			PERIOD OF DIAGNOSIS
	Males	Females	All	
Finland	171	177	348	1978-1984
Mean age (years)	56.5	59.1	57.8	

RELATIVE SURVIVAL (%)

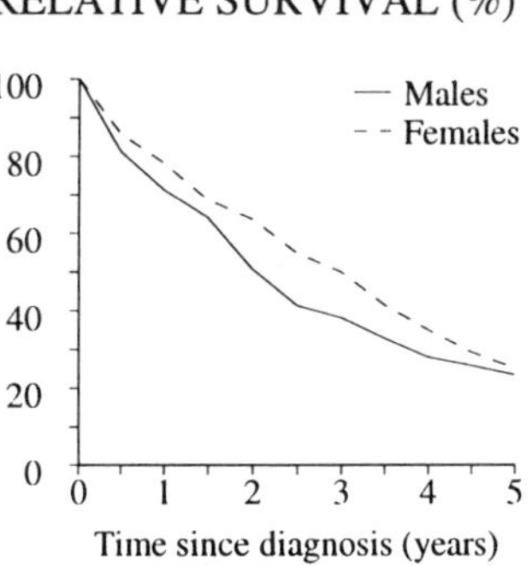

OBSERVED AND RELATIVE SURVIVAL (%) BY AGE AND PERIOD
(Number of cases in parentheses)

	AGE CLASS												PERIOD					
	15-44		45-54		55-64		65-74		75+		All		1978-80		1981-82		1983-85	
	obs	rel	obs	rel	obs	rel	obs	rel	obs	rel	obs	rel	obs	rel	obs	rel	obs	rel
Males	(50)		(27)		(26)		(38)		(30)		(171)		(74)		(53)		(44)	
1 year	82	82	78	78	85	86	53	55	43	50	68	71	70	73	79	81	52	56
3 years	32	32	63	65	62	65	18	22	7	10	34	38	39	44	36	39	23	27
5 years	18	18	41	43	35	39	8	11	3	7	19	24	24	30	19	21	11	15
8 years	7	7	17	18	0	0	3	4	0	0	5	7	7	9	4	5	0	0
10 years	0	0	11	13	0	0	0	0	0	0	2	3	3	4	..	..	0	0
Females	(38)		(26)		(36)		(39)		(38)		(177)		(90)		(39)		(48)	
1 year	89	90	85	85	78	78	85	87	47	52	76	78	81	83	77	79	67	69
3 years	63	63	54	54	47	48	44	47	26	35	46	50	59	63	33	36	33	37
5 years	37	37	31	31	11	12	23	27	11	17	22	25	28	31	10	12	21	25
8 years	29	29	12	12	8	9	2	2	0	0	10	13	14	18	3	3	10	13
10 years	14	15	12	12	3	3	..	..	0	0	6	8	8	10	3	3	..	..
Overall	(88)		(53)		(62)		(77)		(68)		(348)		(164)		(92)		(92)	
1 year	85	85	81	82	81	82	69	72	46	51	72	75	76	79	78	80	60	63
3 years	45	46	58	60	53	55	31	35	18	25	40	44	50	55	35	38	28	32
5 years	26	26	36	37	21	23	16	19	7	13	21	24	26	31	15	17	16	20
8 years	16	17	14	15	5	6	2	3	0	0	8	10	11	14	3	4	7	9
10 years	8	8	12	13	2	2	0	0	0	0	4	6	5	8	3	4	..	..

RELATIVE SURVIVAL (%) BY AGE AND PERIOD

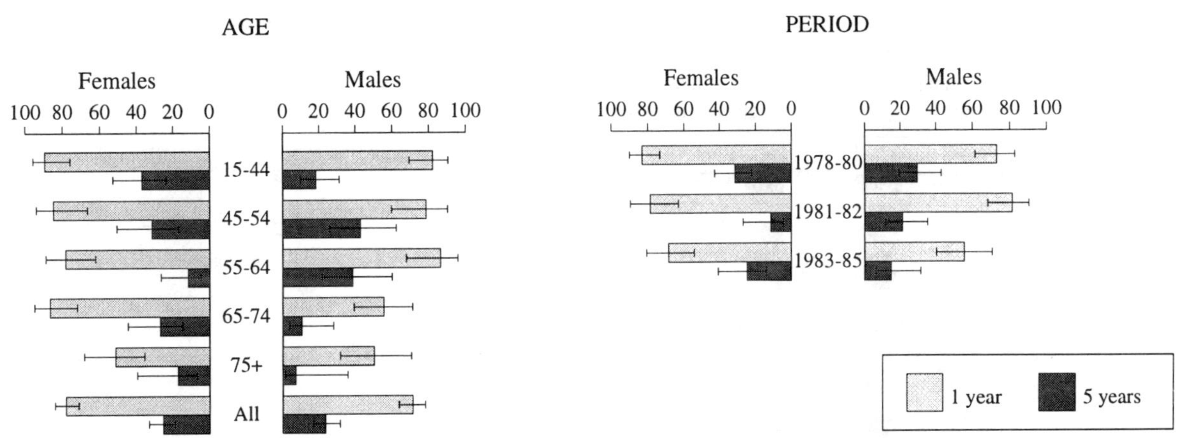

CHRONIC MYELOID LEUKAEMIA

SCOTLAND

REGISTRY	NUMBER OF CASES			PERIOD OF DIAGNOSIS
	Males	Females	All	
Scotland	129	126	255	1978-1982
Mean age (years)	59.1	62.3	60.7	

RELATIVE SURVIVAL (%)

OBSERVED AND RELATIVE SURVIVAL (%) BY AGE AND PERIOD
(Number of cases in parentheses)

	AGE CLASS												PERIOD					
	15-44		45-54		55-64		65-74		75+		All		1978-80		1981-82		1983-85	
	obs	rel	obs	rel	obs	rel	obs	rel	obs	rel	obs	rel	obs	rel	obs	rel	obs	rel
Males	(28)		(18)		(24)		(31)		(28)		(129)		(66)		(63)		(0)	
1 year	82	82	67	67	50	51	55	58	36	41	57	60	53	56	62	65	..	..
3 years	36	36	39	40	33	36	29	35	14	22	29	34	29	33	30	34	..	..
5 years	21	22	11	12	4	5	19	26	4	7	12	16	11	14	14	18	..	..
8 years	17	17	..	..	..	..	6	11	..	..	7	11	5	7	..	..	..	..
10 years	..	..	..	..	..	..	3	7	..	..	4	6	2	4	..	..	..	..
Females	(20)		(20)		(19)		(32)		(35)		(126)		(83)		(43)		(0)	
1 year	85	85	85	85	68	69	66	68	54	60	69	72	70	73	67	70	..	..
3 years	30	30	40	41	47	49	38	42	17	24	33	37	34	38	30	34	..	..
5 years	25	25	25	26	21	22	13	15	6	10	16	19	18	22	12	14	..	..
8 years	15	15	6	7	8	9	0	0	3	8	4	6	5	7	..	..	..	..
10 years	..	..	..	..	..	..	0	0	..	..	..	..	..	..	..	..	..	..
Overall	(48)		(38)		(43)		(63)		(63)		(255)		(149)		(106)		(0)	
1 year	83	83	76	77	58	59	60	63	46	52	63	66	62	65	64	67	..	..
3 years	33	33	39	40	40	42	33	38	16	23	31	35	32	36	30	34	..	..
5 years	23	23	18	19	12	13	16	20	5	9	14	18	15	18	13	16	..	..
8 years	16	17	4	4	5	6	3	5	3	9	5	7	5	7	..	..	..	..
10 years	..	..	..	..	..	..	2	3	..	..	4	6	3	5	..	..	..	..

RELATIVE SURVIVAL (%) BY AGE AND PERIOD

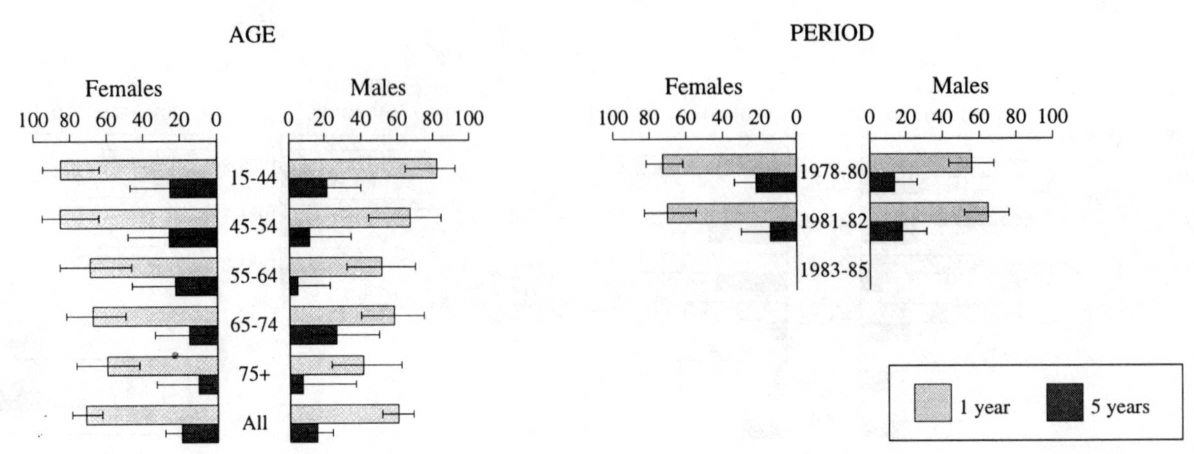

CHRONIC MYELOID LEUKAEMIA

DUTCH REGISTRIES

REGISTRY	NUMBER OF CASES			PERIOD OF DIAGNOSIS
	Males	Females	All	
Eindhoven	46	23	69	1978-1985
Mean age (years)	62.1	65.7	63.3	

RELATIVE SURVIVAL (%)
(Both sexes)

100 80 60 40 20 0
0 1 2 3 4 5
Time since diagnosis (years)

OBSERVED AND RELATIVE SURVIVAL (%) BY PERIOD AND SEX
(Number of cases in parentheses)

	PERIOD						SEX					
	1978-80		1981-82		1983-85		Males		Females		All	
	obs	rel	obs	rel	obs	rel	obs	rel	obs	rel	obs	rel
N. Cases	(23)		(22)		(24)		(46)		(23)		(69)	
1 year	43	45	41	43	50	53	43	46	48	49	45	47
3 years	22	24	14	16	32	38	21	24	25	28	22	25
5 years	9	10	14	17	..	..	8	10	20	24	12	15
8 years	..	..	..	..	..	..	..	..	..	..	..	..
10 years	..	..	..	..	..	..	..	..	..	..	..	..

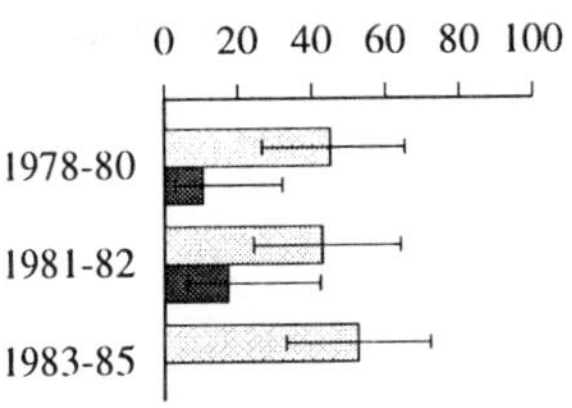

ESTONIA

REGISTRY	NUMBER OF CASES			PERIOD OF DIAGNOSIS
	Males	Females	All	
Estonia	60	55	115	1978-1984
Mean age (years)	58.1	60.7	59.4	

RELATIVE SURVIVAL (%)
(Both sexes)

100 80 60 40 20 0
0 1 2 3 4 5
Time since diagnosis (years)

OBSERVED AND RELATIVE SURVIVAL (%) BY PERIOD AND SEX
(Number of cases in parentheses)

	PERIOD						SEX					
	1978-80		1981-82		1983-85		Males		Females		All	
	obs	rel	obs	rel	obs	rel	obs	rel	obs	rel	obs	rel
N. Cases	(47)		(38)		(30)		(60)		(55)		(115)	
1 year	64	66	74	76	60	62	60	63	73	75	66	68
3 years	49	55	47	51	50	56	42	47	56	61	49	54
5 years	26	31	26	30	33	41	25	31	31	36	28	33
8 years	13	18	14	18	..	..	13	19	16	20	14	20
10 years	5	8	..	..	..	..	9	14	0	0	5	7

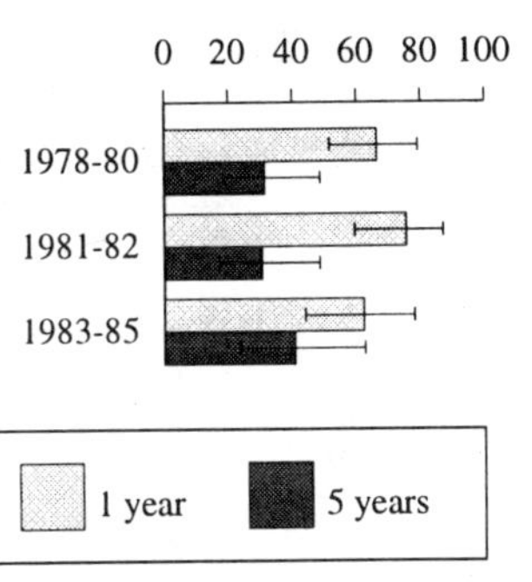

CHRONIC MYELOID LEUKAEMIA

FRENCH REGISTRIES

REGISTRY	NUMBER OF CASES			PERIOD OF DIAGNOSIS
	Males	Females	All	
Côte-d'Or	22	4	26	1980-1984
Mean age (years)	53.0	48.8	52.3	

RELATIVE SURVIVAL (%)
(Both sexes)

Time since diagnosis (years)

OBSERVED AND RELATIVE SURVIVAL (%) BY PERIOD AND SEX
(Number of cases in parentheses)

	PERIOD						SEX					
	1978-80		1981-82		1983-85		Males		Females		All	
	obs	rel	obs	rel	obs	rel	obs	rel	obs	rel	obs	rel
N. Cases	(7)		(9)		(10)		(22)		(4)		(26)	
1 year	86	89	89	90	70	71	82	83	75	76	81	82
3 years	43	47	33	35	60	63	41	44	75	78	46	49
5 years	29	34	22	24	25	28	18	20	75	81	25	28
8 years	14	19	11	13	..	..	9	11	75	85	15	18
10 years	0	0	..	..	..	..	0	0	..	..	..	..

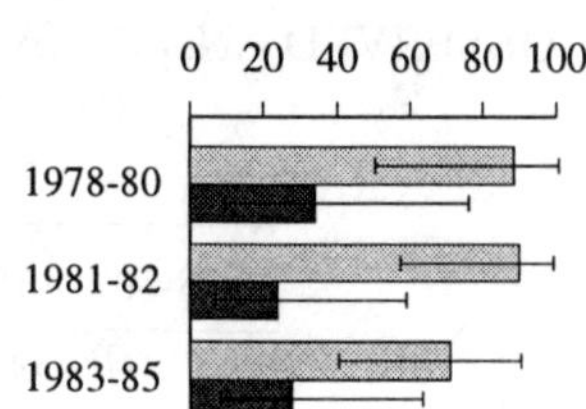

GERMAN REGISTRIES

REGISTRY	NUMBER OF CASES			PERIOD OF DIAGNOSIS
	Males	Females	All	
Saarland	37	34	71	1978-1984
Mean age (years)	56.0	59.9	57.9	

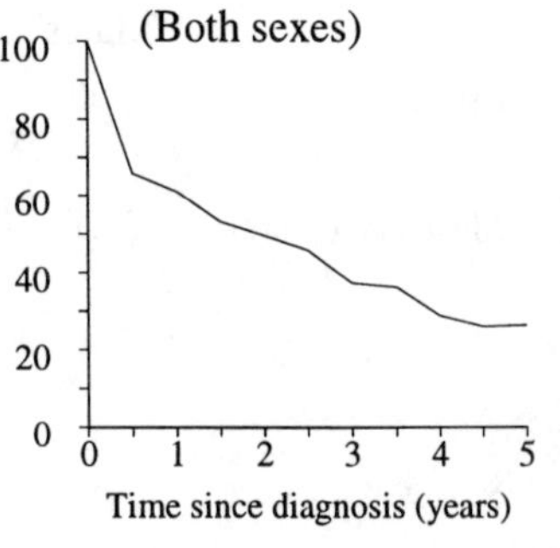

OBSERVED AND RELATIVE SURVIVAL (%) BY PERIOD AND SEX
(Number of cases in parentheses)

	PERIOD						SEX					
	1978-80		1981-82		1983-85		Males		Females		All	
	obs	rel	obs	rel	obs	rel	obs	rel	obs	rel	obs	rel
N. Cases	(31)		(23)		(17)		(37)		(34)		(71)	
1 year	55	57	61	63	65	66	62	65	56	57	59	61
3 years	39	43	26	29	35	38	32	37	35	38	34	37
5 years	26	31	9	10	35	39	19	23	26	30	23	27
8 years	6	9	..	..	..	..	7	10	6	8	6	8
10 years	0	0	..	..	..	..	0	0	0	0	0	0

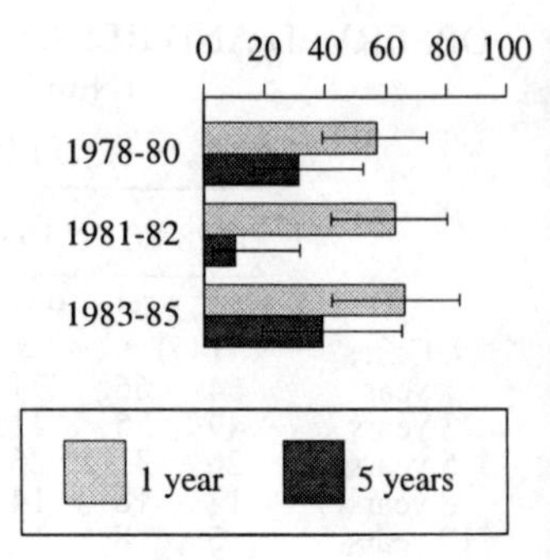

CHRONIC MYELOID LEUKAEMIA

ITALIAN REGISTRIES

REGISTRY	NUMBER OF CASES Males	Females	All	PERIOD OF DIAGNOSIS
Latina	9	2	11	1983-1984
Ragusa	10	5	15	1981-1984
Varese	43	60	103	1978-1984
Mean age (years)	62.1	62.3	62.2	

RELATIVE SURVIVAL (%)
(Both sexes)

OBSERVED AND RELATIVE SURVIVAL (%) BY PERIOD AND SEX
(Number of cases in parentheses)

	PERIOD 1978-80 obs	rel	1981-82 obs	rel	1983-85 obs	rel	SEX Males obs	rel	Females obs	rel	All obs	rel
N. Cases	(55)		(29)		(45)		(62)		(67)		(129)	
1 year	69	72	72	75	71	74	68	71	73	75	71	73
3 years	38	42	41	45	29	33	34	39	37	40	36	40
5 years	27	33	21	24	13	16	19	25	22	26	21	25
8 years	16	22	17	23	7	9	8	12	18	23	14	18
10 years	7	11	..	..	..	..	8	14	6	8	6	10

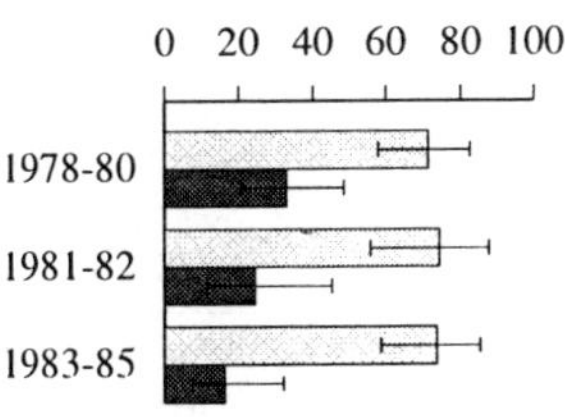

POLISH REGISTRIES

REGISTRY	NUMBER OF CASES Males	Females	All	PERIOD OF DIAGNOSIS
Cracow	14	18	32	1978-1984
Mean age (years)	49.3	55.4	52.8	

RELATIVE SURVIVAL (%)
(Both sexes)

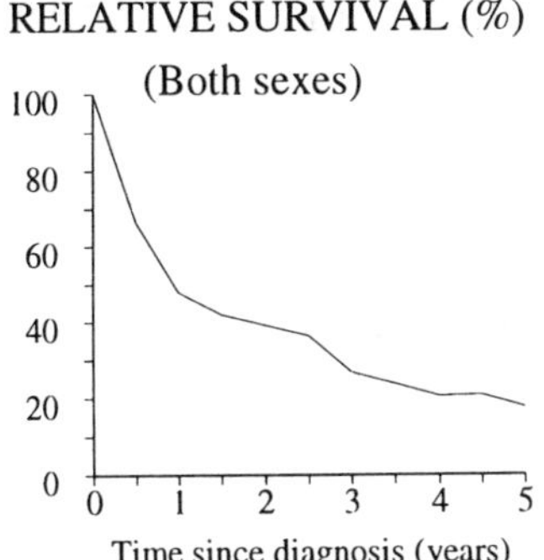

OBSERVED AND RELATIVE SURVIVAL (%) BY PERIOD AND SEX
(Number of cases in parentheses)

	PERIOD 1978-80 obs	rel	1981-82 obs	rel	1983-85 obs	rel	SEX Males obs	rel	Females obs	rel	All obs	rel
N. Cases	(16)		(7)		(9)		(14)		(18)		(32)	
1 year	50	51	71	73	22	23	43	44	50	51	47	48
3 years	31	33	29	30	11	12	14	15	33	36	25	27
5 years	13	14	29	32	11	14	7	8	22	25	16	18
8 years	0	0	0	0	..	..	..	..	0	0	0	0
10 years	0	0	0	0	..	..	..	..	0	0	0	0

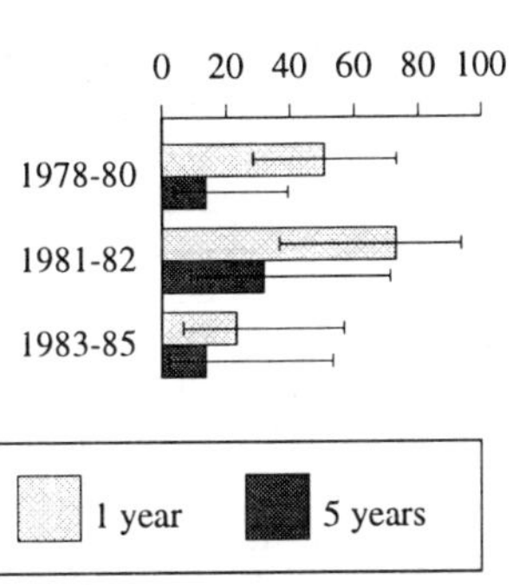

CHRONIC MYELOID LEUKAEMIA

SPANISH REGISTRIES

REGISTRY	NUMBER OF CASES Males	Females	All	PERIOD OF DIAGNOSIS
Tarragona	3	4	7	1985-1985
Mean age (years)	54.0	54.5	54.3	

RELATIVE SURVIVAL (%)

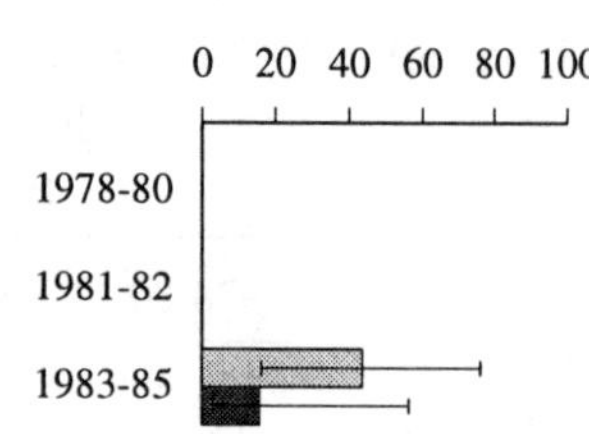

OBSERVED AND RELATIVE SURVIVAL (%) BY PERIOD AND SEX
(Number of cases in parentheses)

	PERIOD 1978-80 obs	rel	1981-82 obs	rel	1983-85 obs	rel	SEX Males obs	rel	Females obs	rel	All obs	rel
N. Cases	(0)		(0)		(7)		(3)		(4)		(7)	
1 year	..	..	..	..	43	44	67	69	25	25	43	44
3 years	..	..	..	..	14	15	33	37	0	0	14	15
5 years	..	..	..	..	14	16	33	40	0	0	14	16
8 years	..	..	..	..	..	..	..	..	0	0	..	..
10 years	..	..	..	..	..	..	..	..	0	0	..	..

0 20 40 60 80 100
1978-80
1981-82
1983-85

SWISS REGISTRIES

REGISTRY	NUMBER OF CASES Males	Females	All	PERIOD OF DIAGNOSIS
Basel	16	11	27	1981-1984
Geneva	30	32	62	1978-1984
Mean age (years)	63.5	67.7	65.6	

RELATIVE SURVIVAL (%)

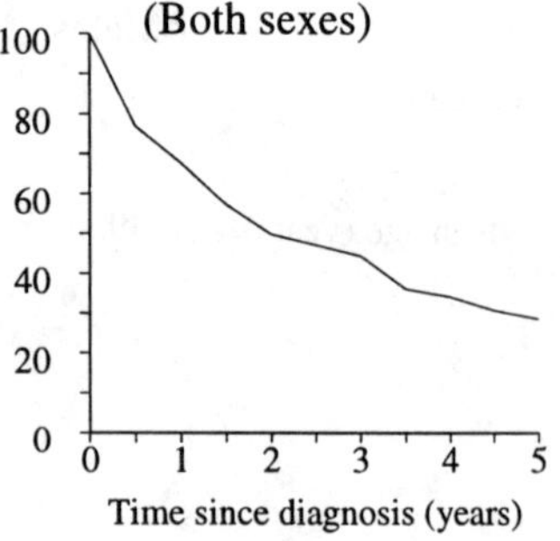

OBSERVED AND RELATIVE SURVIVAL (%) BY PERIOD AND SEX
(Number of cases in parentheses)

	PERIOD 1978-80 obs	rel	1981-82 obs	rel	1983-85 obs	rel	SEX Males obs	rel	Females obs	rel	All obs	rel
N. Cases	(33)		(24)		(32)		(46)		(43)		(89)	
1 year	67	69	53	56	72	75	63	65	67	71	65	68
3 years	39	44	31	37	44	49	31	36	47	53	39	44
5 years	24	29	13	18	28	35	18	23	28	35	23	29
8 years	..	..	0	0	..	..	..	..	..	..	..	..
10 years	..	..	0	0	..	..	..	..	..	..	..	..

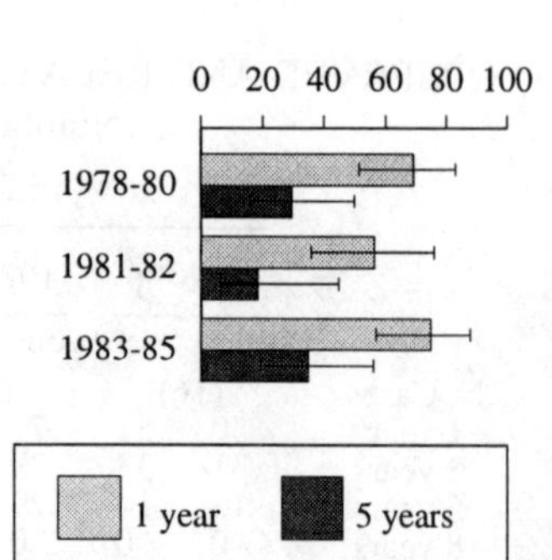

CHRONIC MYELOID LEUKAEMIA

EUROPEAN REGISTRIES

Unweighted analysis

REGISTRY	CASES Males	Females	All
DENMARK	243	185	428
DUTCH REGISTRIES	46	23	69
ENGLISH REGISTRIES	711	614	1325
ESTONIA	60	55	115
FINLAND	171	177	348
FRENCH REGISTRIES	22	4	26
GERMAN REGISTRIES	37	34	71
ITALIAN REGISTRIES	62	67	129
POLISH REGISTRIES	14	18	32
SCOTLAND	129	126	255
SPANISH REGISTRIES	3	4	7
SWISS REGISTRIES	46	43	89
Mean age (years)	60.9	64.3	62.5

RELATIVE SURVIVAL (%)
(Age-standardized)

OBSERVED AND RELATIVE SURVIVAL (%) BY AGE AND PERIOD
(Number of cases in parentheses)

	AGE CLASS												PERIOD					
	15-44		45-54		55-64		65-74		75+		All		1978-80		1981-82		1983-85	
	obs	rel	obs	rel	obs	rel	obs	rel	obs	rel	obs	rel	obs	rel	obs	rel	obs	rel
Males	(297)		(201)		(260)		(419)		(367)		(1544)		(629)		(463)		(452)	
1 year	81	81	73	73	67	68	53	56	32	37	58	61	58	60	61	64	56	59
3 years	45	45	43	44	34	36	24	28	10	15	29	33	29	34	29	33	29	33
5 years	25	25	22	23	17	19	12	15	5	10	15	19	16	20	14	18	14	18
8 years	12	13	10	11	4	5	5	8	2	5	6	9	6	9	6	9	5	8
10 years	8	9	8	9	1	1	3	6	0	0	4	6	4	6	..	..	0	0
Females	(176)		(160)		(248)		(345)		(421)		(1350)		(574)		(386)		(390)	
1 year	89	89	78	78	71	72	63	65	35	39	61	63	61	64	63	65	58	61
3 years	54	55	43	44	41	42	34	37	15	21	33	37	35	39	33	37	31	35
5 years	31	32	26	27	20	21	17	20	6	11	17	21	18	21	16	19	18	22
8 years	19	19	11	11	9	10	5	7	2	5	7	10	7	10	6	9	10	15
10 years	8	8	7	7	1	2	2	3	0	0	3	4	2	4	5	8	..	..
Overall	(473)		(361)		(508)		(764)		(788)		(2894)		(1203)		(849)		(842)	
1 year	84	84	75	75	69	70	57	60	34	38	60	62	59	62	62	65	57	60
3 years	49	49	43	44	38	39	28	32	13	18	31	35	32	36	31	35	30	34
5 years	27	28	24	25	18	20	14	18	6	10	16	20	17	21	15	19	16	20
8 years	15	15	10	11	6	7	5	8	2	5	7	10	7	9	6	9	7	10
10 years	8	8	7	8	1	2	2	4	0	0	3	5	3	5	5	8	0	0

RELATIVE SURVIVAL (%) BY AGE AND PERIOD

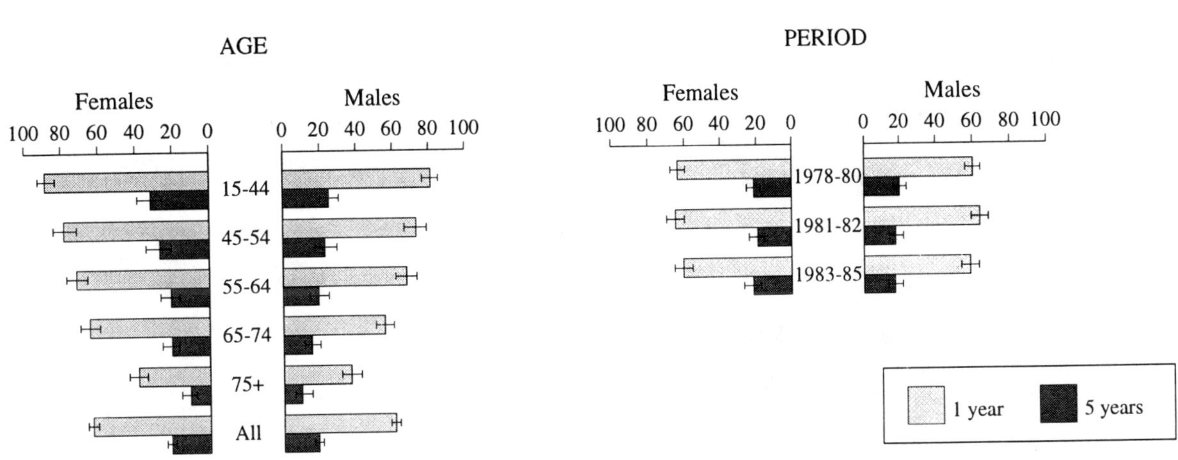

LEUKAEMIA

DENMARK

REGISTRY	NUMBER OF CASES			PERIOD OF DIAGNOSIS
	Males	Females	All	
Denmark	2104	1582	3686	1978-1984
Mean age (years)	65.4	66.7	66.0	

RELATIVE SURVIVAL (%)

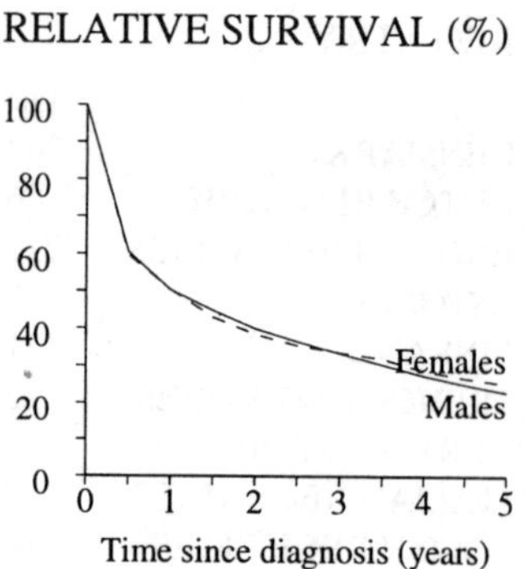

OBSERVED AND RELATIVE SURVIVAL (%) BY AGE AND PERIOD
(Number of cases in parentheses)

	AGE CLASS												PERIOD					
	15-44		45-54		55-64		65-74		75+		All		1978-80		1981-82		1983-85	
	obs	rel	obs	rel	obs	rel	obs	rel	obs	rel	obs	rel	obs	rel	obs	rel	obs	rel
Males	(230)		(160)		(393)		(692)		(629)		(2104)		(878)		(579)		(647)	
1 year	63	63	60	60	58	59	48	50	32	36	48	50	45	47	51	53	49	52
3 years	36	36	41	42	39	41	30	34	14	21	28	33	26	30	31	37	30	35
5 years	23	24	32	33	28	31	17	22	6	11	17	23	16	21	19	25	19	24
8 years	16	16	16	17	14	17	9	14	2	6	9	14	9	14	8	12	..	..
10 years	12	13	6	7	9	11	6	12	1	7	6	11	6	10	..	..	..	..
Females	(160)		(124)		(264)		(480)		(554)		(1582)		(654)		(447)		(481)	
1 year	65	65	65	65	56	57	51	53	34	37	49	50	46	48	51	52	50	52
3 years	33	33	37	38	39	40	35	38	18	24	30	34	28	32	32	36	30	34
5 years	23	23	30	31	30	32	25	29	10	15	21	25	19	23	23	28	22	27
8 years	18	18	15	16	18	21	14	18	5	11	12	17	11	15	10	13	..	..
10 years	14	14	11	12	13	15	9	13	3	10	8	12	7	11	..	..	..	..
Overall	(390)		(284)		(657)		(1172)		(1183)		(3686)		(1532)		(1026)		(1128)	
1 year	64	64	62	62	57	58	49	51	33	37	48	50	45	48	51	53	49	52
3 years	35	35	39	40	39	41	32	36	16	23	29	34	27	31	32	37	30	34
5 years	23	23	31	32	29	31	20	25	7	13	19	24	17	22	20	26	20	26
8 years	17	17	16	17	15	18	11	16	3	9	10	16	10	14	9	13	..	..
10 years	13	13	8	9	10	13	7	12	2	9	7	11	6	11	..	..	..	..

RELATIVE SURVIVAL (%) BY AGE AND PERIOD

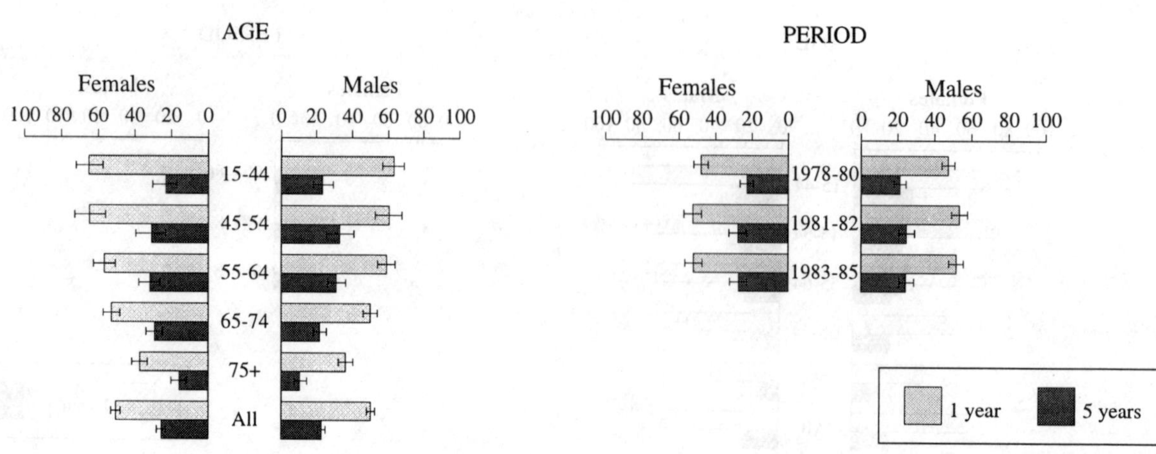

LEUKAEMIA

DUTCH REGISTRIES

REGISTRY	NUMBER OF CASES			PERIOD OF DIAGNOSIS
	Males	Females	All	
Eindhoven	212	146	358	1978-1985
Mean age (years)	62.6	61.6	62.2	

RELATIVE SURVIVAL (%)

OBSERVED AND RELATIVE SURVIVAL (%) BY AGE AND PERIOD
(Number of cases in parentheses)

	AGE CLASS												PERIOD					
	15-44		45-54		55-64		65-74		75+		All		1978-80		1981-82		1983-85	
	obs	rel	obs	rel	obs	rel	obs	rel	obs	rel	obs	rel	obs	rel	obs	rel	obs	rel
Males	(33)		(23)		(40)		(62)		(54)		(212)		(75)		(57)		(80)	
1 year	79	79	57	57	60	61	50	52	37	41	54	56	59	61	46	48	55	58
3 years	37	37	30	31	50	53	35	41	24	34	35	40	37	42	30	34	37	44
5 years	28	29	20	20	33	36	29	39	12	24	25	32	26	32	23	29	22	29
8 years	28	29	20	21	25	30	18	31	8	26	19	28	21	29	..	..	..	..
10 years	..	..	..	..	..	..	..	..	0	0	0	0	0	0	..	..	..	..
Females	(27)		(22)		(18)		(33)		(46)		(146)		(56)		(47)		(43)	
1 year	70	70	41	41	78	78	55	56	30	33	51	52	39	41	53	55	63	64
3 years	44	44	21	21	60	61	42	46	28	36	37	41	29	32	38	42	49	52
5 years	30	30	21	22	47	49	39	45	21	34	31	36	20	24	36	43	43	50
8 years	30	30	..	..	..	..	23	30	15	35	22	30	13	17	..	..	..	..
10 years	..	..	..	..	..	..	..	..	0	0	0	0	0	0	..	..	..	..
Overall	(60)		(45)		(58)		(95)		(100)		(358)		(131)		(104)		(123)	
1 year	75	75	49	49	66	66	52	54	34	37	53	55	50	52	49	51	58	60
3 years	40	40	26	27	53	56	38	43	26	35	36	41	34	38	34	38	41	47
5 years	29	29	20	20	37	40	33	41	17	30	27	34	23	29	29	36	28	35
8 years	29	29	20	20	26	31	20	31	12	33	20	29	17	24	..	..	..	..
10 years	..	..	..	..	..	..	..	..	0	0	0	0	0	0	..	..	..	..

RELATIVE SURVIVAL (%) BY AGE AND PERIOD

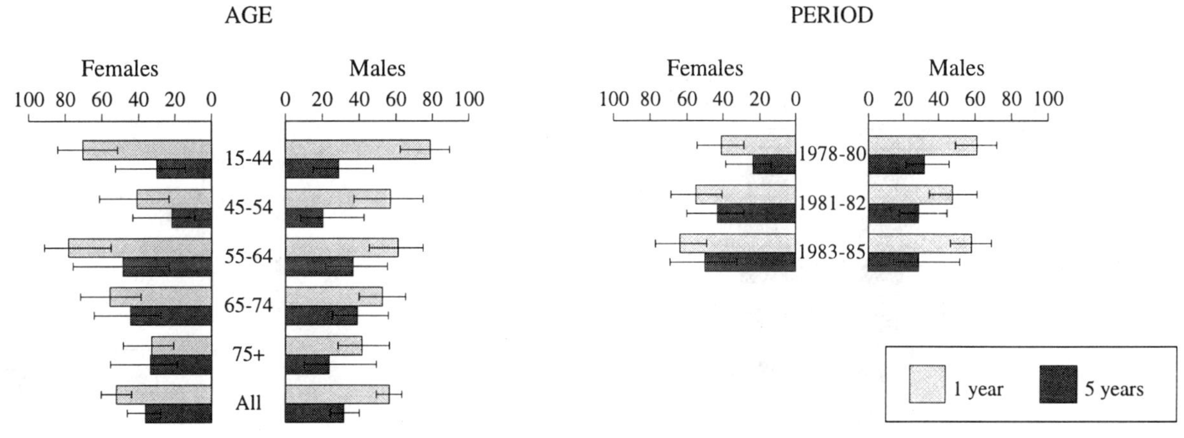

LEUKAEMIA

ENGLISH REGISTRIES

REGISTRY	NUMBER OF CASES			PERIOD OF DIAGNOSIS
	Males	Females	All	
East Anglia	585	412	997	1979-1984
Mersey	700	538	1238	1978-1984
South Thames	1820	1569	3389	1978-1984
Wessex	246	248	494	1983-1984
West Midlands	1173	888	2061	1979-1984
Yorkshire	1019	851	1870	1978-1984
Mean age (years)	64.5	67.4	65.8	

RELATIVE SURVIVAL (%)

100
80
60
40
20
0
0 1 2 3 4 5
Males
Females
Time since diagnosis (years)

OBSERVED AND RELATIVE SURVIVAL (%) BY AGE AND PERIOD
(Number of cases in parentheses)

	AGE CLASS												PERIOD					
	15-44		45-54		55-64		65-74		75+		All		1978-80		1981-82		1983-85	
	obs	rel	obs	rel	obs	rel	obs	rel	obs	rel	obs	rel	obs	rel	obs	rel	obs	rel
Males	(655)		(508)		(1035)		(1740)		(1605)		(5543)		(2180)		(1613)		(1750)	
1 year	62	62	59	59	53	54	43	45	28	31	44	47	44	47	43	45	45	48
3 years	33	33	38	39	34	36	24	28	14	21	25	30	24	29	27	31	26	30
5 years	23	23	26	27	22	25	15	20	7	15	16	21	14	19	18	24	17	22
8 years	17	17	17	19	13	16	8	13	3	11	9	15	8	13	11	17	9	14
10 years	16	16	16	17	9	12	5	11	2	10	7	13	7	12	8	14	..	..
Females	(525)		(314)		(662)		(1158)		(1847)		(4506)		(1744)		(1269)		(1493)	
1 year	60	60	54	55	55	56	47	48	28	31	42	44	42	45	39	41	44	46
3 years	35	35	32	33	33	34	27	30	14	19	24	28	23	27	23	27	25	29
5 years	26	26	23	24	23	24	19	23	8	14	16	21	15	20	16	21	17	22
8 years	21	22	16	17	14	16	11	15	3	9	10	15	9	14	9	14	12	18
10 years	19	19	12	13	12	14	7	11	2	7	8	13	7	12	9	14	..	..
Overall	(1180)		(822)		(1697)		(2898)		(3452)		(10049)		(3924)		(2882)		(3243)	
1 year	61	61	57	57	54	54	44	46	28	31	43	46	43	46	41	44	45	47
3 years	34	34	36	36	33	35	25	29	14	20	25	29	24	28	25	30	25	30
5 years	24	24	25	26	23	25	17	21	8	15	16	21	15	20	17	22	17	22
8 years	19	19	17	18	13	16	9	14	3	10	10	15	9	14	10	16	10	15
10 years	17	18	15	16	11	13	6	11	2	8	7	13	7	12	8	14	..	..

RELATIVE SURVIVAL (%) BY AGE AND PERIOD

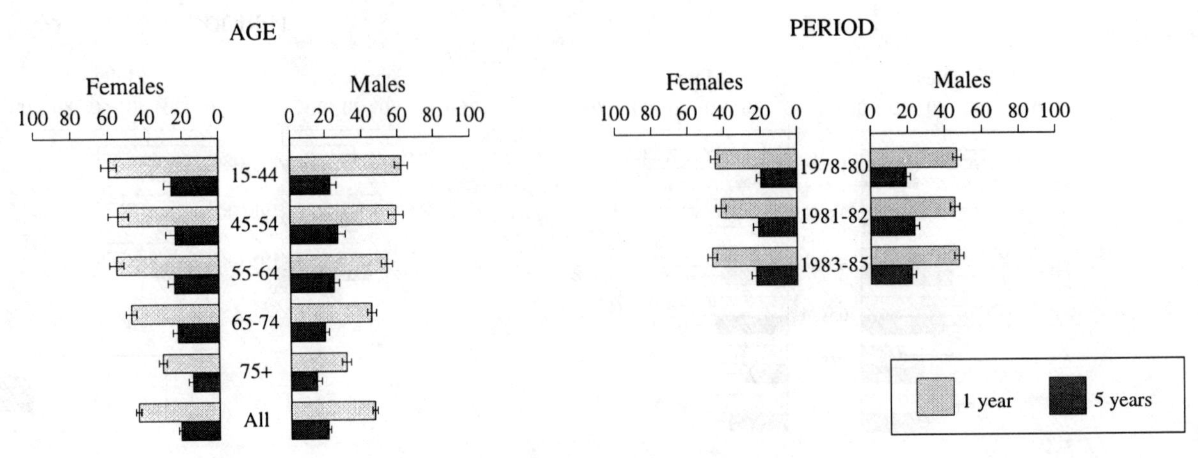

LEUKAEMIA

ESTONIA

REGISTRY	NUMBER OF CASES			PERIOD OF DIAGNOSIS
	Males	Females	All	
Estonia	361	379	740	1978-1984
Mean age (years)	61.5	61.2	61.3	

RELATIVE SURVIVAL (%)

OBSERVED AND RELATIVE SURVIVAL (%) BY AGE AND PERIOD
(Number of cases in parentheses)

	AGE CLASS												PERIOD					
	15-44		45-54		55-64		65-74		75+		All		1978-80		1981-82		1983-85	
	obs	rel	obs	rel	obs	rel	obs	rel	obs	rel	obs	rel	obs	rel	obs	rel	obs	rel
Males	(43)		(57)		(84)		(112)		(65)		(361)		(148)		(95)		(118)	
1 year	37	37	70	71	75	77	56	59	42	47	58	61	56	59	56	59	62	65
3 years	30	31	58	61	61	66	37	45	20	30	42	49	39	44	42	49	46	54
5 years	15	16	43	47	38	45	24	33	15	31	28	36	23	30	31	41	30	39
8 years	13	14	31	36	24	31	13	24	7	25	17	27	13	20	23	37	..	..
10 years	13	14	19	23	13	20	13	29	..	..	13	22	9	16	..	..	..	..
Females	(54)		(55)		(81)		(121)		(68)		(379)		(155)		(106)		(118)	
1 year	46	46	65	66	49	50	58	60	41	46	53	54	50	52	56	57	53	54
3 years	22	22	55	55	40	41	45	50	32	45	40	44	43	47	37	40	39	43
5 years	11	11	44	45	36	38	33	39	22	40	30	35	35	42	20	24	31	37
8 years	0	0	30	31	29	32	28	40	10	30	22	29	25	33	16	21	..	..
10 years	0	0	23	24	29	34	21	35	0	0	17	25	19	27	..	..	..	..
Overall	(97)		(112)		(165)		(233)		(133)		(740)		(303)		(201)		(236)	
1 year	42	42	68	69	62	64	57	59	41	46	55	57	53	55	56	58	57	59
3 years	26	26	56	58	50	53	41	47	26	38	41	46	41	46	39	44	43	48
5 years	13	13	43	46	37	41	28	36	19	36	29	36	30	36	25	32	31	38
8 years	8	8	31	34	26	32	22	34	9	27	20	28	19	27	19	28	..	..
10 years	8	8	21	24	19	25	17	32	0	0	15	24	14	22	..	..	..	..

RELATIVE SURVIVAL (%) BY AGE AND PERIOD

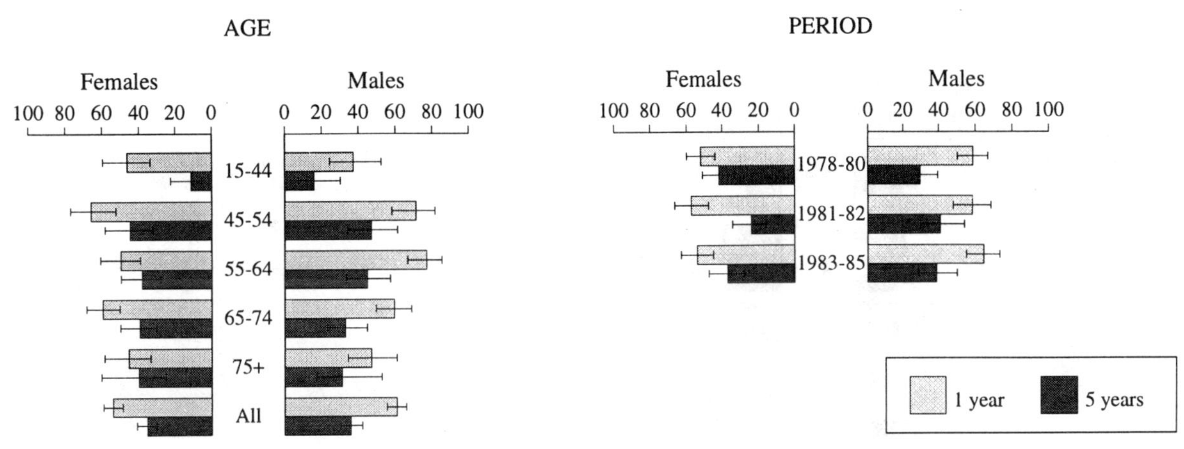

LEUKAEMIA

FINLAND

REGISTRY	NUMBER OF CASES			PERIOD OF DIAGNOSIS
	Males	Females	All	
Finland	1215	1096	2311	1978-1984
Mean age (years)	60.9	64.4	62.5	

RELATIVE SURVIVAL (%)

100
80
60
40
20
0
0 1 2 3 4 5
Females
Males
Time since diagnosis (years)

OBSERVED AND RELATIVE SURVIVAL (%) BY AGE AND PERIOD
(Number of cases in parentheses)

	AGE CLASS												PERIOD					
	15-44		45-54		55-64		65-74		75+		All		1978-80		1981-82		1983-85	
	obs	rel	obs	rel	obs	rel	obs	rel	obs	rel	obs	rel	obs	rel	obs	rel	obs	rel
Males	(210)		(145)		(228)		(359)		(273)		(1215)		(508)		(358)		(349)	
1 year	65	65	69	70	64	66	52	55	41	46	56	59	56	59	60	63	53	56
3 years	28	28	43	44	42	45	31	36	19	28	31	36	29	34	34	39	30	35
5 years	19	19	32	33	29	33	18	24	9	18	20	25	19	25	21	27	19	24
8 years	12	13	17	19	16	19	9	15	3	9	10	15	9	13	12	18	10	15
10 years	11	11	12	14	9	12	3	5	..	..	5	9	5	7	6	10	..	..
Females	(160)		(92)		(191)		(300)		(353)		(1096)		(468)		(316)		(312)	
1 year	69	69	67	68	69	70	56	58	45	49	58	60	59	61	59	61	54	57
3 years	38	38	41	42	41	42	36	39	26	34	34	38	36	40	30	33	36	40
5 years	27	27	28	29	26	27	22	26	13	21	21	25	22	27	17	21	22	28
8 years	21	21	20	20	16	18	7	9	4	10	11	15	12	16	7	10	13	18
10 years	13	13	16	17	10	11	3	4	1	5	6	9	7	10	2	3	..	..
Overall	(370)		(237)		(419)		(659)		(626)		(2311)		(976)		(674)		(661)	
1 year	67	67	68	69	67	68	54	56	43	48	57	59	57	60	59	62	54	56
3 years	32	32	42	43	41	43	33	38	23	32	32	37	33	37	32	36	33	38
5 years	22	23	30	32	27	30	20	25	11	20	20	25	21	26	19	24	20	26
8 years	16	16	18	20	16	19	8	12	3	10	10	15	10	15	10	14	11	17
10 years	11	11	14	15	9	11	3	5	1	4	6	9	6	9	4	6	..	..

RELATIVE SURVIVAL (%) BY AGE AND PERIOD

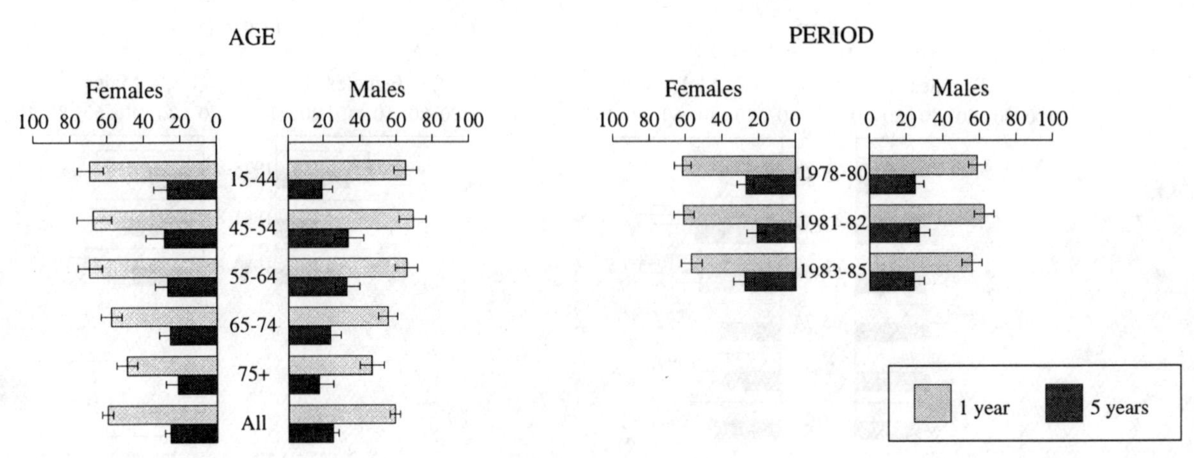

LEUKAEMIA

FRENCH REGISTRIES

REGISTRY	NUMBER OF CASES			PERIOD OF DIAGNOSIS
	Males	Females	All	
Amiens	48	35	83	1983-1984
Côte-d'Or	174	112	286	1980-1984
Doubs	169	120	289	1978-1985
Mean age (years)	63.3	64.5	63.8	

RELATIVE SURVIVAL (%)

100 80 60 40 20 0

Males
Females

0 1 2 3 4 5
Time since diagnosis (years)

OBSERVED AND RELATIVE SURVIVAL (%) BY AGE AND PERIOD
(Number of cases in parentheses)

	AGE CLASS												PERIOD					
	15-44		45-54		55-64		65-74		75+		All		1978-80		1981-82		1983-85	
	obs	rel	obs	rel	obs	rel	obs	rel	obs	rel	obs	rel	obs	rel	obs	rel	obs	rel
Males	(62)		(37)		(71)		(118)		(103)		(391)		(78)		(120)		(193)	
1 year	76	76	75	76	75	76	74	78	44	49	67	70	62	65	69	72	67	70
3 years	48	49	53	54	56	59	49	56	27	39	45	52	39	44	48	55	45	52
5 years	34	34	35	37	45	49	36	46	17	33	32	41	31	38	34	44	31	41
8 years	20	21	35	38	41	48	14	21	0	0	18	27	19	27	15	22	..	..
10 years	..	..	35	39	24	30	9	16	0	0	13	22	14	22	..	..	..	..
Females	(42)		(29)		(36)		(62)		(98)		(267)		(49)		(81)		(137)	
1 year	76	76	66	66	75	75	60	61	52	57	62	65	53	56	64	67	64	66
3 years	49	49	47	48	47	48	46	49	31	41	41	47	41	47	37	42	44	49
5 years	38	38	47	48	41	43	39	44	20	33	33	40	35	43	29	36	35	42
8 years	30	30	37	38	14	15	27	34	12	31	22	31	25	35	20	29	23	31
10 years	..	..	..	..	..	..	27	37	..	..	20	31	22	34	..	..	..	..
Overall	(104)		(66)		(107)		(180)		(201)		(658)		(127)		(201)		(330)	
1 year	76	76	71	71	75	76	69	72	48	53	65	68	59	61	67	70	66	68
3 years	49	49	50	51	53	55	48	54	29	40	43	49	40	45	43	50	45	51
5 years	35	36	40	42	44	47	37	45	18	33	32	41	32	40	32	40	33	41
8 years	24	24	36	38	35	40	18	26	7	19	20	29	21	30	17	25	22	32
10 years	..	..	30	33	21	25	16	25	..	..	16	26	17	26	..	..	..	..

RELATIVE SURVIVAL (%) BY AGE AND PERIOD

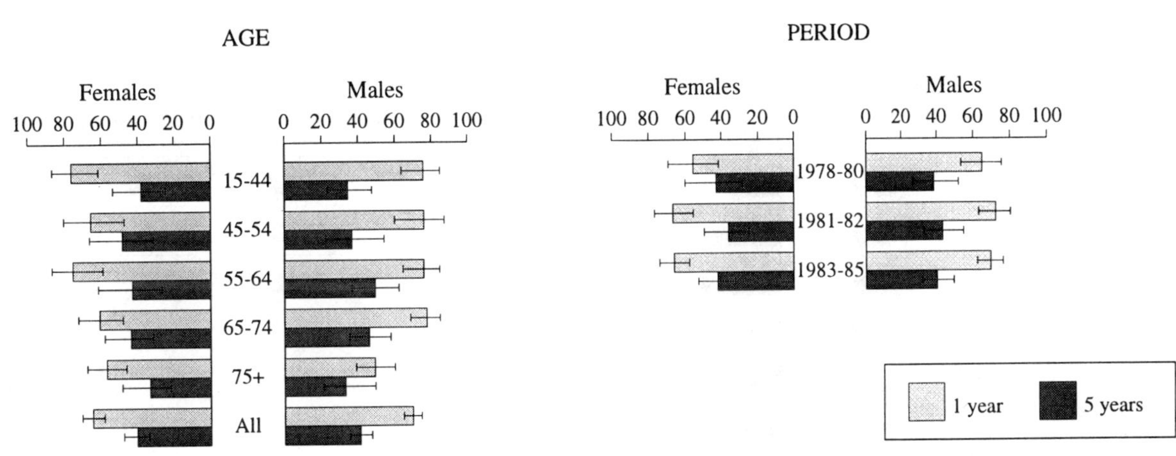

LEUKAEMIA

GERMAN REGISTRIES

REGISTRY	NUMBER OF CASES			PERIOD OF DIAGNOSIS
	Males	Females	All	
Saarland	239	201	440	1978-1984
Mean age (years)	62.2	61.5	61.8	

RELATIVE SURVIVAL (%)

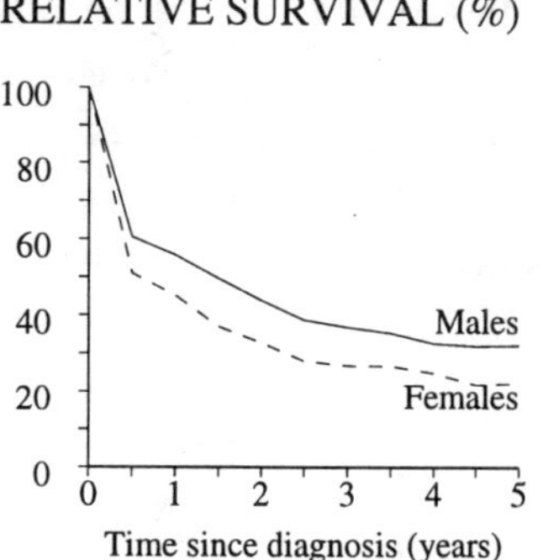

OBSERVED AND RELATIVE SURVIVAL (%) BY AGE AND PERIOD
(Number of cases in parentheses)

	AGE CLASS												PERIOD					
	15-44		45-54		55-64		65-74		75+		All		1978-80		1981-82		1983-85	
	obs	rel	obs	rel	obs	rel	obs	rel	obs	rel	obs	rel	obs	rel	obs	rel	obs	rel
Males	(32)		(35)		(51)		(71)		(50)		(239)		(92)		(66)		(81)	
1 year	69	69	66	66	67	68	44	46	34	39	53	56	51	54	52	54	57	60
3 years	34	35	46	47	41	44	25	31	20	30	32	37	37	43	29	33	28	33
5 years	28	28	40	42	39	44	18	26	8	16	25	32	28	37	21	27	25	31
8 years	16	16	15	16	34	41	14	25	2	7	16	24	15	23	15	23	..	..
10 years	16	17	7	8	27	35	11	25	2	9	13	21	12	20	..	..	..	..
Females	(34)		(24)		(34)		(59)		(50)		(201)		(77)		(57)		(67)	
1 year	47	47	46	46	62	62	39	40	34	37	44	45	36	38	46	47	51	52
3 years	24	24	25	25	41	42	22	24	16	21	24	27	25	27	25	27	24	26
5 years	24	24	21	21	32	34	12	14	14	22	19	22	19	23	18	21	19	22
8 years	11	12	0	0	13	14	8	11	6	13	8	11	8	10	9	12	..	..
10 years	8	8	0	0	..	..	5	8	..	..	5	8	5	7	..	..	..	..
Overall	(66)		(59)		(85)		(130)		(100)		(440)		(169)		(123)		(148)	
1 year	58	58	58	58	65	66	42	43	34	38	49	51	44	46	49	51	54	56
3 years	29	29	37	38	41	43	24	28	18	25	28	32	31	36	27	31	26	29
5 years	26	26	32	33	36	40	15	20	11	20	22	27	24	30	20	24	22	27
8 years	13	14	9	10	27	32	11	17	4	10	12	18	12	17	12	17	..	..
10 years	11	11	5	5	22	27	8	15	4	14	9	15	9	14	..	..	..	..

RELATIVE SURVIVAL (%) BY AGE AND PERIOD

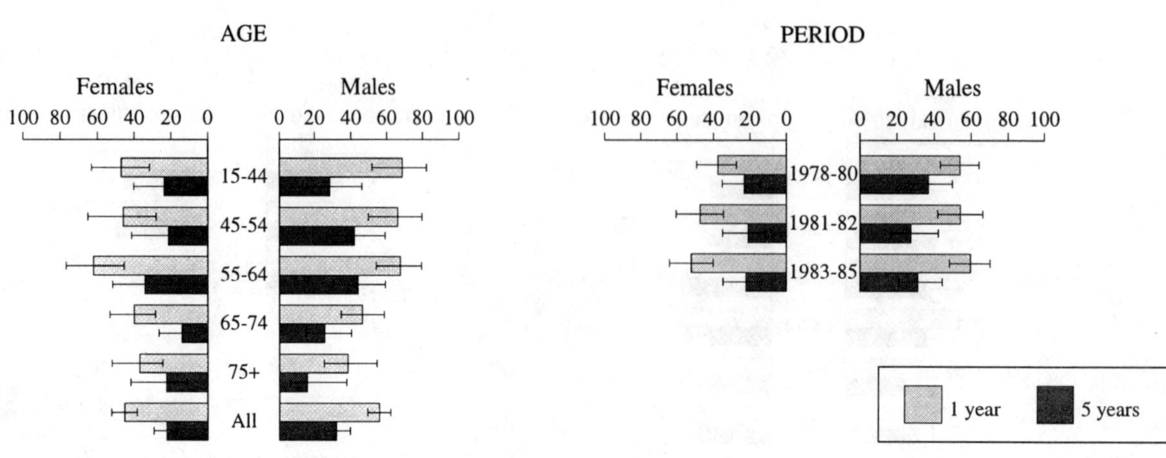

LEUKAEMIA

ITALIAN REGISTRIES

REGISTRY	NUMBER OF CASES			PERIOD OF DIAGNOSIS
	Males	Females	All	
Florence	26	17	43	1985-1985
Latina	42	20	62	1983-1984
Ragusa	48	34	82	1981-1984
Varese	250	230	480	1978-1984
Mean age (years)	61.5	61.9	61.7	

RELATIVE SURVIVAL (%)

100
80
60
40
20
0
Females
Males
0 1 2 3 4 5
Time since diagnosis (years)

OBSERVED AND RELATIVE SURVIVAL (%) BY AGE AND PERIOD
(Number of cases in parentheses)

	AGE CLASS												PERIOD					
	15-44		45-54		55-64		65-74		75+		All		1978-80		1981-82		1983-85	
	obs	rel	obs	rel	obs	rel	obs	rel	obs	rel	obs	rel	obs	rel	obs	rel	obs	rel
Males	(63)		(44)		(56)		(112)		(91)		(366)		(99)		(94)		(173)	
1 year	56	56	57	57	55	56	52	54	31	35	48	51	54	56	53	56	43	45
3 years	37	37	36	37	36	38	29	34	12	18	28	33	27	32	31	36	27	31
5 years	32	32	16	17	27	30	23	30	7	13	20	26	19	25	22	29	20	24
8 years	19	19	11	11	19	23	16	25	4	12	13	19	12	18	14	21	10	14
10 years	15	15	11	12	19	25	12	22	2	8	10	17	9	15	13	22	..	..
Females	(48)		(42)		(43)		(90)		(78)		(301)		(105)		(85)		(111)	
1 year	58	58	60	60	65	66	57	58	36	39	53	55	58	60	58	60	45	47
3 years	31	31	40	41	47	48	30	32	18	24	31	34	37	41	34	38	23	25
5 years	19	19	36	36	28	29	22	25	14	24	22	26	30	35	22	26	15	18
8 years	19	19	30	31	26	28	15	20	6	16	17	22	24	31	16	21	11	14
10 years	11	11	26	27	19	21	13	18	2	8	13	18	18	26	5	7	..	..
Overall	(111)		(86)		(99)		(202)		(169)		(667)		(204)		(179)		(284)	
1 year	57	57	58	58	60	60	54	56	33	37	51	53	56	58	55	58	44	45
3 years	34	34	38	39	40	42	30	33	15	21	29	33	32	37	32	37	25	29
5 years	26	26	26	26	27	30	23	28	10	18	21	26	25	30	22	28	18	22
8 years	19	19	20	21	22	25	16	23	5	14	15	21	18	26	15	21	11	15
10 years	13	14	18	19	18	22	12	20	2	8	11	17	14	21	9	14	..	..

RELATIVE SURVIVAL (%) BY AGE AND PERIOD

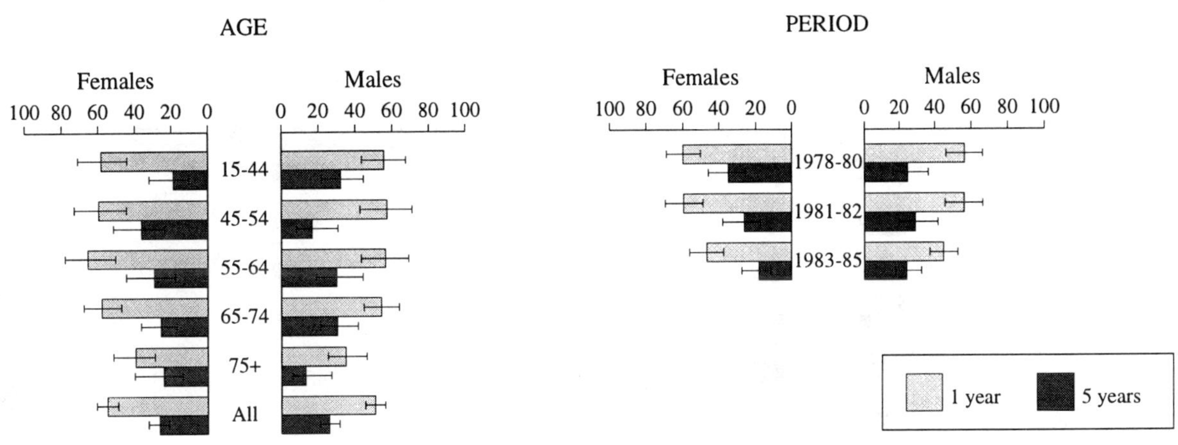

LEUKAEMIA

POLISH REGISTRIES

REGISTRY	NUMBER OF CASES			PERIOD OF DIAGNOSIS
	Males	Females	All	
Cracow	127	115	242	1978-1984
Mean age (years)	57.7	57.8	57.7	

RELATIVE SURVIVAL (%)

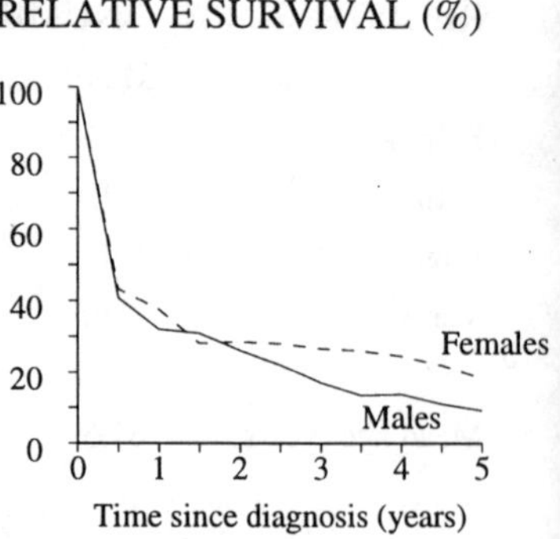

OBSERVED AND RELATIVE SURVIVAL (%) BY AGE AND PERIOD
(Number of cases in parentheses)

	AGE CLASS												PERIOD					
	15-44		45-54		55-64		65-74		75+		All		1978-80		1981-82		1983-85	
	obs	rel	obs	rel	obs	rel	obs	rel	obs	rel	obs	rel	obs	rel	obs	rel	obs	rel
Males	(25)		(25)		(28)		(34)		(15)		(127)		(53)		(37)		(37)	
1 year	28	28	38	39	38	39	26	28	20	22	31	32	35	36	23	24	33	34
3 years	9	9	17	18	30	33	9	11	7	10	15	17	16	17	9	10	21	23
5 years	5	5	9	9	15	18	3	4	7	13	8	9	6	7	6	7	12	14
8 years	..	..	9	10	4	5	0	0	..	..	3	4	4	5	0	0	..	..
10 years	..	..	9	10	4	6	0	0	..	..	3	4	4	6	0	0	..	..
Females	(26)		(18)		(18)		(26)		(27)		(115)		(51)		(27)		(37)	
1 year	42	42	44	45	56	56	35	36	15	16	37	38	41	42	33	34	32	34
3 years	23	23	33	34	39	40	27	30	7	10	24	27	25	28	26	27	22	24
5 years	12	12	28	29	28	30	19	23	0	0	16	18	16	18	22	25	11	13
8 years	8	8	7	8	11	13	8	11	0	0	7	8	4	5	15	18	4	6
10 years	8	8	..	..	..	..	8	12	0	0	7	9	4	5	15	18	..	..
Overall	(51)		(43)		(46)		(60)		(42)		(242)		(104)		(64)		(74)	
1 year	35	36	41	41	45	46	30	31	17	18	34	35	38	39	27	28	33	34
3 years	17	17	24	25	34	36	17	19	7	10	20	22	20	23	16	18	21	24
5 years	8	8	17	18	20	23	10	13	2	4	11	14	11	13	13	15	11	14
8 years	6	6	7	8	7	8	3	5	..	..	5	6	4	5	6	9	4	6
10 years	6	6	7	8	7	9	3	6	..	..	5	7	4	6	6	9	..	..

RELATIVE SURVIVAL (%) BY AGE AND PERIOD

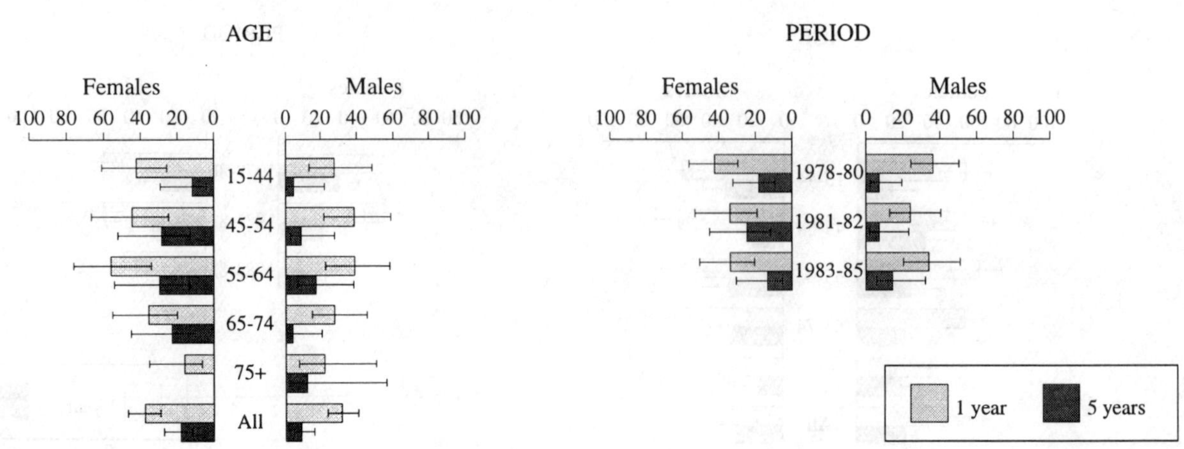

LEUKAEMIA

SCOTLAND

REGISTRY	NUMBER OF CASES			PERIOD OF DIAGNOSIS
	Males	Females	All	
Scotland	981	808	1789	1978-1982
Mean age (years)	63.6	66.4	64.8	

RELATIVE SURVIVAL (%)

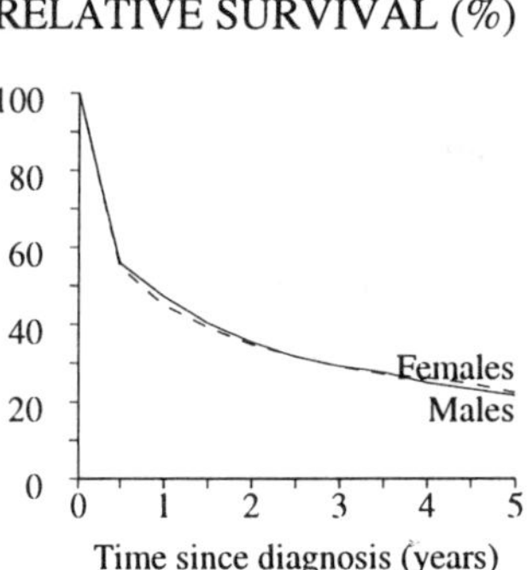

OBSERVED AND RELATIVE SURVIVAL (%) BY AGE AND PERIOD
(Number of cases in parentheses)

	AGE CLASS												PERIOD					
	15-44		45-54		55-64		65-74		75+		All		1978-80		1981-82		1983-85	
	obs	rel	obs	rel	obs	rel	obs	rel	obs	rel	obs	rel	obs	rel	obs	rel	obs	rel
Males	(129)		(107)		(164)		(313)		(268)		(981)		(581)		(400)		(0)	
1 year	58	58	58	58	54	55	40	42	33	38	45	47	44	46	46	49	..	..
3 years	29	30	31	32	38	41	22	26	14	22	24	29	22	27	28	33	..	..
5 years	22	22	24	26	23	26	15	21	7	14	16	22	14	19	19	25	..	..
8 years	18	18	17	19	17	21	6	11	1	4	9	15	8	13	..	..	..	..
10 years	..	..	11	12	..	..	5	12	0	0	7	13	6	12	..	..	..	..
Females	(98)		(66)		(118)		(227)		(299)		(808)		(482)		(326)		(0)	
1 year	64	64	53	53	44	45	46	47	31	34	43	45	42	44	44	46	..	..
3 years	35	35	27	28	31	32	31	35	15	20	25	29	24	29	26	30	..	..
5 years	32	32	20	20	24	26	21	25	8	14	18	23	18	23	17	21	..	..
8 years	22	22	14	14	16	18	11	15	2	6	10	15	10	15	..	..	..	..
10 years	22	22	..	..	16	19	4	6	2	9	6	10	6	11	..	..	..	..
Overall	(227)		(173)		(282)		(540)		(567)		(1789)		(1063)		(726)		(0)	
1 year	61	61	56	57	50	51	42	44	32	36	44	46	43	45	45	48	..	..
3 years	32	32	29	30	35	37	26	30	14	21	25	29	23	28	27	31	..	..
5 years	26	26	23	24	23	26	17	23	7	14	17	22	16	21	18	23	..	..
8 years	20	20	15	17	16	19	8	13	2	6	9	15	9	14	..	..	..	..
10 years	20	20	11	13	16	21	4	8	1	4	6	11	6	11	..	..	..	..

RELATIVE SURVIVAL (%) BY AGE AND PERIOD

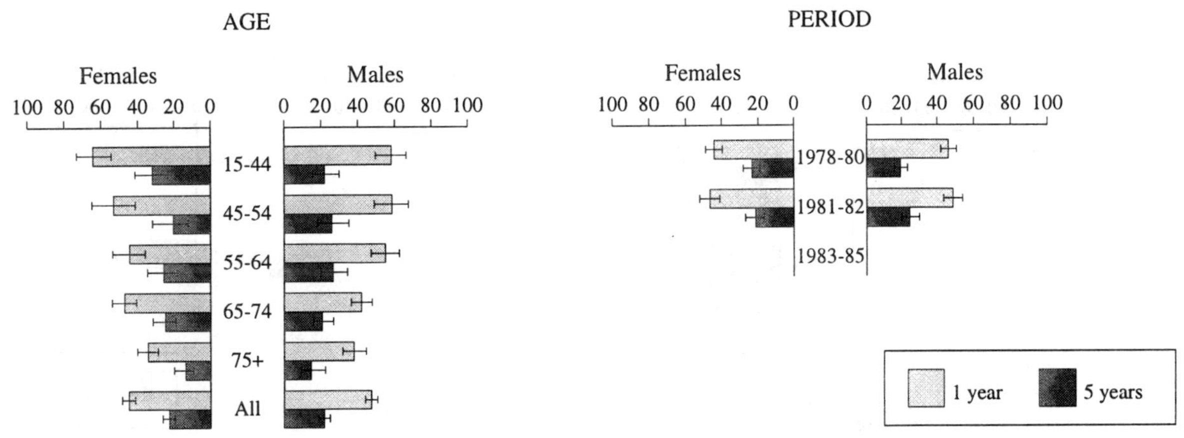

LEUKAEMIA

SPANISH REGISTRIES

REGISTRY	NUMBER OF CASES			PERIOD OF DIAGNOSIS
	Males	Females	All	
Tarragona	19	10	29	1985-1985
Mean age (years)	56.8	61.8	58.5	

RELATIVE SURVIVAL (%)

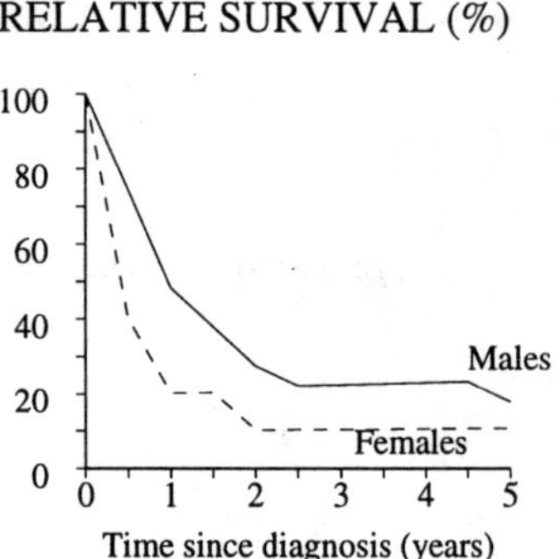

OBSERVED AND RELATIVE SURVIVAL (%) BY AGE AND PERIOD
(Number of cases in parentheses)

	AGE CLASS												PERIOD					
	15-44		45-54		55-64		65-74		75+		All		1978-80		1981-82		1983-85	
	obs	rel	obs	rel	obs	rel	obs	rel	obs	rel	obs	rel	obs	rel	obs	rel	obs	rel
Males	(4)		(2)		(5)		(6)		(2)		(19)		(0)		(0)		(19)	
1 year	75	75	50	50	40	40	33	34	50	54	47	48	..	..	..	..	47	48
3 years	25	25	0	0	40	42	0	0	50	62	21	22	..	..	..	..	21	22
5 years	25	25	0	0	40	43	0	0	0	0	16	18	..	..	..	..	16	18
8 years	..	..	0	0	..	..	0	0	0	0	..	..	..	..	..	..	..	..
10 years	..	..	0	0	..	..	0	0	0	0	..	..	..	..	..	..	..	..
Females	(1)		(1)		(3)		(5)		(0)		(10)		(0)		(0)		(10)	
1 year	100	100	0	0	0	0	20	20	..	..	20	20	..	..	..	..	20	20
3 years	0	0	0	0	0	0	20	21	..	..	10	10	..	..	..	..	10	10
5 years	0	0	0	0	0	0	20	22	..	..	10	11	..	..	..	..	10	11
8 years	0	0	0	0	0	0	..	..	..	..	..	..	..	..	..	..	..	..
10 years	0	0	0	0	0	0	..	..	..	..	..	..	..	..	..	..	..	..
Overall	(5)		(3)		(8)		(11)		(2)		(29)		(0)		(0)		(29)	
1 year	80	80	33	33	25	25	27	28	50	54	38	39	..	..	..	..	38	39
3 years	20	20	0	0	25	26	9	10	50	62	17	18	..	..	..	..	17	18
5 years	20	20	0	0	25	26	9	10	0	0	14	15	..	..	..	..	14	15
8 years	..	..	0	0	..	..	..	..	0	0	..	..	..	..	..	..	..	..
10 years	..	..	0	0	..	..	..	..	0	0	..	..	..	..	..	..	..	..

RELATIVE SURVIVAL (%) BY AGE AND PERIOD

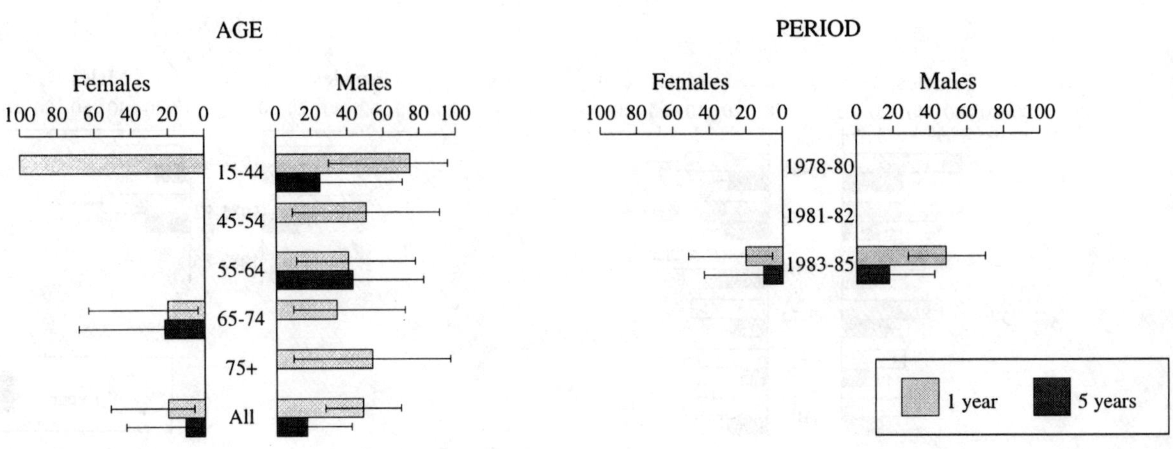

LEUKAEMIA

SWISS REGISTRIES

REGISTRY	NUMBER OF CASES			PERIOD OF DIAGNOSIS
	Males	Females	All	
Basel	78	69	147	1981-1984
Geneva	116	128	244	1978-1984
Mean age (years)	64.2	66.3	65.3	

OBSERVED AND RELATIVE SURVIVAL (%) BY AGE AND PERIOD
(Number of cases in parentheses)

	AGE CLASS												PERIOD					
	15-44		45-54		55-64		65-74		75+		All		1978-80		1981-82		1983-85	
	obs	rel	obs	rel	obs	rel	obs	rel	obs	rel	obs	rel	obs	rel	obs	rel	obs	rel
Males	(24)		(21)		(32)		(55)		(62)		(194)		(45)		(66)		(83)	
1 year	54	54	80	81	84	86	73	75	45	50	64	67	64	68	60	63	67	70
3 years	38	38	60	61	59	62	53	59	24	33	44	50	44	52	36	41	49	56
5 years	33	34	50	52	53	58	38	47	11	20	33	41	29	38	26	33	40	50
8 years	28	28	0	0	43	50	21	31	..	..	22	33	..	..	19	28	..	..
10 years	..	..	0	0	..	..	0	0	..	..	..	..	..	..	..	..	..	..
Females	(22)		(19)		(31)		(52)		(73)		(197)		(57)		(69)		(71)	
1 year	68	68	63	63	61	62	63	65	53	58	60	62	54	56	57	59	68	70
3 years	36	36	41	41	52	53	50	53	32	41	41	46	32	35	39	44	50	56
5 years	31	31	29	29	39	40	40	45	16	27	29	35	25	30	25	32	36	42
8 years	..	..	..	..	..	..	29	36	16	38	24	33	..	..	20	29	..	..
10 years	..	..	..	..	..	..	..	..	..	..	..	..	..	..	..	..	..	..
Overall	(46)		(40)		(63)		(107)		(135)		(391)		(102)		(135)		(154)	
1 year	61	61	72	72	73	74	68	70	50	54	62	65	59	61	58	61	68	70
3 years	37	37	51	51	56	58	51	56	28	38	42	48	37	43	37	43	50	56
5 years	32	32	40	41	46	49	39	46	14	24	31	38	26	33	26	33	38	46
8 years	29	29	0	0	40	45	25	33	14	35	23	33	..	..	19	29	..	..
10 years	..	..	0	0	..	..	..	..	..	..	..	..	..	..	..	..	..	..

RELATIVE SURVIVAL (%) BY AGE AND PERIOD

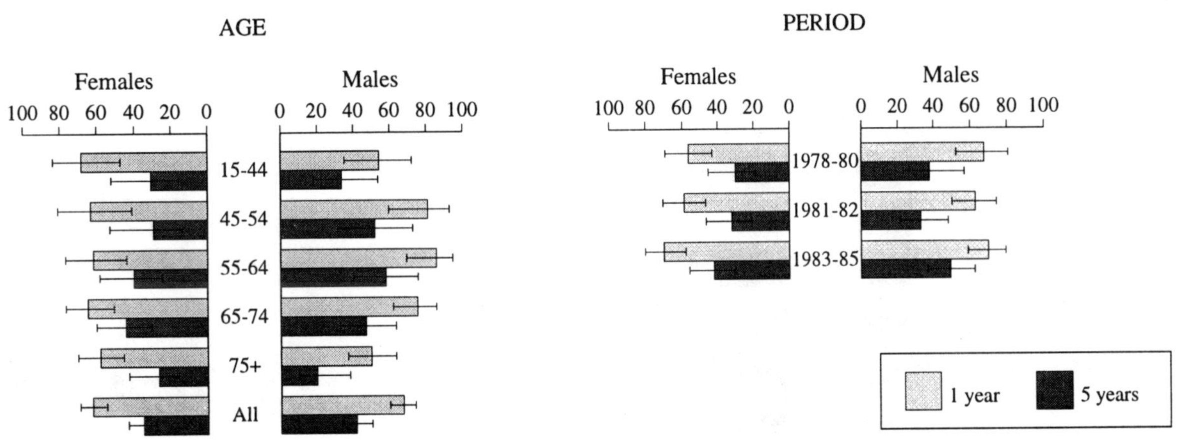

LEUKAEMIA

EUROPEAN REGISTRIES
Weighted analysis

REGISTRY	WEIGHTS (Yearly expected cases in the country) Males	Females	All
DENMARK	330	244	574
DUTCH REGISTRIES	665	515	1180
ENGLISH REGISTRIES	2510	1927	4437
ESTONIA	58	58	116
FINLAND	195	177	372
FRENCH REGISTRIES	3205	2497	5702
GERMAN REGISTRIES	3273	2876	6149
ITALIAN REGISTRIES	3348	2363	5711
POLISH REGISTRIES	1146	880	2026
SCOTLAND	218	178	396
SPANISH REGISTRIES	1391	1097	2488
SWISS REGISTRIES	301	306	607

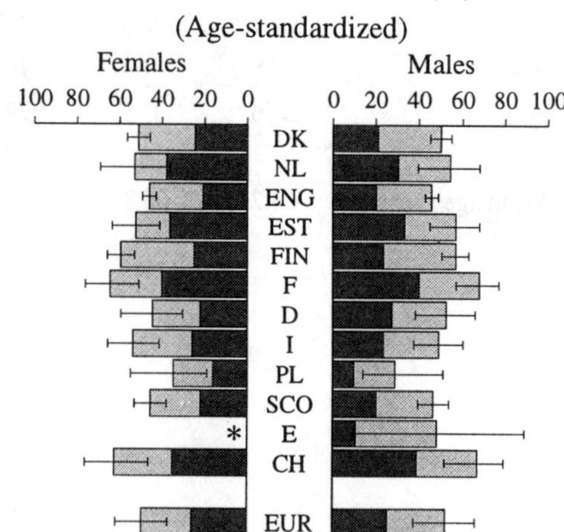

* Not enough cases for reliable estimation

OBSERVED AND RELATIVE SURVIVAL (%) BY AGE AND PERIOD

	AGE CLASS 15-44 obs	15-44 rel	45-54 obs	45-54 rel	55-64 obs	55-64 rel	65-74 obs	65-74 rel	75+ obs	75+ rel	All obs	All rel	PERIOD 1978-80 obs	1978-80 rel	1981-82 obs	1981-82 rel	1983-85 obs	1983-85 rel
Males																		
1 year	64	64	61	62	59	60	50	52	35	39	51	54	52	55	52	55	52	54
3 years	35	35	38	39	42	44	28	33	21	29	31	35	31	36	32	37	31	35
5 years	27	27	25	27	33	37	20	27	9	17	22	28	22	28	23	29	22	28
8 years	19	19	17	18	25	30	11	18	2	7	14	20	13	20	13	19	10	14
10 years	15	16	14	16	19	24	8	15	1	6	10	16	9	15	9	16	..	..
Females																		
1 year	63	63	50	51	59	59	47	48	36	40	47	49	47	49	51	53	48	50
3 years	31	31	32	33	39	40	31	34	20	26	29	32	31	35	30	34	28	31
5 years	23	24	28	29	29	31	23	27	13	22	22	26	24	29	22	27	21	26
8 years	18	18	17	18	15	16	15	20	7	17	14	20	15	21	14	19	14	20
10 years	10	11	11	11	13	15	12	17	2	6	10	15	11	17	8	11	..	..
Overall																		
1 year	63	63	56	57	59	60	49	51	36	39	50	52	50	52	51	54	50	52
3 years	33	33	35	36	41	42	30	33	20	28	30	34	31	35	31	36	30	34
5 years	25	26	27	28	31	34	22	27	11	20	22	27	23	29	22	28	22	27
8 years	18	18	17	18	21	24	13	19	4	12	14	20	14	20	13	19	12	16
10 years	13	13	13	14	16	20	10	16	1	6	10	16	10	16	8	14	..	..

RELATIVE SURVIVAL (%) BY AGE AND PERIOD

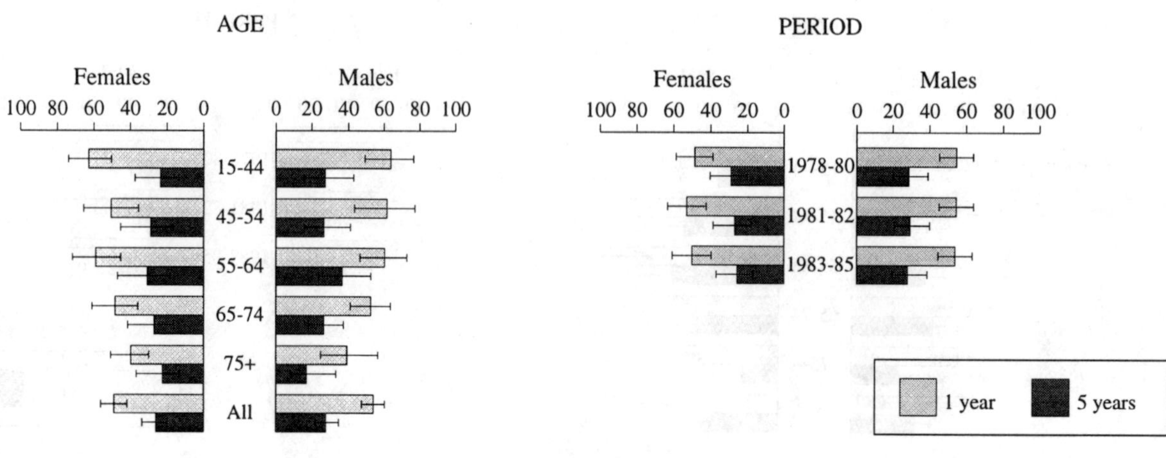

NASOPHARYNX

EUROPEAN REGISTRIES *Children*

Unweighted analysis

REGISTRY	CASES		
	Males	Females	All
DENMARK	2	1	3
ENGLISH REGISTRIES	11	6	17
ESTONIA	0	1	1
FINLAND	1	0	1
FRENCH REGISTRIES	1	0	1
ITALIAN REGISTRIES	5	2	7
MAINZ (GERMANY)	8	6	14
SCOTLAND	2	1	3
Mean age (years)	9.8	9.1	9.5

OBSERVED AND RELATIVE SURVIVAL (%) BY AGE
(Number of cases in parentheses)

	AGE CLASS							
	0-4		5-9		10-14		All	
	obs	rel	obs	rel	obs	rel	obs	rel
Males	(3)		(9)		(18)		(30)	
1 year	67	67	100	100	100	100	97	97
3 years	33	33	78	78	72	72	70	70
5 years	33	33	67	67	72	72	67	67
8 years	33	34	67	67	59	59	59	59
10 years	..	..	44	45	59	59	44	44
Females	(5)		(2)		(10)		(17)	
1 year	100	100	50	50	90	90	88	88
3 years	60	60	50	50	70	70	65	65
5 years	60	60	50	50	59	59	59	59
8 years	60	60	..	..	59	59	59	59
10 years	..	..	..	..	59	59	59	59
Overall	(8)		(11)		(28)		(47)	
1 year	88	88	91	91	96	96	94	94
3 years	50	50	73	73	71	71	68	68
5 years	50	50	64	64	68	68	64	64
8 years	50	50	64	64	59	59	59	59
10 years	..	..	42	43	59	59	47	47

RELATIVE SURVIVAL (%) BY AGE

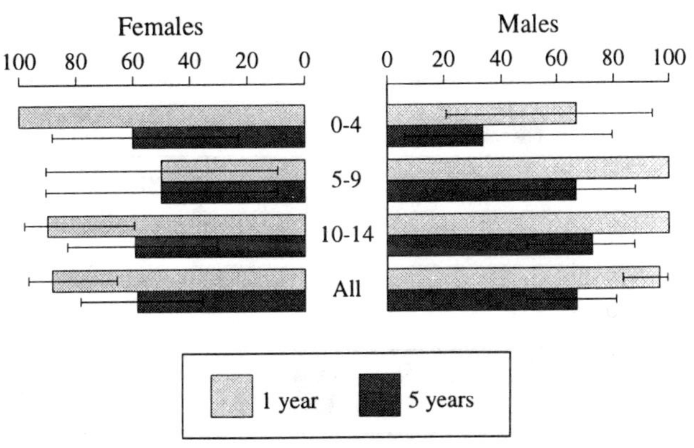

BONE

EUROPEAN REGISTRIES

Children

Unweighted analysis

REGISTRY	CASES		
	Males	Females	All
DENMARK	17	29	46
DUTCH REGISTRIES	6	6	12
ENGLISH REGISTRIES	81	98	179
ESTONIA	3	7	10
FINLAND	33	15	48
FRENCH REGISTRIES	8	5	13
ITALIAN REGISTRIES	28	28	56
MAINZ (GERMANY)	140	121	261
POLISH REGISTRIES	1	3	4
SCOTLAND	19	22	41
SWISS REGISTRIES	5	2	7
Mean age (years)	10.5	10.3	10.4

OBSERVED AND RELATIVE SURVIVAL (%) BY AGE
(Number of cases in parentheses)

	AGE CLASS							
	0-4		5-9		10-19		All	
	obs	rel	obs	rel	obs	rel	obs	rel
Males	(23)		(83)		(235)		(341)	
1 year	87	87	79	79	85	85	84	84
3 years	58	58	59	59	52	52	54	54
5 years	41	42	55	55	44	45	47	47
8 years	41	42	52	52	41	42	44	44
10 years	..	..	44	44	41	42	42	43
Females	(32)		(82)		(222)		(336)	
1 year	90	90	84	84	83	83	84	84
3 years	63	63	54	54	49	49	51	51
5 years	54	54	45	45	42	42	44	44
8 years	54	54	38	38	38	38	39	39
10 years	..	..	38	38	35	35	37	37
Overall	(55)		(165)		(457)		(677)	
1 year	89	89	82	82	84	84	84	84
3 years	61	61	56	56	50	51	53	53
5 years	49	49	50	50	43	43	45	45
8 years	49	49	45	45	40	40	41	42
10 years	..	..	41	41	38	38	39	40

RELATIVE SURVIVAL (%) BY AGE

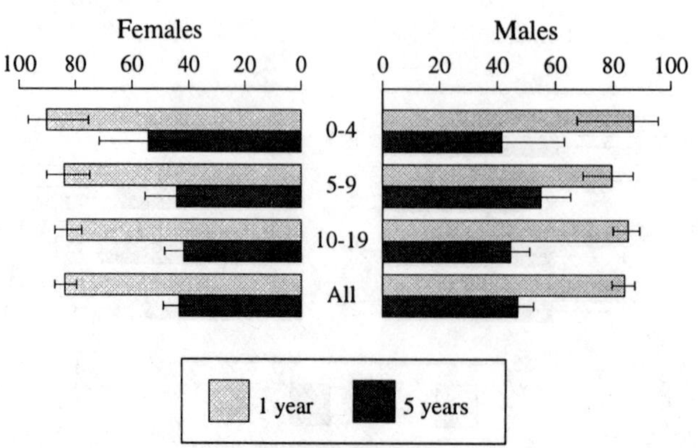

OVARY

EUROPEAN REGISTRIES

Children

Unweighted analysis

REGISTRY	CASES
DENMARK	10
DUTCH REGISTRIES	1
ENGLISH REGISTRIES	35
ESTONIA	2
FINLAND	7
ITALIAN REGISTRIES	7
MAINZ (GERMANY)	21
POLISH REGISTRIES	2
SCOTLAND	5
SPANISH REGISTRIES	1
Mean age (years)	11.0

OBSERVED AND RELATIVE SURVIVAL (%) BY AGE
(Number of cases in parentheses)

	AGE CLASS							
	0-4		5-9		10-14		All	
	obs	rel	obs	rel	obs	rel	obs	rel
Females	(7)		(15)		(69)		(91)	
1 year	86	86	80	80	87	87	85	85
3 years	71	71	73	73	73	73	73	73
5 years	57	57	73	73	70	70	69	70
8 years	..	..	73	73	70	70	69	70
10 years	..	..	73	73	70	70	69	70

RELATIVE SURVIVAL (%) BY AGE

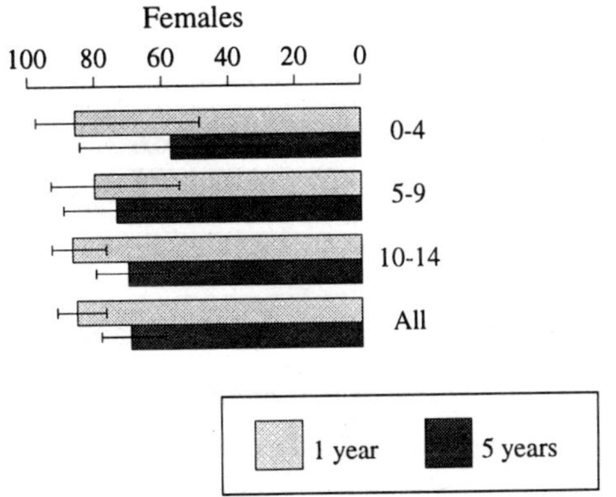

TESTIS

EUROPEAN REGISTRIES
Unweighted analysis

Children

REGISTRY	CASES
DENMARK	9
DUTCH REGISTRIES	3
ENGLISH REGISTRIES	32
ESTONIA	2
FINLAND	6
FRENCH REGISTRIES	1
ITALIAN REGISTRIES	1
MAINZ (GERMANY)	10
POLISH REGISTRIES	1
SCOTLAND	9
SPANISH REGISTRIES	1
Mean age (years)	3.5

OBSERVED AND RELATIVE SURVIVAL (%) BY AGE
(Number of cases in parentheses)

	AGE CLASS							
	0-4		5-9		10-14		All	
	obs	rel	obs	rel	obs	rel	obs	rel
Males	(56)		(8)		(11)		(75)	
1 year	95	95	100	100	82	82	93	94
3 years	83	84	100	100	73	73	84	84
5 years	83	84	100	100	64	64	82	82
8 years	83	84	100	100	64	64	82	83
10 years	83	84	100	100	64	64	82	83

RELATIVE SURVIVAL (%) BY AGE

AGE

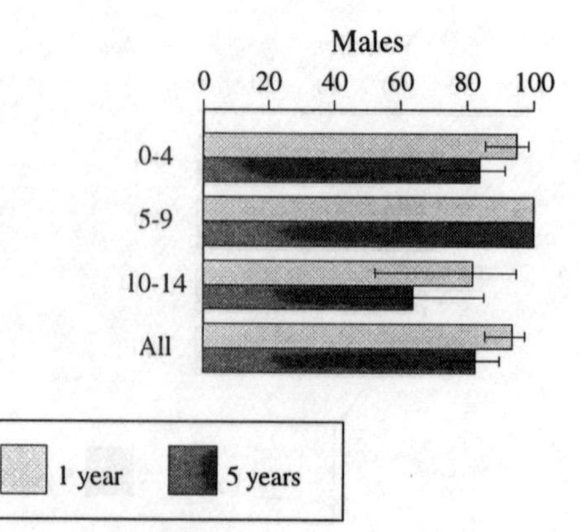

KIDNEY

EUROPEAN REGISTRIES

Children

Unweighted analysis

REGISTRY	CASES		
	Males	Females	All
DENMARK	27	28	55
DUTCH REGISTRIES	8	2	10
ENGLISH REGISTRIES	68	66	134
ESTONIA	11	16	27
FINLAND	32	18	50
FRENCH REGISTRIES	2	5	7
ITALIAN REGISTRIES	23	26	49
MAINZ (GERMANY)	131	122	253
POLISH REGISTRIES	2	4	6
SCOTLAND	16	22	38
SWISS REGISTRIES	1	3	4
Mean age (years)	3.3	3.3	3.3

OBSERVED AND RELATIVE SURVIVAL (%) BY AGE
(Number of cases in parentheses)

	AGE CLASS							
	0-4		5-9		10-14		All	
	obs	rel	obs	rel	obs	rel	obs	rel
Males	(241)		(70)		(10)		(321)	
1 year	86	86	93	93	79	79	87	87
3 years	78	78	74	74	79	79	77	77
5 years	75	76	71	71	79	80	74	75
8 years	74	74	71	71	64	64	73	73
10 years	67	68	71	71	64	64	68	69
Females	(233)		(70)		(9)		(312)	
1 year	86	86	88	88	89	89	87	87
3 years	78	79	72	73	66	66	77	77
5 years	77	77	71	71	66	66	75	75
8 years	75	75	67	67	66	66	73	73
10 years	72	73	67	67	66	66	71	72
Overall	(474)		(140)		(19)		(633)	
1 year	86	86	91	91	84	84	87	87
3 years	78	78	73	73	73	73	77	77
5 years	76	76	71	71	73	73	75	75
8 years	75	75	69	69	64	64	73	73
10 years	70	70	69	69	64	64	70	70

RELATIVE SURVIVAL (%) BY AGE

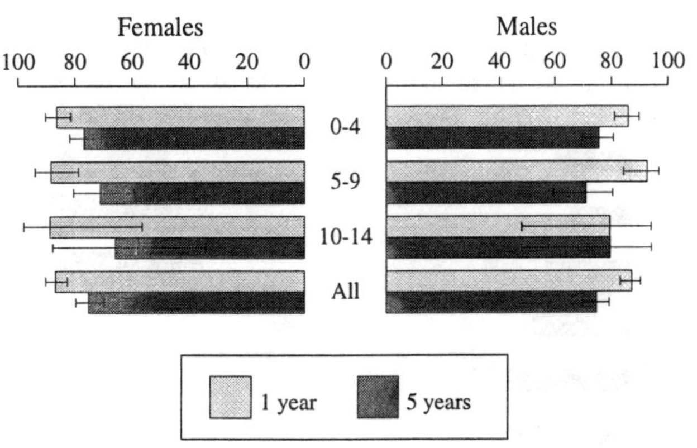

BRAIN

ENGLISH REGISTRIES

Children

REGISTRY	NUMBER OF CASES Males	Females	All	PERIOD OF DIAGNOSIS
East Anglia	27	20	47	1979-1984
Mersey	38	34	72	1978-1984
South Thames	90	64	154	1978-1984
Wessex	11	11	22	1983-1984
West Midlands	73	62	135	1979-1984
Yorkshire	63	47	110	1978-1984
Mean age (years)	7.2	7.0	7.1	

RELATIVE SURVIVAL (%)

100
80
60
40
20
0
Females
Males
0 1 2 3 4 5
Time since diagnosis (years)

OBSERVED AND RELATIVE SURVIVAL (%) BY AGE AND PERIOD
(Number of cases in parentheses)

	AGE CLASS 0-4 obs	0-4 rel	0-1 obs	0-1 rel	2-4 obs	2-4 rel	5-9 obs	5-9 rel	10-14 obs	10-14 rel	All obs	All rel	PERIOD 1978-80 obs	1978-80 rel	1981-82 obs	1981-82 rel	1983-85 obs	1983-85 rel
Males	(93)		(31)		(62)		(106)		(103)		(302)		(116)		(83)		(103)	
1 year	61	61	52	52	66	66	70	70	78	78	70	70	70	70	69	69	71	71
3 years	38	39	29	29	43	43	53	53	60	60	51	51	46	46	51	51	56	56
5 years	37	38	29	29	42	42	50	50	56	56	48	48	45	46	45	45	54	55
8 years	34	34	22	22	40	40	47	47	48	48	43	43	42	42	40	40	48	48
10 years	34	34	22	22	40	40	43	43	48	48	42	42	41	41	37	37	..	..
Females	(83)		(23)		(60)		(70)		(85)		(238)		(87)		(68)		(83)	
1 year	60	60	43	44	67	67	76	76	70	70	68	68	63	63	67	67	75	75
3 years	53	53	30	31	62	62	63	63	57	57	57	57	52	52	61	61	59	59
5 years	49	49	30	31	56	56	63	63	57	57	56	56	51	51	58	58	59	59
8 years	49	49	30	31	56	57	59	59	51	52	53	53	49	49	53	54	58	58
10 years	49	49	30	31	56	57	55	55	49	50	50	51	47	48	50	50	..	..
Overall	(176)		(54)		(122)		(176)		(188)		(540)		(203)		(151)		(186)	
1 year	61	61	48	48	66	66	72	72	74	74	69	69	67	67	68	68	73	73
3 years	45	45	30	30	52	52	57	57	59	59	54	54	49	49	55	55	58	58
5 years	43	43	30	30	49	49	55	55	57	57	52	52	48	48	51	51	56	57
8 years	41	41	26	26	48	48	52	52	50	50	47	48	45	45	46	46	53	53
10 years	41	41	26	26	48	48	48	48	49	49	45	46	44	44	43	43	..	..

RELATIVE SURVIVAL (%) BY AGE AND PERIOD

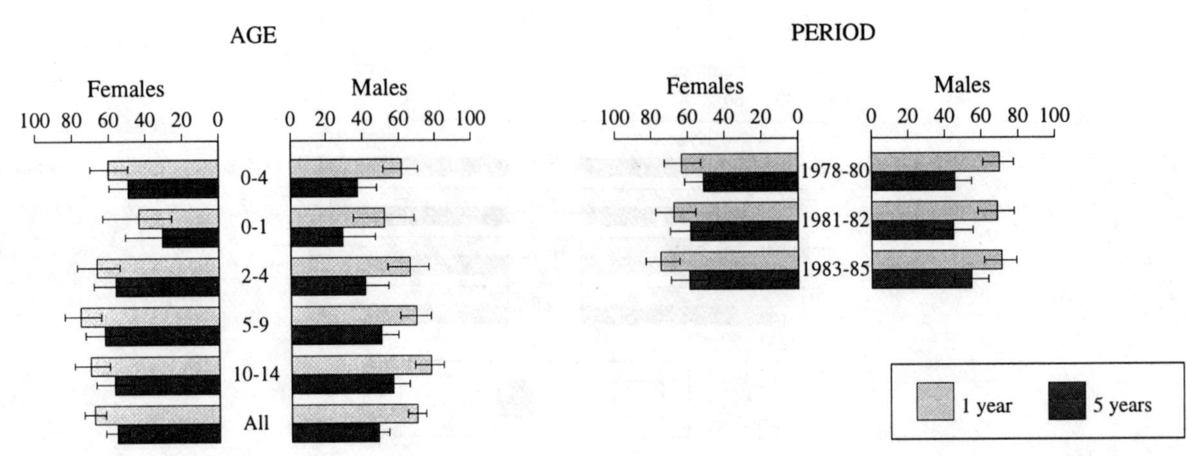

BRAIN

FINLAND

Children

REGISTRY	NUMBER OF CASES			PERIOD OF DIAGNOSIS
	Males	Females	All	
Finland	111	89	200	1978-1984
Mean age (years)	6.9	7.3	7.1	

RELATIVE SURVIVAL (%)

OBSERVED AND RELATIVE SURVIVAL (%) BY AGE AND PERIOD
(Number of cases in parentheses)

	AGE CLASS												PERIOD					
	0-4		0-1		2-4		5-9		10-14		All		1978-80		1981-82		1983-85	
	obs	rel	obs	rel	obs	rel	obs	rel	obs	rel	obs	rel	obs	rel	obs	rel	obs	rel
Males	(40)		(14)		(26)		(33)		(38)		(111)		(51)		(35)		(25)	
1 year	70	70	64	65	73	73	82	82	87	87	79	79	67	67	91	91	88	88
3 years	63	63	64	65	62	62	73	73	82	82	72	72	63	63	80	80	80	80
5 years	52	53	50	50	54	54	67	67	79	79	66	66	59	59	71	72	72	72
8 years	47	47	42	42	50	50	57	57	69	69	58	58	51	51	66	66	34	34
10 years	44	44	31	31	50	50	53	53	69	70	55	55	49	49	62	63	..	..
Females	(27)		(4)		(23)		(32)		(30)		(89)		(41)		(29)		(19)	
1 year	81	82	100	100	78	78	66	66	83	83	76	76	71	71	79	79	84	84
3 years	63	63	75	75	61	61	50	50	63	63	58	58	56	56	52	52	74	74
5 years	59	59	75	75	57	57	47	47	60	60	55	55	54	54	48	48	68	69
8 years	52	52	45	45	52	52	47	47	60	60	53	53	54	54	41	41	68	69
10 years	52	52	45	45	52	52	47	47	60	60	53	53	54	54	41	41	..	..
Overall	(67)		(18)		(49)		(65)		(68)		(200)		(92)		(64)		(44)	
1 year	75	75	72	73	76	76	74	74	85	85	78	78	68	69	86	86	86	86
3 years	63	63	67	67	61	61	62	62	74	74	66	66	60	60	67	67	77	77
5 years	55	55	56	56	55	55	57	57	71	71	61	61	57	57	61	61	70	71
8 years	49	49	42	43	51	51	52	52	65	66	56	56	52	52	55	55	51	51
10 years	47	47	34	34	51	51	50	50	65	66	54	54	51	51	53	53	..	..

RELATIVE SURVIVAL (%) BY AGE AND PERIOD

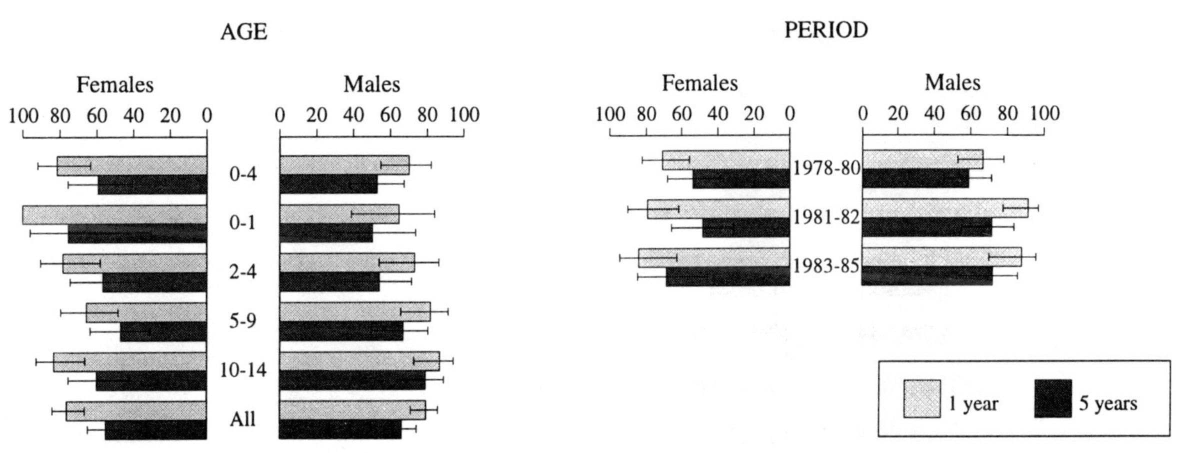

BRAIN

MAINZ (GERMANY)

Children

REGISTRY	NUMBER OF CASES			PERIOD OF DIAGNOSIS
	Males	Females	All	
Mainz	199	155	354	1981-1984
Mean age (years)	6.9	5.7	6.4	

RELATIVE SURVIVAL (%)

100 80 60 40 20 0

Males
Females

0 1 2 3 4 5

Time since diagnosis (years)

OBSERVED AND RELATIVE SURVIVAL (%) BY AGE AND PERIOD
(Number of cases in parentheses)

	AGE CLASS												PERIOD					
	0-4		0-1		2-4		5-9		10-14		All		1978-80		1981-82		1983-85	
	obs	rel	obs	rel	obs	rel	obs	rel	obs	rel	obs	rel	obs	rel	obs	rel	obs	rel
Males	(70)		(25)		(45)		(61)		(68)		(199)		(0)		(98)		(101)	
1 year	67	67	67	67	67	67	76	77	82	82	75	75	..	..	74	74	76	76
3 years	37	38	22	22	46	46	62	62	58	58	52	52	..	..	52	52	52	52
5 years	36	36	22	22	43	43	52	52	55	55	47	47	..	..	48	48	46	46
8 years	36	36	22	22	43	43	40	40	51	51	41	42	..	..	43	43	..	..
10 years	..	..	..	..	..	..	..	..	..	..	..	..	..	..	..	..	..	..
Females	(70)		(28)		(42)		(49)		(36)		(155)		(0)		(71)		(84)	
1 year	67	67	64	65	68	68	77	77	80	80	73	73	..	..	73	73	73	73
3 years	48	48	39	40	54	54	62	62	61	61	55	55	..	..	55	55	56	56
5 years	39	39	35	35	42	42	49	49	53	53	45	46	..	..	37	37	53	53
8 years	39	39	35	35	42	42	42	43	53	53	43	43	..	..	35	35	..	..
10 years	..	..	..	..	..	..	..	..	..	..	..	..	..	..	..	..	..	..
Overall	(140)		(53)		(87)		(110)		(104)		(354)		(0)		(169)		(185)	
1 year	67	67	65	66	68	68	77	77	81	81	74	74	..	..	73	73	75	75
3 years	43	43	32	32	50	50	62	62	59	59	54	54	..	..	53	53	54	54
5 years	38	38	29	30	42	42	51	51	54	54	46	46	..	..	43	43	49	49
8 years	38	38	29	30	42	42	39	39	51	52	42	42	..	..	40	40	..	..
10 years	..	..	..	..	..	..	..	..	..	..	..	..	..	..	..	..	..	..

RELATIVE SURVIVAL (%) BY AGE AND PERIOD

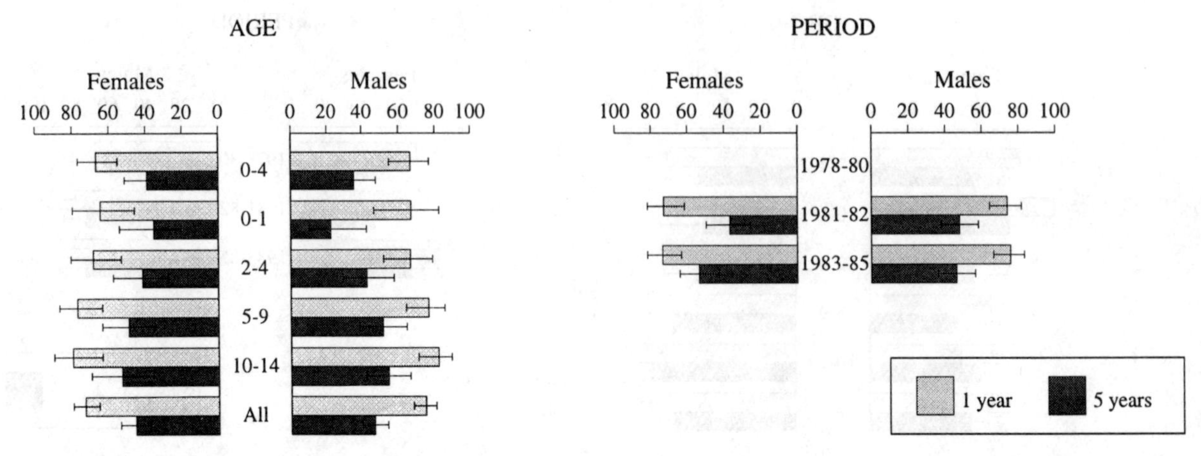

BRAIN

DENMARK

Children

REGISTRY	NUMBER OF CASES			PERIOD OF DIAGNOSIS
	Males	Females	All	
Denmark	92	71	163	1978-1984
Mean age (years)	7.1	6.6	6.8	

RELATIVE SURVIVAL (%)
(Both sexes)

Time since diagnosis (years)

OBSERVED AND RELATIVE SURVIVAL (%) BY PERIOD AND SEX
(Number of cases in parentheses)

	PERIOD						SEX					
	1978-80		1981-82		1983-85		Males		Females		All	
	obs	rel	obs	rel	obs	rel	obs	rel	obs	rel	obs	rel
N. Cases	(76)		(44)		(43)		(92)		(71)		(163)	
1 year	71	71	82	82	72	72	76	76	72	72	74	74
3 years	58	58	66	66	56	56	55	56	65	65	60	60
5 years	53	53	61	61	47	47	49	49	60	60	54	54
8 years	47	48	56	57	..	..	46	46	50	50	48	48
10 years	47	48	..	..	..	..	46	46	50	50	48	48

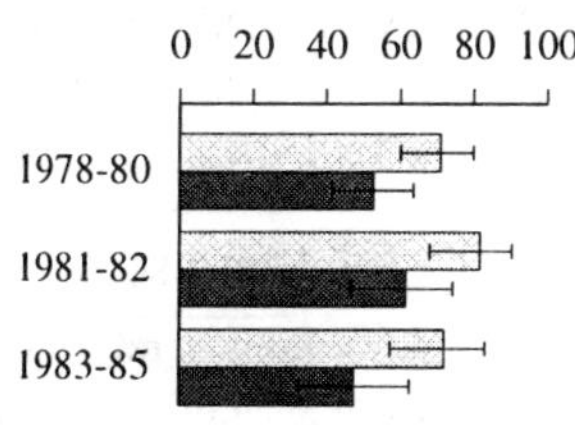

DUTCH REGISTRIES

REGISTRY	NUMBER OF CASES			PERIOD OF DIAGNOSIS
	Males	Females	All	
Eindhoven	20	10	30	1978-1985
Mean age (years)	7.5	9.3	8.1	

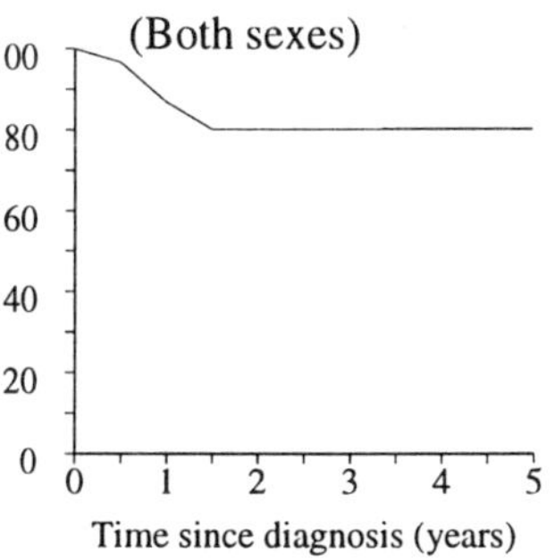

OBSERVED AND RELATIVE SURVIVAL (%) BY PERIOD AND SEX
(Number of cases in parentheses)

	PERIOD						SEX					
	1978-80		1981-82		1983-85		Males		Females		All	
	obs	rel	obs	rel	obs	rel	obs	rel	obs	rel	obs	rel
N. Cases	(13)		(10)		(7)		(20)		(10)		(30)	
1 year	85	85	80	80	100	100	90	90	80	80	87	87
3 years	77	77	70	70	100	100	80	80	80	80	80	80
5 years	77	77	70	70	100	100	80	80	80	80	80	80
8 years	77	77	..	..	..	..	80	80	80	80	80	80
10 years	..	..	..	..	..	..	..	..	..	..	..	..

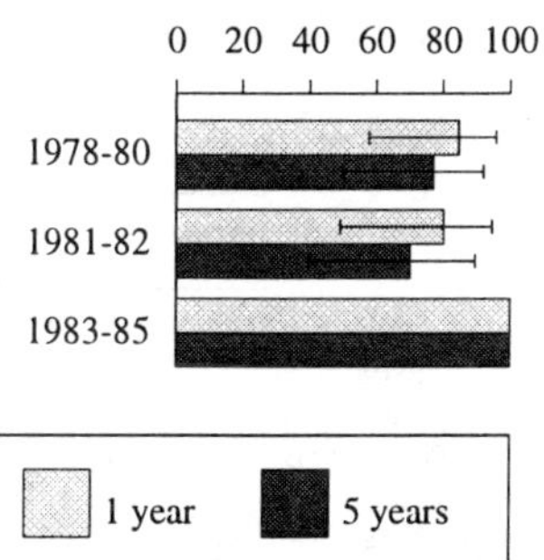

BRAIN

ESTONIA

Children

REGISTRY	NUMBER OF CASES			PERIOD OF DIAGNOSIS
	Males	Females	All	
Estonia	17	25	42	1978-1984
Mean age (years)	7.0	8.1	7.6	

RELATIVE SURVIVAL (%)
(Both sexes)

OBSERVED AND RELATIVE SURVIVAL (%) BY PERIOD AND SEX
(Number of cases in parentheses)

	PERIOD						SEX					
	1978-80		1981-82		1983-85		Males		Females		All	
	obs	rel	obs	rel	obs	rel	obs	rel	obs	rel	obs	rel
N. Cases	(14)		(16)		(12)		(17)		(25)		(42)	
1 year	43	43	50	50	50	50	41	41	52	52	48	48
3 years	21	22	25	25	33	33	24	24	28	28	26	26
5 years	21	22	19	19	33	33	18	18	28	28	24	24
8 years	21	22	19	19	..	..	18	18	28	28	24	24
10 years	21	22	..	..	..	..	18	18	28	28	24	24

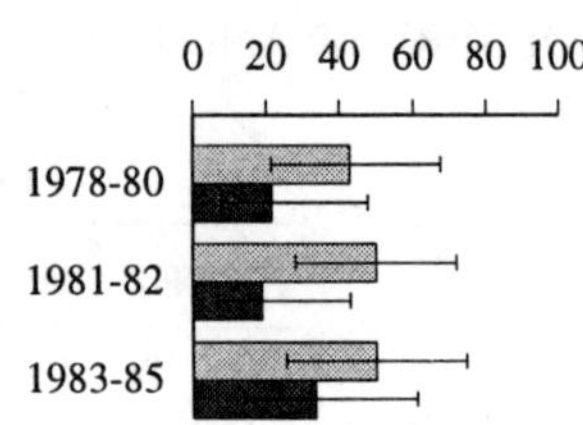

FRENCH REGISTRIES

REGISTRY	NUMBER OF CASES			PERIOD OF DIAGNOSIS
	Males	Females	All	
Amiens	0	1	1	1983-1983
Doubs	10	11	21	1978-1984
Mean age (years)	7.0	7.5	7.3	

RELATIVE SURVIVAL (%)
(Both sexes)

OBSERVED AND RELATIVE SURVIVAL (%) BY PERIOD AND SEX
(Number of cases in parentheses)

	PERIOD						SEX					
	1978-80		1981-82		1983-85		Males		Females		All	
	obs	rel	obs	rel	obs	rel	obs	rel	obs	rel	obs	rel
N. Cases	(9)		(5)		(8)		(10)		(12)		(22)	
1 year	56	56	80	80	60	60	60	60	65	65	63	63
3 years	56	56	60	60	30	30	40	40	56	56	48	48
5 years	44	45	60	60	30	30	30	30	56	56	44	44
8 years	22	22	..	..	30	30	30	30	29	29	31	32
10 years	22	22	..	..	..	..	..	..	29	29	31	32

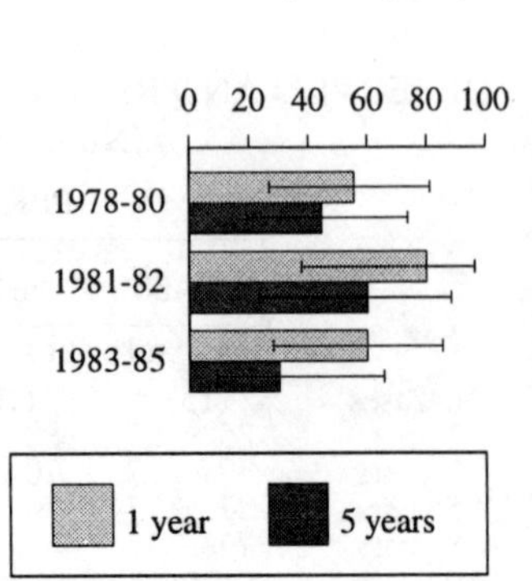

BRAIN

Children

ITALIAN REGISTRIES

REGISTRY	NUMBER OF CASES			PERIOD OF DIAGNOSIS
	Males	Females	All	
Latina	1	3	4	1983-1984
Piedmont	59	50	109	1978-1984
Ragusa	4	2	6	1981-1984
Varese	16	12	28	1978-1984
Mean age (years)	6.9	7.1	7.0	

RELATIVE SURVIVAL (%)
(Both sexes)

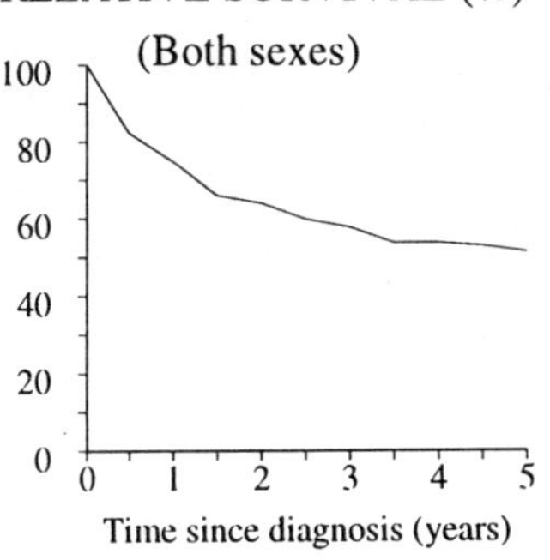

OBSERVED AND RELATIVE SURVIVAL (%) BY PERIOD AND SEX
(Number of cases in parentheses)

	PERIOD						SEX					
	1978-80		1981-82		1983-85		Males		Females		All	
	obs	rel	obs	rel	obs	rel	obs	rel	obs	rel	obs	rel
N. Cases	(58)		(47)		(42)		(80)		(67)		(147)	
1 year	78	78	74	75	71	71	74	74	76	76	75	75
3 years	60	60	60	60	52	52	61	61	54	54	58	58
5 years	55	55	51	51	48	48	53	54	49	49	51	51
8 years	52	52	36	36	48	48	47	47	45	45	46	46
10 years	49	49	36	36	..	..	47	47	41	41	44	44

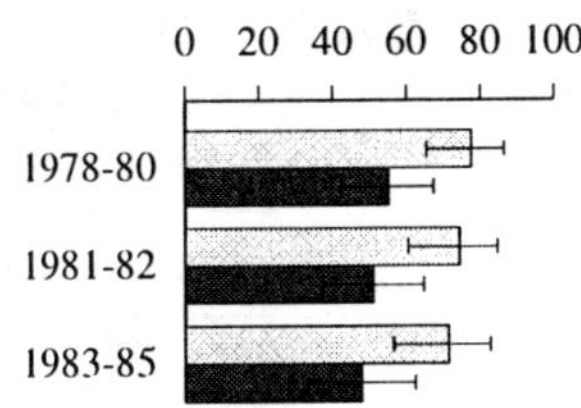

POLISH REGISTRIES

REGISTRY	NUMBER OF CASES			PERIOD OF DIAGNOSIS
	Males	Females	All	
Cracow	13	6	19	1978-1984
Mean age (years)	6.4	8.0	6.9	

RELATIVE SURVIVAL (%)
(Both sexes)

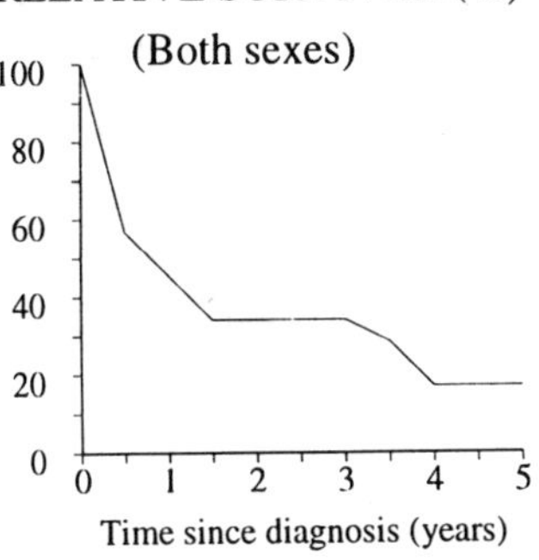

OBSERVED AND RELATIVE SURVIVAL (%) BY PERIOD AND SEX
(Number of cases in parentheses)

	PERIOD						SEX					
	1978-80		1981-82		1983-85		Males		Females		All	
	obs	rel	obs	rel	obs	rel	obs	rel	obs	rel	obs	rel
N. Cases	(6)		(9)		(4)		(13)		(6)		(19)	
1 year	33	33	67	67	0	0	38	39	61	61	45	46
3 years	17	17	56	56	0	0	31	31	41	41	34	34
5 years	17	17	22	22	0	0	23	23	0	0	17	17
8 years	17	17	22	22	0	0	23	23	0	0	17	17
10 years	17	17	..	..	0	0	23	23	0	0	17	17

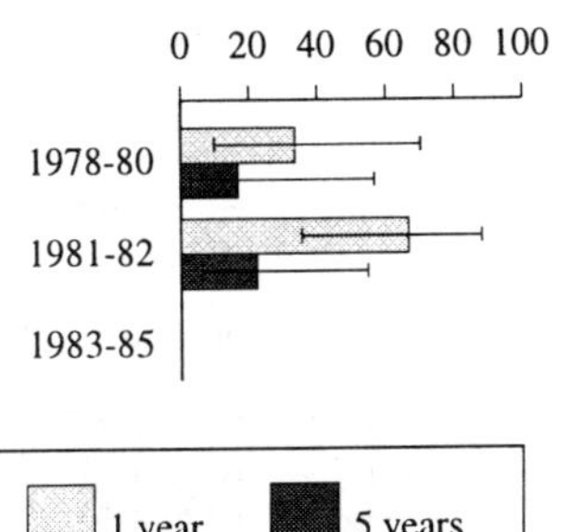

BRAIN

Children

SCOTLAND

REGISTRY	NUMBER OF CASES			PERIOD OF DIAGNOSIS
	Males	Females	All	
Scotland	55	62	117	1978-1982
Mean age (years)	8.2	7.2	7.7	

RELATIVE SURVIVAL (%)

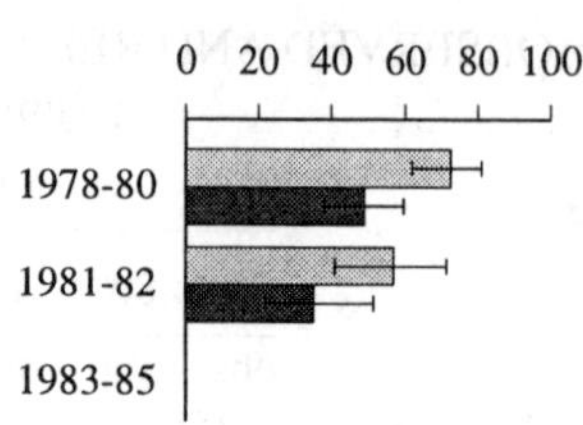

OBSERVED AND RELATIVE SURVIVAL (%) BY PERIOD AND SEX
(Number of cases in parentheses)

	PERIOD						SEX					
	1978-80		1981-82		1983-85		Males		Females		All	
	obs	rel	obs	rel	obs	rel	obs	rel	obs	rel	obs	rel
N. Cases	(80)		(37)		(0)		(55)		(62)		(117)	
1 year	73	73	57	57	..	..	67	67	68	68	68	68
3 years	54	54	35	35	..	..	42	42	53	53	48	48
5 years	49	49	35	35	..	..	38	38	50	50	44	45
8 years	49	49	..	..	..	..	38	38	48	48	43	44
10 years	44	44	..	..	..	..	38	38	40	40	39	39

SWISS REGISTRIES

REGISTRY	NUMBER OF CASES			PERIOD OF DIAGNOSIS
	Males	Females	All	
Basel	1	4	5	1981-1984
Geneva	1	4	5	1978-1983
Mean age (years)	7.5	9.1	8.8	

RELATIVE SURVIVAL (%)

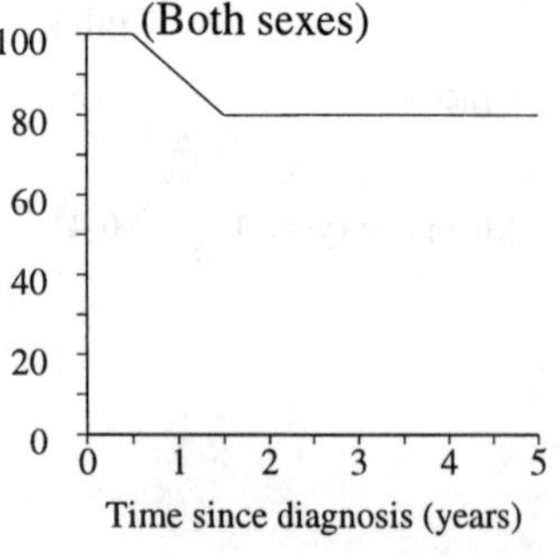

OBSERVED AND RELATIVE SURVIVAL (%) BY PERIOD AND SEX
(Number of cases in parentheses)

	PERIOD						SEX					
	1978-80		1981-82		1983-85		Males		Females		All	
	obs	rel	obs	rel	obs	rel	obs	rel	obs	rel	obs	rel
N. Cases	(2)		(4)		(4)		(2)		(8)		(10)	
1 year	100	100	100	100	75	75	100	100	88	88	90	90
3 years	100	100	100	100	50	50	100	100	75	75	80	80
5 years	100	100	100	100	50	50	100	100	75	75	80	80
8 years	..	..	100	100	..	..	50	50	75	75	68	68
10 years	..	..	..	..	..	..	..	..	..	..	..	..

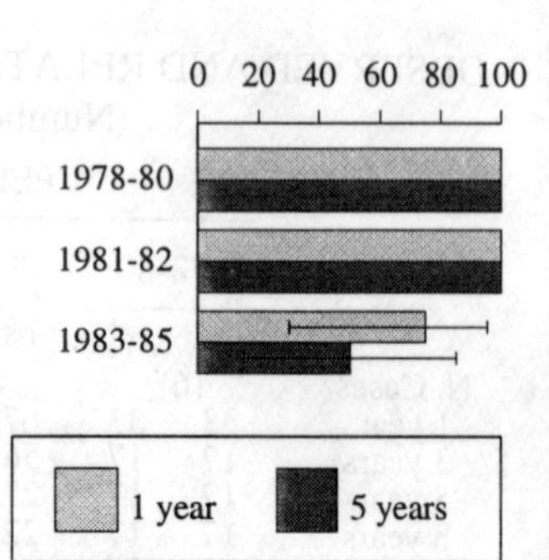

BRAIN

EUROPEAN REGISTRIES — *Children*

Unweighted analysis

REGISTRY	CASES Males	Females	All
DENMARK	92	71	163
DUTCH REGISTRIES	20	10	30
ENGLISH REGISTRIES	302	238	540
ESTONIA	17	25	42
FINLAND	111	89	200
FRENCH REGISTRIES	10	12	22
ITALIAN REGISTRIES	80	67	147
MAINZ (GERMANY)	199	155	354
POLISH REGISTRIES	13	6	19
SCOTLAND	55	62	117
SWISS REGISTRIES	2	8	10
Mean age (years)	7.1	6.9	7.0

RELATIVE SURVIVAL (%)
(Age-standardized)

Females 100 80 60 40 20 0 — Males 0 20 40 60 80 100
ENG
FIN
D
EUR

OBSERVED AND RELATIVE SURVIVAL (%) BY AGE AND PERIOD
(Number of cases in parentheses)

	AGE CLASS 0-4 obs	rel	0-1 obs	rel	2-4 obs	rel	5-9 obs	rel	10-14 obs	rel	All obs	rel	PERIOD 1978-80 obs	rel	1981-82 obs	rel	1983-85 obs	rel
Males	(285)		(98)		(187)		(310)		(306)		(901)		(305)		(313)		(283)	
1 year	63	63	56	56	67	67	75	75	78	78	72	72	69	69	75	75	73	73
3 years	42	42	34	34	47	47	59	59	62	62	55	55	52	52	56	56	56	56
5 years	39	39	29	30	44	44	52	53	57	57	50	50	48	48	51	51	51	51
8 years	36	36	26	26	42	42	47	47	51	51	45	45	44	44	46	46	41	41
10 years	35	35	23	23	42	42	45	45	51	51	44	44	43	43	44	44	..	..
Females	(257)		(79)		(178)		(253)		(233)		(743)		(248)		(243)		(252)	
1 year	66	67	57	57	71	71	71	71	76	76	71	71	69	69	70	70	74	74
3 years	53	53	39	39	59	59	56	56	61	61	56	57	56	56	55	55	58	58
5 years	47	47	34	34	53	53	52	52	59	59	52	52	54	54	47	47	56	56
8 years	45	45	32	32	50	50	47	47	55	55	49	49	51	51	42	42	55	55
10 years	43	43	27	27	50	50	45	45	53	53	47	47	49	49	41	41	..	..
Overall	(542)		(177)		(365)		(563)		(539)		(1644)		(553)		(556)		(535)	
1 year	65	65	56	57	69	69	73	73	77	77	72	72	69	69	73	73	74	74
3 years	47	47	36	36	53	53	58	58	61	61	55	55	54	54	56	56	57	57
5 years	43	43	31	32	48	48	52	52	58	58	51	51	51	51	49	49	53	53
8 years	40	40	28	28	46	46	47	47	53	53	47	47	47	47	44	44	48	48
10 years	39	39	24	25	46	46	45	45	52	52	45	45	46	46	42	43	..	..

RELATIVE SURVIVAL (%) BY AGE AND PERIOD

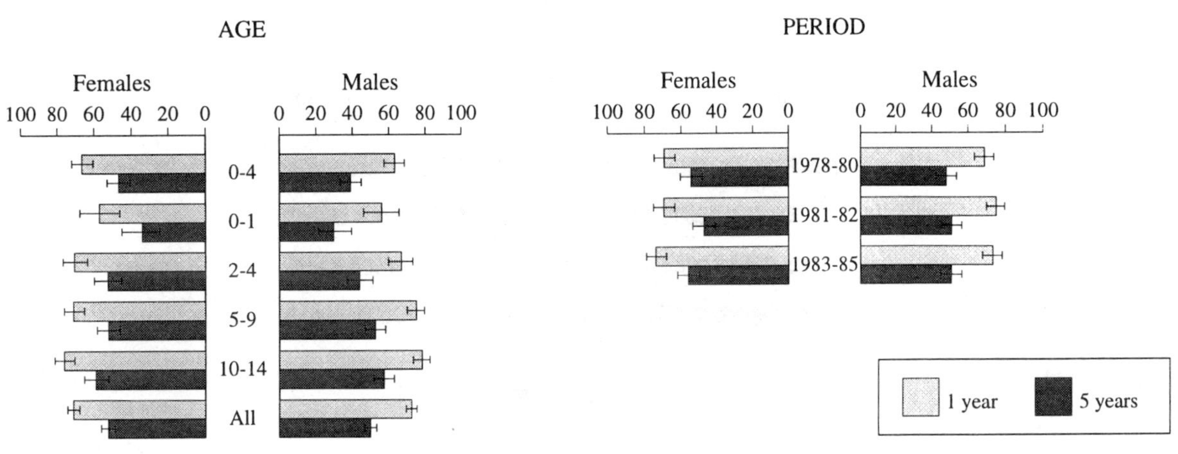

HODGKIN'S DISEASE

EUROPEAN REGISTRIES *Children*

Unweighted analysis

REGISTRY	CASES		
	Males	Females	All
DENMARK	25	16	41
DUTCH REGISTRIES	1	3	4
ENGLISH REGISTRIES	115	43	158
ESTONIA	21	4	25
FINLAND	19	12	31
FRENCH REGISTRIES	4	4	8
ITALIAN REGISTRIES	34	14	48
MAINZ (GERMANY)	152	82	234
POLISH REGISTRIES	3	2	5
SCOTLAND	19	10	29
SPANISH REGISTRIES	2	0	2
SWISS REGISTRIES	5	1	6
Mean age (years)	10.0	11.2	10.4

OBSERVED AND RELATIVE SURVIVAL (%) BY AGE
(Number of cases in parentheses)

	AGE CLASS							
	0-4		5-9		10-14		All	
	obs	rel	obs	rel	obs	rel	obs	rel
Males	(29)		(131)		(240)		(400)	
1 year	93	93	95	95	97	97	96	96
3 years	90	90	94	94	92	92	92	92
5 years	90	90	93	93	88	89	90	90
8 years	90	90	92	92	85	85	88	88
10 years	78	78	89	89	80	81	83	83
Females	(3)		(46)		(142)		(191)	
1 year	100	100	89	89	99	99	96	96
3 years	100	100	87	87	94	94	93	93
5 years	100	100	84	85	93	93	91	91
8 years	100	100	84	85	90	90	89	89
10 years	100	100	84	85	90	90	89	89
Overall	(32)		(177)		(382)		(591)	
1 year	94	94	94	94	97	97	96	96
3 years	91	91	92	92	93	93	92	93
5 years	91	91	91	91	90	90	90	90
8 years	91	91	90	90	87	87	88	88
10 years	80	80	88	88	84	84	84	85

RELATIVE SURVIVAL (%) BY AGE

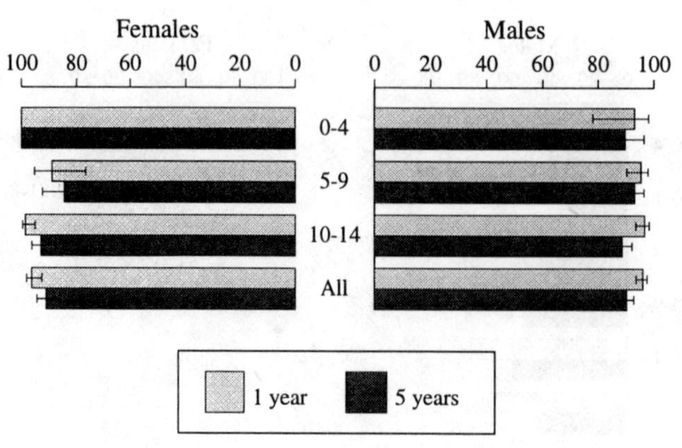

LEUKAEMIA

DENMARK

Children

REGISTRY	NUMBER OF CASES			PERIOD OF DIAGNOSIS
	Males	Females	All	
Denmark	168	119	287	1978-1984
Mean age (years)	6.2	5.6	5.9	

RELATIVE SURVIVAL (%)

OBSERVED AND RELATIVE SURVIVAL (%) BY AGE AND PERIOD
(Number of cases in parentheses)

	AGE CLASS												PERIOD					
	0-4		0-1		2-4		5-9		10-14		All		1978-80		1981-82		1983-85	
	obs	rel	obs	rel	obs	rel	obs	rel	obs	rel	obs	rel	obs	rel	obs	rel	obs	rel
Males	(77)		(18)		(59)		(45)		(46)		(168)		(62)		(51)		(55)	
1 year	84	84	61	61	92	92	89	89	80	80	85	85	92	92	78	78	82	82
3 years	69	69	56	56	73	73	53	53	43	44	58	58	52	52	51	51	71	71
5 years	60	60	39	39	66	66	44	44	38	39	50	50	44	44	41	41	65	66
8 years	58	58	39	39	64	64	40	40	35	35	47	47	42	42	37	37	..	..
10 years	58	58	39	39	64	64	40	40	35	35	47	47	42	42	..	..	..	..
Females	(63)		(21)		(42)		(29)		(27)		(119)		(56)		(28)		(35)	
1 year	83	83	52	53	98	98	90	90	85	85	85	85	82	82	86	86	89	89
3 years	70	70	38	38	86	86	66	66	56	56	66	66	55	55	68	68	80	80
5 years	63	64	38	38	76	76	62	62	52	52	60	60	50	50	61	61	77	77
8 years	61	62	38	38	73	73	62	62	42	42	58	58	46	47	61	61	..	..
10 years	61	62	38	38	73	73	62	62	..	..	58	58	46	47	..	..	..	..
Overall	(140)		(39)		(101)		(74)		(73)		(287)		(118)		(79)		(90)	
1 year	84	84	56	57	94	94	89	89	82	82	85	85	87	87	81	81	84	85
3 years	69	69	46	46	78	78	58	58	48	48	61	61	53	53	57	57	74	75
5 years	61	62	38	39	70	70	51	51	43	43	54	54	47	47	48	48	70	70
8 years	59	60	38	39	68	68	49	49	38	38	51	52	44	44	46	46	..	..
10 years	59	60	38	39	68	68	49	49	38	38	51	52	44	44	..	..	..	..

RELATIVE SURVIVAL (%) BY AGE AND PERIOD

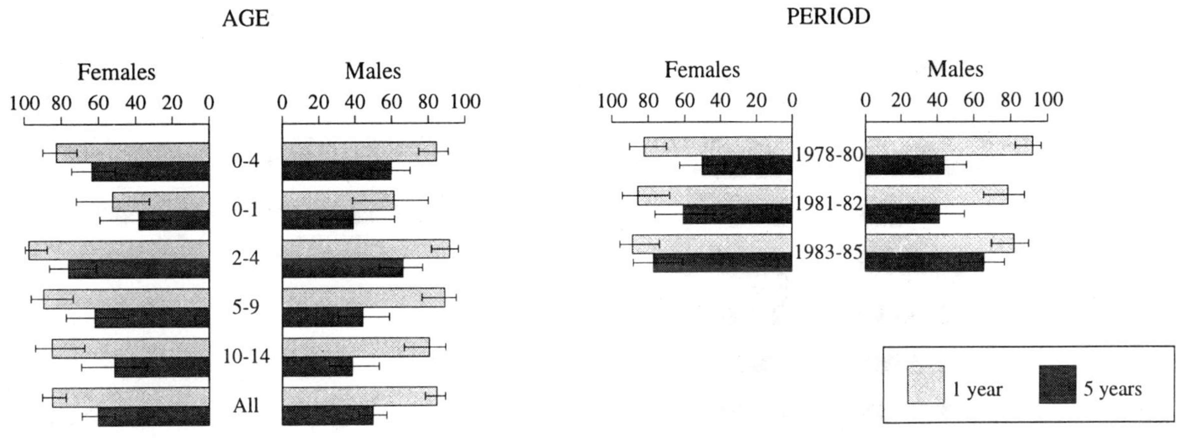

LEUKAEMIA

ENGLISH REGISTRIES

Children

REGISTRY	NUMBER OF CASES			PERIOD OF DIAGNOSIS
	Males	Females	All	
East Anglia	39	34	73	1979-1984
Mersey	71	39	110	1978-1984
South Thames	126	110	236	1978-1984
Wessex	19	20	39	1983-1984
West Midlands	151	91	242	1979-1984
Yorkshire	98	68	166	1978-1984
Mean age (years)	6.1	5.7	6.0	

RELATIVE SURVIVAL (%)

Females
Males
Time since diagnosis (years)

OBSERVED AND RELATIVE SURVIVAL (%) BY AGE AND PERIOD
(Number of cases in parentheses)

	AGE CLASS												PERIOD					
	0-4		0-1		2-4		5-9		10-14		All		1978-80		1981-82		1983-85	
	obs	rel	obs	rel	obs	rel	obs	rel	obs	rel	obs	rel	obs	rel	obs	rel	obs	rel
Males	(237)		(49)		(188)		(142)		(125)		(504)		(197)		(156)		(151)	
1 year	78	78	59	59	83	83	77	77	73	73	77	77	74	74	80	80	76	76
3 years	63	63	45	45	68	68	61	61	44	44	58	58	50	51	63	64	61	61
5 years	56	56	34	34	62	62	52	52	35	35	50	50	39	39	58	58	56	56
8 years	50	51	34	34	55	55	50	50	32	32	46	46	34	34	54	54	54	54
10 years	45	45	34	34	48	48	48	48	26	26	41	41	30	30	51	51	..	..
Females	(181)		(53)		(128)		(97)		(84)		(362)		(134)		(109)		(119)	
1 year	78	79	55	55	88	88	74	74	80	80	78	78	71	71	86	86	77	77
3 years	66	66	34	34	80	80	60	60	61	61	63	63	53	53	75	75	64	64
5 years	60	60	25	25	74	74	55	55	52	52	57	57	45	45	70	70	58	58
8 years	56	57	22	23	70	71	54	54	48	48	54	54	41	41	69	69	55	55
10 years	54	54	22	23	67	67	48	48	32	32	47	47	35	35	66	66	..	..
Overall	(418)		(102)		(316)		(239)		(209)		(866)		(331)		(265)		(270)	
1 year	78	78	57	57	85	85	76	76	76	76	77	77	73	73	83	83	77	77
3 years	65	65	39	39	73	73	60	60	51	51	60	60	52	52	68	68	62	62
5 years	58	58	29	29	67	67	53	53	42	42	53	53	41	41	63	63	57	57
8 years	53	53	28	28	61	61	51	51	38	38	49	49	37	37	60	60	54	54
10 years	48	48	28	28	55	55	48	48	28	28	43	43	32	32	57	57	..	..

RELATIVE SURVIVAL (%) BY AGE AND PERIOD

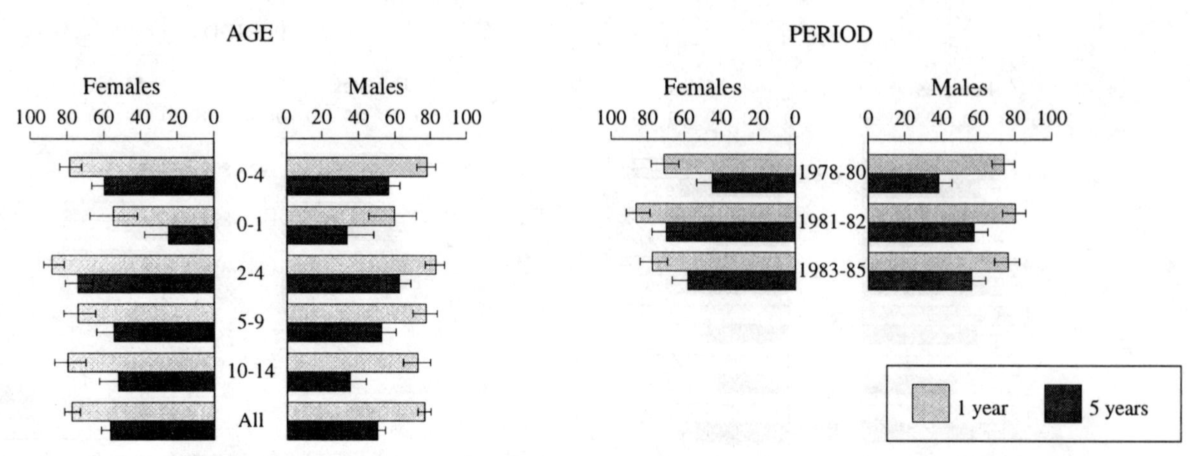

LEUKAEMIA

FINLAND

Children

REGISTRY	NUMBER OF CASES			PERIOD OF DIAGNOSIS
	Males	Females	All	
Finland	155	144	299	1978-1984
Mean age (years)	5.7	5.4	5.5	

RELATIVE SURVIVAL (%)

100 80 60 40 20 0
Females
Males
0 1 2 3 4 5
Time since diagnosis (years)

OBSERVED AND RELATIVE SURVIVAL (%) BY AGE AND PERIOD
(Number of cases in parentheses)

	AGE CLASS														PERIOD					
	0-4		0-1		2-4		5-9		10-14		All		1978-80		1981-82		1983-85	
	obs	rel	obs	rel	obs	rel	obs	rel	obs	rel	obs	rel	obs	rel	obs	rel	obs	rel
Males	(75)		(21)		(54)		(47)		(33)		(155)		(61)		(49)		(45)	
1 year	79	79	52	53	89	89	85	85	73	73	79	79	79	79	78	78	82	82
3 years	55	55	24	24	67	67	66	66	42	42	55	56	52	53	55	55	60	60
5 years	52	52	24	24	63	63	57	58	36	36	50	50	49	49	45	45	58	58
8 years	50	51	24	24	61	61	53	53	27	27	46	46	44	44	43	43	49	49
10 years	48	49	24	24	58	58	53	53	27	27	45	45	43	43	43	43	..	..
Females	(71)		(20)		(51)		(47)		(26)		(144)		(52)		(45)		(47)	
1 year	85	85	70	70	90	90	87	87	73	73	83	83	81	81	84	84	85	85
3 years	69	69	55	55	75	75	66	66	58	58	66	66	60	60	62	62	77	77
5 years	68	68	50	50	75	75	64	64	58	58	65	65	56	56	62	62	77	77
8 years	65	65	50	50	70	70	64	64	58	58	63	63	54	54	60	60	77	77
10 years	65	65	50	50	70	71	64	64	58	58	63	63	54	54	60	60	..	..
Overall	(146)		(41)		(105)		(94)		(59)		(299)		(113)		(94)		(92)	
1 year	82	82	61	61	90	90	86	86	73	73	81	81	80	80	81	81	84	84
3 years	62	62	39	39	70	71	66	66	49	49	61	61	56	56	59	59	68	69
5 years	60	60	37	37	69	69	61	61	46	46	57	57	52	52	53	53	67	67
8 years	57	58	37	37	65	66	58	58	40	40	54	54	49	49	51	51	62	62
10 years	56	56	37	37	64	64	58	58	40	40	54	54	48	48	51	51	..	..

RELATIVE SURVIVAL (%) BY AGE AND PERIOD

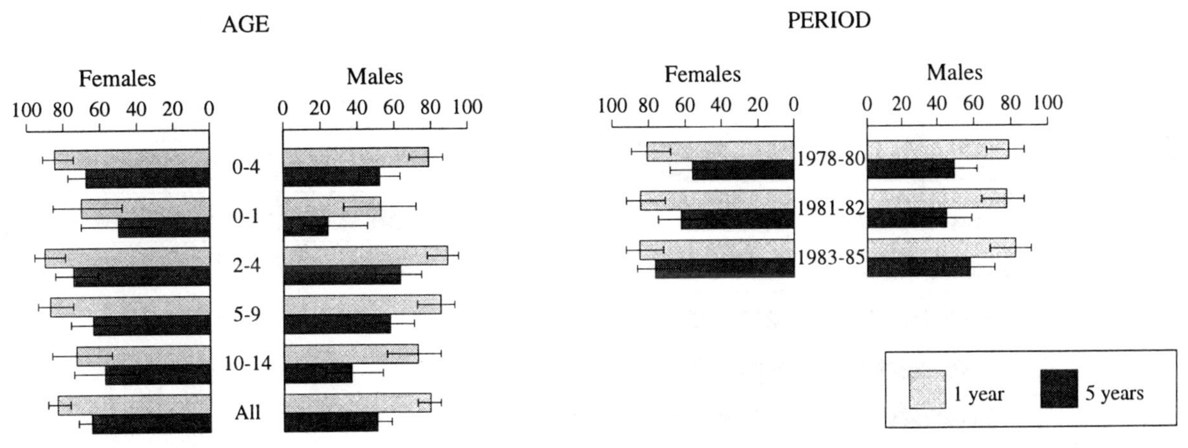

LEUKAEMIA

MAINZ (GERMANY)

Children

REGISTRY	NUMBER OF CASES			PERIOD OF DIAGNOSIS
	Males	Females	All	
Mainz	817	651	1468	1981-1984
Mean age (years)	6.0	5.8	5.9	

RELATIVE SURVIVAL (%)

100
80
60
40
20
0
0 1 2 3 4 5
Females
Males
Time since diagnosis (years)

OBSERVED AND RELATIVE SURVIVAL (%) BY AGE AND PERIOD
(Number of cases in parentheses)

	AGE CLASS												PERIOD					
	0-4		0-1		2-4		5-9		10-14		All		1978-80		1981-82		1983-85	
	obs	rel	obs	rel	obs	rel	obs	rel	obs	rel	obs	rel	obs	rel	obs	rel	obs	rel
Males	(392)		(96)		(296)		(215)		(210)		(817)		(0)		(388)		(429)	
1 year	90	90	78	78	94	94	91	91	79	79	87	87	..	..	87	87	88	88
3 years	77	77	61	62	82	82	76	76	63	63	73	73	..	..	74	74	73	73
5 years	72	72	60	61	76	76	71	71	56	56	67	68	..	..	67	67	68	68
8 years	68	68	54	54	73	73	67	67	51	52	64	64	..	..	63	63	..	..
10 years	..	..	..	..	..	..	..	..	..	..	..	..	..	..	..	..	..	..
Females	(328)		(67)		(261)		(180)		(143)		(651)		(0)		(330)		(321)	
1 year	91	91	82	82	93	93	89	89	81	81	88	88	..	..	86	86	90	90
3 years	81	81	70	71	83	83	78	78	66	66	77	77	..	..	75	75	78	78
5 years	78	78	66	66	81	81	74	74	63	63	73	73	..	..	71	71	75	75
8 years	77	77	66	66	80	80	70	70	58	58	71	71	..	..	69	69	..	..
10 years	..	..	..	..	..	..	..	..	..	..	..	..	..	..	..	..	..	..
Overall	(720)		(163)		(557)		(395)		(353)		(1468)		(0)		(718)		(750)	
1 year	90	90	80	80	93	93	90	90	80	80	88	88	..	..	86	86	89	89
3 years	79	79	65	65	83	83	77	77	64	64	75	75	..	..	74	74	75	75
5 years	75	75	63	63	78	78	72	72	58	59	70	70	..	..	69	69	71	71
8 years	72	72	59	59	76	76	68	68	54	54	67	67	..	..	66	66	..	..
10 years	..	..	..	..	..	..	..	..	..	..	..	..	..	..	..	..	..	..

RELATIVE SURVIVAL (%) BY AGE AND PERIOD

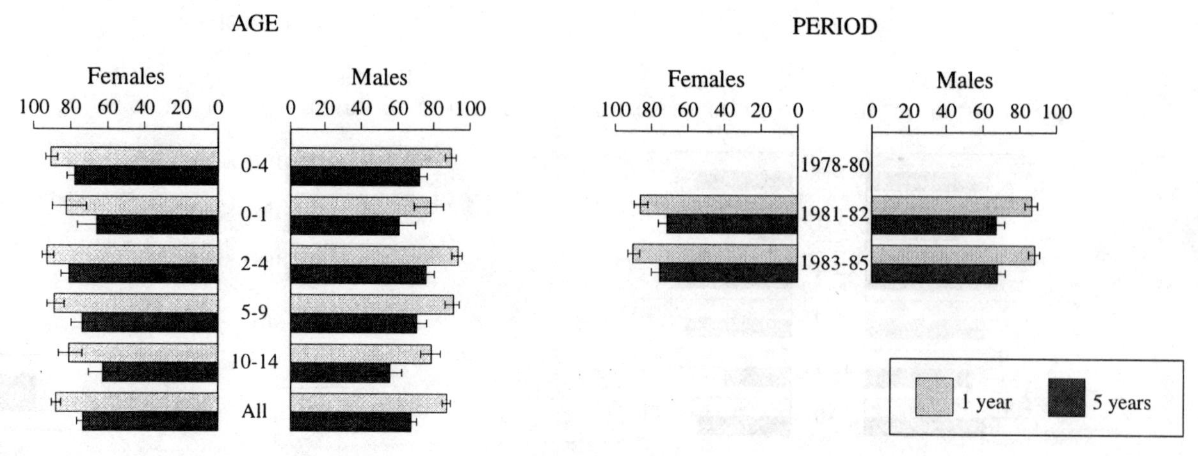

LEUKAEMIA

ITALIAN REGISTRIES

Children

REGISTRY	NUMBER OF CASES Males	Females	All	PERIOD OF DIAGNOSIS
Florence	2	4	6	1985-1985
Latina	3	2	5	1983-1984
Piedmont	136	122	258	1978-1984
Ragusa	8	3	11	1981-1984
Varese	26	28	54	1978-1984
Mean age (years)	6.4	6.4	6.4	

RELATIVE SURVIVAL (%)

Males
Females
Time since diagnosis (years)

OBSERVED AND RELATIVE SURVIVAL (%) BY AGE AND PERIOD
(Number of cases in parentheses)

	AGE CLASS 0-4 obs	rel	0-1 obs	rel	2-4 obs	rel	5-9 obs	rel	10-14 obs	rel	All obs	rel	PERIOD 1978-80 obs	rel	1981-82 obs	rel	1983-85 obs	rel
Males	(68)		(15)		(53)		(58)		(49)		(175)		(79)		(49)		(47)	
1 year	91	91	87	87	92	92	81	81	82	82	85	85	85	85	84	84	87	87
3 years	68	68	40	40	75	76	62	62	55	55	62	62	66	66	59	59	60	60
5 years	61	61	40	40	67	67	49	49	49	49	54	54	57	57	51	51	49	49
8 years	55	55	40	40	58	58	49	49	43	43	50	50	52	52	49	49	49	49
10 years	55	55	40	40	58	58	49	49	43	43	50	50	52	52	49	49	..	..
Females	(67)		(13)		(54)		(55)		(37)		(159)		(70)		(44)		(45)	
1 year	79	79	54	54	85	85	84	84	68	68	78	78	81	81	77	77	73	73
3 years	61	61	15	15	72	72	56	56	46	46	56	56	54	54	59	59	56	56
5 years	56	56	15	15	66	66	47	47	40	41	49	49	43	43	57	57	52	52
8 years	48	48	..	..	56	57	47	47	40	41	46	46	41	42	51	52	..	..
10 years	48	48	..	..	56	57	47	47	40	41	46	46	41	42	51	52	..	..
Overall	(135)		(28)		(107)		(113)		(86)		(334)		(149)		(93)		(92)	
1 year	85	85	71	72	89	89	82	82	76	76	82	82	83	83	81	81	80	80
3 years	64	65	29	29	74	74	59	59	51	51	59	59	60	60	59	59	58	58
5 years	59	59	29	29	67	67	48	48	45	45	52	52	50	50	54	54	51	51
8 years	52	52	29	29	57	57	48	48	41	42	48	48	47	47	50	50	30	31
10 years	52	52	29	29	57	57	48	48	41	42	48	48	47	47	50	50	..	..

RELATIVE SURVIVAL (%) BY AGE AND PERIOD

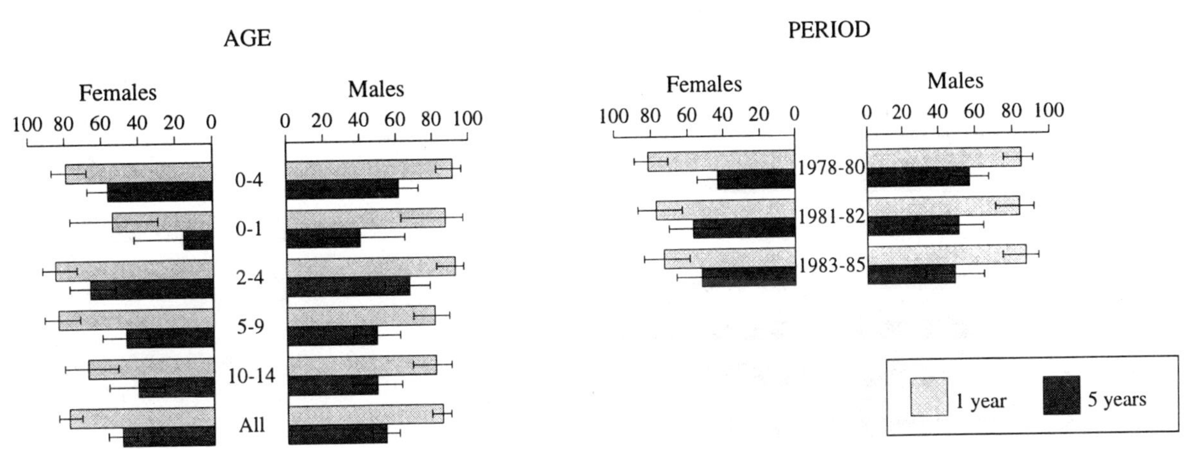

LEUKAEMIA

SCOTLAND

Children

REGISTRY	NUMBER OF CASES			PERIOD OF DIAGNOSIS
	Males	Females	All	
Scotland	111	85	196	1978-1982
Mean age (years)	4.9	5.7	5.3	

RELATIVE SURVIVAL (%)

Females

Males

Time since diagnosis (years)

OBSERVED AND RELATIVE SURVIVAL (%) BY AGE AND PERIOD
(Number of cases in parentheses)

	AGE CLASS												PERIOD					
	0-4		0-1		2-4		5-9		10-14		All		1978-80		1981-82		1983-85	
	obs	rel	obs	rel	obs	rel	obs	rel	obs	rel	obs	rel	obs	rel	obs	rel	obs	rel
Males	(64)		(15)		(49)		(30)		(17)		(111)		(76)		(35)		(0)	
1 year	78	78	60	60	84	84	83	83	82	82	80	80	79	79	83	83	..	..
3 years	55	55	27	27	63	63	50	50	47	47	52	52	47	47	63	63	..	..
5 years	47	47	27	27	53	53	43	43	35	35	44	44	42	42	49	49	..	..
8 years	44	44	27	27	49	50	43	43	25	25	41	42	39	40	..	..	..	..
10 years	44	44	27	27	49	50	43	43	..	..	41	42	39	40	..	..	..	..
Females	(43)		(8)		(35)		(21)		(21)		(85)		(61)		(24)		(0)	
1 year	74	74	50	50	80	80	86	86	86	86	80	80	80	80	79	79	..	..
3 years	67	68	38	38	74	74	71	71	57	57	66	66	66	66	67	67	..	..
5 years	60	61	25	25	69	69	71	71	43	43	59	59	59	59	58	58	..	..
8 years	60	61	..	..	69	69	71	72	27	27	56	56	57	57	..	..	..	..
10 years	60	61	..	..	69	69	54	54	..	..	49	49	51	51	..	..	..	..
Overall	(107)		(23)		(84)		(51)		(38)		(196)		(137)		(59)		(0)	
1 year	77	77	57	57	82	82	84	84	84	84	80	80	80	80	81	81	..	..
3 years	60	60	30	31	68	68	59	59	53	53	58	58	55	56	64	65	..	..
5 years	52	52	26	26	60	60	55	55	39	40	51	51	50	50	53	53	..	..
8 years	51	51	26	26	58	58	55	55	26	26	48	48	47	48	..	..	..	..
10 years	51	51	26	26	58	58	47	47	..	..	46	46	45	45	..	..	..	..

RELATIVE SURVIVAL (%) BY AGE AND PERIOD

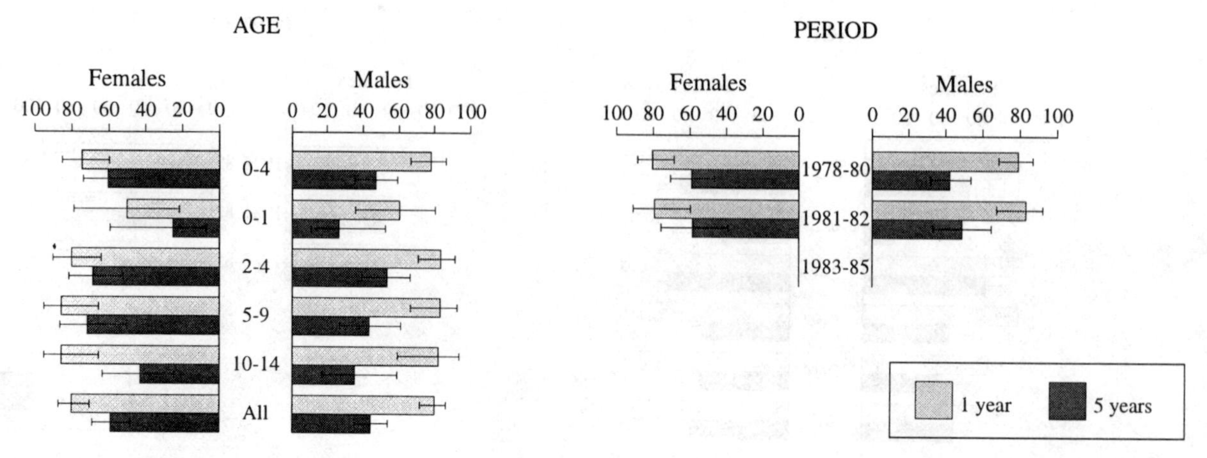

LEUKAEMIA

Children

DUTCH REGISTRIES

REGISTRY	NUMBER OF CASES			PERIOD OF DIAGNOSIS
	Males	Females	All	
Eindhoven	28	21	49	1978-1985
Mean age (years)	4.3	6.2	5.1	

RELATIVE SURVIVAL (%)
(Both sexes)

100
80
60
40
20
0
0 1 2 3 4 5
Time since diagnosis (years)

OBSERVED AND RELATIVE SURVIVAL (%) BY PERIOD AND SEX
(Number of cases in parentheses)

	PERIOD						SEX					
	1978-80		1981-82		1983-85		Males		Females		All	
	obs	rel	obs	rel	obs	rel	obs	rel	obs	rel	obs	rel
N. Cases	(22)		(15)		(12)		(28)		(21)		(49)	
1 year	82	82	73	73	75	75	79	79	76	76	78	78
3 years	64	64	53	53	67	67	57	57	67	67	61	61
5 years	64	64	40	40	58	58	54	54	57	57	55	55
8 years	64	64	33	33	58	58	50	50	57	57	53	53
10 years	64	64	33	33	..	..	50	50	57	57	53	53

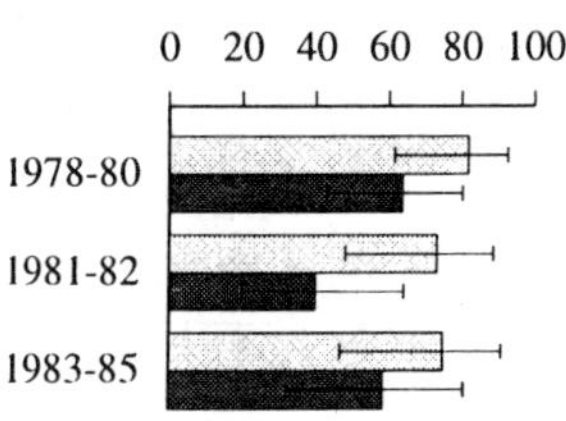

ESTONIA

REGISTRY	NUMBER OF CASES			PERIOD OF DIAGNOSIS
	Males	Females	All	
Estonia	50	30	80	1978-1984
Mean age (years)	5.6	5.5	5.6	

RELATIVE SURVIVAL (%)

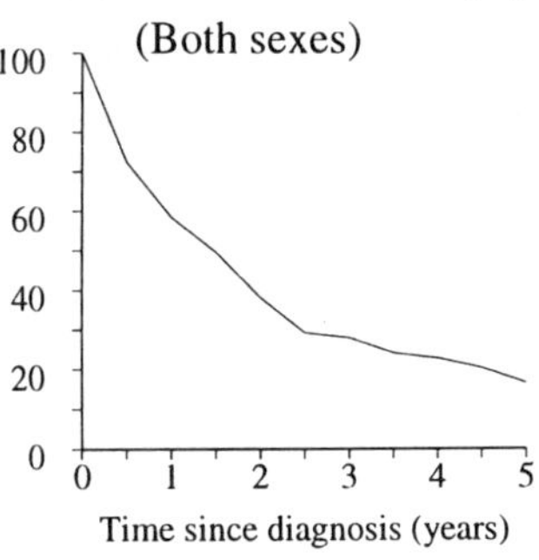

OBSERVED AND RELATIVE SURVIVAL (%) BY PERIOD AND SEX
(Number of cases in parentheses)

	PERIOD						SEX					
	1978-80		1981-82		1983-85		Males		Females		All	
	obs	rel	obs	rel	obs	rel	obs	rel	obs	rel	obs	rel
N. Cases	(30)		(29)		(21)		(50)		(30)		(80)	
1 year	53	53	59	59	66	66	50	50	73	73	58	58
3 years	30	30	28	28	25	25	26	26	31	31	28	28
5 years	17	17	17	17	15	15	14	14	21	21	16	17
8 years	13	13	14	14	..	..	10	10	21	21	14	14
10 years	13	13	..	..	..	..	10	10	21	21	14	14

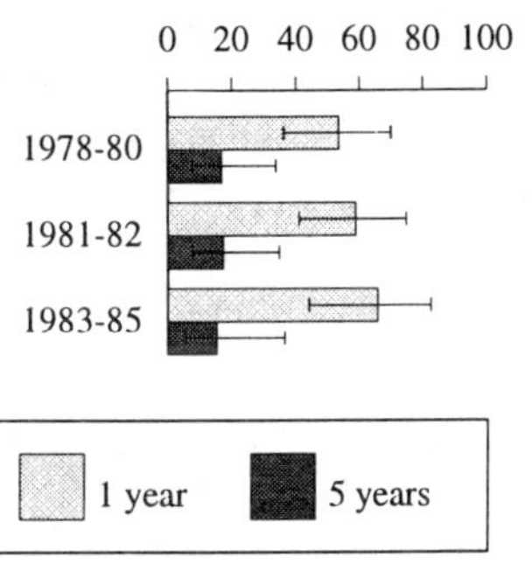

LEUKAEMIA

FRENCH REGISTRIES

Children

REGISTRY	NUMBER OF CASES Males	Females	All	PERIOD OF DIAGNOSIS
Amiens	9	2	11	1983-1984
Côte-d'Or	13	12	25	1980-1984
Doubs	23	12	35	1979-1985
Mean age (years)	6.0	7.0	6.4	

RELATIVE SURVIVAL (%)

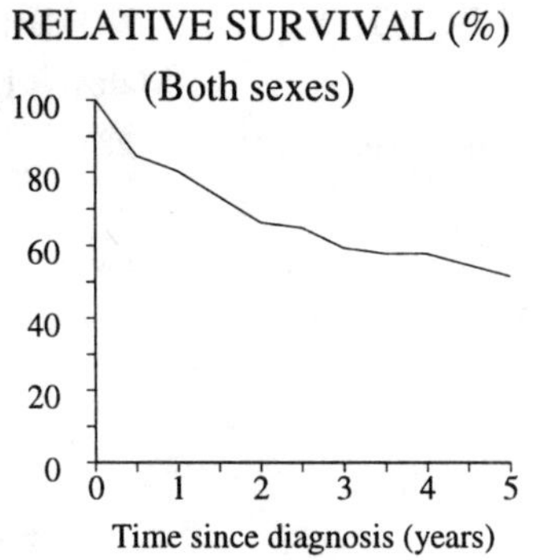

OBSERVED AND RELATIVE SURVIVAL (%) BY PERIOD AND SEX
(Number of cases in parentheses)

	PERIOD						SEX					
	1978-80		1981-82		1983-85		Males		Females		All	
	obs	rel	obs	rel	obs	rel	obs	rel	obs	rel	obs	rel
N. Cases	(15)		(23)		(33)		(45)		(26)		(71)	
1 year	80	80	74	74	85	85	80	80	81	81	80	80
3 years	53	53	65	65	58	58	53	53	69	69	59	59
5 years	40	40	51	51	58	58	49	49	56	56	51	52
8 years	40	40	39	40	58	58	39	39	56	56	46	46
10 years	..	..	..	..	..	..	..	..	..	..	..	..

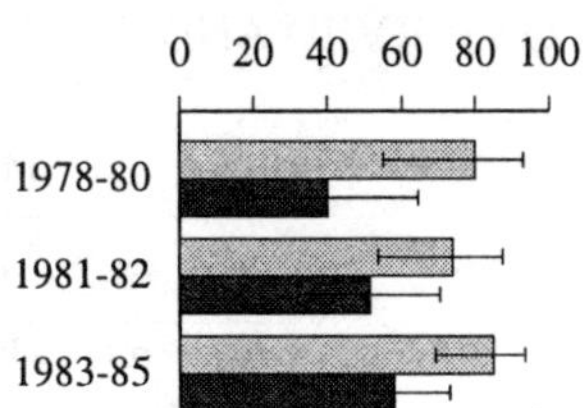

POLISH REGISTRIES

REGISTRY	NUMBER OF CASES Males	Females	All	PERIOD OF DIAGNOSIS
Cracow	17	17	34	1978-1984
Mean age (years)	5.4	5.0	5.2	

RELATIVE SURVIVAL (%)

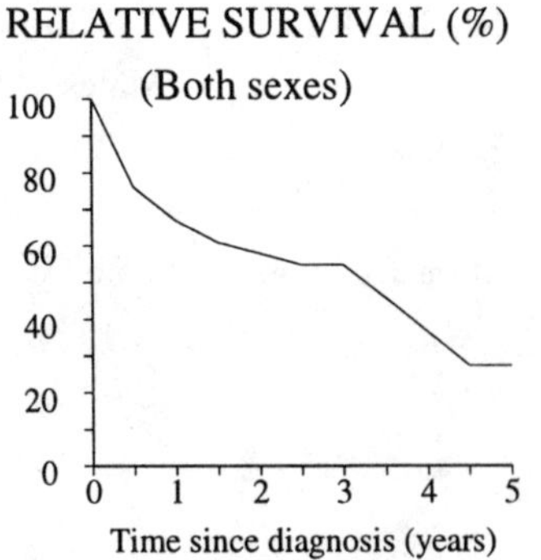

OBSERVED AND RELATIVE SURVIVAL (%) BY PERIOD AND SEX
(Number of cases in parentheses)

	PERIOD						SEX					
	1978-80		1981-82		1983-85		Males		Females		All	
	obs	rel	obs	rel	obs	rel	obs	rel	obs	rel	obs	rel
N. Cases	(13)		(5)		(16)		(17)		(17)		(34)	
1 year	62	62	80	80	67	67	70	70	65	65	67	67
3 years	54	54	60	60	54	54	57	57	53	53	55	55
5 years	8	8	40	40	40	40	19	19	35	35	27	27
8 years	8	8	20	20	..	..	19	19	..	..	24	24
10 years	8	8	20	20	..	..	19	19	..	..	24	24

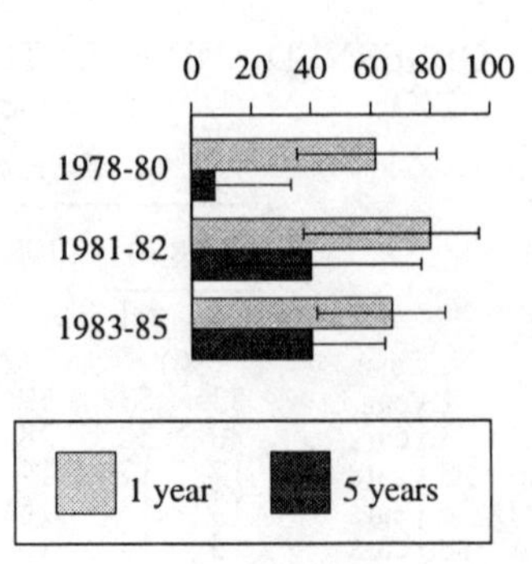

LEUKAEMIA

SPANISH REGISTRIES

Children

REGISTRY	NUMBER OF CASES Males	Females	All	PERIOD OF DIAGNOSIS
Tarragona	4	1	5	1985-1985
Mean age (years)	10.0	12.0	10.4	

RELATIVE SURVIVAL (%)
(Both sexes)

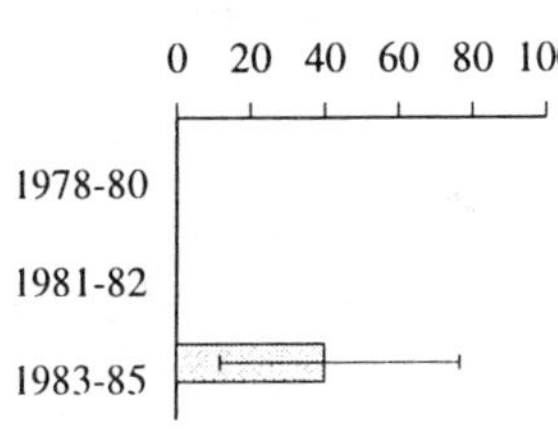

OBSERVED AND RELATIVE SURVIVAL (%) BY PERIOD AND SEX
(Number of cases in parentheses)

	PERIOD						SEX					
	1978-80		1981-82		1983-85		Males		Females		All	
	obs	rel	obs	rel	obs	rel	obs	rel	obs	rel	obs	rel
N. Cases	(0)		(0)		(5)		(4)		(1)		(5)	
1 year	..	..	..	..	40	40	50	50	0	0	40	40
3 years	..	..	..	..	20	20	25	25	0	0	20	20
5 years	..	..	..	..	0	0	0	0	0	0	0	0
8 years	..	..	..	..	0	0	0	0	0	0	0	0
10 years	..	..	..	..	0	0	0	0	0	0	0	0

0 20 40 60 80 100

1978-80

1981-82

1983-85

SWISS REGISTRIES

REGISTRY	NUMBER OF CASES Males	Females	All	PERIOD OF DIAGNOSIS
Basel	5	6	11	1981-1984
Geneva	10	8	18	1978-1984
Mean age (years)	6.3	3.6	5.0	

RELATIVE SURVIVAL (%)
(Both sexes)

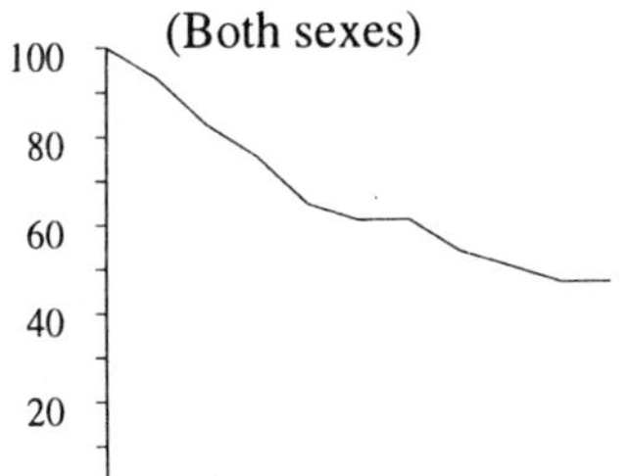

OBSERVED AND RELATIVE SURVIVAL (%) BY PERIOD AND SEX
(Number of cases in parentheses)

	PERIOD						SEX					
	1978-80		1981-82		1983-85		Males		Females		All	
	obs	rel	obs	rel	obs	rel	obs	rel	obs	rel	obs	rel
N. Cases	(9)		(12)		(8)		(15)		(14)		(29)	
1 year	100	100	83	84	63	63	80	80	85	86	83	83
3 years	63	63	67	67	50	50	53	53	70	70	61	61
5 years	50	50	50	50	38	38	40	40	54	54	47	47
8 years	..	..	50	50	..	..	40	40	54	55	47	47
10 years	..	..	..	..	..	..	..	..	..	..	..	..

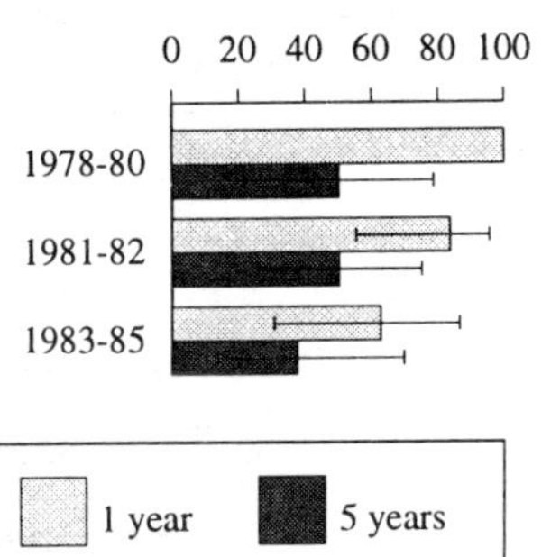

LEUKAEMIA

EUROPEAN REGISTRIES *Children*

Unweighted analysis

REGISTRY	CASES Males	Females	All
DENMARK	168	119	287
DUTCH REGISTRIES	28	21	49
ENGLISH REGISTRIES	504	362	866
ESTONIA	50	30	80
FINLAND	155	144	299
FRENCH REGISTRIES	45	26	71
ITALIAN REGISTRIES	175	159	334
MAINZ (GERMANY)	817	651	1468
POLISH REGISTRIES	17	17	34
SCOTLAND	111	85	196
SPANISH REGISTRIES	4	1	5
SWISS REGISTRIES	15	14	29
Mean age (years)	6.0	5.8	5.9

RELATIVE SURVIVAL (%)
(Age-standardized)

Females 100 80 60 40 20 0 — DK, ENG, FIN, I, D, SCO, EUR — Males 0 20 40 60 80 100

OBSERVED AND RELATIVE SURVIVAL (%) BY AGE AND PERIOD
(Number of cases in parentheses)

	AGE CLASS												PERIOD					
	0-4		0-1		2-4		5-9		10-14		All		1978-80		1981-82		1983-85	
	obs	rel	obs	rel	obs	rel	obs	rel	obs	rel	obs	rel	obs	rel	obs	rel	obs	rel
Males	(997)		(237)		(760)		(574)		(518)		(2089)		(525)		(780)		(784)	
1 year	83	83	68	68	88	88	84	84	77	77	82	82	78	79	82	82	84	84
3 years	67	67	48	48	73	73	65	65	52	52	63	63	52	52	66	66	67	67
5 years	61	61	43	44	66	66	56	57	44	45	56	56	43	43	58	58	61	61
8 years	57	57	41	41	61	61	54	54	39	40	51	52	39	39	54	55	57	57
10 years	53	53	41	41	57	57	53	53	36	37	49	49	37	37	53	54	..	..
Females	(805)		(195)		(610)		(462)		(362)		(1629)		(412)		(612)		(605)	
1 year	84	84	66	66	90	90	84	84	78	78	83	83	77	77	85	85	84	85
3 years	72	72	48	48	79	79	68	68	59	59	68	68	56	56	71	72	72	72
5 years	66	67	42	43	74	74	63	63	54	54	63	63	48	48	66	66	69	69
8 years	64	64	42	42	71	72	61	61	50	50	60	60	46	46	64	64	64	64
10 years	63	63	42	42	70	70	58	58	41	41	57	57	43	43	63	63	..	..
Overall	(1802)		(432)		(1370)		(1036)		(880)		(3718)		(937)		(1392)		(1389)	
1 year	84	84	67	67	89	89	84	84	77	77	82	82	78	78	83	83	84	84
3 years	69	69	48	48	76	76	66	66	55	55	65	65	54	54	68	68	69	69
5 years	63	63	43	43	70	70	59	59	48	48	59	59	45	45	62	62	65	65
8 years	60	60	41	41	66	66	57	57	44	44	55	55	42	42	59	59	60	60
10 years	57	58	41	41	63	63	55	55	38	38	52	52	39	40	57	58	..	..

RELATIVE SURVIVAL (%) BY AGE AND PERIOD

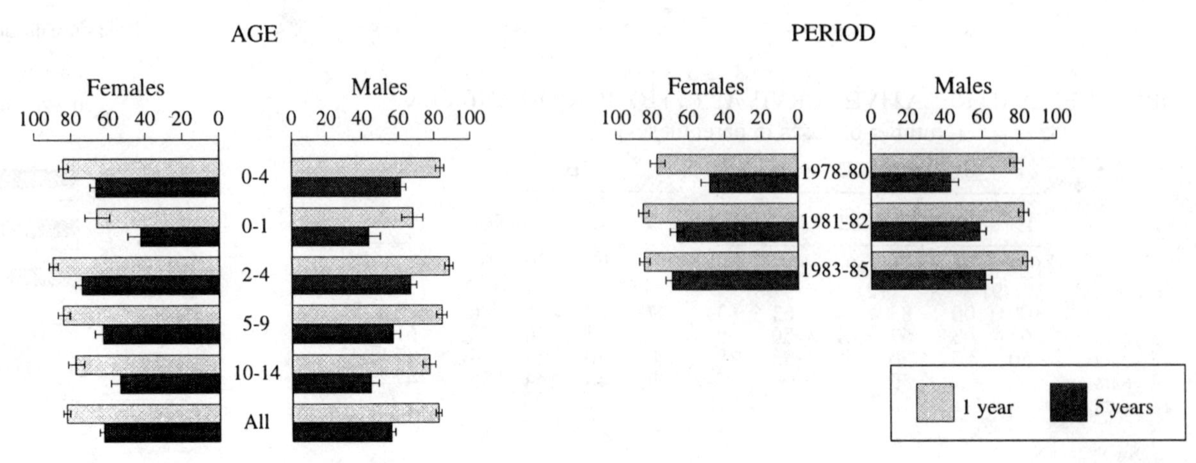

CHAPTER 18

Summary and discussion of results

J.W.W. Coebergh

Introduction

This publication presents the results of the first pan-European study on survival in cancer patients. Thirty population-based cancer registries in 11 European countries contributed data on about 800 000 unselected cancer patients diagnosed during the period 1978-85 and with a minimum follow-up period of five years. Almost 20% of the European population, excluding the former Soviet Union, was covered and the 7600 childhood cases comprised about 35% of the total. The data were analysed in a uniform manner, taking account of major confounding factors, including age at diagnosis. Area-specific general mortality rates, which varied from 6 to 11 per 1000 person-years for all ages, were used to calculate expected and relative survival (Chapter 4).

For each registry and/or country, the data are presented in tabular form according to sex, age and period of diagnosis. Considerable variation in relative survival between countries was found, and possible explanations in terms of the quality of oncological care and major conditioning factors are discussed below.

Differences in relative survival across Europe were not unexpected, in view of previously published results from Denmark (Carstensen *et al.*, 1993), England & Wales (Office of Population Censuses and Surveys and Cancer Research Campaign, 1981), Estonia (Aareleid & Rahu, 1991), Finland (Hakulinen *et al.*, 1981), France (Centre de Lutte contre le Cancer, 1987), south-eastern Netherlands (Coebergh & van der Heijden, 1991), the Cracow area (Pawlega, 1993), Saarland (Dhom *et al.*, 1991; Wiebelt *et al.*, 1991), Scotland (Black *et al.*, 1993) and Switzerland (Registre Genevois des Tumeurs, 1988; Levi *et al.*, 1992a). For children, variation in survival is generally smaller according to various publications (Stiller & Bunch, 1990; Mosso *et al.*, 1992; Haaf *et al.*, 1993).

The differences between these earlier studies, especially for adults, are not easy to interpret, because of variations with respect to detection and definition of disease, inclusion and follow-up criteria, methods of data collection and, last but not least, methods of calculating survival (Hakulinen, 1982, 1983). Thus, artefactual differences in survival of unselected patients, even if estimated in population-based studies, can be considerably biased. Table 18.1 lists the factors that may be responsible for this variation (see also Chapter 1). A single factor rarely fully accounts for a survival difference, but its presence or absence may be an indicator of the presence or absence of other factors. For example, stage at diagnosis, which is a well known prognostic factor for cancer survival, depends on access to and confidence in hospital medicine (Karjalainen *et al.*, 1989), and as such may be related to higher socio-economic status. The relative importance of clinical and pathological factors which affect survival for specific cancers is listed in Table 18.2.

The relevance of different types of therapy according to cancer site is indicated in Table 18.3. For most tumours, the prognosis is clearly stage-dependent regardless of the type of therapy adopted, and differences in quality of care play a relatively small role, except for availability of facilities for early diagnosis. For some tumours, cytotoxic therapy has an independent prognostic value, more or less regardless of stage at diagnosis, and can lower mortality. Finally, the availability of adequately organized medical expertise and facilities, including for supportive care, is crucial; this in turn has geographical and socio-economic components, including distance from specialized centres and the extent of

Table 18.1. Factors known or thought to influence cancer survival

Nature of disease and stage at diagnosis:
- Length of detectable preclinical phase
- Diagnostic criteria and equipment
- Histological type
- Subsite

Host factors:
- Age, birth cohort
- Nutritional status
- Social support

Prevalence of concomitant diseases:
- Independent influence on prognosis
- Limit therapeutic options

Financial and geographical availability of:
- Specialized expertise for diagnosis, treatment and supportive care
- Manpower
- Equipment
- Screening programmes

Registration methods
- Completeness of registration
- Definition of date of diagnosis
- Completeness of follow-up

Selection of patients or registry source population:
- Coverage of selected areas or whole country
- Distribution of social class and occupation
- Social insurance coverage

Indirect factors:
- Gross national product and percentage spent on health care
- Distribution of wealth and education

Table 18.2. Influence of tumour-specific prognostic factors and therapy on cancer survival[a]

Tumour site	Stage	Histology	Subsite	Therapy[b]
Tongue	++	–	+	+
Mouth	++	–	+	+
Pharynx	++	–	++	+
Oesophagus	++	+/–	++	+/–
Stomach	++	+/–	+	+/–
Colon	++	+/–	+	+/–
Rectum	++	–	+/–	+/–
Pancreas	+	–	–	+/–
Nasopharynx	+	+	–	+/–
Larynx	++	–	++	+
Lung	++	++	+	+/–
Bone	++	++	+	+
Breast	++	+/–	–	+
Cervix uteri	++	+/–	–	+/–
Corpus uteri	++	+/–	–	+/–
Ovary	++	+	–	+/–
Vulva	++	–	+	+/–
Testis	+	++	–	++
Penis	++	–	–	+/–
Kidney	+	+	++	+/–
Brain	+	+	+	+/–
Hodgkin's disease	+	+	–	++
Leukaemia	+c	++	+/–	+

–: none, +/–: possible: + certain, ++: major
[a] Derived from Souhami & Tobias (1986)
[b] Regardless of stage, histology and subsite
[c] No. of white blood cells

health insurance coverage. If specialized medical services are insufficient to meet needs, it is the less privileged and elderly who generally experience most difficulty in obtaining access to them (Cella *et al.*, 1991). Inadequate access also perpetuates low expectations for specialist cancer care: the view that "you will die anyway" becomes self-fulfilling (Loehrer *et al.*, 1991). Unfortunately, stage was not registered in a standardized way during the study period in many registries and only indirect evidence is available for the role of stage.

Description of summary tables

Because cancer patients can also die from ("competing") causes other than cancer, the relative survival was computed. This is the ratio of the crude cancer survival, regardless of cause of death, to the expected survival, derived from area-specific general mortality data, which, as seen in Chapter 4, vary markedly across Europe. Table 18.4 ranks the five-year weighted relative survival rates in adult males and females, according to tumour site. In Table 18.5a tumour-specific relative survival rates are presented according to age and period of diagnosis and Table 18.5b provides a separate overview for children. Table 18.6 shows cancer site-specific changes in relative one- and five-year survival over time according to country.

To ensure that results are comparable between countries, whenever the numbers were large enough, one- and five-year relative survival figures have been age-standardized on the age distribution of all patients with a given tumour (Chapter 3). To express between-country variation in survival, the average of the second and third lowest survival rates was subtracted from the average of the second and third highest, and the resulting difference was divided by the European mean, weighted, whenever possible, by the total incidence expected in the participating countries (Table 18.7a). For a few sites, for which

Table 18.3. Relevance of common therapeutic modalities for survival among cancer patients diagnosed 1978–85, according to tumour site[a]

Tumour	Surgery	Irradia-tion	Cyto-toxic	Palliative[b]
Tongue	+++	+		
Mouth	+++	+		
Pharynx	+++	+		
Oesophagus	+	+		++
Stomach	++		+	+
Colon	+++		+	+
Rectum	+++	+		+
Pancreas	+			++
Nasopharynx	+	++		
Larynx	++	++		
Lung – NSC[c]	++	++	+/–	++
– SC[c]	+	+	+++	+
Bone	+++	+	+	
Breast	+++	++	+	
Cervix uteri	+++	++		
Corpus uteri	+++	++		
Ovary	++	+	++	+
Vulva	+++	+		
Testis	++	+	+++	
Penis	+++	+		
Kidney	++		+	+
Brain	++	++		+
Hodgkin's disease	–	++	+++	
Leukaemia	–	+	+++	+

–: no relevance; +: relevant in <25% of patients; ++: in 25–50%; +++: >50% of patients

[a] Derived from Souhami & Tobias (1986)

[b] Reported when >5% of patients receives only palliative care after diagnosis

[c] NSC: non-small-cell; SC: small cell

Table 18.4. Ranked five-year relative survival for adult cancers diagnosed in Europe during 1978–85[a]

Males		Rank	Females	
Testis[b]	85%	1	Corpus uteri	72%
Penis[b]	68%	2	Breast	67%
Hodgkin's disease[b]	66%	3	Hodgkin's disease[b]	67%
Larynx	57%	4	Larynx	62%
CLL[b]	46%	5	Cervix	59%
Kidney	45%	6	Oral cavity[b]	53%
Colon	43%	7	Vulva/vagina[b]	52%
Bone[b]	43%	8	CLL[b]	51%
Oral cavity[b]	43%	9	Kidney	45%
Nasopharynx[b]	38%	10	Bone[b]	45%
Rectum	36%	11	Tongue[b]	43%
Tongue[b]	36%	12	Oropharynx[b]	42%
Oropharynx[b]	29%	13	Colon	41%
CML[b]	19%	14	Rectum	40%
Hypopharynx[b]	19%	15	Nasopharynx[b]	37%
ALL[b]	17%	16	Ovary	32%
Stomach	17%	17	CML[b]	21%
Brain	14%	18	Hypopharynx[b]	20%
Lung	8%	19	ALL[b]	20%
AML[b]	7%	20	Stomach	19%
Oesophagus	5%	21	Brain	15%
Pancreas	3%	22	Lung	10%
		23	AML[b]	7%
		24	Pancreas	5%
		25	Oesophagus	5%

[a] Weighted according to hypothetical cancer incidence in each participating country, except for cancers marked [b] (see Chapter 3 and 16)

[b] Unweighted survival

ALL: acute lymphoid leukaemia, AML: acute myeloid leukaemia, CML: chronic myeloid leukaemia, CLL: chronic lymphoid leukaemia

survival is mainly stage-determined (stomach, colon, cervix and corpus uteri), this was done for two age groups (45–54 and 75+ years) (Table 18.7b). For other sites for which survival is heavily influenced by treatment (testicular cancer, Hodgkin's disease and to some extent breast and ovarian cancer), the difference is shown for the age-groups 15–44 and 65–74 years (Table 18.7c).

The age-standardized five-year relative survival rates for selected cancer sites are compared between countries in Table 18.8. The aim here is to show up patterns in the data. For frequent sites, the three countries with the highest survival figures and the three with the lowest are presented. For less frequent sites, the comparison is restricted to countries for which age-standardized survival rates could be compiled (Chapter 16). The major hypothesized reasons for the differences (from Tables 18.1-3) are also listed and include aspects of quality of care, registry completeness and random variation.

Table 18.5a. One- and five-year relative survival rates (%) in adult European cancer patients diagnosed in 1978–85, according to age and period of diagnosis

Tumour site (Total no. of cases)	Year[a]	Age (years) males and females		Period	
		45–54	75–99	1978–80	1983–85
Head and neck					
Tongue	1	70	52	63	69
(3299)	5	37	29	38	39
Oral cavity	1	78	57	70	74
(4382)	5	53	36	46	48
Oropharynx	1	71	50	64	66
(2457)	5	36	24	33	34
Hypopharynx	1	58	37	50	50
(2199)	5	19	14	18	21
Digestive tract					
Oesophagus	1	28	16	22	26
(18 008)	5	4	3	4	5
Stomach	1	51	24	34	38
(62 600)	5	30	9	16	19
Colon	1	73	50	58	65
(74 826)	5	49	36	39	45
Rectum	1	77	55	64	68
(52 161)	5	43	29	36	41
Pancreas	1	17	12	13	15
(29 733)	5	5	4	4	4
Respiratory tract					
Nasopharynx	1	77	49	68	68
(1078)	5	44	18	38	40
Larynx	1	88	77	80	85
(10 612)	5	68	48	53	59
Lung	1	37	21	28	29
(167 086)	5	13	3	8	9
Female and male genital systems					
Breast	1	94	82	90	91
(119 138)	5	70	61	66	68
Cervix uteri	1	85	57	82	83
(22 119)	5	59	27	56	60
Corpus uteri	1	92	74	85	88
(22 768)	5	85	53	73	74
Ovary	1	73	36	54	62
(24 030)	5	37	20	28	34
Testis	1	94[b]	53	91	93
(5615)	5	86[b]	36	83	87

Table 18.5a. (contd.)

Tumour site (Total no. of cases)	Year[a]	Age (years) males and females		Period	
		45–54	75–99	1978–80	1983–85
Penis	1	90	70	83	83
(1670)	5	78	57	69	64
Miscellaneous					
Bone	1	83	35	62	69
(1560)	5	57	23	42	48
Kidney	1	72	53	62	64
(18 246)	5	55	34	43	45
Brain	1	40	12	34	36
(13 318)	5	12	4	17	16
Haemopoietic system					
Hodgkin's disease	1	94[b]	45	79	85
(6728)	5	81[b]	26	63	71
ALL	1	69[b]	12	51	45
(1247)	5	26[c]	3	17	21
CLL	1	93	62	73	76
(7051)	5	68	34	46	49
AML	1	47[b]	8	23	27
(5822)	5	16[b]	1	5	8
CML	1	84[b]	38	62	60
(2894)	5	28[b]	10	21	20

[a] Since diagnosis

[b] Age group 15–44 years

Discussion

The impact of various forms of bias has been discussed in detail in Chapters 1 and 2. In interpreting the results one has to realize that these data refer to former patients and past health care (i.e. diagnosed 1978-1985 and treated up till 1990); patients were therefore diagnosed nine to sixteen years before 1995, the year of publication. Changes in cancer management affecting survival have occurred in the meantime, examples being earlier detection and more adjuvant therapy of breast cancer and more administration of intensive chemotherapy to patients with ovarian cancer and acute leukaemia.

Sex-differences in five-year relative survival according to tumour site (Table 18.4)

Five-year relative survival rates greater than 50% were found for only four tumour sites in males, accounting for about 5% of all males included in the study, but for eight sites in females, comprising almost 45% of the female patients. Five-year relative survival rates below 10% were found for four sites in both males and females, comprising about 50% of male and 15% of female patients.

Tumour-specific age-standardized five-year relative survival was usually better for females than for males, except for cancers of the kidney, colon, nasopharynx, oesophagus and acute myeloid leukaemia, with similar relative survival rates in both sexes. Superior female survival may be due to a more favourable distribution of subsites (for head and neck cancer) or histology (e.g. women have less squamous cell and more adenocarcinoma of

Table 18.5b. Five-year relative survival rates (%) for European children with cancer (<15 years) diagnosed in 1978–85, according to sex and period of diagnosis

Tumour site (No. of cases)	Year[a]	Sex		Period		Possible explanation for time trend
		Girls	Boys	1978–80	1983–85	
Nasopharynx	1	88	97	93	100	Random variation
(47)	5	59	67	72	59	
Bone[b]	1	84	84	73	91	More complete data
(677)	5	44	47	31	57	Better therapy
Kidney	1	87	87	83	88	Better therapy
(633)	5	75	75	69	76	
Ovary	1	85		82	82	Random variation
(91)	5	70		55	63	Better therapy
Testis	1		94	88	96	Random variation
(75)	5		82	79	86	Better therapy
Brain	1	71	72	69	74	More complete data
(1644)	5	52	50	51	53	Histology & subsite Better therapy
Hodgkin's disease	1	96	96	95	97	Better therapy
(591)	5	91	90	87	94	
Leukaemia	1	83	82	78	84	Better therapy
(3718)	5	63	56	45	65	

[a] Since diagnosis
[b] Age group 0 –19 years

the lung than men). Generally, the stage distribution is more favourable for females, who appear to be more health-conscious than men, leading them to seek medical help sooner (Mechanic, 1978). Gender differences in cancer survival may largely disappear after adjustment for disease-specific prognostic factors (Wiebelt & Hakulinen, 1991). One must bear in mind, furthermore, that the use of relative survival may not eliminate completely the sex-related difference in mortality; factors such as smoking, drinking and occupational exposures, which affect both cancer incidence and competitive mortality, may be much more frequent in male cases than in the general population whose mortality rates are used for computing relative survival; for females, such a difference may be much smaller.

Age-related differences in one- and five-year relative survival rates of adult cancer patients (Table 18.5a)

Relative survival rates were generally highest in young adults, declined after 54 years of age and were distinctly worse for patients over 75. Smaller declines with increasing age were found in patients with cancer of the breast, larynx and corpus uteri (with relatively good prognosis) and cancer of the oesophagus and pancreas (with poor prognoses). The decrease in survival with age was usually most marked in the first year after diagnosis, suggesting an association with stage and treatment or, indirectly, with access to care facilities. Besides the fact that computing relative survival may not correct fully for the increase in prevalence of serious concomitant conditions with increasing age, surgery and cytotoxic agents may either have a negative effect on prognosis of other diseases or be administered less or at lower dosage (Satariano & Ragland, 1994). Also, radiotherapy is administered less often to older patients, even those located close to facilities for irradiation (De Jong *et al.*, 1994). Pattern-of-care studies on breast, colorectal and lung cancer, that are being carried out within the framework of the EUROCARE project, will clarify the reasons for these differences.

Table 18.6. Changes in one- and five-year relative survival rates for adult European cancer patients, according to country, diagnosed over 1978–85

Tumour site	Years[a]	DK	NL	ENG	EST	FIN	F	D	I	PL	SCO	CH
Head & neck	1	=	++	+	=	+	−	+	++	+	++	+
	5	−	−	+	−	++	+	−−	++	−	+	−
Oesophagus	1	=	++	+	+	−	=	=	++	−	+	=
	5	=	+	=	++	+	+	=	++	=	=	+
Stomach	1	+	=	++	=	=	+	+	+	=	+	=
	5	=	=	+	+	+	+	+	+	−	+	−
Colon	1	+	+	++	=	+	++	++	++	−	=	−
	5	=	+	++	+	+	++	++	+	=	=	+
Rectum	1	+	+	++	−−	=	+	=	++	−−	+	+
	5	=	++	++	+	−	+	++	++	=	=	−
Larynx	1	−	−	=	−	−	+	++	++	++	+	−
	5	++	=	=	++	−	++	++	+	=	=	+
Lung	1	=	++	+	−	=	−	=	+	−	=	=
	5	−	+	=	−	=	=	=	++	=	=	+
Breast	1	=	+	=	+	=	+	=	++	++	=	−
	5	=	+	+	++	+	+	=	+	++	=	=
Cervix	1	−	++	+	+	=	=	+	+	−	+	−−
	5	+	++	++	−	−	++	−	+	++	+	−−
Corpus	1	=	=	+	++	+	[b]	++	+	++	=	=
	5	+	++	+	=	+		=	+	++	+	++
Ovary	1	++	++	+	−−	++	++	++	++	++	+	−−
	5	++	++	+	=	+	++	+	+	+	=	−
Testis	1	=	+	+	++	=	++	+	−	−	++	+
	5	=	++	+	++	++	++	++	−−	++	++	++
Kidney	1	=	+	+	−	=	=	++	−−	−−	=	=
	5	=	++	+	=	+	+	+	=	=	=	−−
Brain	1	=	++	=	=	=	−−	++	++	=	=	++
	5	+	++	=	−−	−	−	−	++	−−	=	=
Hodgkin's disease	1	+	−	++	+	++	=	+	++	+	++	+
	5	++	=	++	=	++	−−	++	−−	−−	++	−−
Leukaemia	1	+	++	=	+	−	++	++	−−	−−	+	++
	5	+	++	+	+	=	=	−	−−	=	+	++

= No change
\+ or − : ≥2% absolute change between 1978–80 and 1983–85 (1981–82 for Scotland)
++ or −− : ≥5% absolute change between 1978–80 and 1983–85 (1981–82 for Scotland)
[a] After diagnosis
[b] Numbers too small or no data available

Time trends from 1978-80 to 1983-85 in one- and five-year site-specific relative survival rates in adults (Table 18.5a) and children (Table 18.5b) with cancer; time trends in adults according to country (Table 18.6)

For most cancer sites, relative survival improved from 1978–80 to 1983–85, especially in the first year after diagnosis. Survival failed to improve, however, in adults with chronic myeloid leukaemia, cancer of the tongue, oropharynx, oesophagus, lung, pancreas, corpus uteri, penis or brain.

Improved survival among patients with gastrointestinal tract tumours and cancer of the kidney is probably attributable mainly to earlier diagnosis. Better surgical management, including for example more extensive lymph node removal, may also have contributed, particularly if backed up by

Table 18.7a. Means and trimmed ranges of age-standardized five-year relative survival rates[a] for European adult cancer patients

Tumour site	No. of cases	Relative survival (%)					Major prognostic factors[d]
		Mean	High[c]	Low[c]	Range	As % of mean	
Head & neck and respiratory tract							
Larynx	9099	56	65	50	15	27	S,L,T
Oral cavity	2811	42[b]	47	31	16	38	S,L
Oropharynx	1814	30[b]	34	21	13	43	S,L
Hypopharynx	1481	19[b]	22	13	9	47	S,L
Tongue	2063	36[b]	42	24	18	50	S,L
Lung	129 231	7	11	6	5	71	S,H,C,T
Digestive tract							
Rectum	27 984	34	38	29	9	26	S,L,T
Colon	42 317	41	47	32	15	37	S,L,C
Oesophagus	10 843	4	6	4	2	48	S,L,H,C
Stomach	36 780	14	18	8	10	71	S,L,H,C
Male and female genital systems							
Testis	5615	85[b]	89	73	16	19	H,T,S
Breast	119 139	67	72	60	12	18	S,H,T
Cervix	22 119	58	64	52	12	21	S,T,H
Corpus	22 768	70	77	60	16	24	S,H,T
Ovary	24 030	30	35	25	10	34	S,T,H
Penis	1670	68[b]	83	53	30	44	S,L
Miscellaneous							
Brain	7428	14	17	11	6	44	H,S,T,C
Kidney	10 770	42	47	25	21	51	L,S,H,C
Bone	882	43[b]	51	26	24	57	H,S,T
Haemopoietic system							
Hodgkin's disease	3953	66[b]	77	62	15	23	T,S,H
CLL	4104	46[b]	70	42	28	60	S,T,C
CML	1544	19[b]	28	13	15	81	T,C
AML	3006	7[b]	12	6	6	94	H,T,C
ALL	700	17[b]	31	14	16	95	T,C

[a] Average of five-year relative survival for sex with most cases
[b] Unweighted survival; all others are weighted (see footnote of Table 18.4)
[c] High and Low: average of 2nd and 3rd highest and lowest rates respectively
[d] In order of importance: S= stage, H= histology, L= subsite, T= therapy. C indicates that completeness of registration may also have affected the observed survival

ameliorations in postoperative and supportive care. For cancer of the testis, Hodgkin's disease, and to some extent ovarian cancer, increased application of cytotoxic therapy has improved survival. This also explains the observed decline of mortality relative to incidence (Doll, 1990; Coleman *et al.*, 1993).

Table 18.6 gives an overview of changes in one- and five-year relative survival for certain cancers according to country. With the exception of head and neck, lung, oesophagus, kidney and brain cancer, both one- and five-year relative survival improved in most countries, including tumours with relatively

Table 18.7b. Means and trimmed ranges of one- and five-year relative survival rates from selected cancers with mainly stage-determined prognosis in patients of ages 45–54 and 75+, diagnosed during 1978–1985

			Relative survival				
Tumour site	No. of cases	Year[a]	Mean	High[b]	Low[b]	Range	As % of mean
Age 45–54 years							
Stomach	4905	1	51	59	36	23	44
		5	30	39	17	22	74
Colon	5794	1	72	76	67	10	13
		5	49	52	41	11	22
Cervix	3835	1	85	91	81	10	12
		5	59	68	55	13	22
Corpus	3690	1	92	96	89	7	7
		5	85	92	79	13	15
Age 75+ years							
Stomach	22 620	1	24	32	15	16	67
		5	9	14	6	8	84
Colon	28 437	1	50	63	37	25	50
		5	36	44	25	19	52
Cervix	2395	1	57	73	46	27	47
		5	27	38	18	20	72
Corpus	4343	1	74	81	66	15	20
		5	53	60	40	20	38

[a] Year(s) since diagnosis
[b] High and Low: average of second and third highest and lowest rates respectively

poor prognosis such as stomach, rectum, ovary and leukaemia. Most likely the one-year survival for small cell lung cancer (about 25% of all lung cancers) improved too, but this was not apparent in the overall data. Five-year relative survival increased markedly for several tumours with favourable prognosis, especially for Hodgkin's disease and testicular cancer, but also for colon and ovary. For ovarian cancer, more intensive chemotherapy probably played a significant role since 1980 (Balvert *et al.*, 1991).

Time trends in survival for Hodgkin's disease and testicular cancer are reflected in the marked decrease in mortality rates from these two cancers, despite the increasing incidence of testicular cancer (Coleman *et al.*, 1993; La Vecchia *et al.*, 1992a, b). For other cancers responsive to cytotoxic treatment, such as ovary and breast cancer, the changes in incidence are likely to have been the main determinant of the observed changes in mortality rates, which are decreasing only in younger generations (Geddes *et al.*, 1994) (age-standardized breast cancer mortality is actually increasing in most European countries). The greatest decline in mortality for tumours responsive to chemotherapy was observed in Denmark, the Netherlands, Finland, Germany and Scotland.

Table 18.7c. Means and trimmed ranges of one- and five-year relative survival rates for cancers amenable to cytotoxic therapy in patients of ages 15–44 and 65–74, diagnosed 1978–1985

Tumour site	No. of cases	Year[a]	Relative survival Mean	High[b]	Low[b]	Range	As % of mean
Age 15–44 years							
Breast	15 603	1	96	97	94	4	4
		5	71	78	64	14	20
Ovary	2481	1	83	90	77	13	16
		5	60	70	51	19	32
Testis	4294	1	94	97	92	5	6
		5	86	91	81	10	12
Hodgkin's	3261	1	94	94	92	2	2
disease[d]		5	81	81	78	3	4
Age 65–74 years							
Breast	28 376	1	90	94	87	7	8
		5	66	72	59	13	19
Ovary	6250	1	47	57	37	20	43
		5	21	23	18	5	22
Testis[c]	597	1	93	94	87	7	7
		5	88	90	80	10	12
Hodgkin's	823	1	57	60	55	5	19
disease[d]		5	31	32	26	5	17

[a] Year(s) since diagnosis
[b] High and Low: average of second and third highest and lowest rates respectively
[c] Age group 45–54
[d] Both sexes: range between 2nd and 5th of six countries

Five-year survival improved modestly for most solid childhood tumours. Major improvements in treatment efficacy for most solid childhood cancers occurred largely before the period of the present study (1978–85) (Table 18.5b). The trend was most evident for bone and least so for brain tumours. Changes in histology and subsite distribution may have contributed to these trends. Survival improved markedly for acute leukaemia (mostly lymphocytic). However, compared with American experience (SEER, 1988), the improvement in survival for acute leukaemia is observed later. A possible explanation is the slow centralization of treatment that seems essential for success in childhood leukaemia (Stiller, 1988), for both bureaucratic and professional reasons. Assuming that incidence has not declined, the positive trends in childhood cancer survival are consistent with the observed reduction in mortality (Levi *et al.*, 1992b; Coleman *et al.*, 1993; Carmen Martos & Olsen, 1993).

Differences across Europe in age-standardized one- and five-year site-specific relative cancer survival (Tables 18.7a–c)

As noted previously, between-country variation in survival for each cancer site is expressed as both survival range and the percentage variation of this range with respect to mean European survival. For tumours occurring in both sexes, male figures were used to calculate the range, because of the greater number of male cases and lower random variation. After excluding the highest and lowest survival figures, the difference between the average of the two highest and the two lowest figures was taken as the range, both absolute and relative to the European mean.

Table 18.7a shows the ranges of adult five-year relative survival across-Europe. The major factors probably responsible for these differences (Table 18.2) are indicated in the right-hand column, in order of importance. Absolute differences in survival were small (≤ 6%) for most cancer sites with poor prognosis (oesophagus, lung, brain and acute myeloid leukaemia). Absolute differences were larger (>10%) for cancer sites such as breast, kidney, stomach, colon, rectum, cervix and corpus uteri, and several head and neck sites, for which therapy choice and survival are significantly influenced by stage at diagnosis; it is likely that access to care is an important cause of between-country survival differences for these cancers. Relatively smaller differences were observed for cancers sensitive to cytotoxic therapy (testis, Hodgkin's disease and ovary) especially at younger ages.

In general, among elderly patients, the range of relative survival was larger, especially during the first year after diagnosis (Table 18.7b), in particular for cancers in which stage at diagnosis has an overriding influence on prognosis (e.g. cancer of the head & neck, stomach, colon, cervix and corpus uteri); above anything else, this suggests large across-Europe differences in stage at diagnosis. The one-year survival range was much narrower for the 45–54 than the 75+ age group, suggesting a narrower stage-distribution among younger patients. Because five-year relative survival also varied considerably among patients of middle age, differences in patient management may have played a role.

In Table 18.7c the ranges of one- and five-year relative survival are shown (again divided into two age groups) for tumours generally responsive to cytotoxic therapy: testicular cancer, Hodgkin's disease, and also breast and ovarian cancer, where chemotherapy is adjuvant to surgery. Between-country ranges are narrower in younger patients in the first year after diagnosis, especially for breast and ovarian cancer, indicating that stage at diagnosis has a greater influence on survival for these cancers at older ages. However, for ovarian cancer, variation in five-year survival was greater for younger patients. Besides differences in quality of treatment, a different distribution of morphological types could be responsible.

Differences in five-year relative survival of adult patients between countries (Table 18.8)

An overview of differences in age-standardized five-year relative survival in adults between countries is presented in Table 18.8. For each cancer site, the three countries with the highest survival figures and the three with the lowest are shown. Registries or countries with less than 100 cases of a given tumour in both males and females were excluded, because the random variation was then too great. The last column of this table suggests reasons for the differences (from Tables 18.1 to 18.3). Access to specialized care is often mentioned. For sites where stage at diagnosis is important and cytotoxic therapy is not of much help in advanced cases (e.g., most sites in the gastrointestinal, respiratory and female genital tracts), relative survival rates are generally lower in the areas covered by the registries of Estonia and Poland (Cracow). Survival is also rather low for these tumours in the United Kingdom, except for head and neck cancers, for which, however, the more favourable subsite distribution may explain the relatively good outcomes (Chapter 2).

Survival is frequently at the higher end of the range in the areas covered by the Swiss registries (Geneva, Basel), Finland and the Netherlands (Eindhoven). Survival in Switzerland is likely to be slightly overestimated, because of the censoring of foreign residents who emigrate after diagnosis (Chapter 14). For tumours responsive to cytotoxic therapy (cancer of the ovary, testis and Hodgkin's disease), survival rates in patients from Denmark and England were also in the upper range.

Poor survival in Poland and Estonia appears mainly related to unfavourable stage distribution, which is likely to be related to inadequate availability of specialist care. Unfavourable stage distribution, again probably related to a level of availability of specialist care below the European average, may also explain poor survival especially in the United Kingdom, where the number of consultants per million inhabitants is three to four times lower than in most other Western European countries (Farthing *et al.*, 1993; Schroeder, 1984). It is worth noting that the smaller

Table 18.8. European countries ranked according to relative survival rates (%) from cancer in adult patients diagnosed 1978–1985

Tumour site (No. of cases)	No. of countries[a]	Country/registry age-standardized[b] relative 5-year survival (%) ranking		Suggested explanations for influence of major prognostic factors and health and registration systems[c]
		Highest	Lowest	
Head and neck				
Tongue (3299)	7	Scotland (43) England (39) Finland (37)	French (20 Italian (24) Denmark (31)	Subsite Access to specialized care
Oral cavity (4382)	8	English (44) French (44) Finland (42)	Italian (31) German (31) Swiss (39)	Subsite Access to specialized care
Oropharynx (2457)	4	English (33) Denmark (29)	Italian (21) French (23)	Subsite Access to specialized care
Hypopharynx (2199)	5	Scotland (22) French (20)	Italian (14) Denmark (14)	Subsite Access to specialized care
Digestive tract				
Oesophagus (13 035)	11	German (7) Finland (6) Swiss (6)	Polish (0) Estonia (3) Italian (4)	Access to endoscopy (In)completeness
Stomach (62 887)	12	Swiss (23) German (19) Dutch (18)	Scotland (7) Polish (7) English (8)	Subsite Access to endoscopy (In)completeness
Colon (42 317)	12	Swiss (57) Dutch (47) French (45)	Polish (20) Estonia (33) English (34)	Stage Access to endoscopy (In)completeness
Rectum (52 283)	12	Swiss (49) Finland (41) Dutch (39)	Polish (12) Estonia (28) Scotland (30)	Stage Access to endoscopy (In)completeness
Pancreas (10 559)	11	German (6) Polish (5) Scotland (4)	Estonia (2) English (2) Finland (2)	(In)completeness Access to diagnostic facilities
Respiratory system				
Larynx (10 559)	11	Dutch (72) Scotland (66) English (65)	Estonia (45) French (46) Polish (55)	Subsite Access to specialized care
Lung (167 446)	12	Swiss (12) Dutch (11) Finland (9)	Spanish (5) Polish (5) Estonia (6)	Histology Access to specialized care (In)completeness
Female and male genital system				
Breast (119 533)	12	Swiss (76) Finland (74) French (71)	Polish (44) Estonia (59) Scotland (62)	Access to mammography and radiotherapy Diffusion of adjuvant therapy
Cervix uteri (22 119)	12	Swiss (65) Italian (64) French (64)	Spanish (40) Polish (51) Scotland (52)	Coverage of screening Adequate staging and therapy

Table 18.8. (contd)

Tumour site (No. of cases)	No. of countries[a]	Country/registry age-standardized[b] relative 5-year survival (%) ranking		Suggested explanations for influence of major prognostic factors and health and registration systems[c]
		Highest	Lowest	
Female and male genital system (contd)				
Corpus uteri (22 153)	12	Dutch (78) Finland (77) Swiss (76)	Spanish (53) Polish (57) Estonia (64)	Access to gynaecologists and radiotherapy
Ovary (24 166)	12	Swiss (37) Spanish (36) Finland (34)	Estonia (22) Polish (24) Denmark (26)	Access to gynaecologists Adequate staging and cytotoxic therapy
Testis (5615)	9	Dutch (90) Denmark (88) Italian (87)	German (75) Finland (78) French (80)	Adequate staging and cytotoxic therapy
Penis (1670)	3	Denmark (72)	English (63)	Patient delay
Miscellaneous				
Bone (1560)	3	Finland (43)	English (39)	Subsite/histology Adequate care (In)completeness
Kidney (19 444)	11	German (53) Swiss (47) Italian (47)	Polish (19) Estonia (20) Denmark (31)	(In)completeness Stage
Brain (15 444)	11	Finland (23) Polish (17) German (17)	Scotland (10) Estonia (11) Denmark (11)	Subsite/histology Access to specialized care (In)completeness
Haematopoietic system				
Hodgkin's disease (6728)	6	Denmark (64) English (64) Italian (60)	Estonia (50) Scotland (59) Finland (59)	Adequate staging and chemo- and radiotherapy
ALL (1247)	3	Denmark (18)	Finland (9)	Chemotherapy (In)completeness
CLL (7051)	6	Italian (55) Estonian (51)	Denmark (36) Scotland (41) Finland (41)	Stage (In)completeness
AML (5822)	4	Scotland (7)	Finland (5)	Chemotherapy (In)completeness
CML (2894)	4	Finland (20)	Scotland (15)	Chemotherapy (In)completeness

[a] Number of countries with large enough numbers of patients to be included in the comparison of age-standardized survival

[b] For sites affecting both sexes, only the sex with the most cases (often males, excluding colon) was used for comparisons

[c] (In)completeness' means that some cancer registries may have selectively lost long- or short-term survivors

Table 18.9. General summary of results

After adjustment for age, females survived longer than males for a given tumour site, except for cancer of the oesophagus, hypopharynx, nasopharynx, colon, kidney and acute myeloid leukaemia.
A five-year relative survival of less than 10% was observed for four sites in males and females, however comprising 50% and 15% of all male and female cases included in the study, respectively; a five-year survival rate of more than 50% was observed for four sites among males and eight sites among females, comprising less than 5% and 45% of all male and female cases respectively.
Relative survival declined markedly with age, mainly in the first year of diagnosis; except for the two cancer sites with worst prognosis (oesophagus and pancreas) and, among cancer sites with relatively good prognosis, breast and larynx.
Relative five-year survival generally improved over time, except for the following tumours in adults: chronic myeloid leukaemia, cancer of the tongue and oropharynx, pancreas, lung, corpus uteri, penis and brain, together accounting for about 40% of all cancers.
Between-country differences in relative survival for various tumours were substantial: trimmed differences between high and low rates vary by up to 80% of the mean survival rate; **differences were larger in the first year after diagnosis for tumours whose survival is largely determined by stage at diagnosis and mainly for elderly patients; differences in survival were smaller for tumours amenable to cytotoxic therapy and for young and middle-aged patients.**
Relative survival was generally better in countries with good access to well organized, modern, specialized care and high life-expectancy.

registries, serving restricted parts of certain countries (Italy, France, Netherlands, Germany and Switzerland) are generally located in relatively prosperous areas, whose residents have good access to specialized care. The quality of oncological care may be also relevant here. This depends on a series of factors including level of specialist and postgraduate training, the functioning of both national and regional tumour study groups, participation in clinical trials, but also organization of oncological care, including palliative care. Care is more likely to be suboptimal when specialists are scarce, but also when they are scattered over many small hospitals or do not collaborate in special study groups (Health Council of the Netherlands, 1993).

Although general mortality was accounted for in the calculation of cancer survival in the regions covered by this study, it appears that where cancer survival was low, general mortality was also high (Chapter 17). Exceptions to this were Finland and Denmark, where general mortality was high (especially among Finnish males), and Spain, where male total mortality was low and cancer survival modest.

The relationship between low cancer survival and high general mortality suggests that survival is also linked to the level of health service provision, since general mortality is closely related to wealth. Wealthy countries can devote more resources to health, although this does not always imply a rational organization. Relative cancer survival also seems to correlate with gross national product (GNP) and with the percentage of it that is spent on health services (OECD, 1987). The recent Human Development Index of the United Nations Development Programme may provide a better indicator. For example, general regional mortality rates, which vary widely between EC countries, seem closely related to unemployment rates (Mackenbach & Looman, 1994).

Full explanation for the differences in age-standardized relative survival across Europe cannot be given. Caution is thus required in comparing the EUROCARE data with the results of other population-based survival studies. A crude comparison with the United States Surveillance, Epidemiology and End Results programme (SEER, 1988), for example, suggests that cancer survival rates for whites in the USA are substantially higher than those revealed by EUROCARE for most tumours. However, they are often similar to the higher rates of Table 18.8 and in-depth analysis of the comparability of the data is needed.

With the exception of brain cancer and leukaemia, between-country comparisons were not made for childhood cancers, because the number of cases in most registries was too small (Table 18.5b). A crude comparison with American data on childhood cancer (SEER, 1988) suggests that, in contrast to the results for adults, European survival is broadly similar.

Conclusions

The major results are summarized in Table 18.9. Relative survival for most cancers in adults declined significantly with increasing age, seemed better in females and improved slightly over time in most registries. It is the variation between countries that requires most attention. Why are patterns of relative survival from cancer in Europe not more uniform? Clinical researchers have different experience, because they generally deal with only a small fraction of new cancer patients (less than 10%), most of whom are optimally treated and below the age of 60. The results of the EUROCARE study will presumably come as less of a surprise to general practitioners and specialists familiar with the work of cancer registries, who are already aware of worse survival among the elderly, of problems of access, of differences in treatment strategies, and of the often slow diffusion and learning curves for newer, more efficacious, treatments.

The variations in general mortality and cancer survival across Europe reflect cultural diversity and wealth differences, while variations in social security and in provision of health services may also be important. Availability of specialized health care, and access to it, is vital for timely diagnosis and adequate treatment; this is often a problem in remote and underprivileged areas. Also, public confidence in oncological care in a health system may be a factor. If there is a positive relationship between the quality of oncological care and the availability of a cancer registry as an indicator of cancer awareness, the EUROCARE study may itself be providing an overoptimistic assessment of cancer survival in Europe, because it covers less than 20% of the population. Could the absence of registry-based data on survival in Austria, Belgium, Greece, large parts of West Germany (98%), France (95%), Ireland, Spain (96%), Italy (95%) also reflect deficiencies in oncological care?

Nonetheless, the uniform analysis of data on about 800 000 cancer patients from 30 population-based registries in 12 European countries has given a clear indication of the substantial variation in cancer survival across the continent according to age and period of diagnosis. The results point out areas for further tumour-specific studies of prognostic factors, e.g. histological type, subsite and stage. To determine variation in supply of oncological care related to these factors, analyses of patterns of care are needed for more recent years and such studies are in progress. Separate studies of the elderly are necessary, because clinical trials generally do not include this large group of cancer patients, nor do they include patients with serious intercurrent disease (Charlson *et al.*, 1987; Satariano & Ragland, 1994). The follow-up of the patients diagnosed during 1978–85 is being extended in EUROCARE II, to provide a clearer picture of long-term survival, also in various periods of follow-up (Hankey & Steinhorn, 1982).

An important result of the EUROCARE project is to show that methods of data collection, follow-up and data analysis need to become more standardized. In particular, the standardization of data collection on stage and diagnostic and therapeutic procedures would allow differences in survival between populations to be interpreted with more confidence.

References

Aareleid, T. & Rahu, M. (1991) Survival of cancer in Estonia from 1968 to 1987. *Cancer*, **68**, 2088–2092

Balvert-Locht, H.R., Coebergh, J.W., Hop, W.C., Brölmann, H.A., Crommelin, M.A., van Wijk, D.J. & Verhagen-Teulings, M.Th. (1991) Improved prognosis of ovarian cancer in the Netherlands during the period 1975-85: a population-based study. *Gynecol. Oncol.*, **42**, 3–8

Black, R.J., Sharp L. & Kendrick, S.W. (1993) *Trends in Cancer Survival in Scotland, 1968–1990*. Edinburgh, ISD Publications

Carmen Martos, M. & Olsen, J.H. (1993) Childhood cancer mortality in the European Community. *Eur. J. Cancer*, **29A**, 1783–1789

Carstensen, B., Storm, H.H. & Schou, G. (1993) *Survival of Danish Cancer Patients, 1943–1987*, Copenhagen, Danish Cancer Society, Munksgaard

Cella, D.F., Orav, E.J., Kornblith, A.B., Holland, J.C., Silberfarb, P.M., Kyu Won Lee, Comis, R.L., *et al.* (1991) Socioeconomic status and cancer survival. *J. Clin. Oncol.*, **9,** 1500–1509

Centre de Lutte contre le Cancer (1987) Results and analysis of survival, 1975–1981, Paris, Doin Editeurs

Charlson, M.E., Pompei, P., Ales, K.L. & Mackenzie, C.R. (1987) A new method of classifying prognostic co-morbidity in longitudinal studies: development and validation. *J. Chron. Dis.*, **40,** 373–383

Coebergh, J.W.W. & van der Heijden, L.H. (1991) *Cancer Incidence and Survival in Southeastern Netherlands*, 1975–1987, Eindhoven, Comprehensive Cancer Centre South (IKZ)

Coleman, M.P., Estève, J., Damiecki, P., Arslan, A. & Renard, H. (1993) *Trends in Cancer Incidence and Mortality* (IARC Scientific Publications No. 121), Lyon, IARC

De Jong, B., Coebergh, J.W., Crommelin, M.A. & van der Heijden, L.H. (1994) Patterns of radiotherapy for cancer in Southeastern Netherlands. *Radiother. Oncol.*, **31,** 213–221

Dhom, G., Kaatsch, P., Kolles, H., Michaelis, J., Niemeyer, A.H., Seitz, G. & Ziegler, H. (1991) *Cancer Incidence and Patient Survival*, Baden-Baden, Nomos Verlagsgesellschaft

Doll, R. (1990) Are we winning the fight against cancer? An epidemiological assessment. *Eur. J. Cancer,* **26,** 500–508

Farthing, M.J., Williams, R., Swan, C.H., Burroughs, A., Heading, R.C., Dodge, J.A., Russel, R.I., Venables, C.A., Dick, R., Burnham, R., Leicester, R., Neale, G., Swarbrick, E.T., Fairclough, P.D., Jones, R. & Melia, N.P. (1993) Nature and standards of gastrointestinal and liver services in the United Kingdom. *Gut*, **34,** 1728–1739

Geddes, M., Balzi, D. & Tomatis, L. (1994) Progress in the fight against cancer in EC countries: changes in mortality rates, 1970-90. *Eur. J. Cancer Prev.*, **3,** 31–44

Haaf, H.G., Kaatsch, P. & Michaelis, J. (1993) *Jahresbericht 1991 des Deutschen Kinderkrebsregister*, Mainz, Institut für Medizinische Statistik und Documentation

Hakulinen, T., Pukkala, E., Hakama, M., Lehtonen, M., Saxèn, E. & Teppo, L. (1981) Survival of cancer patients in Finland in 1953–1974. *Ann. Clin. Res.*, **13,** Suppl. 31

Hakulinen, T. (1982) Cancer survival corrected for heterogeneity in patient withdrawal. *Biometrics*, **38,** 933–942

Hakulinen, T. (1983) A comparison of nationwide cancer survival statistics in Finland and Norway. *Wld Hlth Stat. Quart.*, **36,** 35–46

Hankey, B.F. & Steinhorn, S.C. (1982) Long-term patient survival for some of the more frequently occurring cancers. *Cancer*, **50,** 1904–1912

Health Council of the Netherlands (1993) *Advice on the Quality and Allocation of Care in Oncology*, The Hague, Health Council, No. 1993/01 (in Dutch, summary in English)

Karjalainen, S., Aareleid, T., Hakulinen, T., Pukkala, E., Rahu, M. & Tekkel, M. (1989) Survival of female breast cancer patients in Finland and in Estonia — stage at diagnosis important determinant of the differences between countries. *Soc. Sci. Med.*, **28,** 233–238

La Vecchia, C., Lucchini F., Negri, E., Boyle, P., Maisonneuve, P. & Levi, F. (1992a) Trends of cancer mortality in Europe, 1955-1989: III, breast and genital sites. *Eur. J. Cancer,* **28A,** 927–998

La Vecchia, C., Lucchini F., Negri, E., Boyle, P., Maisonneuve, P. & Levi, F. (1992b) Trends of cancer mortality in Europe, 1955-1989: V, lymphohaemopoietic and all cancers. *Eur. J. Cancer*, **28A,** 1509–1581

Levi, F., Randimbison, L., Van Cong Te, Franceschi, S. & La Vecchia, C. (1992a) Trends in cancer survival in Vaud, Switzerland. *Eur. J. Cancer*, **28A,** 1490–1495

Levi, F., La Vecchia, C., Lucchini, F., Negri, E. & Boyle, P. (1992b) Patterns of childhood cancer incidence and mortality in Europe. *Eur. J. Cancer,* **28B,** 2028–2049

Loehrer, P.J., Greger, H.A., Weinberger, M., Musick, B., Miller, M., Nichols, C., Bryan, J., Higgs, D. & Brock, R.N. (1991) Knowledge and beliefs about cancer in a socioeconomically disadvantaged population. *Cancer,* **68,** 1665–1671

Mackenbach, J.P. & Looman, C.W. (1994) Living standards and mortality in the European community. *J. Epidemiol. Commun. Health*, **48,** 140–145

Mechanic, D. (1978) Sex, illness, illness behavior and the use of health services. *Soc. Sci. Med.*, **12b,** 207–214

Mosso, M.L., Colombo, R., Giordano, L., Pastore, G., Terracini, B. & Magnani, C. (1992) Childhood cancer registry of the province of Torino, Italy: survival, incidence and mortality over 20 years. *Cancer*, **69,** 1300–1306

Office of Population Censuses and Surveys and Cancer Research Campaign (1981) *Cancer Statistics: Incidence, Survival and Mortality in England and Wales* (Studies on Medical and Population Subjects No. 43), London, HMSO

OECD (Organization for Economic Cooperation and Development) (1987) *Financing and Delivring Health Care: a Comparative Analysis of OECD-countries*, Paris, OECD

Pawlega, J. (1993) Survival studies: Cracow Cancer Registry experience. *Cancer Prev.*, **17**, 1–10

Registre Genevois des Tumeurs (1988) *Cancer à Genève: Incidence, Mortalité, Survie, 1970–1986*, Geneva, Registre Genevois des Tumeurs

Satariano, W.A. & Ragland, D.R. (1994) The effect of comorbidity on 3-year survival of women with primary breast cancer. *Ann. Intern. Med.*, **120**, 104–110

Schroeder, S.A., (1984) Western European responses to physician oversupply: lessons for the United states. *J. Am. Med. Assoc.*, **252**, 373–384

SEER (Surveillance, Epidemiology and End Results Programme, National Cancer Institute, Division of Cancer Prevention and Control) (1988) *1987 Annual Cancer Statistics Review, Including Cancer Trends 1950-85*, Bethesda, US Department of Health and Human Services, No. 88-2789

Souhami, R. & Tobias, J. (1986) *Cancer and its Management*, Oxford, Blackwell Scientific Publications

Stiller, C.A. (1988) Centralisation of treatment and survival rates for cancer. *Arch. Dis. Child.*, **63**, 23–30

Stiller, C.A. & Bunch, K.J. (1990) Trends in survival for childhood cancer in Britain diagnosed 1971–85. *Br. J. Cancer*, **62**, 806–815

Wiebelt, H. & Hakulinen, T. (1991) Do women survive cancer more frequently than men? *J. Natl Cancer Inst.*, **83**, 579

Wiebelt, H., Hakulinen, T., Ziegler, H. & Stegmaier, C. (1991) Leben die Krebspatienten heute länger als früher? Eine Überlebenszeitanalyse der Krebspatienten im Saarland der Jahre 1972 bis 1986. *Soz. Präventivmed.*, **36**, 86–95

PUBLICATIONS OF THE INTERNATIONAL AGENCY FOR RESEARCH ON CANCER

Scientific Publications Series

(Available from Oxford University Press through local bookshops)

No. 1 **Liver Cancer**
1971; 176 pages (*out of print*)

No. 2 **Oncogenesis and Herpesviruses**
Edited by P.M. Biggs, G. de-Thé and L.N. Payne
1972; 515 pages (*out of print*)

No. 3 ***N*-Nitroso Compounds: Analysis and Formation**
Edited by P. Bogovski, R. Preussman and E.A. Walker
1972; 140 pages (*out of print*)

No. 4 **Transplacental Carcinogenesis**
Edited by L. Tomatis and U. Mohr
1973; 181 pages (*out of print*)

No. 5/6 **Pathology of Tumours in Laboratory Animals, Volume 1, Tumours of the Rat**
Edited by V.S. Turusov
1973/1976; 533 pages (*out of print*)

No. 7 **Host Environment Interactions in the Etiology of Cancer in Man**
Edited by R. Doll and I. Vodopija
1973; 464 pages (*out of print*)

No. 8 **Biological Effects of Asbestos**
Edited by P. Bogovski, J.C. Gilson, V. Timbrell and J.C. Wagner
1973; 346 pages (*out of print*)

No. 9 ***N*-Nitroso Compounds in the Environment**
Edited by P. Bogovski and E.A. Walker
1974; 243 pages (*out of print*)

No. 10 **Chemical Carcinogenesis Essays**
Edited by R. Montesano and L. Tomatis
1974; 230 pages (*out of print*)

No. 11 **Oncogenesis and Herpesviruses II**
Edited by G. de-Thé, M.A. Epstein and H. zur Hausen
1975; Part I: 511 pages
Part II: 403 pages (*out of print*)

No. 12 **Screening Tests in Chemical Carcinogenesis**
Edited by R. Montesano, H. Bartsch and L. Tomatis
1976; 666 pages (*out of print*)

No. 13 **Environmental Pollution and Carcinogenic Risks**
Edited by C. Rosenfeld and W. Davis
1975; 441 pages (*out of print*)

No. 14 **Environmental *N*-Nitroso Compounds. Analysis and Formation**
Edited by E.A. Walker, P. Bogovski and L. Griciute
1976; 512 pages (*out of print*)

No. 15 **Cancer Incidence in Five Continents, Volume III**
Edited by J.A.H. Waterhouse, C. Muir, P. Correa and J. Powell
1976; 584 pages (*out of print*)

No. 16 **Air Pollution and Cancer in Man**
Edited by U. Mohr, D. Schmähl and L. Tomatis
1977; 328 pages (*out of print*)

No. 17 **Directory of On-going Research in Cancer Epidemiology 1977**
Edited by C.S. Muir and G. Wagner
1977; 599 pages (*out of print*)

No. 18 **Environmental Carcinogens. Selected Methods of Analysis. Volume 1: Analysis of Volatile Nitrosamines in Food**
Editor-in-Chief: H. Egan
1978; 212 pages (*out of print*)

No. 19 **Environmental Aspects of *N*-Nitroso Compounds**
Edited by E.A. Walker, M. Castegnaro, L. Griciute and R.E. Lyle
1978; 561 pages (*out of print*)

No. 20 **Nasopharyngeal Carcinoma: Etiology and Control**
Edited by G. de-Thé and Y. Ito
1978; 606 pages (*out of print*)

No. 21 **Cancer Registration and its Techniques**
Edited by R. MacLennan, C. Muir, R. Steinitz and A. Winkler
1978; 235 pages (*out of print*)

No. 22 **Environmental Carcinogens. Selected Methods of Analysis. Volume 2: Methods for the Measurement of Vinyl Chloride in Poly(vinyl chloride), Air, Water and Foodstuffs**
Editor-in-Chief: H. Egan
1978; 142 pages (*out of print*)

No. 23 **Pathology of Tumours in Laboratory Animals. Volume II: Tumours of the Mouse**
Editor-in-Chief: V.S. Turusov
1979; 669 pages (*out of print*)

No. 24 **Oncogenesis and Herpesviruses III**
Edited by G. de-Thé, W. Henle and F. Rapp
1978; Part I: 580 pages, Part II: 512 pages (*out of print*)

Prices, valid for August 1994, are subject to change without notice.

No. 25 **Carcinogenic Risk. Strategies for Intervention**
Edited by W. Davis and C. Rosenfeld
1979; 280 pages (*out of print*)

No. 26 **Directory of On-going Research in Cancer Epidemiology 1978**
Edited by C.S. Muir and G. Wagner
1978; 550 pages (*out of print*)

No. 27 **Molecular and Cellular Aspects of Carcinogen Screening Tests**
Edited by R. Montesano, H. Bartsch and L. Tomatis
1980; 372 pages £30.00

No. 28 **Directory of On-going Research in Cancer Epidemiology 1979**
Edited by C.S. Muir and G. Wagner
1979; 672 pages (*out of print*)

No. 29 **Environmental Carcinogens. Selected Methods of Analysis. Volume 3: Analysis of Polycyclic Aromatic Hydrocarbons in Environmental Samples**
Editor-in-Chief: H. Egan
1979; 240 pages (*out of print*)

No. 30 **Biological Effects of Mineral Fibres**
Editor-in-Chief: J.C. Wagner
1980; **Volume 1:** 494 pages **Volume 2:** 513 pages (*out of print*)

No. 31 ***N*-Nitroso Compounds: Analysis, Formation and Occurrence**
Edited by E.A. Walker, L. Griciute, M. Castegnaro and M. Börzsönyi
1980; 835 pages (*out of print*)

No. 32 **Statistical Methods in Cancer Research. Volume 1. The Analysis of Case-control Studies**
By N.E. Breslow and N.E. Day
1980; 338 pages £18.00

No. 33 **Handling Chemical Carcinogens in the Laboratory**
Edited by R. Montesano *et al.*
1979; 32 pages (*out of print*)

No. 34 **Pathology of Tumours in Laboratory Animals. Volume III. Tumours of the Hamster**
Editor-in-Chief: V.S. Turusov
1982; 461 pages (*out of print*)

No. 35 **Directory of On-going Research in Cancer Epidemiology 1980**
Edited by C.S. Muir and G. Wagner
1980; 660 pages (*out of print*)

No. 36 **Cancer Mortality by Occupation and Social Class 1851-1971**
Edited by W.P.D. Logan
1982; 253 pages (*out of print*)

No. 37 **Laboratory Decontamination and Destruction of Aflatoxins B_1, B_2, G_1, G_2 in Laboratory Wastes**
Edited by M. Castegnaro *et al.*
1980; 56 pages (*out of print*)

No. 38 **Directory of On-going Research in Cancer Epidemiology 1981**
Edited by C.S. Muir and G. Wagner
1981; 696 pages (*out of print*)

No. 39 **Host Factors in Human Carcinogenesis**
Edited by H. Bartsch and B. Armstrong
1982; 583 pages (*out of print*)

No. 40 **Environmental Carcinogens. Selected Methods of Analysis. Volume 4: Some Aromatic Amines and Azo Dyes in the General and Industrial Environment**
Edited by L. Fishbein, M. Castegnaro, I.K. O'Neill and H. Bartsch
1981; 347 pages (*out of print*)

No. 41 ***N*-Nitroso Compounds: Occurrence and Biological Effects**
Edited by H. Bartsch, I.K. O'Neill, M. Castegnaro and M. Okada
1982; 755 pages £50.00

No. 42 **Cancer Incidence in Five Continents, Volume IV**
Edited by J. Waterhouse, C. Muir, K. Shanmugaratnam and J. Powell
1982; 811 pages (*out of print*)

No. 43 **Laboratory Decontamination and Destruction of Carcinogens in Laboratory Wastes: Some *N*-Nitrosamines**
Edited by M. Castegnaro *et al.*
1982; 73 pages £7.50

No. 44 **Environmental Carcinogens. Selected Methods of Analysis. Volume 5: Some Mycotoxins**
Edited by L. Stoloff, M. Castegnaro, P. Scott, I.K. O'Neill and H. Bartsch
1983; 455 pages £32.50

No. 45 **Environmental Carcinogens. Selected Methods of Analysis. Volume 6: *N*-Nitroso Compounds**
Edited by R. Preussmann, I.K. O'Neill, G. Eisenbrand, B. Spiegelhalder and H. Bartsch
1983; 508 pages £32.50

No. 46 **Directory of On-going Research in Cancer Epidemiology 1982**
Edited by C.S. Muir and G. Wagner
1982; 722 pages (*out of print*)

No. 47 **Cancer Incidence in Singapore 1968–1977**
Edited by K. Shanmugaratnam, H.P. Lee and N.E. Day
1983; 171 pages (*out of print*)

No. 48 **Cancer Incidence in the USSR (2nd Revised Edition)**
Edited by N.P. Napalkov, G.F. Tserkovny, V.M. Merabishvili, D.M. Parkin, M. Smans and C.S. Muir
1983; 75 pages (*out of print*)

No. 49 **Laboratory Decontamination and Destruction of Carcinogens in Laboratory Wastes: Some Polycyclic Aromatic Hydrocarbons**
Edited by M. Castegnaro *et al.*
1983; 87 pages (*out of print*)

No. 50 **Directory of On-going Research in Cancer Epidemiology 1983**
Edited by C.S. Muir and G. Wagner
1983; 731 pages (*out of print*)

No. 51 **Modulators of Experimental Carcinogénesis**
Edited by V. Turusov and R. Montesano
1983; 307 pages (*out of print*)

No. 52 **Second Cancers in Relation to Radiation Treatment for Cervical Cancer: Results of a Cancer Registry Collaboration**
Edited by N.E. Day and J.C. Boice, Jr
1984; 207 pages (*out of print*)

No. 53 **Nickel in the Human Environment**
Editor-in-Chief: F.W. Sunderman, Jr
1984; 529 pages (*out of print*)

No. 54 **Laboratory Decontamination and Destruction of Carcinogens in Laboratory Wastes: Some Hydrazines**
Edited by M. Castegnaro *et al.*
1983; 87 pages (*out of print*)

No. 55 **Laboratory Decontamination and Destruction of Carcinogens in Laboratory Wastes: Some *N*-Nitrosamides**
Edited by M. Castegnaro *et al.*
1984; 66 pages (*out of print*)

No. 56 **Models, Mechanisms and Etiology of Tumour Promotion**
Edited by M. Börzsönyi, N.E. Day, K. Lapis and H. Yamasaki
1984; 532 pages (*out of print*)

No. 57 ***N*-Nitroso Compounds: Occurrence, Biological Effects and Relevance to Human Cancer**
Edited by I.K. O'Neill, R.C. von Borstel, C.T. Miller, J. Long and H. Bartsch
1984; 1013 pages (*out of print*)

No. 58 **Age-related Factors in Carcinogenesis**
Edited by A. Likhachev, V. Anisimov and R. Montesano
1985; 288 pages (*out of print*)

No. 59 **Monitoring Human Exposure to Carcinogenic and Mutagenic Agents**
Edited by A. Berlin, M. Draper, K. Hemminki and H. Vainio
1984; 457 pages (*out of print*)

No. 60 **Burkitt's Lymphoma: A Human Cancer Model**
Edited by G. Lenoir, G. O'Conor and C.L.M. Olweny
1985; 484 pages (*out of print*)

No. 61 **Laboratory Decontamination and Destruction of Carcinogens in Laboratory Wastes: Some Haloethers**
Edited by M. Castegnaro *et al.*
1985; 55 pages (*out of print*)

No. 62 **Directory of On-going Research in Cancer Epidemiology 1984**
Edited by C.S. Muir and G. Wagner
1984; 717 pages (*out of print*)

No. 63 **Virus-associated Cancers in Africa**
Edited by A.O. Williams, G.T. O'Conor, G.B. de-Thé and C.A. Johnson
1984; 773 pages (*out of print*)

No. 64 **Laboratory Decontamination and Destruction of Carcinogens in Laboratory Wastes: Some Aromatic Amines and 4-Nitrobiphenyl**
Edited by M. Castegnaro *et al.*
1985; 84 pages (*out of print*)

No. 65 **Interpretation of Negative Epidemiological Evidence for Carcinogenicity**
Edited by N.J. Wald and R. Doll
1985; 232 pages (*out of print*)

No. 66 **The Role of the Registry in Cancer Control**
Edited by D.M. Parkin, G. Wagner and C.S. Muir
1985; 152 pages £10.00

No. 67 **Transformation Assay of Established Cell Lines: Mechanisms and Application**
Edited by T. Kakunaga and H. Yamasaki
1985; 225 pages (*out of print*)

No. 68 **Environmental Carcinogens. Selected Methods of Analysis. Volume 7. Some Volatile Halogenated Hydrocarbons**
Edited by L. Fishbein and I.K. O'Neill
1985; 479 pages (*out of print*)

No. 69 **Directory of On-going Research in Cancer Epidemiology 1985**
Edited by C.S. Muir and G. Wagner
1985; 745 pages (*out of print*)

No. 70 **The Role of Cyclic Nucleic Acid Adducts in Carcinogenesis and Mutagenesis**
Edited by B. Singer and H. Bartsch
1986; 467 pages (*out of print*)

No. 71 **Environmental Carcinogens. Selected Methods of Analysis. Volume 8: Some Metals: As, Be, Cd, Cr, Ni, Pb, Se, Zn**
Edited by I.K. O'Neill, P. Schuller and L. Fishbein
1986; 485 pages (*out of print*)

No. 72 **Atlas of Cancer in Scotland, 1975–1980. Incidence and Epidemiological Perspective**
Edited by I. Kemp, P. Boyle, M. Smans and C.S. Muir
1985; 285 pages (*out of print*)

No. 73 **Laboratory Decontamination and Destruction of Carcinogens in Laboratory Wastes: Some Antineoplastic Agents**
Edited by M. Castegnaro *et al.*
1985; 163 pages £13.50

No. 74 **Tobacco: A Major International Health Hazard**
Edited by D. Zaridze and R. Peto
1986; 324 pages £24.00

No. 75 **Cancer Occurrence in Developing Countries**
Edited by D.M. Parkin
1986; 339 pages £24.00

No. 76 **Screening for Cancer of the Uterine Cervix**
Edited by M. Hakama, A.B. Miller and N.E. Day
1986; 315 pages £31.50

No. 77 **Hexachlorobenzene: Proceedings of an International Symposium**
Edited by C.R. Morris and J.R.P. Cabral
1986; 668 pages (*out of print*)

No. 78 **Carcinogenicity of Alkylating Cytostatic Drugs**
Edited by D. Schmähl and J.M. Kaldor
1986; 337 pages (*out of print*)

No. 79 **Statistical Methods in Cancer Research. Volume III: The Design and Analysis of Long-term Animal Experiments**
By J.J. Gart, D. Krewski, P.N. Lee, R.E. Tarone and J. Wahrendorf
1986; 213 pages £23.50

No. 80 **Directory of On-going Research in Cancer Epidemiology 1986**
Edited by C.S. Muir and G. Wagner
1986; 805 pages (*out of print*)

No. 81 **Environmental Carcinogens: Methods of Analysis and Exposure Measurement. Volume 9: Passive Smoking**
Edited by I.K. O'Neill, K.D. Brunnemann, B. Dodet and D. Hoffmann
1987; 383 pages £37.00

No. 82 **Statistical Methods in Cancer Research. Volume II: The Design and Analysis of Cohort Studies**
By N.E. Breslow and N.E. Day
1987; 404 pages £25.00

No. 83 **Long-term and Short-term Assays for Carcinogens: A Critical Appraisal**
Edited by R. Montesano, H. Bartsch, H. Vainio, J. Wilbourn and H. Yamasaki
1986; 575 pages £37.00

No. 84 **The Relevance of *N*-Nitroso Compounds to Human Cancer: Exposure and Mechanisms**
Edited by H. Bartsch, I.K. O'Neill and R. Schulte-Hermann
1987; 671 pages (*out of print*)

No. 85 **Environmental Carcinogens: Methods of Analysis and Exposure Measurement. Volume 10: Benzene and Alkylated Benzenes**
Edited by L. Fishbein and I.K. O'Neill
1988; 327 pages £42.00

No. 86 **Directory of On-going Research in Cancer Epidemiology 1987**
Edited by D.M. Parkin and J. Wahrendorf
1987; 676 pages (*out of print*)

No. 87 **International Incidence of Childhood Cancer**
Edited by D.M. Parkin, C.A. Stiller, C.A. Bieber, G.J. Draper, B. Terracini and J.L. Young
1988; 401 pages £35.00

No. 88 **Cancer Incidence in Five Continents Volume V**
Edited by C. Muir, J. Waterhouse, T. Mack, J. Powell and S. Whelan
1987; 1004 pages £58.00

No. 89 **Method for Detecting DNA Damaging Agents in Humans: Applications in Cancer Epidemiology and Prevention**
Edited by H. Bartsch, K. Hemminki and I.K. O'Neill
1988; 518 pages £50.00

No. 90 **Non-occupational Exposure to Mineral Fibres**
Edited by J. Bignon, J. Peto and R. Saracci
1989; 500 pages £52.50

No. 91 **Trends in Cancer Incidence in Singapore 1968–1982**
Edited by H.P. Lee , N.E. Day and K. Shanmugaratnam
1988; 160 pages (*out of print*)

No. 92 **Cell Differentiation, Genes and Cancer**
Edited by T. Kakunaga, T. Sugimura, L. Tomatis and H. Yamasaki
1988; 204 pages £29.00

No. 93 **Directory of On-going Research in Cancer Epidemiology 1988**
Edited by M. Coleman and J. Wahrendorf
1988; 662 pages (*out of print*)

No. 94 **Human Papillomavirus and Cervical Cancer**
Edited by N. Muñoz, F.X. Bosch and O.M. Jensen
1989; 154 pages £22.50

No. 95 **Cancer Registration: Principles and Methods**
Edited by O.M. Jensen, D.M. Parkin, R. MacLennan, C.S. Muir and R. Skeet
1991; 288 pages £28.00

No. 96 **Perinatal and Multigeneration Carcinogenesis**
Edited by N.P. Napalkov, J.M. Rice, L. Tomatis and H. Yamasaki
1989; 436 pages £52.50

No. 97 **Occupational Exposure to Silica and Cancer Risk**
Edited by L. Simonato, A.C. Fletcher, R. Saracci and T. Thomas
1990; 124 pages £24.00

No. 98 **Cancer Incidence in Jewish Migrants to Israel, 1961–1981**
Edited by R. Steinitz, D.M. Parkin, J.L. Young, C.A. Bieber and L. Katz
1989; 320 pages £37.00

No. 99 **Pathology of Tumours in Laboratory Animals, Second Edition, Volume 1, Tumours of the Rat**
Edited by V.S. Turusov and U. Mohr
740 pages £90.00

No. 100 **Cancer: Causes, Occurrence and Control**
Editor-in-Chief L. Tomatis
1990; 352 pages £25.50

No. 101 **Directory of On-going Research in Cancer Epidemiology 1989/90**
Edited by M. Coleman and J. Wahrendorf
1989; 818 pages £42.00

No. 102 **Patterns of Cancer in Five Continents**
Edited by S.L. Whelan, D.M. Parkin & E. Masuyer
1990; 162 pages £26.50

No. 103 **Evaluating Effectiveness of Primary Prevention of Cancer**
Edited by M. Hakama, V. Beral, J.W. Cullen and D.M. Parkin
1990; 250 pages £34.00

No. 104 **Complex Mixtures and Cancer Risk**
Edited by H. Vainio, M. Sorsa and A.J. McMichael
1990; 442 pages £40.00

No. 105 **Relevance to Human Cancer of *N*-Nitroso Compounds, Tobacco Smoke and Mycotoxins**
Edited by I.K. O'Neill, J. Chen and H. Bartsch
1991; 614 pages £74.00

No. 106 **Atlas of Cancer Incidence in the Former German Democratic Republic**
Edited by W.H. Mehnert, M. Smans, C.S. Muir, M. Möhner & D. Schön
1992; 384 pages £52.50

No. 107 **Atlas of Cancer Mortality in the European Economic Community**
Edited by M. Smans, C.S. Muir and P. Boyle
1992; 280 pages £35.00

No. 108 **Environmental Carcinogens: Methods of Analysis and Exposure Measurement. Volume 11: Polychlorinated Dioxins and Dibenzofurans**
Edited by C. Rappe, H.R. Buser, B. Dodet and I.K. O'Neill
1991; 426 pages £47.50

No. 109 **Environmental Carcinogens: Methods of Analysis and Exposure Measurement. Volume 12: Indoor Air Contaminants**
Edited by B. Seifert, H. van de Wiel, B. Dodet and I.K. O'Neill
1993; 384 pages £45.00

No. 110 **Directory of On-going Research in Cancer Epidemiology 1991**
Edited by M. Coleman and J. Wahrendorf
1991; 753 pages £40.00

No. 111 **Pathology of Tumours in Laboratory Animals, Second Edition, Volume 2, Tumours of the Mouse**
Edited by V.S. Turusov and U. Mohr
1993; 776 pages; £90.00

No. 112 **Autopsy in Epidemiology and Medical Research**
Edited by E. Riboli and M. Delendi
1991; 288 pages £26.50

No. 113 **Laboratory Decontamination and Destruction of Carcinogens in Laboratory Wastes: Some Mycotoxins**
Edited by M. Castegnaro, J. Barek, J.–M. Frémy, M. Lafontaine, M. Miraglia, E.B. Sansone and G.M. Telling
1991; 64 pages £12.00

No. 114 **Laboratory Decontamination and Destruction of Carcinogens in Laboratory Wastes: Some Polycyclic Heterocyclic Hydrocarbons**
Edited by M. Castegnaro, J. Barek J. Jacob, U. Kirso, M. Lafontaine, E.B. Sansone, G.M. Telling and T. Vu Duc
1991; 50 pages £8.00

No. 115 **Mycotoxins, Endemic Nephropathy and Urinary Tract Tumours**
Edited by M. Castegnaro, R. Plestina, G. Dirheimer, I.N. Chernozemsky and H Bartsch
1991; 340 pages £47.50

No. 116 **Mechanisms of Carcinogenesis in Risk Identification**
Edited by H. Vainio, P.N. Magee, D.B. McGregor & A.J. McMichael
1992; 616 pages £69.00

No. 117 **Directory of On-going Research in Cancer Epidemiology 1992**
Edited by M. Coleman, J. Wahrendorf & E. Démaret
1992; 773 pages £44.50

No. 118 **Cadmium in the Human Environment: Toxicity and Carcinogenicity**
Edited by G.F. Nordberg, R.F.M. Herber & L. Alessio
1992; 470 pages £60.00

No. 119 **The Epidemiology of Cervical Cancer and Human Papillomavirus**
Edited by N. Muñoz, F.X. Bosch, K.V. Shah & A. Meheus
1992; 288 pages £29.50

No. 120 **Cancer Incidence in Five Continents, Volume VI**
Edited by D.M. Parkin, C.S. Muir, S.L. Whelan, Y.T. Gao, J. Ferlay & J.Powell
1992; 1080 pages £120.00

No. 121 **Trends in Cancer Incidence and Mortality**
M.P. Coleman, J. Estève, P. Damiecki, A. Arslan and H. Renard
1993; 806 pages, £120.00

No. 122 **International Classification of Rodent Tumours. Part 1. The Rat**
Editor-in-Chief: U. Mohr
1992/93; 10 fascicles of 60–100 pages, £120.00

No. 123 **Cancer in Italian Migrant Populations**
Edited by M. Geddes, D.M. Parkin, M. Khlat, D. Balzi and E. Buiatti
1993; 292 pages, £40.00

No. 124 **Postlabelling Methods for Detection of DNA Adducts**
Edited by D.H. Phillips, M. Castegnaro and H. Bartsch
1993; 392 pages; £46.00

No. 125 **DNA Adducts: Identification and Biological Significance**
Edited by K. Hemminki, A. Dipple, D. Shuker, F.F. Kadlubar, D. Segerbäck and H. Bartsch
1994; 480 pages; £52.00

No. 127 **Butadiene and Styrene: Assessment of Health Hazards.**
Edited by M. Sorsa, K. Peltonen, H. Vainio and K. Hemminki
1993; 412 pages; £54.00

No. 128 **Statistical Methods in Cancer Research. Volume IV. Descriptive Epidemiology.**
By J. Estève, E. Benhamou & L.Raymond
1994; 302 pages; £25.00

No. 129 **Occupational Cancer in Developing Countries.**
Edited by N. Pearce, E. Matos, H. Vainio, P. Boffetta & M. Kogevinas
1994; 192 pages £20.00

No. 130 **Directory of On-going Research in Cancer Epidemiology 1994**
Edited by R. Sankaranarayanan, J. Wahrendorf and E. Démaret
1994; 792 pages, £46.00

No. 132 **Survival of Cancer Patients in Europe. The EUROCARE Study**
Edited by F. Berrino, M. Sant, A. Verdecchia, R. Capocaccia, T. Hakulinen and J. Estève
1994; 463 pages; £45.00

IARC MONOGRAPHS ON THE EVALUATION OF CARCINOGENIC RISKS TO HUMANS

(Available from booksellers through the network of WHO Sales Agents)

Volume 1 **Some Inorganic Substances, Chlorinated Hydrocarbons, Aromatic Amines, *N*-Nitroso Compounds, and Natural Products**
1972; 184 pages (*out of print*)

Volume 2 **Some Inorganic and Organometallic Compounds**
1973; 181 pages (*out of print*)

Volume 3 **Certain Polycyclic Aromatic Hydrocarbons and Heterocyclic Compounds**
1973; 271 pages (*out of print*)

Volume 4 **Some Aromatic Amines, Hydrazine and Related Substances, *N*-Nitroso Compounds and Miscellaneous Alkylating Agents**
1974; 286 pages Sw. fr. 18.–

Volume 5 **Some Organochlorine Pesticides**
1974; 241 pages (*out of print*)

Volume 6 **Sex Hormones**
1974; 243 pages (*out of print*)

Volume 7 **Some Anti-Thyroid and Related Substances, Nitrofurans and Industrial Chemicals**
1974; 326 pages (*out of print*)

Volume 8 **Some Aromatic Azo Compounds**
1975; 357 pages Sw. fr. 44.–

Volume 9 **Some Aziridines, *N*-, *S*- and *O*-Mustards and Selenium**
1975; 268 pages Sw.fr. 33.–

Volume 10 **Some Naturally Occurring Substances**
1976; 353 pages (*out of print*)

Volume 11 **Cadmium, Nickel, Some Epoxides, Miscellaneous Industrial Chemicals and General Considerations on Volatile Anaesthetics**
1976; 306 pages (*out of print*)

Volume 12 **Some Carbamates, Thiocarbamates and Carbazides**
1976; 282 pages Sw. fr. 41.-

Volume 13 **Some Miscellaneous Pharmaceutical Substances**
1977; 255 pages Sw. fr. 36.–

Volume 14 **Asbestos**
1977; 106 pages (*out of print*)

Volume 15 **Some Fumigants, The Herbicides 2,4-D and 2,4,5-T, Chlorinated Dibenzodioxins and Miscellaneous Industrial Chemicals**
1977; 354 pages (*out of print*)

Volume 16 **Some Aromatic Amines and Related Nitro Compounds - Hair Dyes, Colouring Agents and Miscellaneous Industrial Chemicals**
1978; 400 pages Sw. fr. 60.–

Volume 17 **Some *N*-Nitroso Compounds**
1978; 365 pages Sw. fr. 60.–

Volume 18 **Polychlorinated Biphenyls and Polybrominated Biphenyls**
1978; 140 pages Sw. fr. 24.–

Volume 19 **Some Monomers, Plastics and Synthetic Elastomers, and Acrolein**
1979; 513 pages (*out of print*)

Volume 20 **Some Halogenated Hydrocarbons**
1979; 609 pages (*out of print*)

Volume 21 **Sex Hormones (II)**
1979; 583 pages Sw. fr. 72.–

Volume 22 **Some Non-Nutritive Sweetening Agents**
1980; 208 pages Sw. fr. 30.–

Volume 23 **Some Metals and Metallic Compounds**
1980; 438 pages (*out of print*)

Volume 24 **Some Pharmaceutical Drugs**
1980; 337 pages Sw. fr. 48.–

Volume 25 **Wood, Leather and Some Associated Industries**
1981; 412 pages Sw. fr. 72.–

Volume 26 **Some Antineoplastic and Immunosuppressive Agents**
1981; 411 pages Sw. fr. 75.–

Volume 27 **Some Aromatic Amines, Anthraquinones and Nitroso Compounds, and Inorganic Fluorides Used in Drinking Water and Dental Preparations**
1982; 341 pages Sw. fr. 48.–

Volume 28 **The Rubber Industry**
1982; 486 pages Sw. fr. 84.–

Volume 29 **Some Industrial Chemicals and Dyestuffs**
1982; 416 pages Sw. fr. 72.–

Volume 30 **Miscellaneous Pesticides**
1983; 424 pages Sw. fr. 72.–

Volume 31 **Some Food Additives, Feed Additives and Naturally Occurring Substances**
1983; 314 pages Sw. fr. 66.–

Volume 32 **Polynuclear Aromatic Compounds, Part 1: Chemical, Environmental and Experimental Data**
1983; 477 pages Sw. fr. 88.–

Volume 33 **Polynuclear Aromatic Compounds, Part 2: Carbon Blacks, Mineral Oils and Some Nitroarenes**
1984; 245 pages (*out of print*)

Volume 34 **Polynuclear Aromatic Compounds, Part 3: Industrial Exposures in Aluminium Production, Coal Gasification, Coke Production, and Iron and Steel Founding**
1984; 219 pages Sw. fr. 53.–

Volume 35 **Polynuclear Aromatic Compounds, Part 4: Bitumens, Coal-tars and Derived Products, Shale-oils and Soots**
1985; 271 pages Sw. fr. 77.–

Volume 36 **Allyl Compounds, Aldehydes, Epoxides and Peroxides**
1985; 369 pages Sw. fr. 77.–

Volume 37 **Tobacco Habits Other than Smoking: Betel-quid and Areca-nut Chewing; and some Related Nitrosamines**
1985; 291 pages Sw. fr. 77.–

Volume 38 **Tobacco Smoking**
1986; 421 pages Sw. fr. 83.–

Volume 39 **Some Chemicals Used in Plastics and Elastomers**
1986; 403 pages Sw. fr. 83.–

Volume 40 **Some Naturally Occurring and Synthetic Food Components, Furocoumarins and Ultraviolet Radiation**
1986; 444 pages Sw. fr. 83.–

Volume 41 **Some Halogenated Hydrocarbons and Pesticide Exposures**
1986; 434 pages Sw. fr. 83.–

Volume 42 **Silica and Some Silicates**
1987; 289 pages Sw. fr. 72.

Volume 43 **Man-Made Mineral Fibres and Radon**
1988; 300 pages Sw. fr. 72.–

Volume 44 **Alcohol Drinking**
1988; 416 pages Sw. fr. 83.

Volume 45 **Occupational Exposures in Petroleum Refining; Crude Oil and Major Petroleum Fuels**
1989; 322 pages Sw. fr. 72.–

Volume 46 **Diesel and Gasoline Engine Exhausts and Some Nitroarenes**
1989; 458 pages Sw. fr. 83.–

Volume 47 **Some Organic Solvents, Resin Monomers and Related Compounds, Pigments and Occupational Exposures in Paint Manufacture and Painting**
1989; 535 pages Sw. fr. 94.–

Volume 48 **Some Flame Retardants and Textile Chemicals, and Exposures in the Textile Manufacturing Industry**
1990; 345 pages Sw. fr. 72.–

Volume 49 **Chromium, Nickel and Welding**
1990; 677 pages Sw. fr. 105.-

Volume 50 **Pharmaceutical Drugs**
1990; 415 pages Sw. fr. 93.-

Volume 51 **Coffee, Tea, Mate, Methylxanthines and Methylglyoxal**
1991; 513 pages Sw. fr. 88.-

Volume 52 **Chlorinated Drinking-water; Chlorination By-products; Some Other Halogenated Compounds; Cobalt and Cobalt Compounds**
1991; 544 pages Sw. fr. 88.-

Volume 53 **Occupational Exposures in Insecticide Application and some Pesticides**
1991; 612 pages Sw. fr. 105.-

Volume 54 **Occupational Exposures to Mists and Vapours from Strong Inorganic Acids; and Other Industrial Chemicals**
1992; 336 pages Sw. fr. 72.-

Volume 55 **Solar and Ultraviolet Radiation**
1992; 316 pages Sw. fr. 65.-

Volume 56 **Some Naturally Occurring Substances: Food Items and Constituents, Heterocyclic Aromatic Amines and Mycotoxins**
1993; 600 pages Sw. fr. 95.-

Volume 57 **Occupational Exposures of Hairdressers and Barbers and Personal Use of Hair Colourants; Some Hair Dyes, Cosmetic Colourants, Industrial Dyestuffs and Aromatic Amines**
1993; 428 pages Sw. fr. 75.-

Volume 58 **Beryllium, Cadmium, Mercury and Exposures in the Glass Manufacturing Industry**
1993; 426 pages Sw. fr. 75.-

Volume 59 **Hepatitis Viruses**
1994; 286 pages Sw. fr. 65.-

Volume 60 **Some Industrial Chemicals**
1994; 560 pages Sw. fr. 90.-

Volume 61 **Schistosomes, Liver Flukes and Helicobacter pylori**
1994; 270 pages Sw. fr. 70.-

Supplement No. 1
Chemicals and Industrial Processes Associated with Cancer in Humans (IARC Monographs, Volumes 1 to 20)
1979; 71 pages (*out of print*)

Supplement No. 2
Long-term and Short-term Screening Assays for Carcinogens: A Critical Appraisal
1980; 426 pages Sw. fr. 40.-

Supplement No. 3
Cross Index of Synonyms and Trade Names in Volumes 1 to 26
1982; 199 pages (*out of print*)

Supplement No. 4
Chemicals, Industrial Processes and Industries Associated with Cancer in Humans (IARC Monographs, Volumes 1 to 29)
1982; 292 pages (*out of print*)

Supplement No. 5
Cross Index of Synonyms and Trade Names in Volumes 1 to 36
1985; 259 pages (*out of print*)

Supplement No. 6
Genetic and Related Effects: An Updating of Selected IARC Monographs from Volumes 1 to 42
1987; 729 pages Sw. fr. 80.-

Supplement No. 7
Overall Evaluations of Carcinogenicity: An Updating of IARC Monographs Volumes 1-42
1987; 440 pages Sw. fr. 65.-

Supplement No. 8
Cross Index of Synonyms and Trade Names in Volumes 1 to 46
1990; 346 pages Sw. fr. 60.-

IARC TECHNICAL REPORTS*

No. 1 **Cancer in Costa Rica**
Edited by R. Sierra, R. Barrantes, G. Muñoz Leiva, D.M. Parkin, C.A. Bieber and N. Muñoz Calero
1988; 124 pages Sw. fr. 30.-

No. 2 **SEARCH: A Computer Package to Assist the Statistical Analysis of Case-control Studies**
Edited by G.J. Macfarlane, P. Boyle and P. Maisonneuve
1991; 80 pages (*out of print*)

No. 3 **Cancer Registration in the European Economic Community**
Edited by M.P. Coleman and E. Démaret
1988; 188 pages Sw. fr. 30.-

No. 4 **Diet, Hormones and Cancer: Methodological Issues for Prospective Studies**
Edited by E. Riboli and R. Saracci
1988; 156 pages Sw. fr. 30.-

No. 5 **Cancer in the Philippines**
Edited by A.V. Laudico, D. Esteban and D.M. Parkin
1989; 186 pages Sw. fr. 30.-

No. 6 **La genèse du Centre International de Recherche sur le Cancer**
Par R. Sohier et A.G.B. Sutherland
1990; 104 pages Sw. fr. 30.-

No. 7 **Epidémiologie du cancer dans les pays de langue latine**
1990; 310 pages Sw. fr. 30.-

No. 8 **Comparative Study of Anti-smoking Legislation in Countries of the European Economic Community**
Edited by A. Sasco, P. Dalla Vorgia and P. Van der Elst
1992; 82 pages Sw. fr. 30.-

No. 9 **Epidemiologie du cancer dans les pays de langue latine**
1991 346 pages Sw. fr. 30.-

No. 11 **Nitroso Compounds: Biological Mechanisms, Exposures and Cancer Etiology**
Edited by I.K. O'Neill & H. Bartsch
1992; 149 pages Sw. fr. 30.-

No. 12 **Epidémiologie du cancer dans les pays de langue latine**
1992; 375 pages Sw. fr. 30.-

No. 13 **Health, Solar UV Radiation and Environmental Change**
By A. Kricker, B.K. Armstrong, M.E. Jones and R.C. Burton
1993; 216 pages Sw.fr. 30.–

No. 14 **Epidémiologie du cancer dans les pays de langue latine**
1993; 385 pages Sw. fr. 30.-

No. 15 **Cancer in the African Population of Bulawayo, Zimbabwe, 1963–1977: Incidence, Time Trends and Risk Factors**
By M.E.G. Skinner, D.M. Parkin, A.P. Vizcaino and A. Ndhlovu
1993; 123 pages Sw. fr. 30.-

No. 16 **Cancer in Thailand, 1988–1991**
By V. Vatanasapt, N. Martin, H. Sriplung, K. Vindavijak, S. Sontipong, S. Sriamporn, D.M. Parkin and J. Ferlay
1993; 164 pages Sw. fr. 30.-

No. 18 **Intervention Trials for Cancer Prevention**
By E. Buiatti
1994; 52 pages Sw. fr. 30.-

No. 19 **Comparability and Quality Control in Cancer Registration**
By D.M. Parkin, V.W. Chen, J. Ferlay, J. Galceran, H.H. Storm and S.L. Whelan
1994; 110 pages plus diskette
Sw. fr. 40.-

No. 20 **Epidémiologie du cancer dans les pays de langue latine**
1994; 346 pages Sw. fr. 30.-

No. 21 **ICD Conversion Programs for Cancer**
By J. Ferlay
1994; 24 pages plus diskette
Sw. fr. 30.-

DIRECTORY OF AGENTS BEING TESTED FOR CARCINOGENICITY (Until Vol. 13 Information Bulletin on the Survey of Chemicals Being Tested for Carcinogenicity)*

No. 8 Edited by M.-J. Ghess, H. Bartsch and L. Tomatis
1979; 604 pages Sw. fr. 40.-

No. 9 Edited by M.-J. Ghess, J.D. Wilbourn, H. Bartsch and L. Tomatis
1981; 294 pages Sw. fr. 41.-

No. 10 Edited by M.-J. Ghess, J.D. Wilbourn and H. Bartsch
1982; 362 pages Sw. fr. 42.-

No. 11 Edited by M.-J. Ghess, J.D. Wilbourn, H. Vainio and H. Bartsch
1984; 362 pages Sw. fr. 50.-

No. 12 Edited by M.-J. Ghess, J.D. Wilbourn, A. Tossavainen and H. Vainio
1986; 385 pages Sw. fr. 50.-

No. 13 Edited by M.-J. Ghess, J.D. Wilbourn and A. Aitio 1988; 404 pages Sw. fr. 43.-

No. 14 Edited by M.-J. Ghess, J.D. Wilbourn and H. Vainio
1990; 370 pages Sw. fr. 45.-

No. 15 Edited by M.-J. Ghess, J.D. Wilbourn and H. Vainio
1992; 318 pages Sw. fr. 45.-

No. 16 Edited by M.-J. Ghess, J.D. Wilbourn and H. Vainio
1994; 294 pages Sw. fr. 50.-

NON-SERIAL PUBLICATIONS

Alcool et Cancer†
By A. Tuyns (in French only)
1978; 42 pages Fr. fr. 35.-

Cancer Morbidity and Causes of Death Among Danish Brewery Workers†
By O.M. Jensen
1980; 143 pages Fr. fr. 75.-

Directory of Computer Systems Used in Cancer Registries†
By H.R. Menck and D.M. Parkin
1986; 236 pages Fr. fr. 50.-

Facts and Figures of Cancer in the European Community*
Edited by J. Estève, A. Kricker, J. Ferlay and D.M. Parkin
1993; 52 pages Sw. fr. 10.-

* Available from booksellers through the network of WHO Sales agents.

† Available directly from IARC

Achevé d'mprimer sur rotative
par l'imprimerie Darantiere
en février 1995

Dépôt légal : 1er trimestre 1995
N° d'impression : 940-814